Clinical Handbook of Interstitial Lung Disease

Clinical Handbook of Interstitial Lung Disease

Editor: Arthur Henry

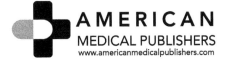

AMERICAN
MEDICAL PUBLISHERS
www.americanmedicalpublishers.com

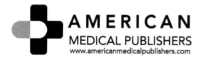

Cataloging-in-Publication Data

Clinical handbook of interstitial lung disease / edited by Arthur Henry.
    p. cm.
Includes bibliographical references and index.
ISBN 978-1-63927-992-0
1. Interstitial lung diseases. 2. Lungs--Diseases. 3. Interstitial lung diseases--Diagnosis.
4. Interstitial lung diseases--Treatment. I. Henry, Arthur.
RC776.I56 C55 2023
616.24--dc23

American Medical Publishers,
41 Flatbush Avenue,
1st Floor, New York,
NY 11217, USA

ISBN 978-1-63927-992-0 (Hardback)

Contents

Preface

Interstitial lung diseases (ILD) or pulmonary fibrosis is a group of lung conditions that involve inflammation and scarring or fibrosis of lung tissues. In this condition, it becomes difficult for the lungs to get enough oxygen. This condition results in shortness of breath and dry cough. The exact cause of ILD is unknown but several factors such as smoking, radiation treatment, certain drugs and medicines, certain connective tissue or collagen diseases, and sarcoidosis may contribute in its development. The common symptoms of ILD include bleeding in the lungs, extreme tiredness and weakness, loss of appetite, unexplained weight loss, and chest discomfort. The most common diagnostic methods used to determine ILD are pulmonary function tests such as spirometry and peak flow monitoring. Chest X-rays, blood tests, and bronchoscopy are some other tests to measure the ability of lungs to move air in and out. Treatment of ILD involves several forms of medications, oxygen therapy, pulmonary rehabilitation, lung transplant and surgery. This book includes some of the vital pieces of work being conducted across the world, on various topics related to the clinical management of interstitial lung disease. For all those who are interested in this medical condition, this book can prove to be an essential guide.

The researches compiled throughout the book are authentic and of high quality, combining several disciplines and from very diverse regions from around the world. Drawing on the contributions of many researchers from diverse countries, the book's objective is to provide the readers with the latest achievements in the area of research. This book will surely be a source of knowledge to all interested and researching the field.

In the end, I would like to express my deep sense of gratitude to all the authors for meeting the set deadlines in completing and submitting their research chapters. I would also like to thank the publisher for the support offered to us throughout the course of the book. Finally, I extend my sincere thanks to my family for being a constant source of inspiration and encouragement.

Editor

Desaturation-Distance Ratio During Submaximal and Maximal Exercise Tests and its Association With Lung Function Parameters in Patients With Lymphangioleiomyomatosis

Douglas Silva Queiroz [1,2], Cibele Cristine Berto Marques da Silva [1],
Alexandre Franco Amaral [3], Martina Rodrigues Oliveira [3], Henrique Takachi Moriya [4],
Carlos Roberto Ribeiro Carvalho [3], Bruno Guedes Baldi [3] and Celso R. F. Carvalho [1]*

[1] Departament of Physical Therapy, School of Medicine, University of São Paulo, São Paulo, Brazil, [2] Hospital Israelita Albert Einstein, São Paulo, Brazil, [3] Divisao de Pneumologia, Instituto do Coracao, Hospital das Clínicas da Faculdade de Medicina da Universidade de São Paulo, São Paulo, Brazil, [4] Biomedical Engineering Laboratory, Escola Politécnica, Universidade de São Paulo, São Paulo, Brazil

*Correspondence:
Celso R. F. Carvalho
cscarval@usp.br

Background: The desaturation–distance ratio (DDR), the ratio of the desaturation area to the distance walked, is a promising, reliable, and simple physiologic tool for functional evaluation in subjects with interstitial lung diseases. Lymphangioleiomyomatosis (LAM) is a rare neoplastic condition frequently associated with exercise impairment. However, DDR has rarely been evaluated in patients with LAM.

Objectives: To assess DDR during maximal and submaximal exercises and evaluate whether DDR can be predicted using lung function parameters.

Methods: A cross-sectional study was conducted in a cohort of women with LAM. The 6-min walking test (6MWT) and the incremental shuttle walking test (ISWT) were performed, and DDR was obtained from both tests. The functional parameters were assessed at rest using spirometry and body plethysmography. The pulmonary function variables predictive of DDR were also assessed.

Results: Forty patients were included in this study. The mean age was 46 ± 10 years. Airway obstruction, reduced DL_{CO}, and air trapping were found in 60, 57, and 15% of patients, respectively. The distance walked and the DDR for the 6MWT and ISWT were, respectively, 517 ± 65 and 443 ± 127 m; and 6.6 (3.8–10.9) and 8.3 (6.2–12.7). FEV_1 (airway obstruction) and reduced DL_{CO} and RV/TLC (air trapping) were independent variables predictive of DDR during exercises field tests [$DDR_{6MWT} = 18.66–(0.06 \times FEV_{1\%pred})–(0.10 \times DL_{CO\%pred}) + (1.54 \times$ air trapping), $R^2_{adjust} = 0.43$] and maximal [$DDR_{ISWT} = 18.84–(0.09 \times FEV_{1\%pred})–(0.05 \times DL_{CO\%pred}) + (3.10 \times$ air trapping), $R^2_{adjust} = 0.33$].

Conclusion: Our results demonstrated that DDR is a useful tool for functional evaluation during maximal and submaximal exercises in patients with LAM, and it can be predicted using airway obstruction, reduced DL_{CO}, and air trapping.

Keywords: lymphangioleiomyomatosis, exercise tests, respiratory function tests, lung volume measurements, lung diseases

INTRODUCTION

Lymphangioleiomyomatosis (LAM) is a rare neoplastic cystic lung disease that affects, mainly women, ~5 persons per million (1). It is characterized by the proliferation of abnormal smooth muscle-like LAM cells, resulting in vascular and airway obstruction and cyst formation (2). LAM's main clinical features are progressive dyspnea, pneumothorax, and chylothorax (3). An obstructive pattern, with air trapping, and a reduction in the diffusion capacity of the lungs for carbon monoxide (DL_{CO}) are the most common abnormalities found during pulmonary function tests (PFTs) (4, 5). Functional impairment in subjects with LAM is frequently associated with exercise limitation (6, 7) that seems multifactorial, including ventilatory and gas exchange abnormalities, cardiovascular dysfunction, and muscle fatigue (7–9).

The 6-min walk test (6MWT) is a submaximal exercise test that is widely used to objectively assess the functional exercise capacity in patients with moderate-to-severe pulmonary disease (10), including LAM (7, 11). Although the distance walked is the primary outcome obtained during the 6MWT, other indexes that incorporate desaturation during the test, such as the desaturation–distance ratio (DDR), have been developed. The DDR is the ratio of the desaturation area to the distance walked. DDR has been considered predictive of morbidity and mortality in patients with other respiratory conditions, such as chronic pulmonary obstructive disease (COPD), pulmonary arterial hypertension, idiopathic pulmonary fibrosis, LAM, and those on the waiting list for lung transplantation (12–14). In addition, DDR is associated with pulmonary function and peripheral oxygen saturation (SpO_2) in patients with interstitial lung diseases (ILDs) (15).

The incremental shuttle walk test (ISWT) is a field test that has been commonly used to quantify maximal exercise capacity. It is already known that 6-min walking distance (6MWD) has a good linear relationship with maximal exercise capacity (VO_2peak); however, most patients reach a ceiling effect during 6MWT (16). Likewise, previous studies demonstrated that 6MWT might not properly evaluate physical capacity in patients with LAM (7, 11, 17). Therefore, other field tests should be tested in this population. The ISWT is a more standardized test that has been used to quantify exercise capacity in patients with chronic respiratory diseases leading to similar physiological responses than the cardiopulmonary exercise test (CPET) (10). However, the performance of patients with LAM and DDR values during the ISWT remains unknown. Therefore, our objectives were to assess DDR during ISWT and 6MWT and evaluate whether DDR is associated with lung function parameters.

METHODS

Trial Design and Participants

This cross-sectional single-center study was conducted from September 2018 to January 2020 in a cohort of women with LAM from the ILD outpatient clinic of the Pulmonary Division from a tertiary university hospital in São Paulo, Brazil. The diagnosis of LAM was based on the current guidelines (3, 18) that include pulmonary function, computed tomography, and serum analysis. The protocol was approved by the Hospital Research Ethics Committee (90196617.1.0000.0068), and all patients signed an informed consent form. The patients were clinically stable (no exacerbation/hospitalization for the last 6 weeks) (18), and they maintained peripheral resting oxygen saturation (SpO_2) of $\geq$ 88% in room air. The exclusion criteria were: supplementary oxygen use, other chronic respiratory diseases, musculoskeletal disorders or uncontrolled heart disease, pregnancy, lung transplantation, or any other disabling condition that could interfere with the tests.

Experimental Design

The patients were evaluated during two nonconsecutive visits (maximum 7 days apart). During visit 1, the clinical and anthropometric data were obtained, and the subjects performed PFTs. After recovery, subjects were randomly assigned (http://www.randomization.com) for 6MWT or ISWT by an investigator not involved in the assessments. The allocations were sealed in opaque envelopes. If the subject performed the 6MWT during visit 1, the ISWT was performed during visit 2, and vice versa. DDR was evaluated during both tests.

Measurements

Clinical and Anthropometric Evaluations

The following data were obtained: age, weight, height, identification and contact information, pathological antecedents, presence of comorbidities, and medication use.

Pulmonary Function Tests

Spirometry and body plethysmography (Bodystik Geratherm Respiratory GmbH, Bad Kissingen, Germany) were performed to obtain lung volumes (forced expiratory volume in 1 s, FEV_1, and residual volume, RV), capacities (inspiratory capacity, IC; forced vital capacity, FVC; functional residual capacity, FRC and total lung capacity, TLC), and DL_{CO}. The predicted values were based on the Brazilian population (19–21). The obstructive pattern, air trapping, and reduced DL_{CO} were defined according to the American Thoracic Society/European Respiratory Society criteria (22).

Peripheral Muscle Strength

Quadriceps strength was measured with a load cell integrated into a circuit in a chair fixed on a wooden plank. The load cell was previously calibrated and attached to the base of the chair with an inextensible strap. One side of the strap was fixed in the right ankle and the other in the load cell, keeping the knee flexed at 90°. During the test, the patient was asked to cross the arms on the chest and extend the knee. Three consecutive 5-s efforts were made at 30-s intervals, with visual feedback and verbal encouragement from the investigator. The maximum value was used in the analysis (23).

Dyspnea and Leg Fatigue Perception

The modified Borg scale was used to evaluate the intensity of dyspnea and leg fatigue, by quantifying the effort during the exercise—within a range from 0 to 10 points, where 0 indicated the absence of symptoms and 10 indicated the worst perception of dyspnea and leg fatigue (24).

Field Exercise Tests

Six-Minute Walking Test

The patient was asked to walk as far as possible along a 30-m corridor for 6-min. The 6-min walk distance (6MWD) was obtained at the end of the test (25). The predicted values for the distance walked were based on the Brazilian population (26). The tests were discontinued if SpO_2 decreased below 80% (10). Before and after the test, heart rate (HR), blood pressure (BP), minimum SpO_2 maintained for at least 10 s, dyspnea, and fatigue symptoms (Borg scale) were assessed. It was considered desaturation if SpO_2 decreased by 4% from the basal level (27).

Incremental Shuttle Walking Test

The ISWT was conducted in an unobstructed and quiet 10-m corridor. The walking speed was determined using a standardized audio signal (beep) that started at 0.5 m/s and was progressively increased by 0.17 m/s every minute for a maximum of 20-min. The ISWT was terminated when the patient indicated that she could not continue or if the operator observed that the patient could not sustain the speed and cover the distance to the cone before the beep (28). SpO_2 < 80% was considered as the criterion for test discontinuation (10). Before and after the test, the HR, BP, minimum SpO_2 maintained for at least 10 s, dyspnea, and fatigue symptoms (Borg scale) were assessed. Desaturation was characterized by a decrease in SpO_2 of 4% from the basal level (27).

Desaturation–Distance Ratio

The DDR was the ratio of the desaturation area to the distance walked during the exercise tests. DDR was previously described by Pimenta et al. (15), who considered desaturation and distance walked as equally important variables for pulmonary functional assessment. During the 6MWT and ISWT, the patient used at pulse Holter oximeter (Nonin WristOxH 3100, Plymouth, MN, USA) to record SpO_2 and HR every 2 s. All SpO_2 values were obtained and recorded using software (nVISIONH, Plymouth, MN, USA). The desaturation area graph was plotted (DAO_2, desaturation vs. time). DDR was calculated as the ratio of oxygen desaturation area (area under the curve) to the distance walked by the patient (DAO_2/distance walked; **Figures 1A,B**). The patients who performed worst during the tests had higher DDR values.

Statistical Analysis

Data are reported as the mean ± SD for variables with a parametric distribution or as the median (25–75% interquartile range) for the variables with a non-parametric distribution. The Pearson correlation coefficient was used to evaluate the association between the DDRs during the 6MWT (6MWT-DDR) and ISWT (ISWT-DDR) (dependent variables) and selected functional parameters (FEV_1/FVC, FEV_1/FVC%pred, FVCliters, FVC%pred, FEV_1liters, FEV_1%pred, FEV_1/FVC%, TLCliters,

TLC%pred, Ratio RV/TLC and RV/TLC%pred, DL_{CO} absolute, DL_{CO}%pred). The linear correlation (r) was considered weak (from −0.3 to 0.3), moderate (from −0.5 to −0.31 or 0.31 to 0.5), strong (from −0.9 to −0.51 or 0.51 to 0.9), or very strong (from −1.0 to −0.91 or 0.91 to 1.0), according to Cohen's classification (29). A forward multiple linear regression analysis was performed, involving variables with linear correlation ($p <$ 0.2). The best predictive models were constructed using the best independent coefficient. Receiver operating characteristic (ROC) curves were used to evaluate the sensitivity and specificity of the DDR for every field test. The optimal cut-point was calculated to predict airway obstruction (%FEV_1 < 80%) (19), reduced DL_{CO} (DL_{CO} < 75%) (22), and air trapping (RV/TLC > 120%) (22). The optimum cutoff points were defined according to the Youden index (30). The level of significance was set at 5% ($p <$ 0.05). The data were analyzed using Sigma Stat version 3.5 (Systat Software, Inc., San Jose, CA).

RESULTS

Sixty women were invited. Twenty declined to participate because they lived far from the hospital and would not honor the second appointment. Therefore, 40 women were included, and their clinical, anthropometric, and functional data are presented in **Table 1**. On average, patients showed peripheral muscle strength weakness (58.7% of the predicted). Obstructive pattern, air trapping, and reduced DL_{CO} were found in 60, 57, and 15% of patients, respectively. Twenty-seven patients (67%) were considered as "desaturators" (decrease of >4% from basal SpO_2) during the 6MWT, and 36 patients (90%) presented with desaturation during the ISWT. Nineteen (47.5%) patients were not able to reach the speed imposed by the audio signal during the ISWT, and 21 (52.5%) patients were limited by their symptoms (16 due to dyspnea and 5 due to fatigue). The DDRs obtained during the 6MWT and ISWT were 6.6 (3.8–10.9) and 8.3 (6.2–12.7), respectively.

There were significant linear correlation between the DDR during the 6MWT and ISWT and the independent variables FEV_1 ($r = −0.54$, $p <$ 0.001, and $r = −0.58$, $p <$ 0.001, respectively), DL_{CO} ($r = −0.62$, $p <$ 0.001, and $r = −0.50$, $p <$ 0.001, respectively), and RV/TLC ($r = 0.34$, $p = 0.03$, and $r = 0.49$, $p <$ 0.001, respectively; **Figures 2A–F**).

The results of the ROC analysis show a high accuracy (area under the ROC curve [AUC] > 0.7) of 6MWT-DDR and ISWT-DDR for predicting airway obstruction (%FEV_1 < 80%), reduced lung diffusion (D_{LCO} < 75%), and air trapping (RV/TLC > 120%; **Table 2**).

The best multivariate association models were constructed using the variables with the best independent coefficients of determination (R^2). DDRs during 6MWT (DDR_{6MWT}) and ISWT (DDR_{ISWT}) for both models included only FEV_1 (%pred) and DL_{CO} (%pred) and air trapping as a dichotomic variable (where RV/TLC>120% = 1; RV/TLC<120% = 0) were independent variables. In a stepwise multiple linear regression model, the derived prediction equations were as follows:

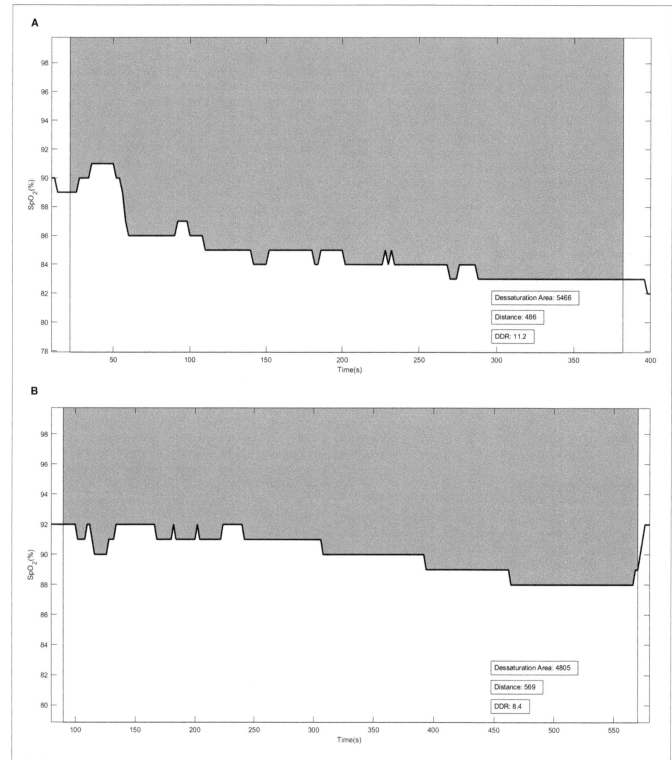

FIGURE 1 | Illustrative figures of the Desaturation-Distance Ratio (DDR) during the 6-min walking test (6MWT) **(A)** and incremental shuttle walking test (ISWT) **(B)**. The solid line represents the oxygen desaturation during the test. DDR was calculated using the ratio between DAO_2 [the gray area—obtained by subtraction between each recorded SpO_2 at every 2 s from 100% (maximal SpO_2)] and the distance walked. Distance in meters.

TABLE 1 | Baseline anthropometrical, clinical, and functional characteristics of the patients with LAM.

Variables	N = 40	
Anthropometric data		
Age (years)	46.60 (1.07)	
Weight (kg)	67.40 (14.4)	
Height (m)	1.60 (0.06)	
BMI (kg/m^2)	26.60 (5.30)	
Peripheral muscle strength		
Quadriceps strength (kgf)	24.58 (8.21)	
Quadriceps strength (%)	58.7 (18.80)	
Pulmonary function tests		
FEV$_1$ (l)	2.14 (0.54)	
FEV$_1$ (% pred) and FVC (% pred)	75.45 (19.33)	
FVC (l)	2.95 (0.58)	
FEV1 (% pred) and FVC (% pred)	88.2 (19.27)	
FEV$_1$/FVC (%)	72.63 (12.34)	
DL$_{CO}$ (ml/min/mmHg)	17.31 (4.93)	
DL$_{CO}$ (%pred)	72.12 (20.65)	
RV (l)	1.85 (1.00)	
RV (%pred)	112.5 (44.57)	
RV/TLC (%)	36.61 (10.83)	
RV/TLC (%pred)	121.82 (37.16)	
Field exercise tests	**6MWT**	**ISWT**
Distance (m)	516.70 (63.90)	452.70 (139.30)
Distance (%pred)	95.10 (17.80)	84.70 (22.0)
SpO$_2$ basel (%)	95.60 (1.90)	95.90 (1.90)
SpO$_2$ minimal (%)	89.40 (1.90)	86.20 (5.0)
DDR	6.6 (3.8–10.9)	8.3 (6.2–12.7)
Borg D (score)	2 (0.2–4)	4 (3–7)
Borg F (score)	2 (0.7–3)	3 (2–5)
HR (bpm)	107.10 (21.0)	142.20 (23.0)
Desaturation during test (%/total)	67/40	90/40

Data presented as mean (standard deviation), except DDR and Borg, presented in median (25–75%, interquartile range). BMI, body mass index; FEV$_1$, Forced expiratory volume in the first second; FVC, forced vital capacity; DL$_{CO}$, carbon monoxide lung diffusion; RV, residual volume; TLC, total lung capacity; l, liters; min, minutes; kg, kilograms; m, meters; ml, milliliters; mmHg, millimeters of mercury; pred, predicted; 6MWT, 6-min walk test; ISWT, incremental shuttle walk test; SpO$_2$, peripheral oxygen saturation; DDR, desaturation–distance ratio; Borg D, Borg dyspnea; Borg F, Borg fatigue; HR, heart rate; bpm, beats per minute.

$$\text{DDR}_{6\text{MWT}} = 18.66 - (0.06 \times \text{FEV}_1\%) - (0.10 \times \text{DL}_{CO}\%) +$$
$$(1.54 \times \text{air trapping}),$$

$$R^2_{\text{adjust}} = 0.43$$

$$\text{DDR}_{\text{ISWT}} = 18.84 - (0.09 \times \text{FEV}_1\%) - (0.05 \times \text{DL}_{CO}\%) +$$
$$(3.10 \times \text{air trapping}),$$

$$R^2_{\text{adjust}} = 0.33$$

DISCUSSION

To the best of our knowledge, this is the first study to investigate the roles of DDR in a general population of patients with LAM during 6MWT and ISWT and correlate it with functional parameters. The performance of patients with LAM during ISWT was also evaluated for the first time. Our results demonstrated that DDR obtained during the submaximal (6MWT) and maximal (ISWT) exercise tests were associated with the severity of pulmonary impairment, air trapping, and reduced DL$_{CO}$ in patients with LAM. Additionally, our patients had satisfactory exercise capacities during both tests.

We included 40 women, which can be considered a relevant sample considering that LAM is a rare disease that affects ~5 persons per million adult women (1). Our patients were classified as having good exercise capacities during the 6MWT and ISWT (~95 and 85% of predicted, respectively). The 6MWT performance in our patients was similar to that observed in previous studies, ranging from 89 to 97% of the predicted distance during the 6MWT in patients with LAM with similar disease severity (7, 11). However, no previous study has assessed the performance of patients during the ISWT.

The DDR is based on the two main variables obtained during the 6MWT, the distance walked, and the decrease in SpO$_2$ evaluated at regular intervals during the test (15). DDR is a more informative indicator for assessing exercise performance than oxygen desaturation, or the distance walked in isolation. Other advantages of DDR include its assessment through simple and low-cost tests (6MWT and ISWT), and easy application. DDR has been previously evaluated in patients with ILDs and COPD, and it has demonstrated associations with pulmonary function parameters (13, 15, 31). Fujimoto et al. (13) showed that DDR was highly predictive of the degree of emphysema and the enlargement of the pulmonary artery on computed tomography scans in COPD patients.

Oxygen desaturation during 6MWT is associated with a worse prognosis and greater mortality, and it has a good correlation with functional variables at rest, such as FVC, DL$_{CO}$, and TLC in patients with ILDs (32–34). However, no previous study has evaluated the role of DDR in predicting disease progression and survival in ILDs, including LAM. Pimenta et al. (15) found that DDR was correlated with functional parameters, including DL$_{CO}$ (%pred), FVC (%pred), and FEV$_1$ (%pred). The authors included 15 patients with LAM and DDR in this subgroup, which was similar to that found in our study (6 vs. 6.6, respectively) (15). A previous study demonstrated that DDR was correlated with the severity of pulmonary cysts on high-resolution computed tomography ($r = 0.77$) in patients with LAM, reinforcing its potential role in evaluating disease severity (12). However, no study has assessed the association between DDR and pulmonary function parameters exclusively in LAM.

Our results demonstrated that DDR is associated with airway obstruction (FEV$_1$), air trapping (RV/TLC), and DL$_{CO}$ during the 6MWT and ISWT in patients with LAM. Previous investigations have shown that reduced exercise performance in cardiopulmonary exercise testing (CPET) is associated with such functional abnormalities in LAM (7, 8). The main mechanisms

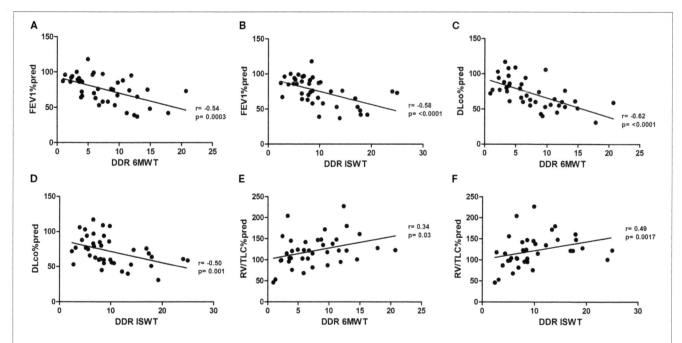

FIGURE 2 | (A) Pearson's correlation between FEV1%pred and DDR 6MWT. **(B)** Pearson's correlation between FEV1%pred and DDR ISWT. **(C)** Pearson's correlation between DL_{CO}%pred and DDR 6MWT. **(D)** Pearson's correlation between DL_{CO}%pred and DDR ISWT. **(E)** Pearson's correlation between RV/LTC%pred and DDR 6MWT. **(F)** Pearson's correlation between RV/LTC%pred and DDR ISWT. FEV1%pred, forced expiratory volume in 1 s as a percentage of predicted; DDR, desaturation distance ratio; 6MWT, 6-min walking test; ISWT, incremental shuttle walking test; DL_{CO}, diffusing capacity of the lung for carbon monoxide as a percentage of predicted; RV, residual volume; TLC, total lung capacity.

TABLE 2 | The optimum cutoff points and ROC curve parameters for prediction of lung function and DDR in patients with LAM.

	Cutoff point	Sensitivity	Specificity	AUC	95%CI
FEV₁ < 80%					
6MWT-DDR	5.9	0.86	0.78	0.85	0.73–0.97
ISWT-DDR	8.5	0.73	0.83	0.85	0.74–0.97
DL_CO < 75%					
6MWT-DDR	6.7	0.82	0.89	0.87	0.74–0.99
ISWT-DDR	9.9	0.59	0.94	0.78	0.64–0.93
RV/TLC > 120%					
6MWT-DDR	7.8	0.62	0.78	0.73	0.57–0.89
ISWT-DDR	7.3	0.91	0.67	0.82	0.68–0.96

ROC, Receiver Operating Characteristic; DDR, Desaturation Distance Ratio; LAM, Lymphangioleiomyomatosis; AUC, Area under the curve; CI, Confidence Interval; FEV₁, Forced Expiratory Volume in the first second of the Expiration (airway obstruction); 6MWT, 6-min walking test; ISWT, Incremental Shuttle Walking Test; DL_CO, Diffusion Capacity of the Lungs for Carbon Monoxid (reduced lung diffusion); RV/LTC, Residual Volume/Lung Total Capacity (air trapping).

determining exercise cessation include ventilatory limitation, gas exchange impairment, peripheral muscle fatigue, and pulmonary hypertension (7, 8). However, no study has compared DDR with data obtained during CPET.

Obstructive pattern and reduced DL_{CO} were commonly observed in our patients, and they were predictors of DDR evaluated during the 6MWT and the ISWT, besides air trapping. Two DDR prediction equations were obtained, DDR-6MWT ($R^2_{adjust} = 0.43$) and DDR-ISWT ($R^2_{adjust} = 0.33$), based on

functional abnormalities that were not previously described. The lung function findings observed in our study were similar to those observed by Li et al. (17) in Chinese patients who presented a mean FVC and FEV_1 of 91%pred and 72%pred, respectively.

In patients with moderate and severe COPD, the distance covered during the ISWT is significantly associated with pulmonary function parameters, such as vital capacity and airway obstruction (FEV_1), as well as health-related quality of life (35). According to Yildiz et al. (36), the ISWT distance is significantly associated with FEV_1 ($r = 0.65$) and FVC ($r = 0.54$) in adults with bronchiectasis. The 6MWT is considered a submaximal field test aimed to assess functional capacity by measuring distance walked within a controlled duration. On the other hand, the ISWT is considered a maximal field test in which patients perform exercises until exhaustion. We are not aware of studies on ISWT in patients with LAM. However, the 6MWT and ISWT presented similar results relative to the predicted values (~90%, **Table 1**). In addition, the association between the 6MWT and ISWT with lung tests were similar.

Our study has some limitations. Our study was performed in only one center; however, our center is a referral center for LAM in Brazil, and it follows patients from different regions with different severities. We included 40 patients that can be considered significant due to the rarity of the disease. Another limitation is the insufficiency of the sample size for stratifying DDR predictions by age, impairment, or physical activity level. Also, no statement can be made regarding patients on oxygen. Finally, it is important to compare the performances during the ISWT and cardiopulmonary exercise testing in patients with LAM.

CONCLUSION

In summary, DDR is useful for functional evaluation during submaximal and maximal exercise tests (6MWT and ISWT) in patients with LAM, and it is associated with functional impairment, reduced DL_{CO}, and air trapping. Future studies are necessary to establish the effectiveness of DDR for evaluating exercises, in comparison with CPET, and predicting disease progression, survival, and response to therapeutic interventions in LAM patients.

ETHICS STATEMENT

The studies involving human participants were reviewed and approved by Comissão em Ética e Pesquisa do Hospital das Clínicas da Faculdade de Medicina da Universidade de São Paulo (CAPPesq). Protocol 90196617.1.0000.0068. The patients/participants provided their written informed consent to participate in this study.

AUTHOR CONTRIBUTIONS

DQ promoted the development of the study design, the scheduling of patient appointments, collecting, analyzing, and interpreting the data, as well as writing the article. CS assisted the research helping develop the study design, scheduling patient appointments, collecting, analyzing, and interpreting the data, as well as improving and developing the article. AA and MO promoted the development of the study design and the scheduling of patient appointments. HM assisted us during the process and interpretation of the DDR data. CRRC greatly contributed to develop the study design, analyse, and interpret the data, as well as to help the elaboration of the article. BB supported us by developing the study design, scheduling patient appointments, analyzing, and interpreting the data, as well as helping the later elaboration of the article. CRFC conducted our research and also provided insight and expertise in all stages of the study, from the concept to the design, data collection and analysis, data interpretation, improvements, and the development of the article. All authors contributed to the article and approved the submitted version.

REFERENCES

1. Harknett EC, Chang WY, Byrnes S, Johnson J, Lazor R, Cohen MM, et al. Use of variability in national and regional data to estimate the prevalence of lymphangioleiomyomatosis. *QJM*. (2011) 104:971–9. doi: 10.1093/qjmed/hcr116
2. Taveira-DaSilva AM, Moss J. Clinical features, epidemiology, and therapy of lymphangioleiomyomatosis. *Clin Epidemiol*. (2015) 7:249–57. doi: 10.2147/CLEP.S50780
3. McCormack FX, Gupta N, Finlay GR, Young LR, Taveira-DaSilva AM, Glasgow CG, et al. Official American Thoracic Society/Japanese Respiratory SocietyClinical Practice Guidelines: lymphangioleiomyomatosis diagnosis and management. *Am J Respir Crit Care Med*. (2016) 194:748–61. doi: 10.1164/rccm.201607-1384ST
4. Ryu JH, Moss J, Beck GJ, Lee JC, Brown KK, Chapman JT, et al. The NHLBI lymphangioleiomyomatosis registry: characteristics of 230 patients at enrollment. *Am J Respir Crit Care Med*. (2006) 173:105–11. doi: 10.1164/rccm.200409-1298OC
5. Taveira-DaSilva AM, Moss J. Epidemiology, pathogenesis and diagnosis of lymphangioleiomyomatosis. *Expert Opin Orphan Drugs*. (2016) 4:369–78. doi: 10.1517/21678707.2016.1148597
6. Crausman RS, Jennings CA, Mortenson RL, Ackerson LM, Irvin CG, King TE Jr. Lymphangioleiomyomatosis - the pathophysiology of diminished exercise capacity. *Am J Respir Crit Care Med*. (1996) 153:1368–76. doi: 10.1164/ajrccm.153.4.8616568
7. Baldi BG, Albuquerque AL, Pimenta SP, Salge JM, Kairalla RA, Carvalho CRR. Exercise performance and dynamic hyperinflation in lymphangioleiomyomatosis. *Am J Respir Crit Care Med*. (2012) 186:341–48. doi: 10.1164/rccm.201203-0372OC
8. Taveira-DaSilva AM, Stylianou MP, Hedin CJ, Kristof AS, Avila NA, Rabel A, et al. Maximal oxygen uptake and severity of disease in lymphangioleiomyomatosis. *Am J Respir Crit Care Med*. (2003) 168:1427–31. doi: 10.1164/rccm.200206-593OC
9. Taveira-DaSilva AM, Hathaway OM, Sachdev V, Shizukuda Y, Birdsall CW, Moss J. Pulmonary artery pressure in lymphangioleiomyomatosis: an echocardiographic study. *Chest*. (2007) 132:1573–8. doi: 10.1378/chest.07-1205
10. Holland AE, Spruit MA, Troosters T, Puhan AM, Pepin V, Saey D, et al. An official European Respiratory Society/American Thoracic Society technical standard: field walking tests in chronic respiratory disease. *Eur Respir J*. (2014) 44:1428–46. doi: 10.1183/09031936.00150314
11. Araujo MS, Baldi BG, Freitas CS, Albuquerque AL, Marques da Silva CC, Kairalla RA, et al. Pulmonary rehabilitation in lymphangioleiomyomatosis: a controlled clinical trial. *Eur Respir J*. (2016) 47:1452–60. doi: 10.1183/13993003.01683-2015
12. Baldi BG, Araujo MS, Freitas CS, da Silva Teles GB, Kairalla RA, Dias OM, et al. Evaluation of the extent of pulmonary cysts and their association with functional variables and serum markers in lymphangioleiomyomatosis (LAM). *Lung*. (2014) 192:967–74. doi: 10.1007/s00408-014-9641-2
13. Fujimoto Y, Oki Y, Kaneko M, Sakai H, Misu S, Yamaguchi T, et al. Usefulness of the desaturation-distance ratio from the six-minute walk test for patients with COPD. *Int J Chron Obstruct Pulmon Dis*. (2017) 12:2669–75. doi: 10.2147/COPD.S143477
14. Agarwala P, Salzman SH. Six-minute walk test: clinical role, technique, coding, and reimbursement. *Chest*. (2020) 157:603–11. doi: 10.1016/j.chest.2019.10.014
15. Pimenta SP, Rocha RB, Baldi BG, Kawasaki AM, Kairalla RA, Carvalho CR. Desaturation - distance ratio: a new concept for a functional assessment of interstitial lung diseases. *Clinics (São Paulo)*. (2010) 65:841–6. doi: 10.1590/S1807-59322010000900005
16. Puente-Maestu L, Stringer W, Casaburi R. Exercise testing to evaluate therapeutic interventions in chronic respiratory diseases. *BRN Rev*. (2018) 4:274–86. doi: 10.23866/BRNRev:2017-0024
17. Li X, Xu W, Zhang L, Zu Y, Li Y, Yang Y, et al. Effects of yoga on exercise capacity in patients with lymphangioleiomyomatosis: a nonrandomized controlled study. *Orphanet J Rare Dis*. (2020) 15:72. doi: 10.1186/s13023-020-1344-6
18. Johnson SR, Cordier JF, Lazor R, Cottin V, Costabel U, Harari S, et al. European Respiratory Society guidelines for the diagnosis and management of lymphangioleiomyomatosis. *Eur Respir J*. (2010) 35:14–26. doi: 10.1183/09031936.00076209
19. Neder JA, Andreoni S, Castelo-Filho A, Nery LE. Reference values for lung function tests. I. Static volumes. *Braz J Med Biol Res*. (1999) 32:703–17. doi: 10.1590/S0100-879X1999000600007
20. Neder JA, Andreoni S, Peres C, Nery LE. Reference values for lung function tests. III. Carbon monoxide diffusing capacity (transfor factor). *Braz J Biol Res*. (1999) 32:729–37. doi: 10.1590/S0100-879X1999000600008
21. Pereira CA, Sato T, Rodrigues SC. New reference values for forced spirometry in white adults in Brazil. *J Bras Pneumol*. (2007) 33:397–406. doi: 10.1590/S1806-37132007000400008

22. Pellegrino R, Viegi G, Brusasco V, Crapo RO, Burgos F, Casaburi R, et al. Series "ATS/ERS Task Force: Standardisation of lung function testing" Edited by V. Brusasco, R. Crapo and G. Viegi Number 5 in this Series Interpretative strategies for lung function tests. *Eur Respir J.* (2005) 26:319–38. doi: 10.1183/09031936.05.00034805

23. Hogel JY, Payan CA, Oliver G, Tanant V, Attarian S, Couillandre A, et al. Development of a French isometric strength normative database for adults using quantitative muscle testing. *Arch Phys Med Rahabil.* (2007) 88, 1289–97. doi: 10.1016/j.apmr.2007.07.011

24. Borg GAV. Psychophysical bases of perceived exertion. *Med Sci Sports Exerc.* (1982) 14:377–81. doi: 10.1249/00005768-198205000-00012

25. American Thoracic Society statement. Guidelines for the six-minute walk test. *Am J Respir Crit Care Med.* (2002) 166:111–7. doi: 10.1164/ajrccm.166.1.at1102

26. Britto RR, Probst VS, de Andrade AF, Samora GA, Hernandes NA, Marinho PE, et al. Reference equations for the six-minute walk distance based on a Brazilian multicenter study. *Braz J Phys Ther.* (2013) 17:556–63. doi: 10.1590/S1413-35552012005000122

27. Puente Maestú L, García de Pedro J. Lung function tests in clinical decision-making. *Arch Bronconeumol.* (2012) 48:161–9. doi: 10.1016/j.arbr.2011.12.007

28. Singh SJ, Morgan MD, Scott S, Walters D, Hardman AE. Development of a shuttle walking test of disability in patients with chronic airways obstruction. *Thorax.* (1992) 47:1019–24. doi: 10.1136/thx.47.12.1019

29. Cohen L. Power primer. *Psychol Bull.* (1992) 112:155–9. doi: 10.1037/0033-2909.112.1.155

30. Youden WJ. An index for rating diagnostic tests. *Cancer.* (1950) 3:32–5. doi: 10.1002/1097-0142 (1950) 3:1<32::AID-CNCR2820030106>3.0.CO;2-3

31. Ijiri N, Kanazawa H, Yoshikawa T, Hirata K. Application of a new parameter in the 6-minute walk test for manifold analysis of exercise capacity in patients with COPD. *Int J Chron Obstruct Pulmon Dis.* (2014) 9:1235–40. doi: 10.2147/COPD.S71383

32. Chetta A, Aiello M, Foresi A, Marangio E, D'Ippolito R, Castagnaro A, et al. Relationship between outcome measures of six-minute walk test and baseline lung function in patients with interstitial lung disease. *Sarcoidosis Vasc Diffuse Lung Dis.* (2001) 18:170–5.

33. Lama VN, Flaherty KR, Toews GB, Colby TV, Travis WD, Long Q, et al. Prognostic value of desaturation during a 6-minute walk test in idiopathic interstitial pneumonia. *Am J Respir Crit Care Med.* (2003) 168:1084–90. doi: 10.1164/rccm.200302-219OC

34. Flaherty KR, Andrei AC, Murray S, Fraley C, Colby TV, Travis WD, et al. Idiopathic pulmonary Fibrosis: prognostic value of changes in physiology and Six-minute-walk test. *Am J Respir Crit Care Med.* (2006) 174:803–9. doi: 10.1164/rccm.200604-488OC

35. Ushiki A, Nozawa S, Yasuo M, Urushihata K, Yamamoto H, Hanaoka M, et al. Associations between the distance covered in the incremental shuttle walk test and lung function and health status in patients with chronic obstructive pulmonary disease. *Respir Investig.* (2017) 55:33–8. doi: 10.1016/j.resinv.2016.08.004

36. Yildiz S, Inal-Ince D, Calik-Kutukcu E, Vardar-Yagli N, Saglam M, Arikan H, et al. Clinical determinants of incremental shuttle walk test in adults with bronchiectasis. *Lung.* (2018) 196:343–9. doi: 10.1007/s00408-018-0094-x

Biologic Treatments in Interstitial Lung Diseases

Theodoros Karampitsakos[1], Argyro Vraka[2], Demosthenes Bouros[2], Stamatis-Nick Liossis[3] and Argyris Tzouvelekis[2]*

[1] 5th Department of Pneumonology, General Hospital for Thoracic Diseases Sotiria, Athens, Greece, [2] First Academic Department of Pneumonology, Hospital for Thoracic Diseases, Sotiria Medical School, National and Kapodistrian University of Athens, Athens, Greece, [3] Division of Rheumatology, Department of Internal Medicine, Patras University Hospital, University of Patras Medical School, Patras, Greece

*Correspondence:
Argyris Tzouvelekis
argyrios.tzouvelekis@fleming.gr

Interstitial lung diseases (ILD) represent a group of heterogeneous parenchymal lung disorders with complex pathophysiology, characterized by different clinical and radiological patterns, ultimately leading to pulmonary fibrosis. A considerable proportion of these disease entities present with no effective treatment, as current therapeutic regimens only slow down disease progression, thus leaving patients, at best case, with considerable functional disability. Biologic therapies have emerged and are being investigated in patients with different forms of ILD. Unfortunately, their safety profile has raised many concerns, as evidence shows that they might cause or exacerbate ILD status in a subgroup of patients. This review article aims to summarize the current state of knowledge on their role in patients with ILD and highlight future perspectives.

Keywords: interstitial lung diseases, biologic treatments, pulmonary fibrosis, treatment, safety

INTRODUCTION

Interstitial lung diseases (ILD) are a group of heterogeneous parenchymal lung disorders, characterized by different clinical and radiological patterns (1, 2). Despite an exponential increase in our knowledge and the advent of novel therapies, treatment remains ineffective for a considerable proportion of patients (3–13). Biologic treatments comprise a wide group of compounds with natural origin produced by biotechnology and other cutting-edge technologies (14); yet, this term mainly refers to the subgroup of complex molecules representing targeted therapy, such as monoclonal antibodies and receptor fusion proteins (15). The last years have seen the emergence of biologic treatments for the treatment of several immune and oncologic disorders (16–18). The most extensively used are tumor necrosis factor-α (TNF-a) inhibitors, B-cell-targeted therapies, T cell co-stimulatory molecule blockers, and immune check point inhibitors. With regards to ILDs, there is established knowledge on the use of biologic therapies in patients with connective tissue disorders (CTD-ILDs) and sarcoidosis (12, 16, 19–21). Despite old skepticism (7, 22–27), there has been recently a shift toward targeting the immune system as a therapeutic option for different forms of interstitial lung inflammation and fibrosis (9, 28–33). Unfortunately, their safety profile has raised many concerns, as evidence shows that they might exacerbate or cause *de novo* development of ILD in a subgroup of patients (34–36) (**Table 1**). This review article aims to summarize the current state of knowledge on their role in patients with ILD and highlight future perspectives.

TABLE 1 | Lung toxicity of biologic treatments.

Biologic treatment	Radiologic findings	References
Anti-TNFα	Aseptic granulomatous pulmonary nodules Interstitial lung infiltrates Incidence of DI-ILD:0.5–3%	(37–40)
Rituximab	Organizing Pneumonia ARDS	(41)
Tocilizumab	Organizing Pneumonia Exacerbation of ILD Pneumonitis	(42–44)
Abatacept	Rarely causes or exacerbates ILD	(45)

ARDS, Acute Respiratory Distress Syndrome; DI-ILD, Drug Induced- Interstitial Lung Disease; TNF, Tumor Necrosis Factor.

SARCOIDOSIS (TABLE 2)

Prednisolone remains the cornerstone of sarcoidosis treatment (55). Biologic therapies currently represent a fruitful therapeutic alternative in sarcoidosis cases refractory to first line immunomodulatory agents including corticosteroids, methotrexate, azathioprine, leflunomide and mycophenolate mofetil (56). TNFα inhibitors in combination with low dose prednisolone or methotrexate have been suggested in: (i) chronic progressive pulmonary disease, (ii) debilitation by lupus pernio, (iii) persistent neurosarcoidosis, (iv) persistent cardiac sarcoidosis (55). Infliximab has shown superior response rates in pulmonary sarcoidosis compared to etanercept and adalimumab (46, 47, 50, 51, 57). In particular, a randomized controlled trial (RCT) enrolling 148 patients with chronic pulmonary sarcoidosis showed that infliximab led to a statistically significant 2.5% improvement in forced vital capacity (FVC%pred) after 24 weeks of treatment (46). Results from other non-randomized trials were rather conflicting (47, 48). Unfortunately, almost 2/3 of patients with sarcoidosis receiving infliximab demonstrated relapse following drug-cessation (49). Adalimumab has shown acceptable tolerability and efficacy profile as indicated by improvements in FVC% pred, 6 Minute-Walk-Distance (6MWD) and Borg scale over a period of 52 weeks in a small cohort of patients with refractory pulmonary sarcoidosis (50). A phase 2 trial of etanercept in patients with pulmonary sarcoidosis was prematurely terminated due to unfavorable outcomes (51). Furthermore, golimumab (TNFα inhibitor) and ustekinumab (a monoclonal antibody targeting both IL-12 and IL-23) failed to show efficacy in patients with pulmonary and/or cutaneous sarcoidosis in an RCT with 173 patients (52). Finally, rituximab had an acceptable safety profile but inconsistent efficacy in a small cohort of patients with different genetic backgrounds and refractory pulmonary sarcoidosis; thus, its use through a personalized medicine approach could be viable in the future (53).

Elevated C-reactive protein (CRP) levels and TNFα Gly308Ala polymorphisms have been found to be predictive of response to anti-TNFα therapy, while soluble IL-2 receptor serum levels $\geq 4,000$ pg·mL^{-1} at start of therapy were predictive of relapse (49,

58). Moreover, ^{18}8F-FDG-PET showed remarkable predictive accuracy in identifying patients that responded or relapsed following infliximab treatment (48, 49).

A broad spectrum of adverse events have been associated with the use of TNF-α inhibitors including anaphylactic reactions, reactivation of latent infections, neurological (i.e., demyelinating diseases) and autoimmune disorders and maybe in some cases malignancy (55, 59, 60). The paradoxical response, denominated sarcoid-like granulomatosis, has also been reported (61).

In conclusion, current evidence based on expert opinion suggests the use of biologic treatments in severe refractory pulmonary sarcoidosis. TNFα-inhibitors are preferred for patients with persistent disease despite treatment with corticosteroids and other second-line immunomodulatory compounds, especially in cases of life-threatening disease. However, such strategies need thorough pre-treatment evaluation and multidisciplinary approaches (12).

IDIOPATHIC PULMONARY FIBROSIS (FIGURE 1, TABLE 3)

The treatment of IPF has been revolutionized by the advent of two novel compounds, pirfenidone and nintedanib (3–11). Nevertheless, both compounds only slow down disease progression; thus, at best leave patients with considerable functional disability. Therefore, the need for alternative therapeutic options remains amenable (75–78).

Biologic agents represent one such option, yet with disappointing results. The clinical trial of carlumab, a monoclonal antibody against CC-chemokine ligand 2 (CCL2), was stopped prematurely as patients in the carlumab-treatment-arm experienced greater functional decline compared to the patients in the placebo-treatment-arm (62). TNFa-blocking agents such as etanercept showed no efficacy in patients with IPF (63). Imatinib, a tyrosine kinase inhibitor with multiple biologic properties, did not affect survival or lung function of patients with IPF (64). The study of simtuzumab, a monoclonal antibody against lysyl oxidase-like 2 (LOXL2), was also a negative study (69). Most recently, two anti-IL-13 monoclonal antibodies have entered the pipeline of clinical trials for IPF. Tralokinumab had an acceptable safety and tolerability profile; yet, key efficacy endpoints were not met (70). Monotherapy with lebrikizumab, another anti-IL-13 monoclonal antibody, did not result in a benefit on lung function or mortality over 52 weeks (65). Combination of lebrikizumab and pirfenidone was well-tolerated but did not meet the primary endpoint of FVC% decline; yet, a trend toward beneficial effects on mortality and acute exacerbations was observed (66, 67). Furthermore, SAR156597, a monoclonal bispecific antibody targeting IL-4 and IL-13, failed to halt disease progression either as monotherapy or in combination with standard-of-care antifibrotics (72). A Phase 2 open label trial of pamrevlumab (FG-3019), a monoclonal antibody blocking the downstream effects of connective tissue growth factor (CTGF), showed an acceptable safety and efficacy profile and thus a phase III clinical trial is currently anticipated (68, 79, 80). Safety and efficacy of VAY736, a monoclonal antibody against the cytokine

TABLE 2 | Biologic treatments in pulmonary sarcoidosis.

Study	Biologic agent	Mechanism of action	Number of patients/Outcome	References
Baughman et al.	Infliximab	Chimeric monoclonal antibody against TNF	148 patients Improvement of 2.5% in FVC over 24 weeks	(46)
Rossman et al.	Infliximab	Chimeric monoclonal antibody against TNF	19 patients No significant improvement over 6 and 14 weeks	(47)
Vorselaars et al.	Infliximab	Chimeric monoclonal antibody against TNF	56 patients Improvement of 6.6% in FVC Uptake value on ^{18}F-FDG-PET predictive of response	(48)
Vorselaars et al.	Infliximab	Chimeric monoclonal antibody against TNF	47 patients Relapse 62% Increased SUV, IL-2r predictors	(49)
Sweiss et al.	Adalimumab	Humanized monoclonal antibody against TNF	11 patients Improvement in FVC (4), stabilization in FVC (7), improvement in 6MWD (5), improvement in Borg (9) over 24/52 weeks	(50)
Utz et al.	Etanercept	Receptor antagonist of TNF	17 patients Excessive treatment failure	(51)
Judson et al.	Ustekinumab/ golimumab	Humanized monoclonal antibody against IL12,IL23/and against TNF, respectively	173 patients (pulmonary or cutaneous) No significant improvement over 28 weeks	(52)
Sweiss et al.	Rituximab	Humanized monoclonal antibody against CD20	10 patients >5% improvement in FVC (5) improvement by >30 m in 6MWD (5) over 24/52 weeks	(53)
NCT02888080	Canakinumab	Human monoclonal antibody against IL-1 b	Change in PFTs from baseline to week 24/Recruiting	(54)

CD, Cluster of Differentiation; IL, interleukin; ^{18}F-FDG-PET, Fludeoxyglucose (^{18}F) Positron Emission Tomography; FVC, Forced Vital Capacity; PFTs, Pulmonary Function Tests; SUV, Standardized Uptake Value; TNF, Tumor Necrosis Factor; 6MWD, 6 Minute Walk Distance.

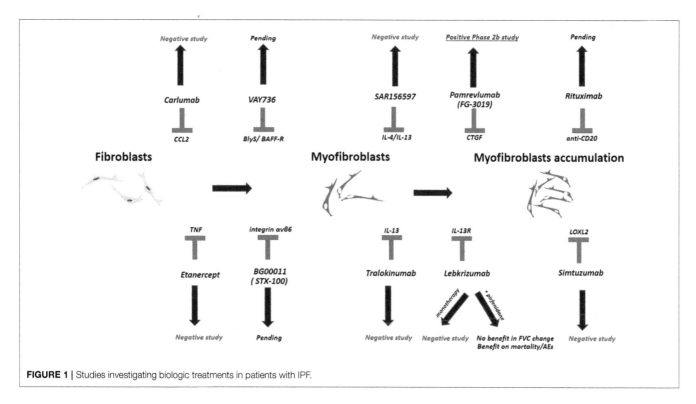

FIGURE 1 | Studies investigating biologic treatments in patients with IPF.

BlyS, a B cell activating factor, is also currently being tested in a phase 2 study (71). BG00011 (STX-100), a humanized monoclonal antibody against integrin αvβ6, demonstrated an acceptable safety profile and its efficacy is currently investigated in a phase 2b study (66, 81). Finally, rituximab ± intravenous immunoglobulin showed 1-year survival benefit in a small cohort of patients with IPF undergoing acute exacerbation compared to historical controls (82). A Phase 2 trial of rituximab in IPF aiming to reduce titers of autoantibodies to HEp-2 Cells over a 9-months period of follow up, has been recently

TABLE 3 | Phase 2 clinical trials for biologic treatments in patients with IPF.

Biologic agent	Mechanism of action	Outcome	References
Carlumab	CCL2 inhibitor	Negative study	NCT00786201 (62)
Etanercept	Receptor antagonist of TNF	Negative study	NCT00063869 (63)
Imatinib	Tyrosine kinase inhibitor	Negative study	NCT00131274 (64)
Lebrikizumab	anti- IL13	Monotherapy: Negative study Combination with pirfenidone: Trend for benefit on AE/mortality	NCT01872689 (65–67)
Pamrevlumab (FG-3019)	Monoclonal antibody against CTGF	Positive phase 2 open label trial	NCT01262001 (68)
simtuzumab	Anti-LOXL2	Negative study	NCT01769196 (69)
Tralokinumab	Anti-IL13	Negative study	NCT01629667 (70)
BG00011 (STX-100)	Humanized monoclonal antibody against integrin $\alpha v \beta 6$	Pending	NCT01371305 (66)
VAY736	Monoclonal antibody against BlyS/ BAFF-R	Pending	NCT03287414 (71)
SAR156597	Bispecific monoclonal antibody against IL-4 and IL-13	Negative study	NCT02921971 (72)
Rituximab	anti-CD20	Pending	NCT01969409 NCT03286556 (73, 74)

BAFF-R, B cell activating factor; CCL2, chemokine (C-C motif) ligand 2; CTGF, Connective Tissue Growth Factor; IL, interleukin; LOXL2, Lysyl oxidase homolog 2; RCT, Randomized Controlled Trial; TNF, Tumor Necrosis Factor.

completed (73, 83). In addition, the results of autoantibody reduction for acute exacerbations of IPF (STRIVE-IPF) are greatly anticipated (74).

CONNECTIVE TISSUE DISEASE-ASSOCIATED INTERSTITIAL LUNG DISEASE (CTD-ILD) RHEUMATOID ARTHRITIS

Pulmonary complications represent an important extra-articular feature of rheumatoid arthritis and a major cause of mortality and worse quality of life (16). The decision to treat them requires a multidisciplinary approach weighting: (i) the disease severity and patients' clinical status, (ii) the potential benefits of early therapy (i.e., treatment of inflammation before fibrosis is established) and (iii) the risk of adverse events (i.e., immunosuppression especially for patients with established fibrosis or severe bronchiectatic lesions). Given the lack of consensus over clinical trials, management is currently based on expert opinion. The recent emergence of novel anti-fibrotic compounds for the IPF-UIP-lung holds promise for the RA-UIP-lung (84–87) and the first randomized trial of antifibrotics in RA-ILD (TRAIL trial) is currently under investigation (84). To this end, biologic treatments may present with beneficial outcomes in a proportion of patients with refractory RA-ILD.

Rituximab represents the most widely used biologic treatment in patients with rapidly progressive RA-ILD who are unresponsive to first line therapeutic compounds including corticosteroids and methotrexate (88). Unfortunately, evidence is based on small observational studies and thus further data is required (89–97). A recent prospective, observational cohort study enrolling 43 patients on rituximab and 309 patients on TNF-α inhibitors, demonstrated better long-term survival in

patients receiving rituximab than in those receiving TNF-α inhibitor, as event rates were 53.0 and 94.8 per 1,000 person years, respectively (98).

The use of TNF-α inhibitors yielded controversial safety and efficacy results in patients with RA-ILD. Caveats following their use in CTD-ILD parallel those previously described in sarcoidosis. Despite their effectiveness in improving clinical status and slowing down articular disease progression, lung toxicity remains a major concern (99–103). Small case series of patients with RA-ILD have shown that infliximab and etanercept could improve dyspnea and cough, as well as stabilize disease functional status (104–107). On the other hand, safety concerns have been raised for current TNF-α inhibitors infliximab (108–111), etanercept (112–116), adalimumab (117–121), golimumab (90), and certolizumab (37, 122, 123) considering reports for ILD exacerbation. Importantly, TNF- induced ILD could be rapidly progressive and even fatal, especially in patients with preexisting ILD (34, 124–127). Nonetheless, large cohorts of patients with RA reported no association between anti-TNF agents and ILD development or progression (128, 129). Caution should be used for elderly patients, as they represent a high-risk and frail group of patients (100).

Data for other agents including abatacept, tocilizumab and anakinra are still scarce. Abatacept has shown an acceptable safety and efficacy profile, as assessed by dyspnea, functional indicators and radiological extent of inflammation, in both large RCTs (130) and smaller case studies (45, 90, 102, 131, 132). The use of tocilizumab yielded conflicting results and it seems to be beneficial only in a small subgroup of patients with RA-ILD (42, 90, 102, 126, 133–137). Isolated cases of ILD-exacerbation following treatment with tocilizumab have been described (138). Finally, anakinra, an IL-1 receptor antagonist, is rarely, if ever, employed in the treatment of patients with RA-ILD (126, 139).

SCLERODERMA

Until recently, the standard treatment for systemic sclerosis-associated ILD (SSc-ILD) was considered to be cyclophosphamide, based on the results of Scleroderma Lung Study (140). However, previously reported data from small-scale studies depicted beneficial effects of mycophenolate mofetil in SSc-ILD (141–143). The recently reported large-scale, randomized, double-blind Scleroderma Lung Study II comparing head-to-head cyclophosphamide vs. mycophenolate mofetil disclosed that mycophenolate mofetil was as effective as cyclophosphamide but with a better safety profile. Thus, mycophenolate mofetil has been established as the current standard of care for SSc-ILD (144). The statistically significant but clinically rather small benefit from the use of such treatment along with the commonly resistant nature of SSc-ILD, clearly underscores the need for novel treatments. Biologic agents, particularly rituximab, have been evaluated in small-scale studies in a minority of patients with progressive, treatment-resistant disease (145). The results of a multicenter, open label, comparative study evaluating rituximab on top of standard treatment ($n = 33$) vs. standard treatment alone ($n = 18$) showed that patients in the rituximab group had a 6% increase of FVC compared to baseline values at 2 years of treatment, a benefit that apparently was preserved later on; however, the number of patients at 7 years of treatment was too small for safe conclusions (146). Direct comparison between the rituximab group and the standard-treatment group disclosed a statistically significant benefit for the rituximab-treated patients. Other studies have reported results along the same lines (19, 20, 145, 147–149). Nevertheless, formal, multicenter, large-scale studies are clearly needed to evaluate the value of B-cell depletion treatment(s) in patients with SSc-ILD. A phase III trial evaluating the effects of the anti-IL-6 receptor monoclonal antibody tocilizumab was terminated despite relatively promising results in the earlier phase trials (150, 151) and the results from the use of belimumab, an anti-BLyS monoclonal antibody, have been evaluated only in one study with a small number of patients ($n = 9$) with clinically non-significant SSc-ILD (152).

MYOSITIS/ ANTISYNTHETASE SYNDROME

ILDs represent a major cause of mortality in dermatomyositis (DM), polymyositis (PM) and antisynthetase syndrome. Most common antibodies in patients with myositis-ILD include anti-EJ, anti-PL12, anti-PL7, anti-Jo1, anti-OJ and anti-KS (153). Biologics have been used in cases of myositis-associated-ILD refractory to more commonly used immunomodulatory agents such as corticosteroids, azathioprine and mycophenolate mofetil (92, 153). Data derived from case series, case reports and retrospective studies suggested clinical, functional and radiologic benefits from rituximab in patients with progressive ILD associated with PM/DM/ antisynthetase syndrome (92, 154–161). Basiliximab, a monoclonal antibody blocking the alpha chain (CD25) of the IL-2 receptor complex, resulted in radiologic and functional improvement in three out of four cases of clinically amyopathic dermatomyositis (CADM) with anti-MDA5 positivity and rapidly progressive ILD (162). However, prior to the application of such therapies, exclusion of other causes of lung function deterioration such as drug-induced pneumonitis, superimposed infection and respiratory muscle weakness is mandatory.

FUTURE PERSPECTIVES AND CONCLUDING REMARKS (TABLE 3)

ILDs represent disease paradigms of unknown pathogenesis, unpredictable clinical course and relatively ineffective therapeutic approaches. Biologic therapies may offer an effective alternative in progressive and refractory cases. Early identification of these patients is of paramount importance. Unfortunately, current physiologic biomarkers neither provide mechanistic insights in disease endotypes nor they predict disease clinical course. While ILDs are associated with several underlying mechanisms, currently applied regimens target specific pathways and thus there is still an amenable need for novel compounds. The development of biologics for the treatment of fibrotic lung diseases may hold promise considering the potential for disease modulation (163).

Biologic agents have shown to have a major impact in severe refractory cases of sarcoidosis. Furthermore, canakinumab, a human monoclonal antibody against IL-1 b, has entered the pipeline of clinical trials for sarcoidosis and the results are greatly anticipated (54). Unfortunately, the majority of biologic agents in IPF have, so far, led to disappointing results mainly due to the fact that they target immune-mediated inflammation and not fibrosis. Application of oncologic and personalized medicine approaches represent crucial steps toward successful implementation of biologic agents in lung fibrosis (164). The advent and implementation of high-throughput computational tools could identify biomarkers able to distinguish patients' endotypes and thus predict the subgroup of patients which are more likely to benefit from specific biologic interventions (165, 166). Biologic enrichment of future clinical trials and implementation of biomarkers as end-points could have a crucial impact toward this direction. Systematic pre-treatment assessment for latent infections and immunocompromise is mandatory prior treatment initiation to avoid undesirable adverse-events. Thoughtful monitoring and multi-disciplinary care with rheumatologists and pulmonologists are strongly encouraged.

AUTHOR CONTRIBUTIONS

TK and AV wrote the manuscript. The manuscript was significantly modified by DB, S-NL, and AT. All authors offered intellectual contribution.

REFERENCES

1. Travis WD, Costabel U, Hansell DM, King TE Jr, Lynch DA, Nicholson AG, et al. An official American Thoracic Society/European Respiratory Society statement: Update of the international multidisciplinary classification of the idiopathic interstitial pneumonias. *Am J Resp Critic Care Med.* (2013) 188:733–48. doi: 10.1164/rccm.201308-1483ST

2. Raghu G, Rochwerg B, Zhang Y, Garcia CA, Azuma A, Behr J, et al. An official ATS/ERS/JRS/ALAT clinical practice guideline: treatment of idiopathic pulmonary fibrosis. An update of the 2011 clinical practice guideline. *Am J Resp Critic Care Med.* (2015) 192:e3–19. doi: 10.1164/rccm.201506-1063ST

3. Tzouvelekis A, Karampitsakos T, Kontou M, Granitsas A, Malliou I, Anagnostopoulos A, et al. Safety and efficacy of nintedanib in idiopathic pulmonary fibrosis: a real-life observational study. *Pulm Pharmacol Ther.* (2018) 49:61–6. doi: 10.1016/j.pupt.2018.01.006

4. Tzouvelekis A, Karampitsakos T, Ntolios P, Tzilas V, Bouros E, Markozannes E, et al. Longitudinal "real-world" outcomes of pirfenidone in idiopathic pulmonary fibrosis in greece. *Front Med.* (2017) 4:213. doi: 10.3389/fmed.2017.00213

5. Tzouvelekis A, Ntolios P, Karampitsakos T, Tzilas V, Anevlavis S, Bouros E, et al. Safety and efficacy of pirfenidone in severe Idiopathic Pulmonary Fibrosis: a real-world observational study. *Pulm Pharmacol Ther.* (2017) 46:48–53. doi: 10.1016/j.pupt.2017.08.011

6. Noble PW, Albera C, Bradford WZ, Costabel U, Glassberg MK, Kardatzke D, et al. Pirfenidone in patients with idiopathic pulmonary fibrosis (CAPACITY): two randomised trials. *Lancet.* (2011) 377:1760–9. doi: 10.1016/S0140-6736(11)60405-4

7. Fletcher S, Jones MG, Spinks K, Sgalla G, Marshall BG, Limbrey R, et al. The safety of new drug treatments for idiopathic pulmonary fibrosis. *Expert Opin Drug Safety.* (2016) 15:1483–9. doi: 10.1080/14740338.2016.1218470

8. King TE Jr, Bradford WZ, Castro-Bernardini S, Fagan EA, Glaspole I, Glassberg MK, et al. A phase 3 trial of pirfenidone in patients with idiopathic pulmonary fibrosis. *N Engl J Med.* (2014) 370:2083–92. doi: 10.1056/NEJMoa1402582

9. Richeldi L, Costabel U, Selman M, Kim DS, Hansell DM, Nicholson AG, et al. Efficacy of a tyrosine kinase inhibitor in idiopathic pulmonary fibrosis. *N Engl J Med.* (2011) 365:1079–87. doi: 10.1056/NEJMoa1103690

10. Richeldi L, du Bois RM, Raghu G, Azuma A, Brown KK, Costabel U, et al. Efficacy and safety of nintedanib in idiopathic pulmonary fibrosis. *N Engl J Med.* (2014) 370:2071–82. doi: 10.1056/NEJMoa1402584

11. Richeldi L, Cottin V, du Bois RM, Selman M, Kimura T, Bailes Z, et al. Nintedanib in patients with idiopathic pulmonary fibrosis: combined evidence from the TOMORROW and INPULSIS® trials. *Respir Med.* (2016) 113:74–9. doi: 10.1016/j.rmed.2016.02.001

12. Spagnolo P, Rossi G, Trisolini R, Sverzellati N, Baughman RP, Wells AU. Pulmonary sarcoidosis. *Lancet Respir Med.* (2018) 6:389–402. doi: 10.1016/S2213-2600(18)30064-X

13. Wells AU, Denton CP. Interstitial lung disease in connective tissue disease–mechanisms and management. *Nat Rev Rheumatol.* (2014) 10:728–39. doi: 10.1038/nrrheum.2014.149

14. https://www.fda.gov/aboutfda/centersoffices/officeofmedicalproductsandtobacco/cber/ucm133077.htm.

15. Rønholt K, Iversen L. Old and new biological therapies for psoriasis. *Int J Mol Sci.* (2017) 18:18112297. doi: 10.3390/ijms18112297

16. Sfikakis PP, Bournia VK, Sidiropoulos P, Boumpas DT, Drosos AA, Kitas GD, et al. Biologic treatment for rheumatic disease: real-world big data analysis from the Greek country-wide prescription database. *Clin Exp Rheumatol.* (2017) 35:579–85.

17. Zugazagoitia J, Molina-Pinelo S, Lopez-Rios F, Paz-Ares L. Biological therapies in nonsmall cell lung cancer. *Eur Respir J.* (2017) 49:2016. doi: 10.1183/13993003.01520-2016

18. Noel MS. Biologics in bowel cancer. *J Gastrointestinal Oncol.* (2017) 8:449–56. doi: 10.21037/jgo.2017.05.03

19. Daoussis D, Liossis SN, Tsamandas AC, Kalogeropoulou C, Kazantzi A, Sirinian C, et al. Experience with rituximab in scleroderma: results from a 1-year, proof-of-principle study. *Rheumatology.* (2010) 49:271–80. doi: 10.1093/rheumatology/kep093

20. Daoussis D, Liossis SN, Tsamandas AC, Kalogeropoulou C, Paliogianni F, Sirinian C, et al. Effect of long-term treatment with rituximab on pulmonary function and skin fibrosis in patients with diffuse systemic sclerosis. *Clin Exp Rheumatol.* (2012) 30:S17–22.

21. Daoussis D, Liossis SN, Yiannopoulos G, Andonopoulos AP. B-cell depletion therapy in systemic sclerosis: experimental rationale and update on clinical evidence. *Int J Rheumatol.* (2011) 2011:214013. doi: 10.1155/2011/214013

22. Herazo-Maya JD, Sun J, Molyneaux PL, Li Q, Villalba JA, Tzouvelekis A, et al. Validation of a 52-gene risk profile for outcome prediction in patients with idiopathic pulmonary fibrosis: an international, multicentre, cohort study. *Lancet Respir Med.* (2017) 5:857–68. doi: 10.1016/S2213-2600(17)30349-1

23. Luzina IG, Todd NW, Iacono AT, Atamas SP. Roles of T lymphocytes in pulmonary fibrosis. *J Leukocyte Biol.* (2008) 83:237–44. doi: 10.1189/jlb.0707504

24. Idiopathic Pulmonary Fibrosis Clinical Research N, Raghu G, Anstrom KJ, King TE Jr, Lasky JA, Martinez FJ. Prednisone, azathioprine, and N-acetylcysteine for pulmonary fibrosis. *N Engl J Med.* (2012) 366:1968–77. doi: 10.1056/NEJMoa1113354

25. Antoniou KM, Nicholson AG, Dimadi M, Malagari K, Latsi P, Rapti A, et al. Long-term clinical effects of interferon gamma-1b and colchicine in idiopathic pulmonary fibrosis. *Eur Respir J.* (2006) 28:496–504. doi: 10.1183/09031936.06.00032605

26. Raghu G, Brown KK, Bradford WZ, Starko K, Noble PW, Schwartz DA, et al. A placebo-controlled trial of interferon gamma-1b in patients with idiopathic pulmonary fibrosis. *N Engl J Med.* (2004) 350:125–33. doi: 10.1056/NEJMoa030511

27. Bouros D, Antoniou KM, Tzouvelekis A, Siafakas NM. Interferon-gamma 1b for the treatment of idiopathic pulmonary fibrosis. *Expert Opin Biol Ther.* (2006) 6:1051–60. doi: 10.1517/14712598.6.10.1051

28. Karampitsakos T, Woolard T, Bouros D, Tzouvelekis A. Toll-like receptors in the pathogenesis of pulmonary fibrosis. *Eur J Pharmacol.* (2017) 808:35–43. doi: 10.1016/j.ejphar.2016.06.045

29. Wuyts WA, Agostini C, Antoniou KM, Bouros D, Chambers RC, Cottin V, et al. The pathogenesis of pulmonary fibrosis: a moving target. *Eur Respir J.* (2013) 41:1207–18. doi: 10.1183/09031936.00073012

30. Karampitsakos T, Tzilas V, Tringidou R, Steiropoulos P, Aidinis V, Papiris SA, et al. Lung cancer in patients with idiopathic pulmonary fibrosis. *Pulm Pharmacol Ther.* (2017) 45:1–10. doi: 10.1016/j.pupt.2017.03.016

31. Karampitsakos T, Tzouvelekis A, Chrysikos S, Bouros D, Tsangaris I, Fares WH. Pulmonary hypertension in patients with interstitial lung disease. *Pulm Pharmacol Ther.* (2018) 22:292–301. doi: 10.1016/j.pupt.2018.03.002

32. Papaioannou O, Karampitsakos T, Barbayianni I, Chrysikos S, Xylourgidis N, Tzilas V, et al. Metabolic disorders in chronic lung diseases. *Front Med.* (2017) 4:246. doi: 10.3389/fmed.2017.00246

33. Tzouvelekis A, Zacharis G, Oikonomou A, Mikroulis D, Margaritopoulos G, Koutsopoulos A, et al. Increased incidence of autoimmune markers in patients with combined pulmonary fibrosis and emphysema. *BMC Pulm Med.* (2013) 13:31. doi: 10.1186/1471-2466-13-31

34. Panopoulos ST, Sfikakis PP. Biological treatments and connective tissue disease associated interstitial lung disease. *Curr Opin Pulm Med.* (2011) 17:362–7. doi: 10.1097/MCP.0b013e3283483ea5

35. Chen J, Chi S, Li F, Yang J, Cho WC, Liu X. Biologics-induced interstitial lung diseases in rheumatic patients: facts and controversies AU - Chen, Juan. *Exp Opin Biol Ther.* (2017) 17:265–83. doi: 10.1080/14712598.2017.1287169

36. Yunt ZX, Solomon JJ. Lung disease in rheumatoid arthritis. *Rheumat Dis Clin N Am.* (2015) 41:225–36. doi: 10.1016/j.rdc.2014.12.004

37. Glaspole IN, Hoy RF, Ryan PF. A case of certolizumab-induced interstitial lung disease in a patient with rheumatoid arthritis. *Rheumatology.* (2013) 52:2302–4. doi: 10.1093/rheumatology/ket175

38. Atzeni F, Boiardi L, Salli S, Benucci M, Sarzi-Puttini P. Lung involvement and drug-induced lung disease in patients with rheumatoid arthritis. *Exp Rev Clin Immunol.* (2013) 9:649–57. doi: 10.1586/1744666X.2013.811173

39. Toussirot E, Berthelot JM, Pertuiset E, Bouvard B, Gaudin P, Wendling D, et al. Pulmonary nodulosis and aseptic granulomatous lung disease occurring in patients with rheumatoid arthritis receiving tumor necrosis factor-alpha-blocking agent: a case series. *J Rheumatol.* (2009) 36:2421–7. doi: 10.3899/jrheum.090030

40. Peno-Green L, Lluberas G, Kingsley T, Brantley S. Lung injury linked to etanercept therapy. *Chest.* (2002) 122:1858–60. doi: 10.1378/chest.122.5.1858

41. Liote H, Liote F, Seroussi B, Mayaud C, Cadranel J. Rituximab-induced lung disease: a systematic literature review. *Eur Resp J.* (2010) 35:681–7. doi: 10.1183/09031936.00080209

42. Kawashiri SY, Kawakami A, Sakamoto N, Ishimatsu Y, Eguchi K. A fatal case of acute exacerbation of interstitial lung disease in a patient with rheumatoid arthritis during treatment with tocilizumab. *Rheum Int.* (2012) 32: 4023–6. doi: 10.1007/s00296-010-1525-z

43. Ikegawa K, Hanaoka M, Ushiki A, Yamamoto H, Kubo K. A case of organizing pneumonia induced by tocilizumab. *Internal Med.* (2011) 50:2191–3. doi: 10.2169/internalmedicine.50.5497

44. Nishimoto N, Yoshizaki K, Miyasaka N, Yamamoto K, Kawai S, Takeuchi T, et al. Treatment of rheumatoid arthritis with humanized anti-interleukin-6 receptor antibody: a multicenter, double-blind, placebo-controlled trial. *Arthrit Rheum.* (2004) 50:1761–9. doi: 10.1002/art.20303

45. Wada T, Akiyama Y, Yokota K, Sato K, Funakubo Y, Mimura T. A case of rheumatoid arthritis complicated with deteriorated interstitial pneumonia after the administration of abatacept. *Japan J Clin Immunol.* (2012) 35:433–8.

46. Baughman RP, Drent M, Kavuru M, Judson MA, Costabel U, du Bois R, et al. Infliximab therapy in patients with chronic sarcoidosis and pulmonary involvement. *Am J Respir Critic Care Med.* (2006) 174:795–802. doi: 10.1164/rccm.200603-402OC

47. Rossman MD, Newman LS, Baughman RP, Teirstein A, Weinberger SE, Miller W Jr, et al. A double-blinded, randomized, placebo-controlled trial of infliximab in subjects with active pulmonary sarcoidosis. *Sarcoidosis Vasc Diffuse Lung Dis.* (2006) 23:201–8.

48. Vorselaars AD, Crommelin HA, Deneer VH, Meek B, Claessen AM, Keijsers RG, et al. Effectiveness of infliximab in refractory FDG PET-positive sarcoidosis. *Eur Respir J.* (2015) 46:175–85. doi: 10.1183/09031936.002 27014

49. Vorselaars AD, Verwoerd A, van Moorsel CH, Keijsers RG, Rijkers GT, Grutters JC. Prediction of relapse after discontinuation of infliximab therapy in severe sarcoidosis. *Eur Respir J.* (2014) 43:602–9. doi: 10.1183/09031936.00055213

50. Sweiss NJ, Noth I, Mirsaeidi M, Zhang W, Naureckas ET, Hogarth DK, et al. Efficacy results of a 52-week trial of adalimumab in the treatment of refractory sarcoidosis. *Sarcoidosis Vasc Diffuse Lung Dis.* (2014) 31:46–54.

51. Utz JP, Limper AH, Kalra S, Specks U, Scott JP, Vuk-Pavlovic Z, et al. Etanercept for the treatment of stage II and III progressive pulmonary sarcoidosis. *Chest.* (2003) 124:177–85. doi: 10.1378/chest.124.1.177

52. Judson MA, Baughman RP, Costabel U, Drent M, Gibson KF, Raghu G, et al. Safety and efficacy of ustekinumab or golimumab in patients with chronic sarcoidosis. *Eur Respir J.* (2014) 44:1296–307. doi: 10.1183/09031936.00000914

53. Sweiss NJ, Lower EE, Mirsaeidi M, Dudek S, Garcia JG, Perkins D, et al. Rituximab in the treatment of refractory pulmonary sarcoidosis. *Eur Respir J.* (2014) 43:1525–8. doi: 10.1183/09031936.00224513

54. ClinicalTrials.gov. *Study of Efficacy, Safety and Tolerability of ACZ885 (Canakinumab) in Patients With Pulmonary Sarcoidosis.* Available online at: https://clinicaltrials.gov/ct2/show/NCT02888080

55. Baughman RP, Grutters JC. New treatment strategies for pulmonary sarcoidosis: antimetabolites, biological drugs, and other treatment approaches. *Lancet Respir Med.* (2015) 3:813–22. doi: 10.1016/S2213-2600(15)00199-X

56. Cremers JP, Drent M, Bast A, Shigemitsu H, Baughman RP, Valeyre D, et al. Multinational evidence-based World Association of Sarcoidosis and Other Granulomatous Disorders recommendations for the use of methotrexate in sarcoidosis: integrating systematic literature research and expert opinion of sarcoidologists worldwide. *Curr Opin Pulm Med.* (2013) 19:545–61. doi: 10.1097/MCP.0b013e3283642a7a

57. Maneiro JR, Salgado E, Gomez-Reino JJ, Carmona L. Efficacy and safety of TNF antagonists in sarcoidosis: data from the Spanish registry of biologics BIOBADASER and a systematic review. *Semin Arthr Rheumat.* (2012) 42:89–103. doi: 10.1016/j.semarthrit.2011.12.006

58. Wijnen PA, Cremers JP, Nelemans PJ, Erckens RJ, Hoitsma E, Jansen TL, et al. Association of the TNF-alpha G-308A polymorphism with TNF-inhibitor response in sarcoidosis. *Eur Respir J.* (2014) 43:1730–9. doi: 10.1183/09031936.00169413

59. Pereira R, Lago P, Faria R, Torres T. Safety of anti-TNF therapies in immune-mediated inflammatory diseases: focus on infections and malignancy. *Drug Dev Res.* (2015) 76:419–27. doi: 10.1002/ddr.21285

60. Saketkoo LA, Baughman RP. Biologic therapies in the treatment of sarcoidosis. *Expert Rev Clin Immunol.* (2016) 12:817–25. doi: 10.1080/1744666X.2016.1175301

61. Tong D, Manolios N, Howe G, Spencer D. New onset sarcoid-like granulomatosis developing during anti-TNF therapy: an under-recognised complication. *Int Med J.* (2012) 42:89–94. doi: 10.1111/j.1445-5994.2011.02612.x

62. Raghu G, Martinez FJ, Brown KK, Costabel U, Cottin V, Wells AU, et al. CC-chemokine ligand 2 inhibition in idiopathic pulmonary fibrosis: a phase 2 trial of carlumab. *Eur Respir J.* (2015) 46:1740–50. doi: 10.1183/13993003.01558-2014

63. Raghu G, Brown KK, Costabel U, Cottin V, du Bois RM, Lasky JA, et al. Treatment of idiopathic pulmonary fibrosis with etanercept: an exploratory, placebo-controlled trial. *Am J Respir Critic Care Med.* (2008) 178:948–55. doi: 10.1164/rccm.200709-1446OC

64. Daniels CE, Lasky JA, Limper AH, Mieras K, Gabor E, Schroeder DR, et al. Imatinib treatment for idiopathic pulmonary fibrosis: randomized placebo-controlled trial results. *Am J Respir Critic Care Med.* (2010) 181:604–10. doi: 10.1164/rccm.200906-0964OC

65. Ogura T, Scholand MB, Glaspole I, Maher TM, Kardatzke D, Kaminski J, et al. The RIFF study (cohort A): a phase II, randomized, double-blind, placebo-controlled trial of Lebrikizumab as monotherapy in patients with idiopathic pulmonary fibrosis. *D12 Immunother Lung Dis.* 197:A6168.

66. ClinicalTrials.gov. *STX-100 in Patients With Idiopathic Pulmonary Fibrosis (IPF).* Available online at: https://clinicaltrials.gov/ct2/show/NCT01371305

67. Kondoh Y, Corte TJ, Glassberg MK, Costabel U, Lancaster LH, Kardatzke D, et al. The RIFF study (Cohort B): A phase II, randomized, double-blind, placebo-controlled trial of lebrikizumab in combination with pirfenidone in patients with idiopathic pulmonary fibrosis. *D12 Immunother Lung Dis.* 197:A6168.

68. Raghu G, Scholand MB, de Andrade J, Lancaster L, Mageto Y, Goldin J, et al. FG-3019 anti-connective tissue growth factor monoclonal antibody: results of an open-label clinical trial in idiopathic pulmonary fibrosis. *Eur Resp J.* (2016) 47:1481–91. doi: 10.1183/13993003.01030-2015

69. Raghu G, Brown KK, Collard HR, Cottin V, Gibson KF, Kaner RJ, et al. Efficacy of simtuzumab versus placebo in patients with idiopathic pulmonary fibrosis: a randomised, double-blind, controlled, phase 2 trial. *Lancet Respir Med.* (2017) 5:22–32. doi: 10.1016/S2213-2600(16)30421-0

70. Parker JM, Glaspole IN, Lancaster LH, Haddad TJ, She D, Roseti SL, et al. A phase 2 randomized controlled study of tralokinumab in subjects with idiopathic pulmonary fibrosis. *Am J Resp Crit Care Med.* (2018) 197:94–103. doi: 10.1164/rccm.201704-0784OC

71. ClinicalTrials.gov. *Study of Pharmacodynamics, Pharmacokinetics, Safety and Tolerability of VAY736 in Patients With Idiopathic Pulmonary Fibrosis.* Available online at: https://clinicaltrials.gov/ct2/show/NCT03287414

72. Raghu G, Richeldi L, Crestani B, Wung P, Bejuit R, Esperet C, Soubrane C. Safety and efficacy of SAR156597 in idiopathic pulmonary fibrosis (IPF): a phase 2, randomized, double-blind, placebo-controlled study. A93 ILD: *Clin Trail.* 197:A2441.

73. ClinicalTrials.gov. *Autoantibody Reduction Therapy in Patients With Idiopathic Pulmonary Fibrosis (ART-IPF).* (2014). Available online at: https://clinicaltrials.gov/ct2/show/NCT01969409

74. ClinicalTrials.gov. *Autoantibody Reduction for Acute Exacerbations of Idiopathic Pulmonary Fibrosis (STRIVE-IPF).* (2018). Available online at: https://clinicaltrials.gov/ct2/show/NCT03286556

75. Yu G, Tzouvelekis A, Wang R, Herazo-Maya JD, Ibarra GH, Srivastava A, et al. Thyroid hormone inhibits lung fibrosis in mice by improving epithelial mitochondrial function. *Nat Med.* (2018) 24:39–49. doi: 10.1038/nm.4447

76. Tzouvelekis A, Yu G, Lino Cardenas CL, Herazo-Maya JD, Wang R, Woolard T, et al. SH2 domain-containing phosphatase-2 is a novel antifibrotic regulator in pulmonary fibrosis. *Am J Respir Crit Care Med.* (2017) 195:500–14. doi: 10.1164/rccm.201602-0329OC

77. Albert RK, Schwartz DA. Revealing the secrets of idiopathic pulmonary fibrosis. *N Engl J Med.* (2019) 380:94–6. doi: 10.1056/NEJMcibr1811639

78. Spagnolo P, Tzouvelekis A, Bonella F. The management of patients with idiopathic pulmonary fibrosis. *Front Med.* (2018) 5:148. doi: 10.3389/fmed.2018.00148

79. Raghu G, Scholand M, Andrade JDE, Lancaster L, Mageto YN, Goldin JG, et al. Safety and efficacy of anti-CTGF monoclonal antibody FG-3019 for the treatment of idiopathic pulmonary fibrosis (IPF): results of Phase 2 clinical trial two years after initiation. *Am J Resp Crit Care Med.* (2014) 189:A1426.

80. ClinicalTrials.gov. Evaluate the Safety and Efficacy of FG-3019 in Patients With Idiopathic Pulmonary Fibrosis. Available online at: https://clinicaltrials.gov/ct2/show/NCT01890265

81. Mouded M, Culver DA, Hamblin MJ, Golden JA, Veeraraghavan S, Enelow RI, et al. Randomized, double-blind, placebo-controlled, multiple dose, dose-escalation study of BG00011 (Formerly STX-100) in patients with idiopathic pulmonary fibrosis (IPF). *D14 ILD Clin Res.* 197:A7785.

82. Donahoe M, Valentine VG, Chien N, Gibson KF, Raval JS, Saul M, et al. Autoantibody-targeted treatments for acute exacerbations of idiopathic pulmonary fibrosis. *PLoS ONE.* (2015) 10: e0127771. doi: 10.1371/journal.pone.0127771

83. Duncan SR, Gibson KF. *Rituximab Therapy in Patients with IPF.* (2013). Available online at: http://grantome.com/grant/NIH/R01-HL119960-02

84. ClinicalTrials.gov. *Phase ll Study of Pirfenidone in Patients With RAILD (TRAIL1).* (2017). Available online at: https://clinicaltrials.gov/ct2/show/NCT02808871

85. ClinicalTrials.gov. *Efficacy and Safety of Nintedanib in Patients With Progressive Fibrosing Interstitial Lung Disease (PF-ILD) (INBUILD®).* (2017). Available online at: https://clinicaltrials.gov/ct2/show/NCT02999178

86. Redente EF, Aguilar MA, Black BP, Edelman B, Bahadur A, Humphries SM, et al. Nintedanib reduces pulmonary fibrosis in a model of rheumatoid arthritis-associated interstitial lung disease. *Am J Physiol Lung Cell Mol Physiol.* (2018) 314:L998–L1009. doi: 10.1152/ajplung.00304.2017

87. Meyer KC, Decker CA. Role of pirfenidone in the management of pulmonary fibrosis. *Therap Clin Risk Manage.* (2017) 13:427–37. doi: 10.2147/TCRM.S81141

88. Sharp C, Dodds N, Mayers L, Millar AB, Gunawardena H, Adamali H. The role of biologics in treatment of connective tissue disease-associated interstitial lung disease. *QJM Int J Med.* (2015) 108:683–8. doi: 10.1093/qjmed/hcv007

89. Franzen D, Ciurea A, Bratton DJ, Clarenbach CF, Latshang TD, Russi EW, et al. Effect of rituximab on pulmonary function in patients with rheumatoid arthritis. *Pulm Pharmacol Ther.* (2016) 37:24–9. doi: 10.1016/j.pupt.2016.02.002

90. Hadjinicolaou AV, Nisar MK, Bhagat S, Parfrey H, Chilvers ER, Ostor AJ. Non-infectious pulmonary complications of newer biological agents for rheumatic diseases–a systematic literature review. *Rheumatology.* (2011) 50:2297–305. doi: 10.1093/rheumatology/ker289

91. Matteson EBT, Ryu J, Crowson C, Hartman T, Dellaripa P. Open-label, pilot study of the safety and clinical effects of rituximab in patients with rheumatoid arthritis-associated interstitial pneumonia. *Open J Rheumatol Autoimmune.* (2012) 2:53–8. doi: 10.4236/ojra.2012.23011

92. Sharp C, McCabe M, Dodds N, Edey A, Mayers L, Adamali H, et al. Rituximab in autoimmune connective tissue disease-associated interstitial lung disease. *Rheumatology.* (2016) 55:1318–24. doi: 10.1093/rheumatology/kew195

93. Kabia AMYM, Dass S, Vital E, Beirne P, Emery P. Efficacy and safety of rituximab in rheumatoid arthritis patients with concomitant interstitial lung disease: 10-year experience at single centre. *Rheumatology.* (2015) 54:i86. doi: 10.1093/rheumatology/kev088.092

94. Braun-Moscovici Y, Butbul-Aviel Y, Guralnik L, Toledano K, Markovits D, Rozin A, et al. Rituximab: rescue therapy in life-threatening complications or refractory autoimmune diseases: a single center experience. *Rheumatol Int.* (2013) 33:1495–504. doi: 10.1007/s00296-012-2587-x

95. Hartung W, Maier J, Pfeifer M, Fleck M. Effective treatment of rheumatoid arthritis-associated interstitial lung disease by B-cell targeted therapy with rituximab. *Case Reports Immunol.* (2012) 2012:272303. doi: 10.1155/2012/272303

96. Md Yusof MY, Kabia A, Darby M, Lettieri G, Beirne P, Vital EM, et al. Effect of rituximab on the progression of rheumatoid arthritis-related interstitial lung disease: 10 years' experience at a single centre. *Rheumatology.* (2017) 56:1348–57. doi: 10.1093/rheumatology/kex072

97. Fernández-Díaz C, Martin-Lopez M, Carrasco-Cubero M, Reina-Sanz D, Rubio-Mu-oz P, Urruticoechea-Arana A, et al. FRI0226 Rituximab in rheumatoid arthritis with interstitial lung disease: a multicenter study. *Ann Rheum Dis.* (2017) 76:569–70.

98. Druce KL, Iqbal K, Watson KD, Symmons DPM, Hyrich KL, Kelly C. Mortality in patients with interstitial lung disease treated with rituximab or TNFi as a first biologic. *RMD Open.* (2017) 3:e000473. doi: 10.1136/rmdopen-2017-000473

99. Perez-De-Lis M, Retamozo S, Flores-Chavez A, Kostov B, Perez-Alvarez R, Brito-Zeron P, et al. Autoimmune diseases induced by biological agents. A review of 12,731 cases (BIOGEAS Registry). *Expert Opin Drug Saf.* (2017) 16:1255–71. doi: 10.1080/14740338.2017.1372421

100. Perez-Alvarez R, Perez-de-Lis M, Diaz-Lagares C, Pego-Reigosa JM, Retamozo S, Bove A, et al. Interstitial lung disease induced or exacerbated by TNF-targeted therapies: analysis of 122 cases. *Semin Arthrit Rheumat.* (2011) 41:256–64. doi: 10.1016/j.semarthrit.2010.11.002

101. Dixon WG, Hyrich KL, Watson KD, Lunt M, Symmons DP, BSRBR Control Centre Consortium, et al. Influence of anti-TNF therapy on mortality in patients with rheumatoid arthritis-associated interstitial lung disease: results from the British Society for Rheumatology Biologics Register. *Ann Rheum Dis.* (2010) 69:1086–91. doi: 10.1136/ard.2009.120626

102. Jani M, Hirani N, Matteson EL, Dixon WG. The safety of biologic therapies in RA-associated interstitial lung disease. *Nat Rev Rheumatol.* (2014) 10:284–94. doi: 10.1038/nrrheum.2013.197

103. Komiya K, Ishii H, Fujita N, Oka H, Iwata A, Sonoda H, et al. Adalimumab-induced interstitial pneumonia with an improvement of pre-existing rheumatoid arthritis-associated lung involvement. *Int Med.* (2011) 50:749–51. doi: 10.2169/internalmedicine.50.4748

104. Vassallo R, Matteson E, Thomas CF Jr. Clinical response of rheumatoid arthritis-associated pulmonary fibrosis to tumor necrosis factor-alpha inhibition. *Chest.* (2002) 122:1093–6. doi: 10.1378/chest.122.3.1093

105. Antoniou KM, Mamoulaki M, Malagari K, Kritikos HD, Bouros D, Siafakas NM, et al. Infliximab therapy in pulmonary fibrosis associated with collagen vascular disease. *Clin Exp Rheumatol.* (2007) 25:23–8.

106. Bargagli E, Galeazzi M, Rottoli P. Infliximab treatment in a patient with rheumatoid arthritis and pulmonary fibrosis. *Eur Resp J.* (2004) 24:708. doi: 10.1183/09031936.04.00076904

107. Wang Y, Xu SQ, Xu JH, Ding C. Treatment with etanercept in a patient with rheumatoid arthritis-associated interstitial lung disease. *Clin Med Insights Case Reports.* (2011) 4:49–52. doi: 10.4137/CCRep.S8150

108. Mori S, Imamura F, Kiyofuji C, Sugimoto M. Development of interstitial pneumonia in a rheumatoid arthritis patient treated with infliximab, an anti-tumor necrosis factor alpha-neutralizing antibody. *Modern Rheumatol.* (2006) 16:251–5. doi: 10.3109/s10165-006-0491-5

109. Ostor AJ, Chilvers ER, Somerville MF, Lim AY, Lane SE, Crisp AJ, et al. Pulmonary complications of infliximab therapy in patients with rheumatoid arthritis. *J Rheumatol.* (2006) 33:622–8.

110. Takeuchi T, Tatsuki Y, Nogami Y, Ishiguro N, Tanaka Y, Yamanaka H, et al. Postmarketing surveillance of the safety profile of infliximab in 5000 Japanese patients with rheumatoid arthritis. *Ann Rheum Dis.* (2008) 67:189–94. doi: 10.1136/ard.2007.072967

111. Taki H, Kawagishi Y, Shinoda K, Hounoki H, Ogawa R, Sugiyama E, et al. Interstitial pneumonitis associated with infliximab therapy without methotrexate treatment. *Rheumatol Int.* (2009) 30:275–76. doi: 10.1007/s00296-009-0931-6

112. Lindsay K, Melsom R, Jacob BK, Mestry N. Acute progression of interstitial lung disease: a complication of etanercept particularly in the presence of rheumatoid lung and methotrexate treatment. *Rheumatology.* (2006) 45:1048–9. doi: 10.1093/rheumatology/kel090

113. Hagiwara K, Sato T, Takagi-Kobayashi S, Hasegawa S, Shigihara N, Akiyama O. Acute exacerbation of preexisting interstitial lung disease after administration of etanercept for rheumatoid arthritis. *J Rheumatol.* (2007) 34: 1151-1154.

114. Tournadre A, Ledoux-Eberst J, Poujol D, Dubost JJ, Ristori JM, Soubrier M. Exacerbation of interstitial lung disease during etanercept therapy: two cases. *Joint Bone Spine Revue Rhum.* (2008) 75:215–8. doi: 10.1016/j.jbspin.2007.04.028

115. Koike T, Harigai M, Inokuma S, Inoue K, Ishiguro N, Ryu J, et al. Postmarketing surveillance of the safety and effectiveness of etanercept in Japan. *J Rheumatol.* (2009) 36:898–906. doi: 10.3899/jrheum.080791

116. Horai Y, Miyamura T, Shimada K, Takahama S, Minami R, Yamamoto M, et al. Eternacept for the treatment of patients with rheumatoid arthritis and concurrent interstitial lung disease. *J Clin Pharm Therap.* (2012) 37:117–21. doi: 10.1111/j.1365-2710.2010.01234.x

117. Schoe A, van der Laan-Baalbergen NE, Huizinga TW, Breedveld FC, van Laar JM. Pulmonary fibrosis in a patient with rheumatoid arthritis treated with adalimumab. *Arthrit Rheumat.* (2006) 55:157–9. doi: 10.1002/art.21716

118. Dascalu C, Mrejen-Shakin K, Bandagi S. Adalimumab-induced acute pneumonitis in a patient with rheumatoid arthritis. *J Clin Rheumatol.* (2010) 16:172–4. doi: 10.1097/RHU.0b013e3181df8361

119. Yamazaki H, Isogai S, Sakurai T, Nagasaka K. A case of adalimumab-associated interstitial pneumonia with rheumatoid arthritis. *Modern Rheumatol.* (2010) 20:518–21. doi: 10.3109/s10165-010-0308-4

120. Koike T, Harigai M, Ishiguro N, Inokuma S, Takei S, Takeuchi T, et al. Safety and effectiveness of adalimumab in Japanese rheumatoid arthritis patients: postmarketing surveillance report of the first 3,000 patients. *Modern Rheumatol.* (2012) 22:498–508. doi: 10.3109/s10165-011-0541-5

121. Dias OM, Pereira DA, Baldi BG, Costa AN, Athanazio RA, Kairalla RA, et al. Adalimumab-induced acute interstitial lung disease in a patient with rheumatoid arthritis. *J Brasil Pneumol.* (2014) 40:77–81. doi: 10.1590/S1806-37132014000100012

122. Lager J, Hilberg O, Lokke A, Bendstrup E. Severe interstitial lung disease following treatment with certolizumab pegol: a case report. *Eur Resp Rev* (2013) 22:414–6. doi: 10.1183/09059180.00002013

123. Pearce F, Johnson SR, Courtney P. Interstitial lung disease following certolizumab pegol. *Rheumatology.* (2012) 51:578–80. doi: 10.1093/rheumatology/ker309

124. Nakashita T, Ando K, Kaneko N, Takahashi K, Motojima S. Potential risk of TNF inhibitors on the progression of interstitial lung disease in patients with rheumatoid arthritis. *BMJ Open.* (2014) 4:e005615. doi: 10.1136/bmjopen-2014-005615

125. Ramos-Casals M, Brito-Zeron P, Munoz S, Soria N, Galiana D, Bertolaccini L, et al. Autoimmune diseases induced by TNF-targeted therapies: analysis of 233 cases. *Medicine.* (2007) 86:242–51. doi: 10.1097/MD.0b013e318141a68

126. Roubille C, Haraoui B. Interstitial lung diseases induced or exacerbated by DMARDS and biologic agents in rheumatoid arthritis: a systematic literature review. *Semin Arthr Rheum.* (2014) 43:613–26. doi: 10.1016/j.semarthrit.2013.09.005

127. Iqbal K, Kelly C. Treatment of rheumatoid arthritis-associated interstitial lung disease: a perspective review. *Therap Adv Musc Dis.* (2015) 7:247–67. doi: 10.1177/1759720X15612250

128. Herrinton LJ, Harrold LR, Liu L, Raebel MA, Taharka A, Winthrop KL, et al. Association between anti-TNF-alpha therapy and interstitial lung disease. *Pharmacoepidemiol Drug Safe.* (2013) 22:394–402. doi: 10.1002/pds.3409

129. Curtis JR, Sarsour K, Napalkov P, Costa LA, Schulman KL. Incidence and complications of interstitial lung disease in users of tocilizumab, rituximab, abatacept and anti-tumor necrosis factor alpha agents, a retrospective cohort study. *Arthrit Res Ther.* (2015) 17:319. doi: 10.1186/s13075-015-0835-7

130. Fernandez-Diaz C, Loricera J, Castaneda S, Lopez-Mejias R, Ojeda-Garcia C, Olive A, et al. Abatacept in patients with rheumatoid arthritis and interstitial lung disease: A national multicenter study of 63 patients. *Semin Arthr Rheum.* (2018) 48:22–27. doi: 10.1016/j.semarthrit.2017.12.012

131. Nakashita T, Ando K, Takahashi K, Motojima S. Possible effect of abatacept on the progression of interstitial lung disease in rheumatoid arthritis patients. *Resp Invest.* (2016) 54:376–9. doi: 10.1016/j.resinv.2016.03.001

132. Mera-Varela A, Perez-Pampin E. Abatacept therapy in rheumatoid arthritis with interstitial lung disease. *J Clin Rheumatol.* (2014) 20:445–6. doi: 10.1097/RHU.0000000000000084

133. Mohr M, Jacobi AM. Interstitial lung disease in rheumatoid arthritis: response to IL-6R blockade. *Scand J Rheumatol.* (2011) 40:400–1. doi: 10.3109/03009742.2011.599072

134. Shetty A, Hanson R, Korsten P, Shawagfeh M, Arami S, Volkov S, et al. Tocilizumab in the treatment of rheumatoid arthritis and beyond. *Drug Des Devel Ther.* (2014) 8:349–64. doi: 10.2147/DDDT.S41437

135. Picchianti Diamanti A, Markovic M, Argento G, Giovagnoli S, Ricci A, Lagana B, et al. Therapeutic management of patients with rheumatoid arthritis and associated interstitial lung disease: case report and literature review. *Ther Adv Respir Dis.* (2017) 11:64–72. doi: 10.1177/1753465816668780

136. Wendling D, Vidon C, Godfrin-Valnet M, Rival G, Guillot X, Prati C. Exacerbation of combined pulmonary fibrosis and emphysema syndrome during tocilizumab therapy for rheumatoid arthritis. *Joint Bone Spine Revue du Rhum.* (2013) 80:670–1. doi: 10.1016/j.jbspin.2013.03.009

137. Fernández-Díaz C, Narvaez-García J, Martín-López M, Rubio-Muñoz P, Castañeda-Sanz S, Vegas-Revenga N, et al. THU0134 Interstitial lung disease and rheumatoid arthritis. multicenter study with tocilizumab. *Ann Rheum Dis.* (2017) 76:251–2. doi: 10.1136/annrheumdis-2017-eular.3580

138. Akiyama M, Kaneko Y, Yamaoka K, Kondo H, Takeuchi T. Association of disease activity with acute exacerbation of interstitial lung disease during tocilizumab treatment in patients with rheumatoid arthritis: a retrospective, case-control study. *Rheumatol Int.* (2016) 36:881–9. doi: 10.1007/s00296-016-3478-3

139. Cohen SB. The use of anakinra, an interleukin-1 receptor antagonist, in the treatment of rheumatoid arthritis. *Rheum Dis Clin North Am.* (2004) 30:365–80. doi: 10.1016/j.rdc.2004.01.005

140. Tashkin DP, Elashoff R, Clements PJ, Goldin J, Roth MD, Furst DE, et al. Cyclophosphamide versus placebo in scleroderma lung disease. *N Engl J Med.* (2006) 354:2655–66. doi: 10.1056/NEJMoa055120

141. Liossis SN, Bounas A, Andonopoulos AP. Mycophenolate mofetil as first-line treatment improves clinically evident early scleroderma lung disease. *Rheumatology.* (2006) 45:1005–8. doi: 10.1093/rheumatology/kei211

142. Fischer A, Brown KK, Du Bois RM, Frankel SK, Cosgrove GP, Fernandez-Perez ER, et al. Mycophenolate mofetil improves lung function in connective tissue disease-associated interstitial lung disease. *J Rheumatol.* (2013) 40:640–6. doi: 10.3899/jrheum.121043

143. Kowal-Bielecka O, Landewe R, Avouac J, Chwiesko S, Miniati I, Czirjak L, et al. EULAR recommendations for the treatment of systemic sclerosis: a report from the EULAR Scleroderma Trials and Research group (EUSTAR). *Ann Rheum Dis.* (2009) 68:620–8. doi: 10.1136/ard.2008.096677

144. Tashkin DP, Roth MD, Clements PJ, Furst DE, Khanna D, Kleerup EC, et al. Mycophenolate mofetil versus oral cyclophosphamide in scleroderma-related interstitial lung disease (SLS II): a randomised controlled, double-blind, parallel group trial. *Lancet Resp Med.* (2016) 4:708–19. doi: 10.1016/S2213-2600(16)30152-7

145. Giuggioli D, Lumetti F, Colaci M, Fallahi P, Antonelli A, Ferri C. Rituximab in the treatment of patients with systemic sclerosis. Our experience and review of the literature. *Autoimmun Rev.* (2015) 14:1072–8. doi: 10.1016/j.autrev.2015.07.008

146. Daoussis D, Melissaropoulos K, Sakellaropoulos G, Antonopoulos I, Markatseli TE, Simopoulou T, et al. A multicenter, open-label, comparative study of B-cell depletion therapy with Rituximab for systemic sclerosis-associated interstitial lung disease. *Semin Arthr Rheum.* (2017) 46:625–31. doi: 10.1016/j.semarthrit.2016.10.003

147. Keir GJ, Maher TM, Hansell DM, Denton CP, Ong VH, Singh S, et al. Severe interstitial lung disease in connective tissue disease: rituximab as rescue therapy. *Eur Resp J.* (2012) 40:641–8. doi: 10.1183/09031936.00163911

148. Bosello SL, De Luca G, Rucco M, Berardi G, Falcione M, Danza FM, et al. Long-term efficacy of B cell depletion therapy on lung and skin involvement in diffuse systemic sclerosis. *Semin Arthr Rheum.* (2015) 44:428–36. doi: 10.1016/j.semarthrit.2014.09.002

149. Jordan S, Distler JH, Maurer B, Huscher D, van Laar JM, Allanore Y, et al. Effects and safety of rituximab in systemic sclerosis: an analysis

from the European Scleroderma Trial and Research (EUSTAR) group. *Ann Rheum Dis.* (2015) 74:1188–94. doi: 10.1136/annrheumdis-2013-204522

150. Khanna D, Denton CP, Jahreis A, van Laar JM, Frech TM, Anderson ME, et al. Safety and efficacy of subcutaneous tocilizumab in adults with systemic sclerosis (faSScinate): a phase 2, randomised, controlled trial. *Lancet.* (2016) 387:2630–40. doi: 10.1016/S0140-6736(16)00232-4

151. Khanna D, Denton CP, Lin CJF, van Laar JM, Frech TM, Anderson ME, et al. Safety and efficacy of subcutaneous tocilizumab in systemic sclerosis: results from the open-label period of a phase II randomised controlled trial (faSScinate). *Ann Rheum Dis.* (2018) 77:212–20. doi: 10.1136/annrheumdis-2017-211682

152. Gordon JK, Martyanov V, Franks JM, Bernstein EJ, Szymonifka J, Magro C, et al. Belimumab for the treatment of early diffuse systemic sclerosis: results of a randomized, double-blind, placebo-controlled, pilot trial. *Arthr Rheumatol.* (2018) 70:308–16. doi: 10.1002/art.40358

153. Watanabe K, Handa T, Tanizawa K, Hosono Y, Taguchi Y, Noma S, et al. Detection of antisynthetase syndrome in patients with idiopathic interstitial pneumonias. *Respir Med.* (2011) 105:1238–47. doi: 10.1016/j.rmed.2011.03.022

154. Lambotte O, Kotb R, Maigne G, Blanc FX, Goujard C, Delfraissy JF. Efficacy of rituximab in refractory polymyositis. *J Rheumatol.* (2005) 32:1369–70.

155. Brulhart L, Waldburger JM, Gabay C. Rituximab in the treatment of antisynthetase syndrome. *Ann Rheum Dis.* (2006) 65:974–5. doi: 10.1136/ard.2005.045898

156. Andersson H, Sem M, Lund MB, Aalokken TM, Gunther A, Walle-Hansen R, et al. Long-term experience with rituximab in anti-synthetase syndrome-related interstitial lung disease. *Rheumatology.* (2015) 54:1420–8. doi: 10.1093/rheumatology/kev004

157. Zappa MC, Trequattrini T, Mattioli F, Rivitti R, Vigliarolo R, Marcoccia A, et al. Rituximab treatment in a case of antisynthetase syndrome with severe interstitial lung disease and acute respiratory failure. *Multidiscip Res Med.* (2011) 6:183–8. doi: 10.1186/2049-6958-6-3-183

158. Vandenbroucke E, Grutters JC, Altenburg J, Boersma WG, ter Borg EJ, van den Bosch JM. Rituximab in life threatening antisynthetase syndrome. *Rheumatol Int.* (2009) 29:1499–502. doi: 10.1007/s00296-009-0859-x

159. Dasa O, Ruzieh M, Oraibi O. Successful Treatment of life-threatening interstitial lung disease secondary to antisynthetase syndrome using rituximab: a case report and review of the literature. *Am J Ther.* (2016) 23:e639–45. doi: 10.1097/MJT.0000000000000245

160. Marie I, Dominique S, Janvresse A, Levesque H, Menard JF. Rituximab therapy for refractory interstitial lung disease related to antisynthetase syndrome. *Respir Med.* (2012) 106:581–7. doi: 10.1016/j.rmed.2012.01.001

161. Keir GJ, Maher TM, Ming D, Abdullah R, de Lauretis A, Wickremasinghe M, et al. Rituximab in severe, treatment-refractory interstitial lung disease. *Respirology.* (2014) 19:353–9. doi: 10.1111/resp.12214

162. Zou J, Li T, Huang X, Chen S, Guo Q, Bao C. Basiliximab may improve the survival rate of rapidly progressive interstitial pneumonia in patients with clinically amyopathic dermatomyositis with anti-MDA5 antibody. *Ann Rheum Dis.* (2014) 73:1591–3. doi: 10.1136/annrheumdis-2014-205278

163. Karampitsakos T CS, Tzilas V, Dimakou K, Bouros D, Tzouvelekis A. Idiopathic pulmonary fibrosis. Time to get personal. *Pneumon.* (2018) 31:71–80.

164. Doyle TJ, Lee JS, Dellaripa PF, Lederer JA, Matteson EL, Fischer A, et al. A roadmap to promote clinical and translational research in rheumatoid arthritis-associated interstitial lung disease. *Chest.* (2014) 145:454–63. doi: 10.1378/chest.13-2408

165. Spagnolo P, Tzouvelekis A, Maher TM. Personalized medicine in idiopathic pulmonary fibrosis: facts and promises. *Curr Opin Pulm Med.* (2015) 21:470–8. doi: 10.1097/MCP.0000000000000187

166. Tzouvelekis A, Herazo-Maya J, Sakamoto K, Bouros D. Biomarkers in the evaluation and management of idiopathic pulmonary fibrosis. *Curr Topics Med Chem.* (2016) 16:1587–98. doi: 10.2174/1568026616666150930120959

Comorbidities of Patients With Idiopathic Pulmonary Fibrosis in Four Latin American Countries: Are There Differences by Country and Altitude?

Mauricio Gonzalez-Garcia[1], Emily Rincon-Alvarez[1], Maria Laura Alberti[2], Mauricio Duran[1], Fabian Caro[2], Maria del Carmen Venero[3], Yuri Edison Liberato[4] and Ivette Buendia-Roldan[5]*

[1] Fundación Neumológica Colombiana, Bogotá, Colombia, [2] Hospital María Ferrer, Buenos Aires, Argentina, [3] Hospital Nacional Arzobispo Loayza, Lima, Peru, [4] Hospital Belén de Trujillo, Trujillo, Peru, [5] Instituto Nacional de Enfermedades Respiratorias Ismael Cosío Villegas, Ciudad de México, Mexico

*Correspondence:
Ivette Buendia-Roldan
ivettebu@yahoo.com.mx

Background: Comorbidities in idiopathic pulmonary fibrosis (IPF) affect quality of life, symptoms, disease progression and survival. It is unknown what are the comorbidities in patients with IPF in Latin America (LA) and if there are differences between countries. Our objective was to compare IPF comorbidities in four countries and analyze possible differences by altitude.

Methods: Patients with IPF according 2012 ATS/ERS/JRS/ALAT guidelines, from two cities with an altitude of $\geq 2,250$ m: Mexico City (Mexico) and Bogotá (Colombia) and from three at sea level: Buenos Aires (Argentina) and Lima and Trujillo (Peru). Comorbidities and pulmonary function tests were taken from clinical records. Possible pulmonary hypertension (PH) was defined by findings in the transthoracic echocardiogram of systolic pulmonary arterial pressure (sPAP) >36 mmHg or indirect signs of PH in the absence of other causes of PH. Emphysema as the concomitant finding of IPF criteria on chest tomography plus emphysema in the upper lobes. ANOVA or Kruskal Wallis and χ^2-tests were used for comparison.

Results: Two hundred and seventy-six patients were included, 50 from Argentina, 86 from Colombia, 91 from Mexico and 49 from Peru. There prevalence of PH was higher in Colombia and Mexico ($p < 0.001$), systemic arterial hypertension in Argentina ($p < 0.015$), gastro-esophageal reflux and dyslipidemia in Colombia and Argentina ($p < 0.001$) and diabetes mellitus in Mexico ($p < 0.007$). Other comorbidities were obesity (28.4%), coronary artery disease (15.2%) and emphysema (14.9%), with no differences between countries. There was more PH in the altitude cities than those at sea level (51.7 vs. 15.3%, $p < 0.001$). In patients from Bogotá and Mexico City, arterial oxygen pressure, saturation ($p < 0.001$) and carbon monoxide diffusing capacity ($p = 0.004$) were significantly lower than in cities at sea level.

Conclusions: In this study with a significant number of patients, we were able to describe and compare the comorbidities of IPF in four LA countries, which contributes to the epidemiological data of this disease in the region. The main results were the differences in comorbidities between the countries and more PH in the subjects residing in the cities of higher altitude, a finding that should be validated in future studies.

Keywords: idiopathic pulmonary fibrosis, comorbidities, Latin America, altitude, pulmonary hypertension

INTRODUCTION

Idiopathic pulmonary fibrosis (IPF) is a specific form of chronic fibrosante interstitial disease, progressive, unknown-cause, which occurs mainly in older adults and is limited to the lung (1). Among idiopathic interstitial pneumonias is the most common, with an incidence of 3–9 cases per 100,000 and a prevalence of 18–20 cases per 100,000 (2–4). The natural history of IPF is of progressive decline in lung function, with an average survival of 3–5 years from diagnosis (2, 3, 5, 6).

Respiratory and non-respiratory comorbidities have been identified in IFP, some also associated with aging, being the most common are sleep apnea, pulmonary hypertension (PH) and gastroesophageal reflux (GER). These comorbidities affect patients' quality of life, can increase symptoms, contribute to disease progression and increase mortality (7, 8).

In Latin America there are no studies on the comorbidities associated with IPF. Taking into account the differences between the countries in terms of the prevalence of risk factors and comorbidities in the general population, we consider that there could be differences in the comorbidities of IPF. Additionally, in cities located at high altitude such as Mexico City (2,240 m) and Bogotá (2,640 m), due to the decrease in barometric pressure (PB) and inspired oxygen pressure, the alveolar (PAO_2) and arterial oxygen pressure (PaO_2) are lower compared to sea level. This PaO_2 decreases even more with age (9, 10) and in subjects with lung disease (6, 11–13). Although the decreased PAO_2 causes hypoxic pulmonary vasoconstriction, which can increase pulmonary artery pressure at less advanced stages of respiratory disease (14, 15), there are no studies reporting more PH in patients with IPF living at high altitude.

The respiratory and non-respiratory comorbidities of patients with IPF in Latin America are less known and whether they differ between countries in the region. Taking this into account and the fact that there are no comparative studies that have shown more pulmonary hypertension in patients with IPF living at high altitudes, our objective was to describe and compare IPF comorbidities in four Latin American countries and analyze possible differences by altitude.

Abbreviations: IPF, idiopathic pulmonary fibrosis; PH, pulmonary hypertension; TE, transthoracic echocardiogram; sPAP, systolic pulmonary arterial pressure; GER, gastroesophageal reflux; SAH, systemic arterial hypertension; CAD, coronary artery disease; DM, diabetes mellitus; CVD, cerebrovascular disease; CKD, chronic kidney disease; COAD, chronic occlusive arterial disease; A-aPO₂, alveolar-arterial oxygen tension gradient.

METHODS

Participants

Retrospective study in four Latin American countries. Expert groups on interstitial disease from five cities were asked for demographic data, respiratory function tests, echocardiography, and comorbidities of patients with IPF that meet the diagnostic criteria of the 2011 ATS/ERS/JRS/ALAT guidelines (1). The study included patients diagnosed between 2014 and 2018. The cities included and their altitude were: Bogotá, Colombia (2,640 m); Buenos Aires, Argentina (25 m); Mexico City, Mexico (2,240 m); Lima, Peru (150 m), and Trujillo, Peru (34 m). The study was approved by the Research Ethics Committee of the FNC (Approval Number 201902-24111) and the participants were asked for their authorization to be included in the study by signing an informed consent, maintaining the confidentiality of their data.

Clinical Data and Comorbidities

Clinical records were reviewed to establish the presence of comorbidities at the time of IPF diagnosis. The body mass index (BMI) was used to define obesity (≥ 30) and underweight (< 18.5). Emphysema was defined as the concomitant finding of IPF signs on chest tomography (CT) plus emphysema in the upper lobes. Possible PH was defined by findings in the transthoracic echocardiogram (TE) of systolic pulmonary arterial pressure (sPAP) > 36 mm Hg or indirect signs of PH in the absence of other causes of PH: left ventricular systolic dysfunction with ejection fraction $< 40\%$, diastolic dysfunction greater than grade I or valvular disease greater to moderate (16). At the time of collecting the information on comorbidities in the clinical records of the patients, it was recorded whether the patients had died. Age, physiology, and comorbidities were used to calculate the TORVAN index, a validated predictive mortality index in IPF (17).

Pulmonary Function Test

Data of forced vital capacity (FVC), forced expiratory volume in the first second (FEV_1), FEV_1/FVC ratio, diffusion of carbon monoxide (DLCO), arterial blood gases, meters walked and oxygen saturation (SpO_2) during SMWT, were registered. To compare lung function between countries, the reference values for spirometry and DLCO were calculated in all participants using Crapo's equations (18, 19). The alveolar-arterial oxygen tension gradient (A-aPO₂) was calculated with the simplified alveolar gas equation using the BP of each city.

Data Analysis

In continuous variables, the assumption of normality was evaluated by the Kolmogorov Smirnov-test and they are presented as means and standard deviation or medians and interquartile ranges. In the qualitative variables, proportions were calculated. The ANOVA-test or the non-parametric Kruskall Wallis-test was used to compare demographic data, pulmonary function tests and TORVAN index among the four countries, and the χ^2-test was used to compare the proportions.

To evaluate possible differences in pulmonary hypertension due to altitude, participants with TE from the highest cities (Bogotá and Mexico) were compared with those from sea-level cities (Buenos Aires, Lima, and Trujillo). The Student's t-test or the Mann-Whitney-test was used for continuous variables, depending on the distribution of the data, and the χ^2-test for categorical variables. All p-values were two-tailed and values <0.05 were considered statistically significant. SPSS version 17 statistical software was used.

RESULTS

Participants

Two hundred and seventy-six patients were included, 50 from Argentina, 86 from Colombia, 91 from Mexico and 49 from Peru, with a mean age of 68.7 ± 8.8 years. Hundred percentage had the requested data, except for the TE result, which could not be obtained in 53 patients (19%). In 83.7% of cases, the pattern on chest CT was definitive UIP and in the remaining 16.3%, a surgical biopsy was performed to confirm the diagnosis. Eighty-one percentage of the total sample were men, with a lower percentage in Peru (59.2%) than other countries ($p < 0.001$). Patients from Argentina had a higher BMI than those from other countries ($p = 0.002$). The smoking index was higher in Argentina ($p < 0.001$) and the years of exposure to wood smoke was higher in Peru ($p < 0.001$). The FVC in the total group was 68.1 ± 19.3 with the highest values in the patients from Colombia ($p < 0.001$). The lowest DLCO values were in patients from Colombia and Mexico ($p < 0.001$). The other demographic data and respiratory function tests are in **Table 1**.

Comorbidities

The most frequent comorbidities in the four countries were PH, systemic arterial hypertension (SAH), GER and obesity (**Table 2**). There were significant differences between countries, with a higher prevalence of PH in Colombia and Mexico ($p < 0.001$), of SAH in Argentina ($p < 0.015$), of GER and dyslipidemia in Colombia and Argentina ($p < 0.001$) and of diabetes mellitus (DM) in Mexico ($p > 0.007$). 28.4% of the patients were obese, with no differences between countries ($p = 0.166$) and only 8 subjects (3.0%) of the total sample were underweight (BMI < 18.5). Other comorbidities such as coronary artery disease and the presence of emphysema on chest CT were also frequent, with no differences between countries (**Figure 1**). The presence of cerebrovascular disease, chronic kidney disease, atrial fibrillation, chronic occlusive arterial disease, and lung cancer was documented in <5% of the participants.

The median number of comorbidities per patient in Colombia and Argentina was two and in Mexico and Peru one ($P < 0.001$; **Table 2**). In the population studied, there were 60 patients (21.7%) without comorbidities, 62 (22.5%) with one comorbidity, 121 (43.8%) with two to three and 33 (12.0%) with four or more. The country with the highest percentage of patients without comorbidities was Peru (46.9%) and the countries with the highest percentage of patients with two or three comorbidities were Colombia and Argentina (56%) ($p < 0.001$; **Figure 2**).

At the time of collecting the information, 23.4% of the patients had died. This percentage of deceased patients was significantly higher in Mexico (47.3%) than in Colombia (23.4%), Argentina (10.9%) and Peru (6.1%) ($p < 0.001$). In the total group, the median TORVAN index was 16.0 (12.0–19.0) and it was significantly higher in Mexico than in Colombia, Argentina and Peru ($p < 0.001$; **Table 2**). Most of the patients in Mexico were classified in TORVAN stages III and V and in Argentina, Colombia and Peru in stages I and II ($p < 0.001$; **Figure 3**).

Differences by Altitude

Of the total of participants, 223 had TE (81%), 73% in cities at sea level and 85% in those of higher altitude. There were no differences in age ($p = 0.680$), sex ($p = 0.755$), or in FVC ($p = 0.392$) between patients with and without TE. The percentage of PH was significantly higher in cities with higher altitude than in those located at sea level, (51.7 vs. 15.3%, $p < 0.001$) (**Figure 4**). In patients with IPF from Bogotá and Mexico City, PaO_2, arterial carbon dioxide pressure ($PaCO_2$), SpO_2 at rest and during exercise, and DLCO were significantly lower than in cities at sea level (**Table 3**). In the cities of higher altitude there was more smoking (67.2 vs. 44.4%, $p < 0.001$), DM (23.7 vs. 13.3%, $p = 0.038$) and coronary heart disease (19.2 vs. 8.1%, $p = 0.014$) and there were no differences in the percentage of patients with emphysema on CT ($p = 0.103$).

DISCUSSION

In this study with a significant number of patients, we were able to describe and compare the comorbidities of IPF in four Latin American countries, which contributes to the epidemiological data of this disease in the region. The main results were the differences in comorbidities between the countries and the higher percentage of PH in the subjects residing in the cities of higher altitude.

As expected in IPF, most of the patients were men (81.5%) and with a high percentage of smoking (59.1%), higher than in the general population of these same countries (20–23). The number of comorbidities per patient was lower and the percentage of patients without comorbidities greater than that described in a previous study in Europa (24), although in the total group, 55.8% of the patients had 2 or more comorbidities. As relevant data, there were differences between countries in the number of comorbidities, being significantly higher in Argentina and Colombia.

TABLE 1 | Participants characteristics and lung function tests.

	Total $N = 276$	Colombia $N = 86$	Mexico $N = 91$	Argentina $N = 50$	Peru $N = 49$	p
Age, years	68.7 ± 8.8	69.7 ± 10.6	67.1 ± 7.7	68.5 ± 8.4	69.8 ± 7.8	0.180
Male sex	225 (81.5)	68 (79.1)	84 (92.3)	44 (88.0)	29 (59.2)	<0.001
BMI, kg/m²	26.9 ± 4.5	26.6 ± 3.9	26.6 ± 3.9	29.1 ± 5.0	25.6 ± 5.5	0.002
Lung biopsy	45 (16.3)	13 (15.1)	22 (24.2)	9 (18.0)	1 (2.0)	0.009
Smoking history	163 (59.1)	63 (73.3)	56 (61.5)	39 (78.0)	5 (10.2)	<0.001
Smoking, pack-years	11.0 (2.5–30.0)	7.0 (1.0–30.0)	8.0 (2.3–20.0)	20.0 (12.0–40.0)	6.0 (3.0–30.0)	<0.001
Wood smoke exposure, years	10.0 (9.0–25.0)	7.0 (6.0–30.0)	10.0 (9.0–15.5)	-	20.0 (10.0–30.0)	0.362
FVC, % predicted	68.1 ± 19.3	75.8 ± 16.4	63.0 ± 19.1	66.5 ± 16.4	65.7 ± 22.7	<0.001
FEV₁, % predicted	72.6 ± 19.9	79.2 ± 18.1	67.1 ± 19.7	71.5 ± 16.3	72.5 ± 22.9	0.001
FEV₁/FVC, %	84.2 ± 7.8	82.0 ± 8.1	84.3 ± 7.7	84.4 ± 7.3	87.7 ± 6.6	0.001
DLCO, % predicted	47.0 ± 17.8	50.0 ± 13.6	40.4 ± 18.5	52.5 ± 18.7	58.9 ± 23.9	<0.001
PaCO₂, mmHg	35.4 ± 4.9	34.9 ± 3.3	32.3 ± 4.4	38.9 ± 3.9	42.0 ± 6.2	<0.001
PaO₂, mmHg	60.2 ± 14.2	52.5 ± 7.7	55.7 ± 9.0	83.2 ± 9.6	72.6 ± 5.5	<0.001
SaO₂, %	88.3 ± 5.9	86.4 ± 4.9	86.6 ± 6.1	94.9 ± 1.8	92.9 ± 3.2	<0.001
A-aPO₂, mmHg	15.0 ± 8.9	11.5 ± 7.1	16.6 ± 9.0	17.9 ± 10.5	23.3 ± 6.6	<0.001
SMWT						
Distance, m	425.1 ± 119.4	471.8 ± 111.1	419.8 ± 131.3	403.9 ± 97.2	356.1 ± 113.6	0.001
SpO₂ at the end of the test, %	92.1 ± 3.6	88.9 ± 3.0	92.4 ± 2.6	94.8 ± 2.4	94.7 ± 2.2	<0.001
SpO₂ end of the test, %	82.8 ± 7.7	77.7 ± 6.1	81.9 ± 6.7	87.4 ± 6.7	89.2 ± 6.0	<0.001

P = differences between countries. Values as mean ± SD, median (P25–P75) or N (%).
BMI, body mass index; FVC, forced vital capacity; FEV₁, forced expiratory volume in the first second; DLCO, carbon monoxide diffusing capacity; PaO₂, arterial oxygen pressure; PaCO₂, carbon dioxide arterial pressure; HCO₃, bicarbonate; SaO₂, oxygen arterial saturation; A-aPO₂, alveolar-arterial oxygen tension gradient; SMWT, six-minute walking test; SpO₂, oxygen saturation by pulse oximetry.

TABLE 2 | Comorbidities by country.

	Total $N = 276$	Colombia $N = 86$	Mexico $N = 91$	Argentina $N = 50$	Peru $N = 49$	p
Number of comorbidities	2.0 (1.0–3.0)	2.0 (1.0–3.0)	1.0 (0.0–2.0)	2.0 (1.0–3.0)	1.0 (0.0–2.0)	<0.001
Pulmonary hypertension	89 (39.9)	38 (47.5)	40 (56.3)	5 (10.4)	6 (25.0)	<0.001
SAH	105 (38.0)	36 (41.9)	25 (27.5)	27 (54.0)	17 (34.7)	0.015
GER	93 (33.9)	37 (43.0)	14 (15.4)	34 (70.8)	8 (16.3)	<0.001
Obesity	77 (28.4)	22 (25.6)	23 (25.3)	19 (42.2)	13 (26.5)	0.166
Diabetes	55 (20.0)	13 (15.1)	29 (31.9)	7 (14.3)	6 (12.2)	0.007
Dyslipidemia	52 (19.3)	27 (31.4)	7 (7.7)	16 (36.4)	2 (4.2)	<0.001
Coronary artery disease	42 (15.2)	17 (19.8)	17 (18.7)	5 (10.0)	3 (6.1)	0.093
Emphysema	41 (14.9)	17 (19.8)	14 (15.4)	8 (16.3)	2 (4.1)	0.101
Hypothyroidism	30 (10.9)	22 (25.6)	1 (1.1)	6 (12.0)	1 (2.0)	<0.001
Cerebrovascular disease	11 (4.0)	2 (2.3)	4 (4.4)	4 (8.2)	1 (2.0)	0.379
Chronic kidney disease	7 (2.5)	4 (4.7)	1 (1.1)	0 (0.0)	2 (4.1)	0.056
Atrial fibrillation	5 (1.8)	2 (2.3)	0 (0.0)	1 (2.0)	2 (4.1)	0.212
COAD	4 (1.5)	0 (0.0)	1 (1.1)	1 (2.0)	2 (4.1)	0.231
Lung cancer	1 (0.4)	1 (1.2)	0.0 (0.0)	0 (0.0)	0 (0.0)	0.505
TORVAN index, points	16.0 (12.0–19.0)	16.0 (13.0–18.0)	19.0 (16.0–22.0)	13.5 (9.0–18.0)	14.0 (9.0–16.0)	<0.001

Values as N (%) or median (P25–P75). P: differences between countries.
SAH, systemic arterial hypertension; GER, gastroesophageal reflux; COAD, chronic occlusive arterial disease.

The most frequent respiratory comorbidities in the four countries were PH and emphysema. The percentage of patients with PH was 39.9%, similar to previous studies. In the systematic review by Raghu (7), the informed prevalence of PH was between 3 and 86%, although most of the data were between 30 and 50%. In 22 (51.2%) of the 43 studies analyzed in this review,

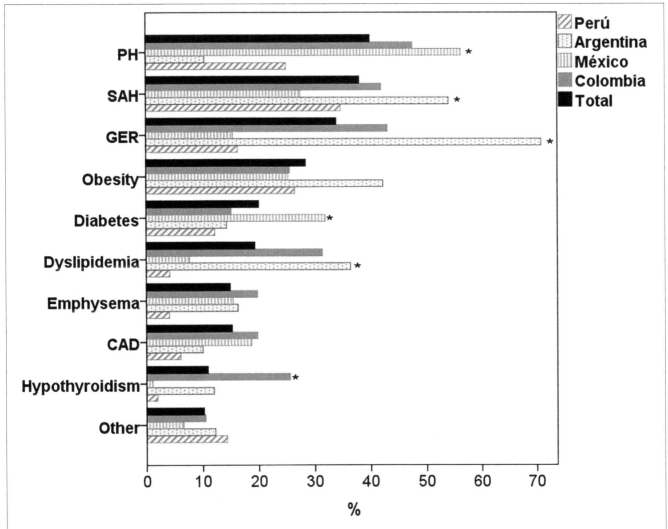

FIGURE 1 | Comorbidities in patients with IPF by country. PH, pulmonary hypertension; SAH, systemic arterial hypertension; GER, gastroesophageal reflux; CAD, coronary artery disease. *$p < 0.05$ for differences between countries.

the prevalence was estimated by sPAP values in the TE with cut-off points between 35 and 40 mmHg, similar to that used in this study. In the studies in which right catheterization was used, which is considered the gold standard for the diagnosis of pulmonary hypertension, the reported prevalence was between 29 and 46% (25).

We highlight the higher percentage of subjects with PH in the TE in the cities of higher altitude (51.7 vs. 15.3%, $p < 0.001$). The mechanism of hypoxic vasoconstriction with a secondary increase in pulmonary vascular resistance triggered by lower PAO$_2$ values at altitude, the pulmonary artery remodeling described in long-term exposure to hypoxia and the erythrocytosis described in altitude in healthy subjects and in patients with respiratory disease (10, 26), could explain the development of PH in these patients (14, 15). Along the same lines of our data, in previous studies in Mexico City and Bogotá, high prevalence of PH have been described in patients with chronic respiratory disease (27, 28).

As expected, there were differences in arterial blood gases between cities of different altitude. In patients from Bogotá and Mexico City, PaCO$_2$ was lower, explained by the adaptive mechanism of hyperventilation at altitude (10, 29). Due to the decrease in PAO$_2$, PaO$_2$ and saturation at rest and during exercise were significantly lower in patients from higher altitude cities. Although the DLCO decrease is a characteristic functional finding of IPF, it was even lower in patients from higher altitude cities, despite having less involvement of the FVC and not having greater emphysema on chest CT, which could be explained due to possible PH in these patients.

Similar to the studies in PH, different definitions have been used to establish the prevalence of emphysema in IPF, such as disease diagnosis codes, questionnaires, pathology findings or CT scan (7). In the studies that have used CT with the definition of the presence or absence of emphysema, without its quantification, the reported prevalence is from 19 to 67% and in those that used the quantification of the extent of

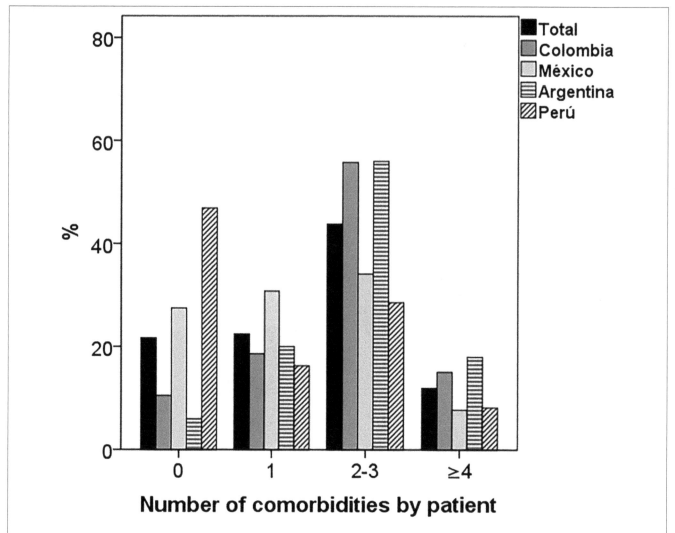

FIGURE 2 | Number of comorbidities per patient by country. There were significant differences in the distribution of comorbidities by country. Most of the patients from Peru and Mexico had one or no comorbidity and those from Colombia and Argentina two or three ($p < 0.001$).

emphysema from 8 to 28%. In this study, the prevalence of emphysema was lower (14.9%) and there were no differences between countries, although there were differences in exposure to tobacco and wood smoke. The smoking rate was higher in Argentina and the years of exposure to wood smoke was higher in Peru.

The most frequent non-respiratory comorbidities in the four countries were SAH, GER, obesity, and DM. The prevalence of SAH in these patients was high (38.0%), although it was similar to some series of patients with IPF (7, 24). The highest percentage of SAH was in Argentina, a country with a higher prevalence of this disease in the general population compared to what was described in Colombia, Mexico and Peru (20–23). 28.4% of the patients were obese, similar to that described in other IPF studies (7, 30). Compared with the general population of these countries, this percentage of obesity was higher than that reported in Peru and Colombia, but lower than that described in Argentina and Mexico (20–23).

Using the cut-off point of BMI ≥ 30 to define obesity, there were no significant differences between countries ($P = 0.166$), but there were differences in BMI, which was significantly higher in patients from Argentina ($P = 0.002$). A low percentage of the study patients (3.0%) were underweight, a factor that has been related to a poor prognosis of the disease, as well as weight loss during follow-up (30, 31). The prevalence of DM (20%) was similar to that reported in other studies (10–40%) (7, 32). We highlight that the prevalence of 31.9% of DM in IPF patients from Mexico was significantly higher than the other countries ($p < 0.001$), despite the fact that the prevalence in the general population in the four countries, including Mexico, is <15% (20–23).

The prevalence of GER reported in IPF is highly variable, with values up to 90%, which could be related to the definition used. In the four countries it was 33.9%, but with significant differences between countries, with the highest prevalence in Argentina (70.8%) and the lowest in Mexico and Peru. Hypothyroidism

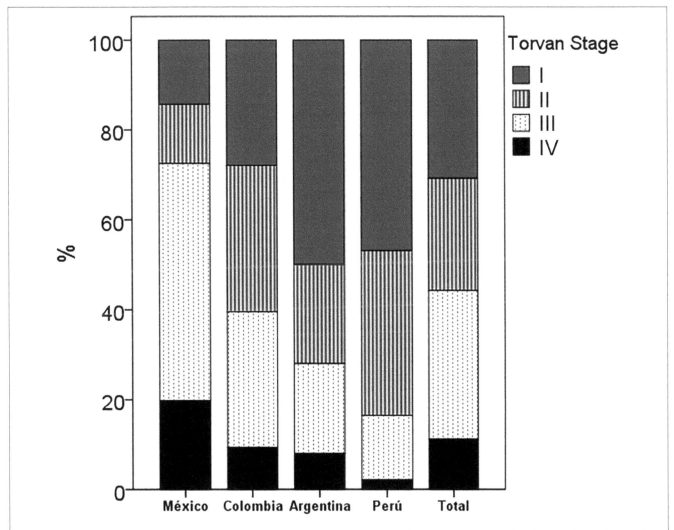

FIGURE 3 | Proportion of patients in the TORVAN states in the total group and in each country. In Mexico, there were more patients in stages III-IV and in Argentina, Colombia and Peru in stages I-II ($p < 0.001$).

is another comorbidity of IPF associated with higher mortality (33). The prevalence of 10.9% in these patients was similar to that reported in other IPF studies and higher than that of the general population reported in studies from other countries (7, 32, 33).

The other comorbidities included in the study had a low frequency, such as cerebrovascular disease, chronic kidney disease, atrial fibrillation, chronic occlusive arterial disease, valvular heart disease and lung cancer, which were present in <5% of the participants. It is noteworthy that in the subjects of these four countries, the percentage of lung cancer was very low (0.4%) and lower than that reported in the literature (4 to 23%) (7, 34), which is probably explained by the significantly lower incidence of lung cancer in the general population of Latin American countries compared to the United States, Europe and Asia (35, 36). Among the patients from the four countries, there were no differences in age, a factor related to greater morbidity, mortality, and use of health resources in patients with IPF (37). Additionally, aging and smoking are part of the pathophysiology

of IPF and other coexisting diseases such as emphysema and lung cancer (8, 38, 39).

Although we were unable to perform a mortality analysis that included comorbidities, we observed differences between countries with a significantly higher percentage of dead patients in Mexico. Similarly, the TORVAN mortality prediction index had the same trend between countries. Patients from Mexico had a significantly higher TORVAN score than in the other countries and most of these patients were classified into TORVAN stages III and IV, unlike patients from Colombia, Argentina, and Peru, who were mostly classified as stage I and II. Taking into account that the patients were of similar age, the differences in TORVAN between countries could be explained by a greater functional compromise (lower DLCO and FVC) and a higher percentage of PH and DM in patients from Mexico than in other countries.

The differences in the frequency of comorbidities, between the study countries and with that described in the literature, could be explained by the differences in the lifestyle and diet

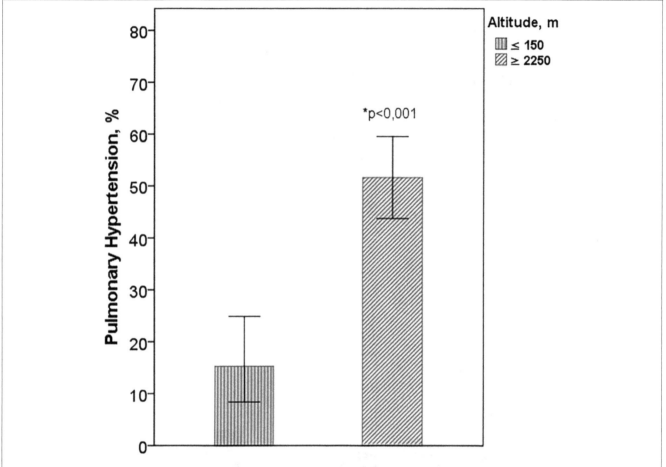

FIGURE 4 | Pulmonary hypertension according to altitude. Altitude: ≥2,250 m Mexico City and Bogotá; ≤150 m: Buenos Aires, Lima, and Trujillo. *Difference between the cities of higher altitude with those of sea level.

of the populations, the history of exposure to tobacco and the prevalence of these comorbidities in general population. Although the study countries belong to the same geographic region, there are important differences between them in the comorbidities reported in national studies of risk factors in the general population (20–23). On the other hand, the differences in comorbidities reported in studies from Europe and the United States can be related to the aforementioned differences in lifestyles, diet and comorbidities in the general population, and probably in the used methodology; as differences in diagnostic methods, the lack of standardized definitions of some comorbidities such as the percentage of extension of emphysema on CT or differences in the diagnostic method used for others such as GER, and the prospective design of several of these studies (7, 25, 40).

As strengths of this work, we highlight that it is the first study in Latin America with a significant number of patients that describes the comorbidities in IPF and the differences between countries, as well as the presence of more pulmonary hypertension in patients with IPF living at altitude. Although this finding could be expected due to the explained pathophysiological mechanisms related to low

PAO_2, hypoxic vasoconstriction, increased pulmonary vascular resistance, pulmonary artery remodeling and erythrocytosis, there are no previous studies that have demonstrated a higher prevalence of PH in patients with IPF who live at high altitudes compared to those who live at sea level. We believe that this study contributes to the knowledge of the clinical behavior of IPF and the epidemiology of this disease in the region. Although the TE is not a confirmatory examination of PH, it is accepted that it is a useful tool to establish a diagnosis of possible PH and, as already commented, most of the studies that have established the prevalence of PH in IPF were based on a methodology similar to that used in this study, which allowed us to compare our results (7). It should be noted that due to the age and functional characteristics of patients with IPF, it is generally difficult to perform right catheterization in these patients.

This study has several weaknesses related to the retrospective design based on the clinical reports of the patients. Unlike prospective studies, the possibility of underreporting comorbidities is greater. In addition, we did not have information on the treatment of comorbidities, which may have an impact on the outcomes of the disease, and on the improvement of the quality of life and symptoms of the patients. It is important to

Comorbidities of Patients With Idiopathic Pulmonary Fibrosis in Four Latin American Countries: Are There Differences...

27

TABLE 3 | Characteristics of participants with echocardiogram by altitude.

	Total	Altitude ≤150 m	Altitude ≥ 2,250 m	p
	N = 223	N = 72	N = 151	
Age, years	68.6 ± 9.1	69.3 ± 8.3	68.3 ± 9.5	0.461
BMI, kg/m^2	27.2 ± 4.4	27.5 ± 5.5	27.0 ± 3.8	0.504
Pulmonary hypertension	89 (39.9)	11 (15.3)	78 (51.7)	<0.001
sPAP, mmHg	43.5 ± 19.7	31.9 ± 15.7	47.5 ± 19.5	<0.001
FVC, % predicted	68.7 ± 18.3	64.1 ± 17.0	70.7 ± 18.5	0.014
FEV$_1$, % predicted	73.1 ± 19.0	70.2 ± 17.6	74.3 ± 19.5	0.140
FEV$_1$/FVC, %	84.0 ± 7.9	86.1 ± 7.2	83.0 ± 8.1	0.006
DLCO, % predicted	48.3 ± 17.7	55.0 ± 18.9	46.3 ± 16.9	0.004
PaCO$_2$, mmHg	35.9 ± 4.9	40.3 ± 5.1	34.4 ± 3.9	<0.001
HCO$_3$, meq/L	23.4 ± 2.9	25.5 ± 3.0	22.6 ± 2.5	<0.001
PaO$_2$, mmHg	59.4 ± 15.0	81.3 ± 9.4	52.6 ± 8.1	<0.001
SaO$_2$, %	87.9 ± 6.2	94.2 ± 2.7	85.9 ± 5.6	<0.001
A-aPO$_2$, mmHg	15.1 ± 9.8	18.0 ± 8.8	13.7 ± 8.7	0.060
SMWT				
Distance, m	428.7 ± 121.3	396.7 ± 103.4	448.0 ± 127.8	0.021
SpO$_2$ at the end of the test, %	92.1 ± 3.8	95.0 ± 2.4	90.5 ± 3.5	<0.001
SpO$_2$ end of the test, %	82.9 ± 7.8	88.3 ± 6.4	79.8 ± 6.7	<0.001

Values as mean ± SD, or N (%).
P: differences by altitude.
BMI, body mass index; sPAP, systolic pulmonary arterial pressure; FVC, forced vital capacity; FEV$_1$, forced expiratory volume in the first second; DLCO, carbon monoxide diffusing capacity; PaO$_2$, arterial oxygen pressure; PaCO$_2$, carbon dioxide arterial pressure; HCO$_3$, bicarbonate; SaO$_2$, oxygen arterial saturation; A-aPO$_2$, alveolar-arterial oxygen tension gradient; SMWT, six-minute walking test; SpO$_2$, oxygen saturation by pulse oximetry.
Altitude: ≥2,250 m Mexico City and Bogotá; ≤150 m: Buenos Aires, Lima, and Trujillo.

highlight that in some comorbidities, such as GER, the effect of antacid therapy on disease progression and mortality has been studied. Although benefit in these outcomes has been suggested with proton pump inhibitors (41), most studies have not shown an impact on the progression or survival of IPF (42–44).

An important limitation of the study is that we were unable to perform a multivariate analysis of mortality that included comorbidities. Even so, we found significant differences between countries in the percentage of mortality, which correlated well with the result of the TORVAN index. Also, the evaluation of various IPF comorbidities was not possible. First of all, we do not have data on sleep apnea, a comorbidity described in up

to 90% of IPF patients (7, 32), which has been associated with greater cardiovascular comorbidity and risk of death due to intermittent nocturnal hypoxemia (45, 46). Another comorbidity not evaluated was pulmonary embolism, an entity related to higher mortality, but with a low prevalence in IPF (7, 8, 32).

The importance of comorbidities in the clinical course of patients with IPF is clearly recognized, so their identification, treatment and management are part of the comprehensive evaluation of these patients (8, 17, 24, 25). In Latin America, prospective studies are required that include all IPF comorbidities, with standardized definitions, which allow evaluating the impact of these comorbidities on clinical outcomes such as disease progression and mortality.

CONCLUSION

In this study with a significant number of patients, we were able to describe and compare the comorbidities of the IPF in four LA countries, which contributes to the epidemiological data of this disease in the region. The main results were the differences in comorbidities between the countries and the higher percentage of PH in the patients residing in the cities of higher altitude, a finding that should be validated in future prospective studies.

ETHICS STATEMENT

The studies involving human participants were reviewed and approved by Fundación Neumologica Colombiana Research Ethics Committee. The patients/participants provided their written informed consent to participate in this study.

AUTHOR CONTRIBUTIONS

MG-G, ER-Á, and IB-R contributed to the conceptualization and design of the study. MG-G drafted the initial manuscript and guarantor of this work. All authors contributed to data abstraction and analysis, contributed to manuscript writing, and approved the submission of the final manuscript.

ACKNOWLEDGMENTS

To doctors Vicente Girón Atoche, Jorge Gave Zarate, Isabel Bertha Jaramillo Peralta, Víctor Oswaldo Lizarbe Castro, Shanery Gonzales Vargas from the Arzobispo Loayza National Hospital (Lima, Peru) and Tania Chavez Bazan and Sandra Ruiz Armas from the Hospital Belén de Trujillo (Trujillo, Peru), for their collaboration in the inclusion of participants in the study and in data collection.

REFERENCES

1. Raghu G, Collard HR, Egan JJ, Martinez FJ, Behr J, Brown KK, et al. An official ATS/ERS/JRS/ALAT statement: idiopathic pulmonary fibrosis: evidence-based guidelines for diagnosis and management. *Am J Respir Crit Care Med.* (2011) 183:788–824. doi: 10.1164/rccm.2009-040GL

2. Hutchinson J, Fogarty A, Hubbard R, McKeever T. Global incidence and mortality of idiopathic pulmonary fibrosis: a systematic review. *Eur Respir J.* (2015) 46:795–806. doi: 10.1183/09031936.00185114

3. Hopkins RB, Burke N, Fell C, Dion G, Kolb M. Epidemiology and survival of idiopathic pulmonary fibrosis from national data in Canada. *Eur Respir J.* (2016) 48:187–95. doi: 10.1183/13993003.01504-2015

4. Raghu G, Chen SY, Hou Q, Yeh WS, Collard HR. Incidence and prevalence of idiopathic pulmonary fibrosis in US adults 18-64 years old. *Eur Respir J.* (2016) 48:179–86. doi: 10.1183/13993003.01653-2015

5. Ley B, Collard HR, King TE, Jr. Clinical course and prediction of survival in idiopathic pulmonary fibrosis. *Am J Respir Crit Care Med.* (2011) 183:431–40. doi: 10.1164/rccm.201006-0894CI

6. Gonzalez-Garcia M, Chamorro J, Jaramillo C, Casas A, Maldonado D. Survival of patients with idiopathic pulmonary fibrosis at the altitude of Bogota (2640 m). *Acta Med Colomb.* (2014) 39:15–20.

7. Raghu G, Amatto VC, Behr J, Stowasser S. Comorbidities in idiopathic pulmonary fibrosis patients: a systematic literature review. *Eur Respir J.* (2015) 46:1113–30. doi: 10.1183/13993003.02316-2014

8. Buendia-Roldan I, Mejia M, Navarro C, Selman M. Idiopathic pulmonary fibrosis: clinical behavior and aging associated comorbidities. *Respir Med.* (2017) 129:46–52. doi: 10.1016/j.rmed.2017.06.001

9. Rico FG, Urias P, Barquera S, Jiménez L, Navarro M, Guzman L, et al. Valores espirométricos y gasométricos en una población geriátrica sana, a diferentes alturas sobre el nivel del mar, en la República Mexicana. *Estudio multicéntrico Rev Inst Nal Enf Resp Mex.* (2001) 14:90–98.

10. Gonzalez-Garcia M, Maldonado D, Barrero M, Casas A, Perez-Padilla R, Torres-Duque CA. Arterial blood gases and ventilation at rest by age and sex in an adult Andean population resident at high altitude. *Eur J Appl Physiol* (2020) 120:2729–36. doi: 10.1007/s00421-020-04498-z

11. Gonzalez-Garcia M, Barrero M, Maldonado D. Exercise limitation in patients with chronic obstructive pulmonary disease at the altitude of Bogota (2640 m). Breathing pattern and arterial gases at rest and peak exercise. *Arch Bronconeumol.* (2004) 40:54–61. doi: 10.1016/S1579-2129(06)60195-X

12. Maldonado D, Gonzalez M, Barrero M, Jaramillo C, Casas A. Exercise endurance in hypoxemic COPD patients at an altitude of 2640m breathing air and oxygen (FIO2 28 and 35%). *Chest.* (2007) 132:454a. doi: 10.1378/chest.132.4_MeetingAbstracts.454a

13. Mejia M, Carrillo G, Rojas-Serrano J, Estrada A, Suarez T, Alonso D, et al. Idiopathic pulmonary fibrosis and emphysema: decreased survival associated with severe pulmonary arterial hypertension. *Chest.* (2009) 136:10–5. doi: 10.1378/chest.08-2306

14. Swenson ER. Hypoxic pulmonary vasoconstriction and chronic lung disease. *Adv Pulm Hypertens.* (2013) 12:135–44. doi: 10.21693/1933-088X-12.3.135

15. Nathan SD, Barbera JA, Gaine SP, Harari S, Martinez FJ, Olschewski H, et al. Pulmonary hypertension in chronic lung disease and hypoxia. *Eur Respir J.* (2019) 53:1801914. doi: 10.1183/13993003.01914-2018

16. Galie N, Hoeper MM, Humbert M, Torbicki A, Vachiery JL, Barbera JA, et al. Guidelines for the diagnosis and treatment of pulmonary hypertension: the Task Force for the Diagnosis and Treatment of Pulmonary Hypertension of the European Society of Cardiology (ESC) and the European Respiratory Society (ERS), endorsed by the International Society of Heart and Lung Transplantation (ISHLT). *Eur Heart J.* (2009) 30:2493–537. doi: 10.1093/eurheartj/ehp297

17. Torrisi SE, Ley B, Kreuter M, Wijsenbeek M, Vittinghoff E, Collard HR, et al. The added value of comorbidities in predicting survival in idiopathic pulmonary fibrosis: a multicentre observational study. *Eur Respir J.* (2019) 53:1801587. doi: 10.1183/13993003.01587-2018

18. Crapo RO, Morris AH, Gardner RM. Reference spirometric values using techniques and equipment that meet ATS recommendations. *Am Rev Respir Dis.* (1981) 123:659–64.

19. Macintyre N, Crapo RO, Viegi G, Johnson DC, van der Grinten CP, Brusasco V, et al. Standardisation of the single-breath determination of carbon monoxide uptake in the lung. *Eur Respir J.* (2005) 26:720–35. doi: 10.1183/09031936.05.00034905

20. Instituto Nacional de Salud Pública, Instituto Nacional de Estadística y Geografía. *Encuesta Nacional de Salud y Nutrición (ENSANUT).* Ciudad de México, México (2018). Available online at: https://ensanut.insp.mx/encuestas/ensanut2018/doctos/informes/ensanut_2018_presentacion_resultados.pdf (accessed October 30, 2020).

21. Instituto Nacional de Estadistica e Informática. *Encuesta Demográfica y de Salud Familiar.* Lima, Perú (2019). Available online at: http://www.inei.gob.pe/ (accessed October 30, 2020).

22. Instituto Nacional de Estadística y Censos (INDEC) - Secretaréa de Gobierno de Salud. *4 Encuesta Nacional de Factores de Riesgo.* Buenos Aires (2019). Available online at: http://www.msal.gob.ar/images/stories/bes/graficos/0000001622cnt-2019-10_4ta-encuesta-nacionalfactores-riesgo.pdf (accessed March 2020).

23. Ministerio de Salud y Protección Social. Análisis de Situación de Salud. Bogotá (2019). Available online at: https://www.minsalud.gov.co/salud/publica/epidemiologia/Paginas/analisis-de-situacion-de-salud-.aspx (accessed on October 30, 2020).

24. Kreuter M, Ehlers-Tenenbaum S, Palmowski K, Bruhwyler J, Oltmanns U, Muley T, et al. Impact of comorbidities on mortality in patients with idiopathic pulmonary fibrosis. *PLoS ONE.* (2016) 11:e0151425. doi: 10.1371/journal.pone.0151425

25. Caminati A, Lonati C, Cassandro R, Elia D, Pelosi G, Torre O, et al. Comorbidities in idiopathic pulmonary fibrosis: an underestimated issue. *Eur Respir Rev.* (2019) 28:190044. doi: 10.1183/16000617.0044-2019

26. Perez-Padilla R, Salas J, Carrillo G, Selman M, Chapela R. Prevalence of high hematocrits in patients with interstitial lung disease in Mexico City. *Chest.* (1992) 101:1691–3. doi: 10.1378/chest.101.6.1691

27. Aguirre C, Torres-Duque C, Salazar G, Gonzalez-Garcia M, Jaramillo C, Casas A, et al. "Prevalence of pulmonary hypertension in patients with chronic obstructive pulmonary disease living at high altitude. In *D59. COPD Epidemiology: Risk Factors, Trends, Comorbidities. American Thoracic Society International Conference Abstracts.* San Francisco, CA (2012). p. A6883.

28. Briceño C, Sepulveda C, Melo J, Linacre V, Dreyse J. Hipertensión pulmonar en pacientes con fibrosis pulmonar y sobrevida post-trasplante pulmonar. *Rev Chil Enferm Respir.* (2016) 32:13–7. doi: 10.4067/S0717-73482016000100003

29. West JB. The physiologic basis of high-altitude diseases. *Ann Intern Med.* (2004) 141:789–800. doi: 10.7326/0003-4819-141-10-200411160-00010

30. Alakhras M, Decker PA, Nadrous HF, Collazo-Clavell M, Ryu JH. Body mass index and mortality in patients with idiopathic pulmonary fibrosis. *Chest.* (2007) 131:1448–53. doi: 10.1378/chest.06-2784

31. Nakatsuka Y, Handa T, Kokosi M, Tanizawa K, Puglisi S, Jacob J, et al. The clinical significance of body weight loss in idiopathic pulmonary fibrosis patients. *Respiration.* (2018) 96:338–47. doi: 10.1159/000490355

32. Oldham JM, Collard HR. Comorbid conditions in idiopathic pulmonary fibrosis: recognition and management. *Front Med (Lausanne).* (2017) 4:123. doi: 10.3389/fmed.2017.00123

33. Oldham JM, Kumar D, Lee C, Patel SB, Takahashi-Manns S, Demchuk C, et al. Thyroid disease is prevalent and predicts survival in patients with idiopathic pulmonary fibrosis. *Chest.* (2015) 148:692–700. doi: 10.1378/chest.14-2714

34. Tomassetti S, Gurioli C, Ryu JH, Decker PA, Ravaglia C, Tantalocco P, et al. The impact of lung cancer on survival of idiopathic pulmonary fibrosis. *Chest.* (2015) 147:157–64. doi: 10.1378/chest.14-0359

35. Wong MCS, Lao XQ, Ho KF, Goggins WB, Tse SLA. Incidence and mortality of lung cancer: global trends and association with socioeconomic status. *Sci Rep.* (2017) 7:14300. doi: 10.1038/s41598-017-14513-7

36. Sung H, Ferlay J, Siegel RL, Laversanne M, Soerjomataram I, Jemal A, et al. Global cancer statistics 2020: GLOBOCAN estimates of incidence and mortality worldwide for 36 cancers in 185 countries. *CA Cancer J Clin.* (2021) 71:209–49. doi: 10.3322/caac.21660

37. Mortimer K, Hartmann N, Chan C, Norman H, Wallace L, Enger C. Characterizing idiopathic pulmonary fibrosis patients using US Medicare-advantage health plan claims data. *BMC Pulm Med.* (2019) 19:11. doi: 10.1186/s12890-018-0759-5

38. Selman M, Buendia-Roldan I, Pardo A. Aging and pulmonary fibrosis. *Rev Invest Clin.* (2016) 68:75–83.

39. Spella M, Lilis I, Stathopoulos GT. Shared epithelial pathways to lung repair and disease. *Eur Respir Rev.* (2017) 26:170048. doi: 10.1183/16000617.0048-2017

40. Cottin V. Combined pulmonary fibrosis and emphysema: bad and ugly all the same? *Eur Respir J.* (2017) 50:1700846. doi: 10.1183/13993003.00846-2017

41. Lee JS, Collard HR, Anstrom KJ, Martinez FJ, Noth I, Roberts RS, et al. Anti-acid treatment and disease progression in idiopathic pulmonary fibrosis: an analysis of data from three randomised controlled trials. *Lancet Respir Med.* (2013) 1:369–76. doi: 10.1016/S2213-2600(13)70105-X

42. Kreuter M, Wuyts W, Renzoni E, Koschel D, Maher TM, Kolb M, et al. Antacid therapy and disease outcomes in idiopathic pulmonary fibrosis: a pooled analysis. *Lancet Respir Med.* (2016) 4:381–9. doi: 10.1016/S2213-2600(16)00067-9

43. Kreuter M, Spagnolo P, Wuyts W, Renzoni E, Koschel D, Bonella F, et al. Antacid therapy and disease progression in patients with idiopathic pulmonary fibrosis who received pirfenidone. *Respiration.* (2017) 93:415–23. doi: 10.1159/000468546

44. Tran T, Assayag D, Ernst P, Suissa S. Effectiveness of proton pump inhibitors in idiopathic pulmonary fibrosis: a population-based cohort study. *Chest.* (2021) 159:673–82. doi: 10.1016/j.chest.2020.08.2080

45. Kolilekas L, Manali E, Vlami KA, Lyberopoulos P, Triantafillidou C, Kagouridis K, et al. Sleep oxygen desaturation predicts survival in idiopathic pulmonary fibrosis. *J Clin Sleep Med.* (2013) 9:593–601. doi: 10.5664/jcsm.2758

46. Gille T, Didier M, Boubaya M, Moya L, Sutton A, Carton Z, et al. Obstructive sleep apnoea and related comorbidities in incident idiopathic pulmonary fibrosis. *Eur Respir J.* (2017) 49:1601934. doi: 10.1183/13993003.01934-2016

4

Methotrexate-Associated Pneumonitis and Rheumatoid Arthritis-Interstitial Lung Disease: Current Concepts for the Diagnosis and Treatment

George E. Fragoulis [1,2], Elena Nikiphorou [3], Jörg Larsen [4], Peter Korsten [5] and Richard Conway [6*]

[1] First Department of Propaedeutic Internal Medicine, National and Kapodistrian University of Athens, Laiko General Hospital, Athens, Greece, [2] Institute of Infection, Immunity and Inflammation, University of Glasgow, Glasgow, United Kingdom, [3] Department of Inflammation Biology, Faculty of Life Sciences & Medicine, Centre for Rheumatic Diseases, School of Immunology and Microbial Sciences, King's College London, London, United Kingdom, [4] Department of Diagnostic and Interventional Radiology, University Medical Center Göttingen, Göttingen, Germany, [5] Department of Nephrology and Rheumatology, University Medical Center Göttingen, Göttingen, Germany, [6] Department of Rheumatology, Blackrock Clinic, Dublin, Ireland

*Correspondence:
Richard Conway
drrichardconway@gmail.com

Rheumatoid arthritis (RA) is a type of inflammatory arthritis that affects ~1% of the general population. Although arthritis is the cardinal symptom, many extra-articular manifestations can occur. Lung involvement and particularly interstitial lung disease (ILD) is among the most common. Although ILD can occur as part of the natural history of RA (RA-ILD), pulmonary fibrosis has been also linked with methotrexate (MTX); a condition also known as MTX-pneumonitis (M-pneu). This review aims to discuss epidemiological, diagnostic, imaging and histopathological features, risk factors, and treatment options in RA-ILD and M-pneu. M-pneu, usually has an acute/subacute course characterized by cough, dyspnea and fever. Several risk factors, including genetic and environmental factors have been suggested, but none have been validated. The diagnosis is based on clinical and radiologic findings which are mostly consistent with non-specific interstitial pneumonia (NSIP), more so than bronchiolitis obliterans organizing pneumonia (BOOP). Histological findings include interstitial infiltrates by lymphocytes, histiocytes, and eosinophils with or without non-caseating granulomas. Treatment requires immediate cessation of MTX and commencement of glucocorticoids. RA-ILD shares the same symptomatology with M-pneu. However, it usually has a more chronic course. RA-ILD occurs in about 3–5% of RA patients, although this percentage is significantly increased when radiologic criteria are used. Usual interstitial pneumonia (UIP) and NSIP are the most common radiologic patterns. Several risk factors have been identified for RA-ILD including smoking, male gender, and positivity for anti-citrullinated peptide antibodies and rheumatoid factor. Diagnosis is based on clinical and radiologic findings while pulmonary function tests may demonstrate a restrictive pattern. Although no clear guidelines exist for RA-ILD treatment, glucocorticoids and conventional disease modifying antirheumatic drugs (DMARDs) like MTX or leflunomide, as well as treatment with biologic DMARDs can be effective. There is limited evidence that rituximab, abatacept, and tocilizumab are better options compared to TNF-inhibitors.

Keywords: rheumatoid arthritis, interstitial lung disease, methotrexate, biologics, immunosuppressive therapies

INTRODUCTION

Rheumatoid arthritis (RA) is the most common inflammatory arthritis with a worldwide prevalence of about 1% and a female predominance of about 3:1 (1). While there are numerous synthetic and biologic disease-modifying antirheumatic drugs (DMARDs) that can halt progression of the articular manifestations of the disease, data on extraarticular manifestations are less conclusive. Over the past few years, the lung has become a major focus in terms of pathophysiology and overall prognosis (2). In clinical practice, there are perceived discrepancies regarding pulmonary toxicity between pulmonologists and rheumatologists, especially regarding methotrexate (MTX) and the potential risks of long-term pulmonary fibrosis. Over the past few years, more evidence has evolved adding to the controversy. To make matters more complex, the pulmonary toxicity of biological therapies is less clear. Therefore, rheumatologists are frequently faced with the situation of how to treat joint manifestations effectively in the presence of interstitial lung disease (ILD) since evidence regarding pulmonary safety is sparse. In this review article, we aim to summarize the available evidence regarding MTX-associated pneumonitis (M-pneu), RA-ILD, and discuss treatment options based on available evidence.

METHODS AND LITERATURE SELECTION

A focused literature review including the keywords "methotrexate," "pneumonitis," "interstitial lung disease," and "rheumatoid arthritis" was performed. In addition, articles from the personal archives of the authors or references from key papers were included if deemed relevant by the authors.

PULMONARY DISEASE PATTERNS IN RHEUMATOID ARTHRITIS

Methotrexate-Associated Pneumonitis
Epidemiology
The frequency of M-pneu has been reported to range between 0.3 and 11.6% (3–6), depending on the methodology used and the criteria applied for M-pneu diagnosis. Interestingly, since 2001, no cases of M-pneu have been reported in randomized clinical trials of MTX in RA (7). M-pneu generally has an acute or subacute course and is usually observed within the first year of treatment (8). However, cases of late-onset M-pneu have been also described (9, 10).

Clinical Symptomatology and Laboratory Findings
Symptomatology mainly pertains to dry cough and dyspnea observed in more than 80% of the patients. Fever also occurs in more than 60% of them (3, 11, 12). Some authors have suggested that mild peripheral blood eosinophilia is present in about 25–40% of patients with sub-acute M-pneu (4, 9–11). Also, in case-series from patients with M-pneu it was demonstrated that peripheral blood lymphocytes dropped at the time of M-pneu and went back to normal after recovery (13). These findings, although very useful in everyday clinical practice, remain to be confirmed in larger studies.

Pathogenesis and Risk Factors for the Development of M-Pneu
Pathogenic mechanisms underlying M-pneu are unclear. It is considered by many investigators to be a hypersensitivity reaction, while interleukin-8 has been implicated in the pathogenesis (14). It should also be noted that patients receiving MTX are also at an increased risk for developing MTX-related lymphoproliferative disorder (LPD) (15). Interestingly, LPD regresses in many cases after the withdrawal of MTX (15, 16). Recent studies investigating the clinical and histopathologic characteristics of these patients have shown that in half of these cases this is linked to Epstein-Barr virus infection (15, 17) with p38 MAP kinase, PI3 kinase, and MEK pathways being implicated (18). The lung can also be involved in the context of MTX-related LPD (15, 16, 19, 20): Cases of lung lymphomatoid granulomatosis, a rare entity characterized histologically by multiple nodular lesions and vessel wall infiltration by lymphoid cells, have been described (16, 19, 20).

Several risk factors have been identified (**Table 1**), but it is remains uncertain to what extent they contribute to the occurrence of M-pneu. These factors include: age more than 60 years, diabetes mellitus, hypoalbuminemia, previous use of DMARDs), renal dysfunction, male gender, increased Health Assessment Questionnaire (HAQ) score, decreased pain Visual Analog Scale (VAS) score and pre-existing lung disease (6, 12, 21–23). However, these have not been replicated in other studies (24). Genetic factors might also play a role. In a Japanese population, an association between M-pneu and the HLA-A31:01 haplotype has been described (25). However, in a Genome Wide Association Study in a United Kingdom population, these results were not reproduced, but three Single Nucleotide Polymorphisms (SNPs) have been found to be associated with M-pneu occurrence with borderline significance (26). Environmental factors also possibly contribute. It has been suggested that increased latitude is related to an increased risk for M-pneu development. In fact, Jordan et al. using data from the New Zealand ministry of health showed that

TABLE 1 | Proposed risk factors for the development of methotrexate-associated pneumonitis (M-pneu) and rheumatoid-arthritis-interstitial lung disease (RA-ILD).

Risk factors	
M-pneu	**RA-ILD**
Pre-existing lung disease	Disease activity
Age > 60 years	Age
Male sex	Male gender
Diabetes mellitus	Smoking
High HAQ score, low pain VAS score	Positive rheumatoid factor
Chronic kidney disease	Positive anti-citrullinated peptide antibody
Hypoalbuminemia	MUC5B promoter variant rs35705950
Previous use of DMARDs	
Genetic factors (e.g., HLA-A31:01)*	
Environmental factors (e.g., latitude)	

DMARDs, disease-modifying antirheumatic drugs; HAQ, health assessment questionnaire; HLA, human leukocyte antigen; VAS, visual analog scale.
*Not confirmed in all populations.

the incidence rate ratio for M-pneu was increased by 16% per one degree of increasing latitude (27).

Diagnosis

A diagnosis of M-pneu is based on the clinical and radiologic findings. Other diagnostic modalities like pulmonary function tests (PFTs) and bronchoalveolar lavage (BAL) might prove to be helpful as well. However, the differential diagnosis, which includes infections, like *Pneumocystis jirovecii* pneumonia (PJP), viral and atypical pneumonias, and ILD due to RA (RA-ILD), is difficult to be made (11).

Performance of PFTs routinely for diagnostic or prognostic purposes is still under debate (12). Although some studies have demonstrated only a minor effect of MTX on PFTs (28), two prospective studies have found that there are some alterations: Khadadah et al. (29), describe that after 2 years of treatment of low-dose MTX, patients may develop a restrictive pattern with significant decline in total lung capacity (TLC), functional residual capacity (FRC), forced expiratory volume in 1 s (FEV1), forced vital capacity (FVC), and an increase in the FEV1/FVC ratio. Similarly, Cottin et al. (30), examining 124 patients treated with MTX, described a reduction of FVC, FEV1, and diffusing capacity of the lung for carbon monoxide (DLCO)/alveolar volume (VA). However, these changes could not predict the 3.2% of patients who developed M-pneu in their study (30). On the other hand, Saravanan et al. (8), have suggested that PFT abnormalities [low FEV1, vital capacity (VC) and diffusing transfer of the lung for carbon monoxide (TLCO)] might have a prognostic role, carrying a higher risk for M-pneu development in RA patients.

Of note, in published guidelines for MTX treatment in RA, based on literature review and expert opinion it is stated that PFTs with DLCO should be performed in patients with pre-existing lung disease or current symptoms (low strength of recommendation [D]) (6). In pediatric populations, some studies do not describe any abnormalities in children with juvenile

idiopathic arthritis (JIA) treated with MTX (31, 32), while others conclude that there are some alterations in PFTs, like decrease of the mid-mean expiratory flow (MMEF) and DLCO (33, 34) or an increase in the TLC, FRC and residual volume (RV) (35). However, these are not affected by MTX and they were rather attributed to JIA *per se*. Besides, none of these patients developed clinically significant lung disease in these studies (33).

BAL examination is often performed in these patients. Most investigators agree that a lymphocytic pattern is observed (36), although cases of with BAL neutrophilia have been also reported (10, 37). Lymphocytosis in BAL is not specific for M-pneu as it is also seen in interstitial pneumonitis due to RA (36, 38) and in RA patients treated with MTX without respiratory symptoms (39). A recent systematic literature review examining characteristics of BAL in M-pneu has shown that lymphocytosis was present in the majority (89%) of BAL samples, while high levels of neutrophils were present in only 17% (40). In fact, six cytological patterns were identified (four with predominant lymphocytosis and two in which neutrophilia was the principal finding (40). It has been also suggested that predominance of CD4$^+$ T cells in BAL is suggestive of M-pneu (36) but there is some evidence that an increased CD4/CD8 ratio can also be found in other RA patients, usually those with pulmonary involvement (40). Also, the CD4/CD8 ratio can be found low or normal in about half of the M-pneu patients. Chikura et al. suggested that neutrophils are increased in the BAL of patients with M-pneu having received treatment for <6 months and with a cumulative dose of <300 mg, while the opposite was the case for lymphocyte numbers (41). These results were independent of the indication for which MTX was given (i.e., RA, Primary biliary cholangitis, Psoriatic arthritis, and others). Finally, serum levels of KL-6, a glycoprotein antigen, and surfactant protein D, both expressed mainly by type II pneumocytes, have been proposed as biomarkers for diagnosing and monitoring M-pneu (42). However, they are found to be increased in other lung diseases as well (43), therefore their utility, if any, in the setting of M-pneu remains to be defined.

Transbronchial lung biopsy (TBLB) might also be a useful diagnostic adjunct. In a study evaluating 44 patients with drug-induced lung injury, 75% underwent TBLB (44). TBLB was diagnostically helpful in 75%. Although histopathology alone cannot diagnose M-pneu, it may provide useful supplemental information that can be incorporated with clinical, radiologic, laboratory, and other features in the final diagnosis (44).

Imaging Features

Radiological findings reflect the underlying histopathologic process and include mostly non-specific interstitial pneumonia (NSIP), more so than bronchiolitis obliterans organizing pneumonia (BOOP) (45): on chest radiography, M-pneu gives rise to diffuse heterogeneous opacities in NSIP or bilateral scattered heterogeneous or homogeneous opacities with a peripheral distribution in the upper and lower lobes in BOOP. On CT scanning, scattered or diffuse ground-glass opacities are seen in early NSIP and basal fibrosis in the later stages of the disease. In BOOP, poorly defined nodular consolidations, centrilobular nodules, bronchiolitic (tree-in-bud) changes and

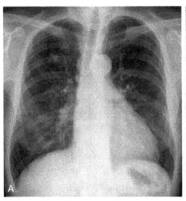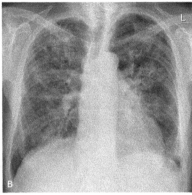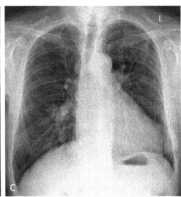

FIGURE 1 | Methotrexate-induced pneumonitis in a 77-year-old man with rheumatoid arthritis. **(A)** Posterior-anterior chest radiograph immediately before the initiation of treatment. Following 10 days of methotrexate, the patient experienced progressive dyspnea and fever. Follow-up chest radiography showed bilateral heterogeneous opacities in all lung zones. **(B)** The patient was transferred to the intensive care unit for supportive treatment. High-dose glucocorticoids were administered and gradually withdrawn following clinical and radiological improvement. Initial high-resolution CT scanning showed diffuse infiltrates and bilateral patchy consolidations with only very limited ground-glass opacities (images not shown). **(C)** Seven months after stopping methotrexate, the changes of pulmonary toxicity had fully resolved.

bronchial dilatation are the dominant features (**Figures 1A–C**) (6, 46). In a study examining CT findings in M-pneu, it was found that in the majority of the patients, these lesions subsided during a mean follow-up period of 31 days (46).

Histologic Findings

The most common histopathological pattern observed includes interstitial infiltrates by lymphocytes, histiocytes, and eosinophils with or without granulomas (36). Granulomas, usually non-caseating, are also identified in some patients, while hyperplastic type II pneumocytes and perivascular inflammation are also commonly seen (47). Other patterns have also been described and often coexist with interstitial pneumonitis, such as diffuse and organized alveolar damage (3, 12, 47). The latter seems to be more frequent in acute cases of M-pneu (47).

Treatment

In suspected M-pneu MTX should be discontinued immediately. Often, treatment with steroids is required (8). Other immunosuppressive drugs, such as cyclophosphamide (CYC), have also been administered successfully (48). Tocilizumab (TCZ), given its efficacy as monotherapy in RA, is also an attractive therapeutic option, since its use has been reported to be beneficial (38).

Prognosis

The prognosis of M-pneu is generally good and most patients recover fully (8), however, mortality is reported to be relatively high reaching 17.6% (6, 11). Other smaller studies have reported even higher figures up to 30% (49). Besides, in a review assessing patients (including individuals with RA) who developed M-pneu, the percentage was 13% (47). Furthermore, a study by Chikura et al. examining 56 RA patients with M-pneu suggested that mortality was more increased in patients who developed pneumonitis after treated with MTX for <6 months compared to those treated for a longer time period (41). It is suggested that this difference in mortality is accompanied by specific histopathologic

features and characteristics in the BAL examination (41). Re-introduction of MTX in patients who have developed M-pneu has led to recurrence of lung injury and in many cases to death (11, 49). There are single cases, however, in which the drug has been re-introduced successfully (50).

Rheumatoid Arthritis Related Interstitial Lung Disease

RA is not merely a disease of the joints. It is a true systemic inflammatory disease with effects on many organs and organ systems. A variety of pulmonary manifestations can be seen in RA including pulmonary nodules, pleural effusions, bronchiectasis, and, most importantly, ILD (2).

Epidemiology

ILD is a frequently under-recognized complication of RA. The estimated prevalence is heavily dependent on the ascertainment method used. Bongartz et al. reported a lifetime risk of 7.7%, a 9-fold increase over the general population (51). Studies using the ERAS and ERAN early arthritis cohorts as well as the ILD specific BRILL study in the UK reported a prevalence of RA-ILD of 3–5% (52, 53) (**Table 2**). All of these studies identified clinical RA-ILD; if screening of asymptomatic individuals with RA is utilized, the prevalence of ILD increases depending on the performance characteristics of the screening methodology used. High resolution CT scanning identifies ILD in 19–67% of RA patients depending on the thresholds for diagnosis employed (54, 55). A study performing unselected histological assessment of pulmonary tissue in RA patients revealed evidence of ILD in 80% of patients (69). For these studies in which ILD was diagnosed based on radiologic and histological data, it should be noted that they probably overestimate clinically relevant RA-ILD. Patients were included irrespective of pulmonary symptoms and many of them had normal PFTs.

TABLE 2 | Comparison of clinical and imaging features in M-pneu vs. RA-ILD.

	MTX-pneu	RA-ILD	References
Frequency in RA	0.3–11.6%	3–5% (clinical diagnosis) 19–67% (radiological diagnosis)	(3–6, 52–55)
Course	Usually acute or sub-acute, within the first year of treatment	Usually chronic*	(8, 10, 38)
Clinical symptoms	Fever, dry cough, dyspnoea	Fever, dry cough, dyspnoea	(3, 11, 12)
Imaging findings	Mostly NSIP No specific predilection New or evolving diffuse interstitial or mixed interstitial and alveolar infiltrates Diffuse and patchy bilateral ground glass opacity with or without reticulation Cellular interstitial infiltrates, granulomas, diffuse alveolar damage	UIP > NSIP Basal and peripheral distribution CXR: punctate and reticulonodular densities and coarse reticulations CT: basal cystic changes (honeycombing, periperheal reticular opacities, bronchioloectasis Lower lobe volume loss in the course of disease	(45–47, 56–58)
Bronchoalveolar lavage	Lymphocytic more common that neutrophilic pattern	Neutrophilic or lymphocytic pattern#	(36, 40, 41, 59)
Histopathology	Interstitial infiltrates by lymphocytes, histiocytes and eosinophils sometimes with non-caseating granulomas	UIP, NSIP > OP and other patterns	(12, 38, 47, 53, 60)
Treatment options	Discontinuation of MTX Glucocorticoids Rarely cyclophosphamide, TCZ	Glucocorticoids MTX or LEF possibly beneficial anti-TNF, ATC, TCZ: inconclusive data rituximab: possibly beneficial	(3, 7, 8, 12, 48, 61–68)

*ATC, abatacept; CT; computed tomography; CXR, chest x-ray; LEF, leflunomide; MTX, methotrexate; NSIP, non-specific interstitial pneumonia; OP, organizing pneumonia; TCZ, tocilizumab; TNF, tumor necrosis factor; UIP, usual interstitial pneumonia. *Cases of fulminant RA-ILD have been described. #It has been suggested that RA patients with clinical/radiologic findings of lung involvement have neutrophilic pattern and those without a lymphocytic pattern.*

Pathogenesis and Risk Factors

Increasing evidence supports a primary role for the lung in initiating RA pathogenesis and RA-ILD may occur prior to the onset of the joint disease (70–72). Known predictors of RA-ILD include RA severity, age, male sex, smoking, and seropositivity for rheumatoid factor or anti-citrullinated peptide antibodies anti-citrullinated peptide antibodies (51, 71) (**Table 1**). In the past several years, biomarkers for RA-ILD have been suggested: Citrullinated isoforms of heat shock protein 90 (hsp90) have been shown to be potentially useful as a biomarker of RA-ILD (73). Hsp90 could also be identified in BAL specimens (74). Recently,

the gain-of-function MUC5B promoter variant rs35705950, has been found to be associated with the development of ILD in RA patients with an Odds Ratio of 3.1 (75). This is especially interesting given that the same MUC5B variant is the strongest known risk factor for idiopathic pulmonary fibrosis (IPF), which shares many similarities with RA-ILD (76).

Clinical Symptomatology and Laboratory Findings

The clinical findings in RA-ILD are similar to those previously described for M-pneu with dyspnoea and non-productive cough with or without fever predominating (7). Most typically, RA-ILD develops insidiously over time and may be present and asymptomatic for a significant period. This diagnostic delay may be further exacerbated by the fact that patient's rheumatoid joint disease may limit their ability to exercise sufficiently to precipitate exertional dyspnea. Clinical examination findings may be absent in early disease but ultimately the majority of patients will have fine bibasal crepitations (77). The majority of those with an usual interstitial pneumonia (UIP) pattern RA-ILD will also develop clubbing, similar to IPF patients (77). Radiologic findings are of little help in distinguishing the two disorders with a significant degree of overlapping features (46). However, a key distinguishing feature can be chronicity. MTX-pneu is typically a fulminant acute process (11) (**Table 2**). A more indolent subacute or chronic development of radiologic findings strongly favors RA-ILD. In this scenario, historic radiologic imaging demonstrating evidence of similar but early ILD changes argues against MTX-pneu. However, RA-ILD may present as a fulminant and potentially fatal process, including early in the disease process (2, 78, 79).

Diagnosis

The diagnosis of RA-ILD can generally be made by a combination of clinical features as described above and congruent findings on chest imaging. It is important to remember that RA patients are, at least equally, and in often cases more likely, to develop other causes of dyspnea and cough than the general population. For example, the risk of infection, including atypical infections, pulmonary emboli, and lung cancer, are all increased in RA patients (80–82). PFTs may provide evidence of restrictive lung disease with a reduced TLCO/DCLO generally being the first manifestation.

Bronchoscopy and BAL may be performed to rule out other diagnoses. BAL is frequently abnormal in RA-ILD, but the findings are non-specific and rarely diagnostically useful. In rare cases open lung biopsy may be needed to confirm a diagnosis, in general when an alternative diagnosis is suspected.

Imaging Features

Apart from treatment-related complications, the thoracic manifestations of RA are plentiful (56) and include pleural changes, large airway involvement and, more so than with other collagen vascular diseases, a usual interstitial pneumonia (UIP) pattern of interstitial lung disease as distinct from a non-specific interstitial pneumonia (NSIP) or other patterns (71, 83) (**Table 2**). Clinically relevant ILD is less common, comprising basal cystic changes (honey combing), peripheral reticular

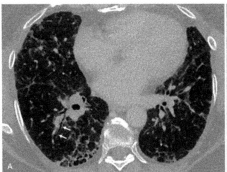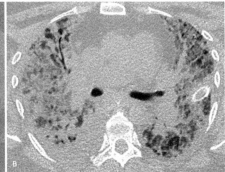

FIGURE 2 | Interstitial lung disease in a 56-year-old woman with rheumatoid arthritis. **(A)** One millimeter transverse axial CT-section through the lung bases show subpleural honeycombing and early traction bronchiectasis (arrows), consistent with a usual interstitial pneumonia pattern. **(B)** Nine months later, the patient developed severe dyspnea at rest and required mechanical ventilation. On bronchoalveolar lavage, influenza A virus was found to be present. A follow-up CT now showed a small right-sided pleural effusion and multifocally confluent consolidation, partially obscuring equally patchy bilateral ground-glass opacification. A few thickened septae (crazy-paving pattern) could be delineated (not shown). These findings were consistent with a viral pneumonia. Despite extracorporeal membrane oxygenation therapy, the patient deceased.

opacities and bronchioloectasis, best seen on CT scanning, and lower lobe volume loss which may advance in the chronic stage (**Figure 2**). Bronchiolitis obliterans has been described in RA, while follicular bronchiolitis is more common, showing small nodular changes on CT. Rheumatoid nodules as large as 5 cm are more likely in men, typically occur in smokers and may be seen prior to the articular manifestation of the disease. Nodules may cavitate, occasionally calcify and rarely rupture.

Histologic Findings
Findings on BAL are generally abnormal but non-specific in RA-ILD. Common findings include some form of neutrophil or lymphocytic predominant leucocytosis, or alterations in T-lymphocyte ratios (36, 41, 59, 84–86). Histologic findings are congruent with those seen with the underlying ILD phenotype, including neutrophilic or lymphocytic infiltrates, and fibrotic changes. A number of histopathological findings have been suggested to aid in the differentiation of MTX-pneu from RA-ILD including type II pneumocyte hyperplasia and fibroblast proliferation (11). However, these features have also been reported in RA-ILD.

Treatment
Glucocorticoids remain an important part of the acute management of RA-ILD. The optimum longer-term management of RA-ILD is uncertain, however, given the known factors predictive of RA-ILD described above it is logical that good RA disease control should be the cornerstone of any strategy (61). This is supported by the significant decline in the reported frequency of RA-ILD as RA treatment options have advanced (87). Given its proven efficacy in RA joint disease there is good reason to expect that MTX may be a justified part of any treatment strategy in an RA patient with ILD; evidence to support this strategy is beginning to emerge (60, 88). Despite previous concerns over potential pulmonary toxicity with leflunomide, this agent also appears to be potentially

beneficial for RA-ILD (62). In the setting of RA-ILD, the choice of biological therapy is not clear: A recent review of the literature identified seven studies and 28 case reports, which showed an increased mortality with the use of tumor necrosis factor-inhibitors (TNF-i) (63). In this analysis, female sex and longer disease duration were associated with ILD onset or worsening (63). The heterogeneity in the reported outcome measures was too large to draw any firm conclusions. Other agents, such as Abatacept (ATC) have been investigated in few studies: In a Japanese study, deterioration of RA-ILD was described in 11 of 131 patients (8.4%) and was associated with concomitant MTX use (Odds Ratio of 12.75) (89). By contrast, a multicentric analysis from Spain concluded that ATC was associated with stable ILD in about two thirds of the patients (64). The role of TCZ in RA-ILD is less clear. A retrospective study in Japan showed worsening of ILD with TCZ in only six of 78 patients (7.7%) (65) or even improvement (38). These findings are in line with data from clinical trials in Systemic sclerosis (90), where it has been shown to preserve lung function, although this was not the primary endpoint.

Preliminary evidence of a particular role for Rituximab (RTX) is beginning to emerge (66, 67, 91, 92). An observational study of 56 patients with RA-ILD treated with RTX showed that 16% improved and 52% remained stable; a particularly impressive response given the aggressive natural history of RA-ILD (11, 66). This is logical given the association of RA-ILD with other known predictors of Rituximab response, in particular seropositivity (68).

Other agents are currently under investigation in the treatment of RA-ILD: The anti-fibrotic tyrosine kinase inhibitor nintedanib has been shown to be effective in an animal model of RA-ILD; the same agent has demonstrable efficacy in RCTs in IPF and, recently, also in systemic sclerosis (93–95). Another anti-fibrotic agent, pirfenidone, has been shown to downregulate profibrotic pathways in a bleomycin-induced mouse model and lung biopsy specimens from RA-ILD patients (96). **Figure 3**

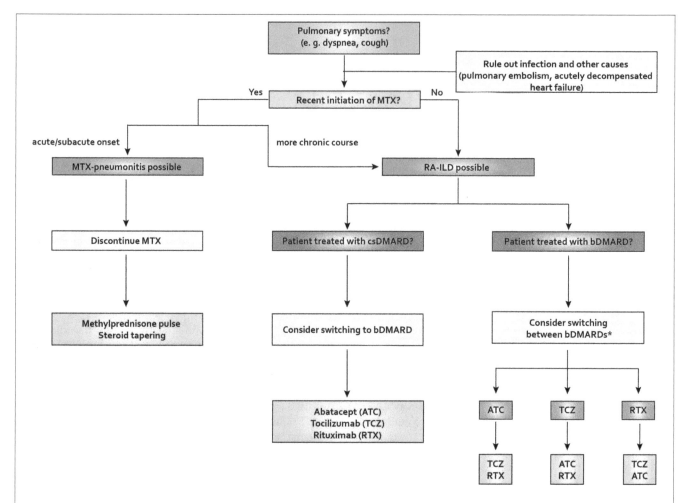

FIGURE 3 | Proposed algorithm for pulmonary symptoms in rheumatoid arthritis. In the setting of recent MTX initiation, MTX-pneu is always a concern, especially if the onset of symptoms is acute or sub-acute. In this case, MTX needs to be stopped and usually glucocorticoid therapy and supportive care in an intensive care unit is required. If the onset is more insidious, RA-ILD is a possibility. After ruling out other causes of pulmonary symptoms, management should depend on various factors, including comorbities, age, disease activity, and others. If a patient is diagnosed as having RA-ILD and receives a csDMARD, switching to a bDMARD may be appropriate. If a patient is already on bDMARD therapy, switching therapies may be required. Many authors tend to avoid TNF-inhibitors in this situation, but the evidence is weak. ATC, abatacept; bDMARD, biological disease-modifying antirheumatic drug; csDMARD, conventional synthetic disease-modifying antirheumatic drug; ILD, interstitial lung disease; MTX, methotrexate; MTX-pneu, MTX-pneumonitis; RA, rheumatoid arthritis; RTX, rituximab; TCZ, tocilizumab. *TNF-inhibitors have been reported to be associated with worsening lung function in RA-ILD (weak evidence level).

depicts our proposed treatment approach to the treatment of pulmonary manifestations in RA.

Prognosis

ILD in general has a poor prognosis, however, this is even more true of RA-ILD, which has an ominous prognosis with a Hazard Ratio (HR) for death of 2.86 (51). Overall, respiratory causes are the second most common cause of death in patients with RA; symptomatic RA-ILD contributes 13% of the excess mortality associated with RA (51, 53, 97). Median survival following a diagnosis of RA-ILD is <3 years (2, 97). Acute fulminant RA-ILD occurring rapidly following disease onset is well-documented and frequently fatal (2, 78, 79). RA-ILD patients with a UIP pattern on imaging have increased mortality compared to other patterns, with a relative risk of 2.39 for UIP compared to NSIP (98). As well as the inherent mortality associated with RA-ILD itself,

these patients are also at significantly increased risk of pulmonary infection (71, **Figure 2**).

CONCLUSIONS AND FUTURE RESEARCH DIRECTIONS

Methotrexate pneumonitis usually presents acutely but its incidence has been decreasing over time. Suspension of MTX and administration of glucocorticoid pulse therapy are usually required. In the long term, MTX therapy may associate with a lower incidence of RA-ILD, thus questioning the fear of progressive pulmonary fibrosis associated with this agent. Regarding bDMARDs, ATC, TCZ, or RTX appear more promising than TNF-i in patients requiring more intense immunosuppression although the evidence base for this remains weak.

Future studies should aim at determining the exact prevalence of RA-ILD in early stage RA patients and will certainly rely on PFTs and imaging with CT at baseline and during the disease course to help identify patients at high risk for progression.

REFERENCES

1. Smolen JS, Aletaha D, Barton A, Burmester GR, Emery P, Firestein GS, et al. Rheumatoid arthritis. *Nat Rev Dis Primers.* (2018) 4:18001. doi: 10.1038/nrdp.2018.1

2. Shaw M, Collins BF, Ho LA, Raghu G. Rheumatoid arthritis-associated lung disease. *Eur Respir Rev.* (2015) 24:1–16. doi: 10.1183/09059180.00008014

3. Atzeni F, Boiardi L, Sallì S, Benucci M, Sarzi-Puttini P. Lung involvement and drug-induced lung disease in patients with rheumatoid arthritis. *Expert Rev Clin Immunol.* (2013) 9:649–57. doi: 10.1586/1744666X.2013.811173

4. Barrera P, Laan RF, van Riel PL, Dekhuijzen PN, Boerbooms AM, van de Putte LB. Methotrexate-related pulmonary complications in rheumatoid arthritis. *Ann Rheum Dis.* (1994) 53:434–9. doi: 10.1136/ard.53.7.434

5. Dawson JK, Graham DR, Desmond J, Fewins HE, Lynch MP. Investigation of the chronic pulmonary effects of low-dose oral methotrexate in patients with rheumatoid arthritis: a prospective study incorporating HRCT scanning and pulmonary function tests. *Rheumatology.* (2002) 41:262–7. doi: 10.1093/rheumatology/41.3.262

6. Pavy S, Constantin A, Pham T, Gossec L, Maillefert J-F, Cantagrel A, et al. Methotrexate therapy for rheumatoid arthritis: clinical practice guidelines based on published evidence and expert opinion. *Joint Bone Spine.* (2006) 73:388–95. doi: 10.1016/j.jbspin.2006.01.007

7. Conway R, Low C, Coughlan RJ, O'Donnell MJ, Carey JJ. Methotrexate and lung disease in rheumatoid arthritis: a meta-analysis of randomized controlled trials. *Arthritis Rheumatol.* (2014) 66:803–12. doi: 10.1002/art.38322

8. Saravanan V, Kelly CA. Reducing the risk of methotrexate pneumonitis in rheumatoid arthritis. *Rheumatology.* (2004) 43:143–7. doi: 10.1093/rheumatology/keg466

9. Salehi M, Miller R, Khaing M. Methotrexate-induced Hypersensitivity Pneumonitis appearing after 30 years of use: a case report. *J Med Case Rep.* (2017) 11:174. doi: 10.1186/s13256-017-1333-0

10. Yamakawa H, Yoshida M, Takagi M, Kuwano K. Late-onset methotrexate-induced pneumonitis with neutrophilia in bronchoalveolar lavage fluid. *BMJ Case Rep.* (2014) 2014:bcr2014206123. doi: 10.1136/bcr-2014-206123

11. Kremer JM, Alarcón GS, Weinblatt ME, Kaymakcian MV, Macaluso M, Cannon GW, et al. Clinical, laboratory, radiographic, and histopathologic features of methotrexate-associated lung injury in patients with rheumatoid arthritis: a multicenter study with literature review. *Arthritis Rheum.* (1997) 40:1829–37. doi: 10.1002/art.1780401016

12. Roubille C, Haraoui B. Interstitial lung diseases induced or exacerbated by DMARDS and biologic agents in rheumatoid arthritis: a systematic literature review. *Semin Arthritis Rheum.* (2014) 43:613–26. doi: 10.1016/j.semarthrit.2013.09.005

13. Inokuma S, Kono H, Kohno Y, Hiramatsu K, Ito K, Shiratori K, et al. Methotrexate-induced lung injury in patients with rheumatoid arthritis occurs with peripheral blood lymphocyte count decrease. *Ann Rheum Dis.* (2006) 65:1113–4. doi: 10.1136/ard.2005.045211

14. Fujimori Y, Kataoka M, Tada S, Takehara H, Matsuo K, Miyake T, et al. The role of interleukin-8 in interstitial pneumonia. *Respirology.* (2003) 8:33–40. doi: 10.1046/j.1440-1843.2003.00420.x

15. Yamakawa H, Yoshida M, Katagi H, Hirooka S, Okuda K, Ishikawa T, et al. Pulmonary and retroperitoneal lesions induced by methotrexate-associated lymphoproliferative disorder in a patient with rheumatoid arthritis. *Mod Rheumatol.* (2016) 26:441–4. doi: 10.3109/14397595.2014.898559

16. Kameda H, Okuyama A, Tamaru J-I, Itoyama S, Iizuka A, Takeuchi T. Lymphomatoid granulomatosis and diffuse alveolar damage associated with methotrexate therapy in a patient with rheumatoid arthritis. *Clin Rheumatol.* (2007) 26:1585–9. doi: 10.1007/s10067-006-0480-2

17. Kurita D, Miyoshi H, Ichikawa A, Kato K, Imaizumi Y, Seki R, et al. Methotrexate-associated lymphoproliferative disorders in patients with rheumatoid arthritis: clinicopathologic features and prognostic factors. *Am J Surg Pathol.* (2019) 43:869–84. doi: 10.1097/PAS.0000000000001271

18. Feng W, Cohen JI, Fischer S, Li L, Sneller M, Goldbach-Mansky R, et al. Reactivation of latent Epstein-Barr virus by methotrexate: a potential contributor to methotrexate-associated lymphomas. *J Natl Cancer Inst.* (2004) 96:1691–702. doi: 10.1093/jnci/djh313

19. Barakat A, Grover K, Peshin R. Rituximab for pulmonary lymphomatoid granulomatosis which developed as a complication of methotrexate and azathioprine therapy for rheumatoid arthritis. *Springerplus.* (2014) 3:751. doi: 10.1186/2193-1801-3-751

20. Shimada K, Matsui T, Kawakami M, Nakayama H, Ozawa Y, Mitomi H, et al. Methotrexate-related lymphomatoid granulomatosis: a case report of spontaneous regression of large tumours in multiple organs after cessation of methotrexate therapy in rheumatoid arthritis. *Scand J Rheumatol.* (2007) 36:64–7. doi: 10.1080/03009740600902403

21. Alarcón GS, Kremer JM, Macaluso M, Weinblatt ME, Cannon GW, Palmer WR, et al. Risk factors for methotrexate-induced lung injury in patients with rheumatoid arthritis. A multicenter, case-control study. Methotrexate-Lung Study Group. *Ann Intern Med.* (1997) 127:356–64. doi: 10.7326/0003-4819-127-5-199709010-00003

22. Ohosone Y, Okano Y, Kameda H, Fujii T, Hama N, Hirakata M, et al. Clinical characteristics of patients with rheumatoid arthritis and methotrexate induced pneumonitis. *J Rheumatol.* (1997) 24:2299–303.

23. Shidara K, Hoshi D, Inoue E, Yamada T, Nakajima A, Taniguchi A, et al. Incidence of and risk factors for interstitial pneumonia in patients with rheumatoid arthritis in a large Japanese observational cohort, IORRA. *Mod Rheumatol.* (2010) 20:280–6. doi: 10.1007/s10165-010-0280-z

24. Carroll GJ, Thomas R, Phatouros CC, Atchison MH, Leslie AL, Cook NJ, et al. Incidence, prevalence and possible risk factors for pneumonitis in patients with rheumatoid arthritis receiving methotrexate. *J Rheumatol.* (1994) 21:51–4.

25. Furukawa H, Oka S, Shimada K, Rheumatoid Arthritis-Interstitial Lung Disease Study Consortium, Tsuchiya N, Tohma S. HLA-A*31:01 and methotrexate-induced interstitial lung disease in Japanese rheumatoid arthritis patients: a multidrug hypersensitivity marker? *Ann Rheum Dis.* (2013) 72:153–5. doi: 10.1136/annrheumdis-2012-201944

26. Bluett J, Owen S-A, Massey J, Alfirevic A, Pirmohamed M, Plant D, et al. HLA-A 31:01 is not associated with the development of methotrexate pneumonitis in the UK population: results from a genome-wide association study. *Ann Rheum Dis.* (2017) 76:e51. doi: 10.1136/annrheumdis-2017-211512

27. Jordan SR, Stevanovic VR, Herbison P, Dockerty J, Highton J. Methotrexate pneumonitis in rheumatoid arthritis: increased prevalence with increasing latitude: an epidemiological study of trends in new zealand. *J Clin Rheumatol.* (2011) 17:356–7. doi: 10.1097/RHU.0b013e3182314e34

28. Beyeler C, Jordi B, Gerber NJ, Im Hof V. Pulmonary function in rheumatoid arthritis treated with low-dose methotrexate: a longitudinal study. *Br J Rheumatol.* (1996) 35:446–52. doi: 10.1093/rheumatology/35.5.446

29. Khadadah ME, Jayakrishnan B, Al-Gorair S, Al-Mutairi M, Al-Maradni N, Onadeko B, et al. Effect of methotrexate on pulmonary function in patients with rheumatoid arthritis–a prospective study. *Rheumatol Int.* (2002) 22:204–7. doi: 10.1007/s00296-002-0227-6

AUTHOR CONTRIBUTIONS

GF, EN, and RC wrote the first draft of the manuscript. PK edited and revised the manuscript and drafted the figures. JL edited the manuscript and contributed figures. All authors revised the manuscript critically and approved the final version of the manuscript.

30. Cottin V, Tébib J, Massonnet B, Souquet PJ, Bernard JP. Pulmonary function in patients receiving long-term low-dose methotrexate. *Chest.* (1996) 109:933–8. doi: 10.1378/chest.109.4.933

31. Graham LD, Myones BL, Rivas-Chacon RF, Pachman LM. Morbidity associated with long-term methotrexate therapy in juvenile rheumatoid arthritis. *J Pediatric.* (1992) 120:468–73. doi: 10.1016/S0022-3476(05)80923-0

32. Wallace CA, Bleyer WA, Sherry DD, Salmonson KL, Wedgwood RJ. Toxicity and serum levels of methotrexate in children with juvenile rheumatoid arthritis. *Arthritis Rheum.* (1989) 32:677–81. doi: 10.1002/anr.1780320604

33. Leiskau C, Thon A, Gappa M, Dressler F. Lung function in children and adolescents with juvenile idiopathic arthritis during long-term treatment with methotrexate: a retrospective study. *Clin Exp Rheumatol.* (2012) 30:302–7.

34. Schmeling H, Stephan V, Burdach S, Horneff G. Pulmonary function in children with juvenile idiopathic arthritis and effects of methotrexate therapy. *Z Rheumatol.* (2002) 61:168–72. doi: 10.1007/s003930200025

35. Camiciottoli G, Trapani S, Castellani W, Ginanni R, Ermini M, Falcini F. Effect on lung function of methotrexate and non-steroid anti-inflammatory drugs in children with juvenile rheumatoid arthritis. *Rheumatol Int.* (1998) 18:11–6. doi: 10.1007/s002960050047

36. Schnabel A, Richter C, Bauerfeind S, Gross WL. Bronchoalveolar lavage cell profile in methotrexate induced pneumonitis. *Thorax.* (1997) 52:377–9. doi: 10.1136/thx.52.4.377

37. Leduc D, De Vuyst P, Lheureux P, Gevenois PA, Jacobovitz D, Yernault JC. Pneumonitis complicating low-dose methotrexate therapy for rheumatoid arthritis. Discrepancies between lung biopsy and bronchoalveolar lavage findings. *Chest.* (1993) 104:1620–3. doi: 10.1378/chest.104.5.1620

38. Picchianti Diamanti A, Markovic M, Argento G, Giovagnoli S, Ricci A, Laganà B, et al. Therapeutic management of patients with rheumatoid arthritis and associated interstitial lung disease: case report and literature review. *Ther Adv Respir Dis.* (2017) 11:64–72. doi: 10.1177/1753465816668780

39. Scherak O, Popp W, Kolarz G, Wottawa A, Ritschka L, Braun O. Bronchoalveolar lavage and lung biopsy in rheumatoid arthritis. *In vivo* effects of disease modifying antirheumatic drugs. *J Rheumatol.* (1993) 20:944–9.

40. D'Elia T. Methotrexate-induced pneumonitis: heterogeneity of bronchoalveolar lavage and differences between cancer and rheumatoid arthritis. *Inflamm Allergy Drug Targets.* (2014) 13:25–33. doi: 10.2174/1871528112666131230013059

41. Chikura B, Sathi N, Lane S, Dawson JK. Variation of immunological response in methotrexate-induced pneumonitis. *Rheumatology.* (2008) 47:1647–50. doi: 10.1093/rheumatology/ken356

42. Taniguchi K, Usui Y, Matsuda T, Suzuki S, Fujiki K, Yakusiji F, et al. Methotrexate-induced acute lung injury in a patient with rheumatoid arthritis. *Int J Clin Pharmacol Res.* (2005) 25:101–5.

43. Miyata M, Sakuma F, Fukaya E, Kobayashi H, Rai T, Saito H, et al. Detection and monitoring of methotrexate-associated lung injury using serum markers KL-6 and SP-D in rheumatoid arthritis. *Intern Med.* (2002) 41:467–73. doi: 10.2169/internalmedicine.41.467

44. Romagnoli M, Bigliazzi C, Casoni G, Chilosi M, Carloni A, Dubini A, et al. The role of transbronchial lung biopsy for the diagnosis of diffuse drug-induced lung disease: a case series of 44 patients. *Sarcoidosis Vasc Diffuse Lung Dis.* (2008) 25:36–45.

45. Rossi SE, Erasmus JJ, McAdams HP, Sporn TA, Goodman PC. Pulmonary drug toxicity: radiologic and pathologic manifestations. *Radiographics.* (2000) 20:1245–59. doi: 10.1148/radiographics.20.5.g00se081245

46. Arakawa H, Yamasaki M, Kurihara Y, Yamada H, Nakajima Y. Methotrexate-induced pulmonary injury: serial CT findings. *J Thorac Imaging.* (2003) 18:231–6. doi: 10.1097/00005382-200310000-00004

47. Imokawa S, Colby TV, Leslie KO, Helmers RA. Methotrexate pneumonitis: review of the literature and histopathological findings in nine patients. *Eur Respir J.* (2000) 15:373–81. doi: 10.1034/j.1399-3003.2000.15b25.x

48. Suwa A, Hirakata M, Satoh S, Mimori T, Utsumi K, Inada S. Rheumatoid arthritis associated with methotrexate-induced pneumonitis: improvement with i.v. cyclophosphamide therapy. *Clin Exp Rheumatol.* (1999) 17:355–8.

49. Bartram SA. Experience with methotrexate-associated pneumonitis in northeastern England: comment on the article by Kremer et al. *Arthritis Rheum.* (1998) 41:1327–8.

50. Cook NJ, Carroll GJ. Successful reintroduction of methotrexate after pneumonitis in two patients with rheumatoid arthritis. *Ann Rheum Dis.* (1992) 51:272–4. doi: 10.1136/ard.51.2.272

51. Bongartz T, Nannini C, Medina-Velasquez YF, Achenbach SJ, Crowson CS, Ryu JH, et al. Incidence and mortality of interstitial lung disease in rheumatoid arthritis: a population-based study. *Arthritis Rheum.* (2010) 62:1583–91. doi: 10.1002/art.27405

52. Kiely P, Busby AD, Nikiphorou E, Sullivan K, Walsh DA, Creamer P, et al. Is incident rheumatoid arthritis interstitial lung disease associated with methotrexate treatment? Results from a multivariate analysis in the ERAS and ERAN inception cohorts. *BMJ Open.* (2019) 9:e028466. doi: 10.1136/bmjopen-2018-028466

53. Kelly CA, Saravanan V, Nisar M, Arthanari S, Woodhead FA, Price-Forbes AN, et al. Rheumatoid arthritis-related interstitial lung disease: associations, prognostic factors and physiological and radiological characteristics–a large multicentre UK study. *Rheumatology.* (2014) 53:1676–82. doi: 10.1093/rheumatology/keu165

54. Bilgici A, Ulusoy H, Kuru O, Celenk C, Unsal M, Danaci M. Pulmonary involvement in rheumatoid arthritis. *Rheumatol Int.* (2005) 25:429–35. doi: 10.1007/s00296-004-0472-y

55. Dawson JK, Fewins HE, Desmond J, Lynch MP, Graham DR. Fibrosing alveolitis in patients with rheumatoid arthritis as assessed by high resolution computed tomography, chest radiography, and pulmonary function tests. *Thorax.* (2001) 56:622–7. doi: 10.1136/thorax.56.8.622

56. Capobianco J, Grimberg A, Thompson BM, Antunes VB, Jasinowodolinski D, Meirelles GSP. Thoracic manifestations of collagen vascular diseases. *Radiographics.* (2012) 32:33–50. doi: 10.1148/rg.321105058

57. Searles G, McKendry RJ. Methotrexate pneumonitis in rheumatoid arthritis: potential risk factors. Four case reports and a review of the literature. *J Rheumatol.* (1987) 14:1164–71.

58. Brown KK. Rheumatoid lung disease. *Proc Am Thorac Soc.* (2007) 4:443–8. doi: 10.1513/pats.200703-045MS

59. Garcia JG, James HL, Zinkgraf S, Perlman MB, Keogh BA. Lower respiratory tract abnormalities in rheumatoid interstitial lung disease. Potential role of neutrophils in lung injury. *Am Rev Respir Dis.* (1987) 136:811–7. doi: 10.1164/ajrccm/136.4.811

60. Rojas-Serrano J, Herrera-Bringas D, Pérez-Román DI, Pérez-Dorame R, Mateos-Toledo H, Mejía M. Rheumatoid arthritis-related interstitial lung disease (RA-ILD): methotrexate and the severity of lung disease are associated to prognosis. *Clin Rheumatol.* (2017) 36:1493–500. doi: 10.1007/s10067-017-3707-5

61. Sparks JA, He X, Huang J, Fletcher EA, Zaccardelli A, Friedlander HM, et al. Rheumatoid arthritis disease activity predicting incident clinically-apparent RA-associated interstitial lung disease: A prospective cohort study. *Arthritis Rheumatol.* (2019) 71:1472–82. doi: 10.1002/art.40904

62. Conway R, Low C, Coughlan RJ, O'Donnell MJ, Carey JJ. Leflunomide use and risk of lung disease in rheumatoid arthritis: a systematic literature review and metaanalysis of randomized controlled trials. *J Rheumatol.* (2016) 43:855–60. doi: 10.3899/jrheum.150674

63. Huang Y, Lin W, Chen Z, Wang Y, Huang Y, Tu S. Effect of tumor necrosis factor inhibitors on interstitial lung disease in rheumatoid arthritis: angel or demon? *Drug Des Devel Ther.* (2019) 13:2111–25. doi: 10.2147/DDDT.S204730

64. Fernández-Díaz C, Loricera J, Castañeda S, López-Mejías R, Ojeda-García C, Olivé A, et al. Abatacept in patients with rheumatoid arthritis and interstitial lung disease: a national multicenter study of 63 patients. *Semin Arthritis Rheum.* (2018) 48:22–7. doi: 10.1016/j.semarthrit.2017.12.012

65. Akiyama M, Kaneko Y, Yamaoka K, Kondo H, Takeuchi T. Association of disease activity with acute exacerbation of interstitial lung disease during tocilizumab treatment in patients with rheumatoid arthritis: a retrospective, case-control study. *Rheumatol Int.* (2016) 36:881–9. doi: 10.1007/s00296-016-3478-3

66. Md Yusof MY, Kabia A, Darby M, Lettieri G, Beirne P, Vital EM, et al. Effect of rituximab on the progression of rheumatoid arthritis-related interstitial lung disease: 10 years' experience at a single centre. *Rheumatology.* (2017) 56:1348–57. doi: 10.1093/rheumatology/kex072

67. Fui A, Bergantini L, Selvi E, Mazzei MA, Bennett D, Pieroni MG, et al. Rituximab therapy in interstitial lung disease associated with rheumatoid arthritis. *Intern Med J.* (2019). doi: 10.1111/imj.14306. [Epub ahead of print].

68. Conway R, Carey JJ. Methotrexate and lung disease in rheumatoid arthritis. *Panminerva Med.* (2017) 59:33–46. doi: 10.23736/S0031-0808.16.03260-2

69. Cervantes-Perez P, Toro-Perez AH, Rodriguez-Jurado P. Pulmonary

involvement in rheumatoid arthritis. *JAMA*. (1980) 243:1715–9. doi: 10.1001/jama.243.17.1715

70. Catrina AI, Svensson CI, Malmström V, Schett G, Klareskog L. Mechanisms leading from systemic autoimmunity to joint-specific disease in rheumatoid arthritis. *Nat Rev Rheumatol*. (2017) 13:79–86. doi: 10.1038/nrrheum.2016.200

71. Zamora-Legoff JA, Krause ML, Crowson CS, Ryu JH, Matteson EL. Patterns of interstitial lung disease and mortality in rheumatoid arthritis. *Rheumatology*. (2017) 56:344–50. doi: 10.1093/rheumatology/kex299

72. Nurmi HM, Purokivi MK, Kärkkäinen MS, Kettunen H-P, Selander TA, Kaarteenaho RL. Variable course of disease of rheumatoid arthritis-associated usual interstitial pneumonia compared to other subtypes. *BMC Pulm Med*. (2016) 16:107. doi: 10.1186/s12890-016-0269-2

73. Harlow L, Rosas IO, Gochuico BR, Mikuls TR, Dellaripa PF, Oddis CV, et al. Identification of citrullinated hsp90 isoforms as novel autoantigens in rheumatoid arthritis-associated interstitial lung disease. *Arthritis Rheum*. (2013) 65:869–79. doi: 10.1002/art.37881

74. Harlow L, Gochuico BR, Rosas IO, Doyle TJ, Osorio JC, Travers TS, et al. Anti-citrullinated heat shock protein 90 antibodies identified in bronchoalveolar lavage fluid are a marker of lung-specific immune responses. *Clin Immunol*. (2014) 155:60–70. doi: 10.1016/j.clim.2014.08.004

75. Juge P-A, Lee JS, Ebstein E, Furukawa H, Dobrinskikh E, Gazal S, et al. MUC5B promoter variant and rheumatoid arthritis with interstitial lung disease. *N Engl J Med*. (2018) 379:2209–19. doi: 10.1056/NEJMoa1801562

76. Seibold MA, Wise AL, Speer MC, Steele MP, Brown KK, Loyd JE, et al. A common MUC5B promoter polymorphism and pulmonary fibrosis. *N Engl J Med*. (2011) 364:1503–12. doi: 10.1056/NEJMoa1013660

77. Rajasekaran BA, Shovlin D, Lord P, Kelly CA. Interstitial lung disease in patients with rheumatoid arthritis: a comparison with cryptogenic fibrosing alveolitis. *Rheumatology*. (2001) 40:1022–5. doi: 10.1093/rheumatology/40.9.1022

78. Ellman P, Ball RE. Rheumatoid disease with joint and pulmonary manifestations. *Br Med J*. (1948) 2:816–20. doi: 10.1136/bmj.2.4583.816

79. Bély M, Apáthy A. Changes of the lung in rheumatoid arthritis—rheumatoid pneumonia. A clinicopathological study. *Acta Morphol Hung*. (1991) 39:117–56.

80. Doran MF, Crowson CS, Pond GR, O'Fallon WM, Gabriel SE. Frequency of infection in patients with rheumatoid arthritis compared with controls: a population-based study. *Arthritis Rheum*. (2002) 46:2287–93. doi: 10.1002/art.10524

81. Chung W-S, Peng C-L, Lin C-L, Chang Y-J, Chen Y-F, Chiang JY, et al. Rheumatoid arthritis increases the risk of deep vein thrombosis and pulmonary thromboembolism: a nationwide cohort study. *Ann Rheum Dis*. (2014) 73:1774–80. doi: 10.1136/annrheumdis-2013-203380

82. Simon TA, Thompson A, Gandhi KK, Hochberg MC, Suissa S. Incidence of malignancy in adult patients with rheumatoid arthritis: a meta-analysis. *Arthritis Res Ther*. (2015) 17:212. doi: 10.1186/s13075-015-0728-9

83. Lee H-K, Kim DS, Yoo B, Seo JB, Rho J-Y, Colby TV, et al. Histopathologic pattern and clinical features of rheumatoid arthritis-associated interstitial lung disease. *Chest*. (2005) 127:2019–27. doi: 10.1378/chest.127.6.2019

84. Mornex JF, Cordier G, Pages J, Vergnon JM, Lefebvre R, Brune J, et al. Activated lung lymphocytes in hypersensitivity pneumonitis. *J Allergy Clin Immunol*. (1984) 74:719–27. doi: 10.1016/0091-6749(84)90236-7

85. Gabbay E, Tarala R, Will R, Carroll G, Adler B, Cameron D, et al. Interstitial lung disease in recent onset rheumatoid arthritis. *Am J Respir Crit Care Med*. (1997) 156:528–35. doi: 10.1164/ajrccm.156.2.9609016

86. Turesson C, Matteson EL, Colby TV, Vuk-Pavlovic Z, Vassallo R, Weyand CM, et al. Increased CD4+ T cell infiltrates in rheumatoid arthritis-associated interstitial pneumonitis compared with idiopathic interstitial pneumonitis. *Arthritis Rheum*. (2005) 52:73–9. doi: 10.1002/art.20765

87. Donaghy C. Rheumatoid arthritis: now and then. *Rheumatology*. (2016) 55:118–8.

88. Rojas-Serrano J, González-Velásquez E, Mejía M, Sánchez-Rodríguez A, Carrillo G. Interstitial lung disease related to rheumatoid arthritis: evolution after treatment. *Reumatol Clin*. (2012) 8:68–71. doi: 10.1016/j.reumae.2011.12.001

89. Mochizuki T, Ikari K, Yano K, Sato M, Okazaki K. Long-term deterioration of interstitial lung disease in patients with rheumatoid arthritis treated with abatacept. *Mod Rheumatol*. (2019) 29:413–7. doi: 10.1080/14397595.2018.1481566

90. Khanna D, Denton CP, Lin CJF, van Laar JM, Frech TM, Anderson ME, et al. Safety and efficacy of subcutaneous tocilizumab in systemic sclerosis: results from the open-label period of a phase II randomised controlled trial (faSScinate). *Ann Rheum Dis*. (2018) 77:212–20. doi: 10.1136/annrheumdis-2017-211682

91. Duarte AC, Porter JC, Leandro MJ. The lung in a cohort of rheumatoid arthritis patients-an overview of different types of involvement and treatment. *Rheumatology*. (2019) kez177. doi: 10.1093/rheumatology/kez177. [Epub ahead of print].

92. Druce KL, Iqbal K, Watson KD, Symmons DPM, Hyrich KL, Kelly C. Mortality in patients with interstitial lung disease treated with rituximab or TNFi as a first biologic. *RMD Open*. (2017) 3:e000473. doi: 10.1136/rmdopen-2017-000473

93. Distler O, Highland KB, Gahlemann M, Azuma A, Fischer A, Mayes MD, et al. Nintedanib for systemic sclerosis-associated interstitial lung disease. *N Engl J Med*. (2019) 380:2518–28. doi: 10.1056/NEJMoa1903076

94. Redente EF, Aguilar MA, Black BP, Edelman BL, Bahadur AN, Humphries SM, et al. Nintedanib reduces pulmonary fibrosis in a model of rheumatoid arthritis-associated interstitial lung disease. *Am J Physiol Lung Cell Mol Physiol*. (2018) 314:L998–1009. doi: 10.1152/ajplung.00304.2017

95. Richeldi L, du Bois RM, Raghu G, Azuma A, Brown KK, Costabel U, et al. Efficacy and safety of nintedanib in idiopathic pulmonary fibrosis. *N Engl J Med*. (2014) 370:2071–82. doi: 10.1056/NEJMoa1402584

96. Wu C, Lin H, Zhang X. Inhibitory effects of pirfenidone on fibroblast to myofibroblast transition in rheumatoid arthritis-associated interstitial lung disease via the downregulation of activating transcription factor 3 (ATF3). *Int Immunopharmacol*. (2019) 74:105700. doi: 10.1016/j.intimp.2019.105700

97. Sokka T, Abelson B, Pincus T. Mortality in rheumatoid arthritis: 2008 update. *Clin Exp Rheumatol*. (2008) 26(5 Suppl. 51):S35–61.

98. Singh N, Varghese J, England BR, Solomon JJ, Michaud K, Mikuls TR, et al. Impact of the pattern of interstitial lung disease on mortality in rheumatoid arthritis: a systematic literature review and meta-analysis. *Semin Arthritis Rheum*. (2019). doi: 10.1016/j.semarthrit.2019.04.005. [Epub ahead of print].

5

Epidemiology, Mortality and Healthcare Resource Utilization Associated With Systemic Sclerosis-Associated Interstitial Lung Disease in France

Vincent Cottin[1]*, Sophie Larrieu[2], Loic Boussel[3,4], Salim Si-Mohamed[3,4], Fabienne Bazin[2], Sébastien Marque[2], Jacques Massol[5], Françoise Thivolet-Bejui[6], Lara Chalabreysse[6], Delphine Maucort-Boulch[7,8,9,10], Stéphane Jouneau[11], Eric Hachulla[12], Julien Chollet[13] and Mouhamad Nasser[1]

[1] Hôpital Louis Pradel, Centre Coordonnateur National de Référence des Maladies Pulmonaires Rares, Hospices Civils de Lyon, UMR754 INRAE and Université Claude Bernard Lyon 1, Member of ERN-LUNG, RespiFil, OrphaLung, Lyon, France, [2] IQVIA – RWS La Défense, Courbevoie, France, [3] Département de Radiologie, Hospices Civils de Lyon, Lyon, France, [4] Université Lyon, INSA-Lyon, Université Claude Bernard Lyon 1, UJM-Saint Etienne, CNRS Inserm, CREATIS UMR 5220, Lyon, France, [5] AIXIAL – Paris, Paris, France, [6] Département d'anatomo-pathologie, Hospices Civils de Lyon, Lyon, France, [7] Hospices Civils de Lyon, Pôle Santé Publique, Service de Biostatistique et Bioinformatique, Lyon, France, [8] Université de Lyon, Lyon, France, [9] Université Lyon 1, Villeurbanne, France, [10] CNRS, UMR 5558, Laboratoire de Biométrie et Biologie Évolutive, Équipe Biostatistique-Santé, Villeurbanne, France, [11] Centre Hospitalier Universitaire de Rennes, Centre de Compétences pour les Maladies Pulmonaires Rares, Univ Rennes, Inserm, EHESP, IRSET (Institut de recherche en santé, environnement et travail), RespiFil, OrphaLung, Rennes, France, [12] Hôpital Claude Huriez, Centre National de Référence des maladies auto-immunes systémiques rares (CeRAINO), CHU de Lille, Lille, France, [13] Boehringer Ingelheim France SAS, Paris, France

*Correspondence:
Vincent Cottin
vincent.cottin@chu-lyon.fr

Objectives: To investigate the clinical characteristics, epidemiology, survival estimates and healthcare resource utilization and associated costs in patients with systemic sclerosis-associated interstitial lung disease (SSc-ILD) in France.

Methods: The French national administrative healthcare database, the Système National des Données de Santé (SNDS), includes data on 98.8% of the French population, including data relating to ambulatory care, hospitalizations and death. In our study, claims data from the SNDS were used to identify adult patients with SSc-ILD between 2010 and 2017. We collected data on clinical features, incidence, prevalence, survival estimates, healthcare resource use and costs.

Results: In total, 3,333 patients with SSc-ILD were identified, 76% of whom were female. Patients had a mean age [standard deviation (SD)] of 60.6 (14.4) years and a mean (SD) individual study duration of 3.9 (2.7) years. In 2016, the estimated overall incidence and prevalence were 0.69/100,000 individuals and 5.70/100,000 individuals, respectively. The overall survival estimates of patients using Kaplan–Meier estimation were 93, 82, and 55% at 1, 3, and 8 years, respectively. During the study, 98.7% of patients had ≥1 hospitalization and 22.3% of patients were hospitalized in an intensive care unit. The total annual mean healthcare cost per patient with SSc-ILD was €25,753, of which €21,539 was related to hospitalizations.

Conclusions: This large, real-world longitudinal study provides important insights into the epidemiology of SSc-ILD in France and shows that the disease is associated with high mortality, healthcare resource utilization and costs. SSc-ILD represents a high burden on both patients and healthcare services.

Clinical Trial Registration: www.ClinicalTrials.gov, identifier: NCT03858842.

Keywords: epidemiology, cost, pulmonary fibrosis, scleroderma, systemic sclerosis

INTRODUCTION

Systemic sclerosis (SSc) is a rare, heterogeneous, chronic, autoimmune disease characterized by fibrosis of the skin and internal organs (1). Interstitial lung disease (ILD) is a common complication of SSc and normally develops early in the disease (1, 2). ILD is estimated to affect between 19 and 90% of patients with SSc (depending on the study), and around 40% have clinically significant ILD (3–7). It is the leading cause of death in patients with SSc (2), with a 4.6-fold increased risk of mortality compared with the general population (8). Risk factors associated with mortality in SSc-associated ILD (SSc-ILD) are male sex, older age, extent of disease on chest high-resolution computed tomography (HRCT), lower forced vital capacity (FVC), diffusing capacity of the lungs for carbon monoxide (DLco) and pulmonary hypertension (PH) (9, 10). PH is a common complication in patients with SSc and SSc-ILD, and causes up to 33% of SSc-related deaths (11–13).

In North America, the prevalence of SSc is estimated to be 13.5–44.3 per 100,000 individuals (5, 14), and the incidence is estimated at 1.4–5.6 per 100,000 individuals (5). Estimates of SSc-ILD prevalence are less common but one US cohort study estimated it to be 9.8 per 100,000 persons (14). In a Canadian study, the prevalence of SSc and SSc-ILD was 19.1 and 2.3 per 100,000 persons, respectively (15). In Europe, the estimates for prevalence and annual incidence of SSc are lower, at 7.2–33.9 and 0.6–2.3 per 100,000 individuals, respectively. For patients who develop SSc-ILD, the prevalence and annual incidence in Europe are 1.7–4.2 and 0.1–0.4 per 100,000 individuals, respectively (5).

SSc has a substantial negative impact on patient quality of life and places a considerable burden on healthcare resources (1, 16). Patients with SSc have greater healthcare costs than unaffected individuals and patients with ILD have increased healthcare costs compared with patients without ILD (17).

Until recently, there were no drugs approved for the treatment of SSc-ILD. Based on the results of randomized controlled trials (18, 19), the anti-inflammatory drugs cyclophosphamide and mycophenolate mofetil (MMF) have often been used where treatment is considered. More recently, the tyrosine kinase inhibitor nintedanib was shown to reduce the rate of pulmonary function decline in patients with SSc-ILD (20) and has been approved for the treatment of SSc-ILD in the US, Europe, Canada, Japan and Brazil (21–23).

There is a lack of large-scale data on epidemiology, mortality and healthcare resource utilization of patients with SSc-ILD in France. The objectives of this retrospective study were to evaluate the prevalence and incidence of SSc-ILD and the clinical characteristics, survival estimates, and the healthcare resource use and associated direct costs of patients with SSc-ILD in France.

METHODS
Database Used

This was a non-interventional, longitudinal, retrospective, cohort study using administrative claim data extracted from the French national administrative healthcare database, Système National des Données de Santé (SNDS), which is managed by the National Health Insurance Fund [Caisse nationale d'assurance maladie (CNAM)]. The SNDS is a real-world, digital data set of French healthcare utilization and is one of the largest data repositories in the world, including 98.8% of the French population of more than 66 million people (24). It contains anonymous, comprehensive information on sociodemographic characteristics, date of death, all out-of-hospital reimbursed healthcare expenditures (from both public and private healthcare), and all hospital discharge summaries with International Classification of Diseases (ICD)-10 codes. In addition, the SNDS contains direct information on medical diagnoses for patients who have full coverage for all medical expenses by the national health security system, as is the case for the majority of patients diagnosed with SSc in France. The SNDS includes, in particular, the country-wide health insurance data related to ambulatory care [Système national d'information interrégimes de l'Assurance Maladie (SNIIRAM) database], hospitalizations [Programme de médicalisation des systèmes d'information (PMSI)] and death (CépiDc).

Patients with SSc and ILD were identified in the SNDS database between 1 January 2010 and 31 December 2017 (the study period) using ICD-10 codes that appeared on medical claims (**Figure 1**; **Supplementary Table 1**).

Patient Selection

To be included in the analysis, patients had to be aged ≥20 years, meet the criteria for a diagnosis of SSc-ILD, have ≥2-year history in the general reimbursement scheme of the SNDS prior to inclusion date (in order to distinguish between incident and prevalent cases) and be affiliated to the general reimbursement scheme in the SNDS. Patients were included if they had a diagnosis of both SSc and ILD where the ILD diagnosis was either any time after, or within 6 months prior to, SSc diagnosis.

In France, the diagnosis of SSc-ILD is made during a short stay of elective hospitalization (≥1 day) in the majority of patients.

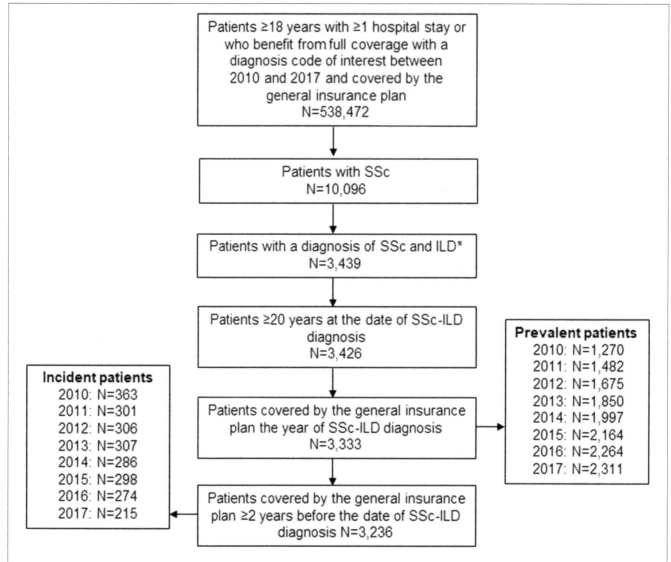

FIGURE 1 | Patient selection. *An eligible adult SSc-ILD patient was defined as a patient with either ≥1 hospital stay with a diagnosis code (principal, related or associated) of lung fibrosis, or ≥1 hospital stay with a diagnosis code (principal, related or associated) of SSc and/or a patient who benefited from full coverage for SSc (patients fully reimbursed for their claims related to SSc). ILD diagnosis could be made after, or within 6 months prior to, SSc diagnosis. ILD, interstitial lung disease; SNDS, Système National des Données de Santé; SSc, systemic sclerosis.

Patients with an SSc-ILD diagnosis before 2010 were included as prevalent patients in 2010. The study period was until the earliest of patient death, end of study (31 December 2017) or last available record (hospitalization or any healthcare reimbursement) in the data source. For patients with a data gap persisting beyond 12 months, the follow-up period was ended at their last record.

The study was approved by the Expert Committee for Health Research, Studies and Assessments [Comité d'expertise pour les recherches, les études et les évaluations dans le domaine de la santé (CEREES)] on 18 August 2018 (TPS 72584) and by the National Commission for Information Technology and Freedoms [Commission Nationale de l'Informatique et des Libertés (CNIL)] on 9 November 2018 (N:918305). The SNDS data are anonymized; therefore, written informed consent is waived for studies analyzing these data sets.

Outcomes

Patients' healthcare resource use was captured under the following categories: medical visits, hospitalizations, tests (laboratory and imaging), pulmonary function tests, pathology, ambulance use, sick leave daily allowances, and drug and non-pharmacologic treatments.

Total and annual costs per patient were estimated in euros during the study period according to the national health insurance perspective. For outpatient healthcare resources [general practitioner (GP) visits, pulmonary specialist visits, nursing and physiologist appointments, laboratory tests, medical procedures and treatments], ambulance use and sick leave daily allowances, the amount reimbursed by the healthcare insurance was directly extracted from the SNDS database. For hospitalizations, costs were valued taking into consideration reimbursement by the national health insurance. The cost of each stay was valued by the diagnosis-related group [Groupe Homogène de Malades (GHM)] using the official tariffs from the French Diagnosis Related Group prospective payment system (source: Agence technique de l'information sur l'hospitalisation, Médecine chirurgie obstétrique et odontologie 2010–2017 tariffs for private and public institutions) (24, 25).

Statistical Analysis

Descriptive data analyses were performed depending on the criteria. Annual incidence rate was calculated as the proportion of subjects who were first identified as having SSc-ILD during the calendar year of interest (i.e., without any diagnosis of SSc-ILD during the 2 previous years) to all enrollees at risk (i.e., excluding prevalent cases) aged ≥20 years. Annual prevalence rate was calculated for each year as the proportion of all subjects identified as prevalent during the year of interest to all enrollees who were ≥20 years old. Patients contributed to annual incidence only once, but could contribute to prevalence during multiple years.

Crude incidence, prevalence and mortality rates were calculated for the total cohort and by the following subgroups: year of diagnosis (2010–2017), age, sex, and presence of lung cancer and PH in the 12 months prior to inclusion (both mortality only). PH was defined as patients with a full coverage or hospitalization for PH (ICD-10 code I270) in the main, related or associated diagnosis. Lung cancer was identified as patients with full coverage or hospitalization for lung cancer (C34 or D02.2 ICD-10 codes) in the main, related or associated diagnosis. Overall survival (OS) was defined as time from date of inclusion (date of presence of SSc and ILD claims) to date of death due to any cause or end of the study period. Patients were considered lost to follow-up if they had no recorded healthcare use during the follow-up and no death was registered. OS analyses were performed using the Kaplan–Meier method (**Supplementary Methods**).

RESULTS

Demographic Characteristics

Of the 9,817 patients with SSc who met the inclusion criteria, 3,333 (34%) had SSc-ILD (**Figure 1**). The majority of patients with SSc-ILD were female (75.6%). The mean [standard deviation (± SD)] age was 60.6 (± 14.4) years. The mean (± SD) individual duration of follow-up was 3.9 (± 2.7) years. The mean (± SD) time from SSc diagnosis to ILD diagnosis was 0.40 (± 1.16) years (**Table 1**). Most patients had comorbidities, the most common of which were hypertension (66.8%) and gastroesophageal reflux disease (65.8%) (**Supplementary Figure 1**).

Incidence and Prevalence of SSc-ILD

Between 2010 and 2017, the estimated incidence was 0.98–0.53 per 100,000 individuals per year, with incident cases varying between 215 and 363 per year. Between 2010 and 2017, the estimated prevalence was 3.42–5.73 per 100,000 individuals per year, with 1,270–2,311 prevalent cases per year (**Supplementary Table 2; Figure 1**).

TABLE 1 | Characteristics of patients with SSc-ILD.

	Patients (N = 3,333)
Sex, n (%)	
Female	2,521 (75.6)
Age, years	
Mean age (SD)	60.6 (14.4)
Median (IQR)	61.0 (50.0–71.0)
Min–max	20.0–97.0
Time between SSc diagnosis and ILD diagnosis, years	
Mean (SD)	0.40 (1.16)
Median (IQR)	0 (0–0.05)
Age category, n (%)	
20–<30 years	73 (2.2)
30–<45 years	378 (11.3)
45–<60 years	1,067 (32.0)
60–<75 years	1,200 (36.0)
≥75 years	615 (18.5)
Individual study period duration, years	
Mean (SD)	3.90 (2.70)
Median (IQR)	3.54 (1.59–6.51)

IQR, interquartile range; SD, standard deviation; SSc-ILD, systemic sclerosis-associated interstitial lung disease.

Survival Estimates of Patients With SSc-ILD

In total, 934 (28.0%) patients died, 2,093 (62.8%) were alive at the end of the study period and 306 (9.2%) patients were lost to follow-up. The OS estimates for all patients at 1, 3, 5 and 8 years were 93.4, 82.2, 70.8, and 55.3%, respectively (**Figure 2A**; **Supplementary Table 3**). At 8 years, the OS estimates were 41.4% for men and 59.7% for women (**Figure 2B**; **Supplementary Table 3**). The median OS for all patients was not reached (**Supplementary Table 3**). Mean (± SD) age at the time of death was 69.1 (± 12.9) years.

Factors associated with mortality were male sex, PH, lung cancer, and older age (age categories 50–<60 years, 60–<75 years and ≥75 years) (**Supplementary Table 4**). For the overall population and for women, more than 50% of patients were alive at the end of follow-up; however, the median OS [95% confidence interval (CI)] for men was 6.9 (6.3–7.6) years (**Supplementary Table 3**). OS estimates at 8 years were higher for younger patients (20–<50 years: 76.9%) compared with patients aged 50–<60 years (63.7%), 60–<75 years (49.6%) and ≥75 years (25.4%) (**Figure 2C**; **Supplementary Table 5**).

OS was also lower for patients with lung cancer or PH [medians (95% CI) of 3.1 (2.5–4.8) and 5.7 (4.7–6.4) years, respectively]. The OS estimates at 1, 3, 5 and 8 years were 78.1, 54.9, 27.7, and 11.1% for patients with lung cancer and 93.6, 82.4, 71.2, and 55.7% for patients without lung cancer. They were 89.2, 68.4, 55.6, and 36.8% in patients with PH and 93.9, 83.5, 72.3, and 57.2% for patients without PH.

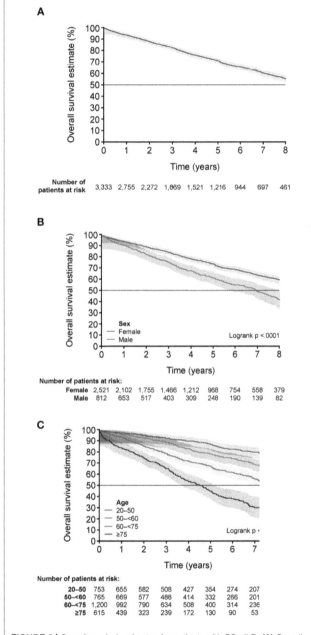

FIGURE 2 | Overall survival estimates for patients with SSc-ILD. **(A)** Overall survival estimates for all patients, **(B)** by sex and **(C)** by age in years. The shading indicates 95% Hall-Wellner band. SSc-ILD, systemic sclerosis-associated interstitial lung disease.

Healthcare Resource Utilization and Cost Evaluation

The healthcare consumption and costs for SSc-ILD patients are shown in **Supplementary Tables 6**, **7** and **Table 2**. The most commonly used drug treatments were glucocorticoids (74.1%), MMF (21.2%) and azathioprine (10.2%) (**Supplementary Table 6**). The annual mean costs (± SD) per patient for drug treatments during the follow-up were €883 (± 8,224) (**Table 2**).

TABLE 2 | Annual costs during the study.

	Cost per patient (€)	
	Mean (SD)	**Median (IQR)**
Total annual cost	25,752.8 (68,911.3)	9,316.4 (3,334.0–23,296.8)
Total drug treatment costs	882.9 (8,224.0)	28.1 (0.6–201.2)
Total non-pharmacologic treatment costs	1,501.1 (11,510.7)	0.0 (0.0–0.0)
Total medical and paramedical costs*	1,682.9 (3,530.6)	641.0 (279.3–1,604.6)
All hospitalization costs	21,538.8 (64,778.0)	6,289.9 (2,025.1–18,116.3)
Total laboratory test costs	56.8 (94.0)	33.8 (0.0–80.7)
Total imaging test** costs	63.4 (347.9)	16.6 (0.0–60.8)
Total pathology costs**	2.2 (26.7)	0.0 (0.0–0.0)
Total pulmonary function test costs**	24.7 (87.7)	0.0 (0.0–24.0)

*Excludes sick leaves, daily allowance and transport costs. **Outpatient only.
IQR, interquartile range; SD, standard deviation.

Nearly all patients (95.7%) had at least one GP visit but only around half (49.4%) were seen by a pulmonary specialist during the study period. 20.7% of patients had sick leave daily allowances (**Supplementary Table 7**). In total, 3,289 (98.7%) patients had ≥1 hospitalization, with a mean (± SD) of 12.6 (± 26.0) hospitalizations during the study. Of all patients, 60.4 and 27.3% were hospitalized due to acute events and PH, respectively, and 22.3% of patients were admitted to an intensive care unit.

The total annual cost of all healthcare use per patient was €25,753, with the highest contributor being hospitalizations costs (€21,539), followed by medical and paramedical costs (€1,683), and non-pharmacologic treatment costs (supplemental oxygen use, palliative care) (€1,501) (**Table 2**).

DISCUSSION

By using a large, real-world database covering most of the population of France, this study provides valuable insights into the epidemiology, mortality, healthcare resource utilization and costs associated with SSc-ILD.

In our study, the majority of patients were female, consistent with other studies (5, 26), and had underlying comorbidities, most commonly hypertension. Most patients were diagnosed with SSc and ILD at the same time, possibly because the majority of patients are diagnosed with SSc-ILD during hospitalization in France and their data are entered into the SNDS when they are hospitalized. Of 9,817 patients with SSc, 3,333 (34%) also had ILD, comparable with the estimate of 35% in Europe in a recent systematic review (5). In a registry of SSc patients in The Netherlands, the percentage of patients with SSc-ILD was 18.8–47.0% depending on the definition used (3). In a Norwegian SSc cohort of 324 patients, 50% of patients had ILD by HRCT (6). The differences may be explained by the different methodologies. In France, it is recommended that patients with SSc are screened for ILD using lung auscultation and chest HRCT (27). Patients with SSc are usually referred to a specialist ILD center where they are initially screened for ILD by chest examination, pulmonary function tests and HRCT. Patients who are not diagnosed with ILD would then be followed up annually at a specialist ILD center, with an annual physical examination, pulmonary function testing and HRCT on a case-by-case basis. In our study, we identified patients with clinically relevant ILD using ILD diagnosis codes for reimbursement. Conversely, the Norwegian study defined ILD using HRCT review only, which may have led to the inclusion of patients with evidence of ILD on HRCT that was not clinically significant at baseline.

The prevalence of SSc in France has been estimated to be 13.2–15.8 per 100,000 persons (5). The overall incidence of SSc-ILD in our study was higher than a prior estimate of 0.1–0.4 in Europe (5). Furthermore, between 2012 and 2017, the reported prevalence of SSc-ILD was also higher than those estimated in a European systematic review and a study in The Netherlands (3, 5). There was an apparent decrease in incidence and increase in prevalence of SSc-ILD during our study. In 2017, the incidence is likely to be under-represented because of non-identification of cases where a patient with one diagnosis of SSc or ILD in 2017 can only be identified as having SSc-ILD after the study end date. Our study was not designed to track changes in prevalence and incidence over time, and thus trends should be interpreted with caution as we cannot exclude any artifact in the methodology and/or algorithm.

Male sex, older age, extent of disease on HRCT, lower FVC and DLco, and PH are known risk factors linked to mortality in SSc-ILD (9). The development of PH in patients with SSc-ILD significantly reduces patient survival (28). In line with previous studies (9), our study showed that male sex, older age, PH, as well as lung cancer, were factors associated with increased mortality in SSc-ILD.

Our study, based on national, real-world healthcare data in France, shows that SSc-ILD is associated with poor prognosis and high mortality. The OS estimate in our study was 55.3% at 8 years. In comparison, 76.9% of patients with SSc-ILD were alive at 9 years in the European Scleroderma Trials and Research (EUSTAR) France SSc-ILD cohort (29). A meta-analysis of SSc studies found a survival estimate from diagnosis of 74.9% at 5 years, although this included all SSc patients rather than those with SSc-ILD (30). In a French multicenter cohort study of SSc patients, the OS at 10 years was 71.7% (31). In addition, in a Spanish SSc cohort, the survival estimate at 10 years was 93%, although the inclusion criteria likely led to recruitment of patients with milder disease compared with the other cohort studies (32). In these cohort studies involving expert centers, there is greater confidence in the diagnoses, although there may be selection bias present. In our nationwide study, selection bias is less likely but patient inclusion is only based on reimbursement. There may also be some differences in study populations that contribute to the different findings; for example, patients in our study were somewhat older, with a mean age of 60.6 years compared with 56.6 years in the EUSTAR France cohort (29). Patients in our study were identified through hospital claims for SSc and ILD, meaning patients had potentially more severe disease than in EUSTAR. Overall, the different findings between our cohort and other cohorts, in particular the lower

OS estimate, may be caused by the differences in methodology leading to selection of different populations of patients.

Nevertheless, our results support other studies showing that SSc-ILD places a considerable burden on patients and healthcare systems (1, 16, 17, 26, 33). Nearly all (98.7%) of the patients in our study were hospitalized at least once and nearly a quarter of patients were hospitalized in an intensive care unit. During the study period, the mean total annual costs of healthcare per patient were substantial at €25,753, with hospitalization costs being the main contributor. In comparison, in a UK retrospective study, the age-weighted median annual healthcare cost per patient with SSc-ILD was £6,375 (26), which is similar to the median total annual healthcare cost of €9,316 in our study. In two US claims database studies, the mean adjusted total direct healthcare cost over 1 year for patients with SSc-ILD was $33,195 (33), and the mean all-cause healthcare cost over 5 years was $191,107 (17).

Our study showed that the most common drug treatment in patients with SSc-ILD was glucocorticoids, even though there is limited evidence for their efficacy, they are associated with scleroderma renal crisis, and they are not recommended as first-line treatments (27, 34–36). In contrast, only 21% of patients received MMF (**Supplementary Table 6**), which is now recommended in SSc-ILD (37). Our study was conducted prior to the approval of nintedanib, a tyrosine kinase inhibitor first indicated for the treatment of idiopathic pulmonary fibrosis (22), by the U.S. Food & Drug Administration and European Medicines Agency for treating adult patients with SSc-ILD (22, 23). However, due to the nature of the data, we do not know what indication or organ involvement in SSc each drug was prescribed for, only that a prescription claim was made.

After diagnosis of SSc-ILD, although the majority of patients with SSc-ILD were seen by a GP during follow-up, only around half were seen by a pulmonary specialist, indicating that many patients were not referred to pulmonologists. This could reflect the lack of treatment options available at the time. In addition, the proportions of patients with diagnostic investigations were lower than expected for some tests; for example, a quarter did not have pulmonary function tests.

A strength of this study is that, in order to identify patients, only those who needed at least one hospitalization with a diagnosis code for SSc or who had full coverage for SSc were included, as per the algorithm for identification of patients in **Supplementary Table 1**. Since the diagnosis of SSc is routinely made in 1-day elective hospitalization, the majority of cases would have been captured. However, patients who had not been hospitalized and who did not have full coverage for SSc during the study period would not have been included. In France, to obtain full coverage for SSc, which means obtaining full reimbursement from the national health security system for claims related to their SSc, patients must submit a claim that has been verified by a physician. Using diagnosis codes and full coverage criteria for SSc allowed us to more accurately identify patients with SSc in our study.

In this large, real-world study, where all-cause mortality data for patients with SSc-ILD in France were collected, there were virtually no missing data despite the large size of the cohort. Although we do not have the causes of death for patients within this study, all-cause mortality data are robust because the national registry of death certificates in France includes exhaustive and accurate all-cause mortality data. Unlike all-cause mortality, disease-related deaths are subject to potential error because they are dependent on the information available to the physician who establishes a patient's cause of death, and their medical interpretation.

There are several limitations of our study. The date of SSc-ILD diagnosis was the first date where both diagnoses were present (i.e., where a patient had diagnostic codes for both SSc and ILD). Thus, we may have underestimated the timing of SSc-ILD diagnosis in patients whose ILD diagnosis preceded the onset of SSc. Our study used administrative claims data to identify patients with SSc-ILD without supporting clinical data such as pulmonary function tests and imaging results. Patient inclusion was dependent on physicians accurately assigning diagnostic codes for both SSc and ILD, meaning there is the possibility of miscoding or undercoding. Patients with subclinical ILD can have mild lung abnormalities detected by HRCT or pulmonary function tests, but may be asymptomatic and undiagnosed (38). Patients with subclinical ILD who did not have full coverage for SSc may not have been included in this study. Physicians did not code each disease manifestation individually, and this may lead to the burden of illness or comorbidities being underestimated (39). Coding systems and practices may also change over time as they are modified to suit scientific evidence and reimbursement purposes rather than medical care. Direct counts from nationwide healthcare databases may not give reliable incidence data (39). As incidence *per se* cannot be measured retrospectively, our results represent estimates of the incidence. The study was designed to estimate the epidemiology and mortality rate of SSc-ILD but not changes over time or causes of death. We also did not have data on occupational or environmental exposures, which could have affected the OS estimates. Patients with other diseases were not excluded, which may have led to lower OS estimates. Therefore, results regarding OS should be interpreted with caution.

In conclusion, this study shows that SSc-ILD is associated with a high burden of disease, as reflected by high mortality, healthcare resource utilization and associated costs. Improving the diagnosis and management of this complex disease is vital to improve the outcomes of patients with SSc-ILD.

REFERENCES

1. Denton CP, Khanna D. Systemic sclerosis. *Lancet.* (2017) 390:1685–99. doi: 10.1016/S0140-6736(17)30933-9
2. Cottin V, Brown KK. Interstitial lung disease associated with systemic sclerosis (SSc-ILD). *Respir Res.* (2019) 20:13. doi: 10.1186/s12931-019-0980-7
3. Vonk MC, Broers B, Heijdra YF, Ton E, Snijder R, van Dijk APJ, et al. Systemic sclerosis and its pulmonary complications in the Netherlands: an epidemiological study. *Ann Rheum Dis.* (2009) 68:961–5. doi: 10.1136/ard.2008.091710
4. Ha Y-J, Lee YJ, Kang EH. Lung involvements in rheumatic diseases: update on the epidemiology, pathogenesis, clinical features, and treatment. *Biomed Res Int.* (2018) 2018:6930297. doi: 10.1155/2018/6930297
5. Bergamasco A, Hartmann N, Wallace L, Verpillat P. Epidemiology of systemic sclerosis and systemic sclerosis-associated interstitial lung disease. *Clin Epidemiol.* (2019) 11:257–73. doi: 10.2147/CLEP.S191418

ETHICS STATEMENT

The study was reviewed and approved by the Expert Committee for Health Research, Studies and Assessments [Comité d'expertise pour les recherches, les études et les évaluations dans le domaine de la santé (CEREES)] on 18 August 2018 (TPS 72584) and by the National Commission for Information Technology and Freedoms [Commission Nationale de l'Informatique et des Libertés (CNIL)] on 9 November 2018 (N:918305). Written informed consent for participation was not required for this study in accordance with the national legislation and the institutional requirements.

AUTHOR CONTRIBUTIONS

MN and VC: study design. SL, MN, and VC: data analysis and interpretation. All authors wrote, read, and approved the manuscript.

FUNDING

This study was supported by Boehringer Ingelheim International GmbH (BI). The authors meet criteria for authorship as recommended by the International Committee of Medical Journal Editors (ICMJE). The authors did not receive payment for the development of the manuscript. IQVIA received financial support from Boehringer Ingelheim France for the design, monitoring, data-management and statistical analysis of the study. Writing, editorial support, and formatting assistance, under the authors' conceptual direction and based on feedback from the authors, was provided by Claire Scott (PhD) of MediTech Media, UK, which was contracted and funded by BI. BI was given the opportunity to review the manuscript for medical and scientific accuracy as well as intellectual property considerations.

ACKNOWLEDGMENTS

We thank Laura Luciani for her help in the study preparatory period. She was an employee of Boehringer Ingelheim.

6. Hoffmann-Vold A-M, Fretheim H, Halse A-K, Seip M, Bitter H, Wallenius M, et al. Tracking impact of interstitial lung disease in systemic sclerosis in a complete nationwide cohort. *Am J Res Cri Care Med.* (2019) 200:1258–66. doi: 10.1164/rccm.201903-0486OC
7. Young A, Vummidi D, Visovatti S, Homer K, Wilhalme H, White ES, et al. Prevalence, treatment, and outcomes of coexistent pulmonary hypertension and interstitial lung disease in systemic sclerosis. *Arthrit Rheumatol.* (2019) 71:1339–49. doi: 10.1002/art.40862
8. Hesselstrand R, Scheja A, Akesson A. Mortality and causes of death in a Swedish series of systemic sclerosis patients. *Ann Rheum Dis.* (1998) 57:682–6. doi: 10.1136/ard.57.11.682
9. Winstone TA, Assayag D, Wilcox PG, Dunne JV, Hague CJ, Leipsic J, et al. Predictors of mortality and progression in scleroderma-associated interstitial lung disease: a systematic review. *Chest.* (2014) 146:422–36. doi: 10.1378/chest.13-2626

10. Chauvelot L, Gamondes D, Berthiller J, Nieves A, Renard S, Catella-Chatron J, et al. Hemodynamic response to treatment and outcome in pulmonary hypertension associated with interstitial lung disease versus pulmonary arterial hypertension in systemic sclerosis. *Arthrit Rheumatol.* (2021) 73:295–304. doi: 10.1002/art.41512

11. Lefevre G, Dauchet L, Hachulla E, Montani D, Sobanski V, Lambert M, et al. Survival and prognostic factors in systemic sclerosis-associated pulmonary hypertension: a systematic review and meta-analysis. *Arthrit Rheum.* (2013) 65:2412–23. doi: 10.1002/art.38029

12. Distler O, Volkmann ER, Hoffmann-Vold AM, Maher TM. Current and future perspectives on management of systemic sclerosis-associated interstitial lung disease. *Exp Rev Clin Immunol.* (2019) 15:1009–17. doi: 10.1080/1744666X.2020.1668269

13. Steen VD, Medsger TA. Changes in causes of death in systemic sclerosis, 1972–2002. *Ann Rheum Dis.* (2007) 66:940–4. doi: 10.1136/ard.2006.066068

14. Li Q, Wallace L, Patnaik P, Alves M, Gahlemann M, Kohlbrenner V, et al. Disease frequency, patient characteristics, comorbidity outcomes and immunosuppressive therapy in systemic sclerosis and systemic sclerosis-associated interstitial lung disease: a US cohort study. *Rheumatology.* (2021) 60:1915–25. doi: 10.1093/rheumatology/keaa547

15. Pope J, Quansah K, Kolb M, Flavin J, Shazia H, Seung SJ. Prevalence and survival of systemic sclerosis (SSc) and associated interstitial lung disease (ILD) in Ontario, Canada over 10 years. *Arthrit Rheumatol.* (2020) 72:0392. Available online at: https://acrabstracts.org/abstract/prevalence-and-survival-of-systemic-sclerosis-ssc-and-associated-interstitial-lung-disease-ild-in-ontario-canada-over-10-years/ (accessed August 17, 2021).

16. Fischer A, Zimovetz E, Ling C, Esser D, Schoof N. Humanistic and cost burden of systemic sclerosis: a review of the literature. *Autoimmun Rev.* (2017) 16:1147–54. doi: 10.1016/j.autrev.2017.09.010

17. Fischer A, Kong AM, Swigris JJ, Cole AL, Raimundo K. All-cause healthcare costs and mortality in patients with systemic sclerosis with lung involvement. *J Rheumatol.* (2018) 45:235–41. doi: 10.3899/jrheum.170307

18. Tashkin DP, Elashoff R, Clements PJ, Goldin J, Roth MD, Furst DE, et al. Cyclophosphamide versus placebo in scleroderma lung disease. *N Engl J Med.* (2006) 354:2655–66. doi: 10.1056/NEJMoa055120

19. Tashkin DP, Roth MD, Clements PJ, Furst DE, Khanna D, Kleerup EC, et al. Mycophenolate mofetil versus oral cyclophosphamide in scleroderma-related interstitial lung disease (SLS II): a randomised controlled, double-blind, parallel group trial. *Lancet Res Med.* (2016) 4:708–19. doi: 10.1016/S2213-2600(16)30152-7

20. Distler O, Highland KB, Gahlemann M, Azuma A, Fischer A, Mayes MD, et al. Nintedanib for systemic sclerosis–associated interstitial lung disease. *N Engl J Med.* (2019) 380:2518–28. doi: 10.1056/NEJMoa1903076

21. Boehringer Ingelheim. *European Commission Approves Nintedanib for the Treatment of Systemic Sclerosis-Associated Interstitial Lung Disease (SSc-ILD).* (2020). Available online at: https://www.boehringer-ingelheim.com/press-release/europeancommissionapprovesnintedanibssc-ild (accessed April 21, 2020).

22. U.S. Food & Drug Administration. *OFEV® (nintedanib): Prescribing Information.* (2020). Available online at: https://www.accessdata.fda.gov/drugsatfda_docs/label/2020/205832s013lbl.pdf (accessed September 24, 2020).

23. European Medicines Agency. *OFEV® (nintedanib): Summary of Product Characteristics.* (2020). Available online at: https://www.ema.europa.eu/en/documents/product-information/ofev-epar-product-information_en.pdf (accessed September 24, 2020).

24. Bezin J, Duong M, Lassalle R, Droz C, Pariente A, Blin P, et al. The national healthcare system claims databases in France, SNIIRAM and EGB: powerful tools for pharmacoepidemiology. *Pharmacoepidemiol Drug Safety.* (2017) 26:954–62. doi: 10.1002/pds.4233

25. Moulis G, Lapeyre-Mestre M, Palmaro A, Pugnet G, Montastruc JL, Sailler L. French health insurance databases: what interest for medical research? *Rev Méd Interne.* (2015) 36:411–7. doi: 10.1016/j.revmed.2014.11.009

26. Gayle A, Schoof N, Alves M, Clarke D, Raabe C, Das P, et al. Healthcare resource utilization among patients in England with systemic sclerosis-associated interstitial lung disease: a retrospective database analysis. *Adv Ther.* (2020) 37:2460–76. doi: 10.1007/s12325-020-01330-0

27. Hachulla E, Agard C, Allanore Y, Avouac J, Bader-Meunier B, Belot A, et al. *National Protocol for Diagnosis and Care on Systemic Scleroderma.* (2020). Available online at: https://www.has-sante.fr/upload/docs/application/pdf/2008-11/pnds__sclerodermie_web.pdf (accessed September 24, 2020).

28. Le Pavec J, Girgis RE, Lechtzin N, Mathai SC, Launay D, Hummers LK, et al. Systemic sclerosis–related pulmonary hypertension associated with interstitial lung disease: impact of pulmonary arterial hypertension therapies. *Arthr Rheum.* (2011) 63:2456–64. doi: 10.1002/art.30423

29. Lescoat A, Hachulla E, Truchetet ME, Mouthon L, Farge D, Granel B, et al. Caractéristiques des patients français atteints de pneumopathie interstitielle diffuse au cours de la sclérodermie systémique (PID-ScS) à partir de la base de données European Scleroderma Trials and Research (EUSTAR). *Rev Malad Res Actualit.* (2020) 12:53–4. doi: 10.1016/j.rmra.2019.11.092

30. Rubio-Rivas M, Royo C, Simeón CP, Corbella X, Fonollosa V. Mortality and survival in systemic sclerosis: systematic review and meta-analysis. *Semin Arthrit Rheum.* (2014) 44:208–19. doi: 10.1016/j.semarthrit.2014.05.010

31. Pokeerbux MR, Giovannelli J, Dauchet L, Mouthon L, Agard C, Lega JC, et al. Survival and prognosis factors in systemic sclerosis: data of a French multicenter cohort, systematic review, and meta-analysis of the literature. *Arthrit Res Ther.* (2019) 21:86. doi: 10.1186/s13075-019-1867-1

32. Simeon-Aznar CP, Fonollosa-Pla V, Tolosa-Vilella C, Espinosa-Garriga G, Campillo-Grau M, Ramos-Casals M, et al. Registry of the Spanish Network for Systemic Sclerosis: survival, prognostic factors, and causes of death. *Medicine.* (2015) 94:e1728. doi: 10.1097/MD.0000000000001728

33. Zhou Z, Fan Y, Thomason D, Tang W, Liu X, Zhou Z-Y, et al. Economic burden of illness among commercially insured patients with systemic sclerosis with interstitial lung disease in the USA: a claims data analysis. *Adv Ther.* (2019) 36:1100–13. doi: 10.1007/s12325-019-00929-2

34. Kowal-Bielecka O, Fransen J, Avouac J, Becker M, Kulak A, Allanore Y, et al. Update of EULAR recommendations for the treatment of systemic sclerosis. *Ann Rheum Dis.* (2017) 76:1327–39. doi: 10.1136/annrheumdis-2016-209909

35. Roofeh D, Jaafar S, Vummidi D, Khanna D. Management of systemic sclerosis-associated interstitial lung disease. *Curr Opin Rheumatol.* (2019) 31:241–9. doi: 10.1097/BOR.0000000000000592

36. Fernandez-Codina A, Walker KM, Pope JE, Scleroderma Algorithm Group. Treatment algorithms for systemic sclerosis according to experts. *Arthrit Rheumatol.* (2018) 70:1820–8. doi: 10.1002/art.40560

37. Hoffmann-Vold A-M, Maher TM, Philpot EE, Ashrafzadeh A, Barake R, Barsotti S, et al. The identification and management of interstitial lung disease in systemic sclerosis: evidence-based European consensus statements. *Lancet Rheumatol.* (2020) 2:e71–83. doi: 10.1016/S2665-9913(19)30144-4

38. Doyle TJ, Hunninghake GM, Rosas IO. Subclinical interstitial lung disease: why you should care. *Am J Respir Crit Care Med.* (2012) 185:1147–53. doi: 10.1164/rccm.201108-1420PP

39. Chatignoux É, Remontet L, Iwaz J, Colonna M, Uhry Z. For a sound use of health care data in epidemiology: evaluation of a calibration model for count data with application to prediction of cancer incidence in areas without cancer registry. *Biostatistics.* (2018) 20:452–67. doi: 10.1093/biostatistics/kxy012

Systemic Sclerosis Associated Interstitial Lung Disease: New Directions in Disease Management

Mehdi Mirsaeidi*, Pamela Barletta and Marilyn K. Glassberg

Division of Pulmonary, Critical Care, and Sleep Medicine, University of Miami Miller School of Medicine, Miami, FL, United States

*Correspondence:
Mehdi Mirsaeidi
msm249@med.miami.edu;
mglassbe@med.miami.edu

A subgroup of patients with systemic sclerosis (SSc) develop interstitial lung disease (ILD), characterized by inflammation and progressive scarring of the lungs that can lead to respiratory failure. Although ILD remains the major cause of death in these individuals, there is no consensus statement regarding the classification and characterization of SSc-related ILD (SSc-ILD). Recent clinical trials address the treatment of SSc-ILD and the results may lead to new disease-altering therapies. In this review, we provide an update to the diagnosis, management and treatment of SSc-ILD.

Keywords: scleroderma, interstitial lung disease, systemic sclerosis, cyclophosphamide, nintedanib, pirfenidone

INTRODUCTION

Scleroderma or systemic sclerosis (SSc) is a systemic multi-organ disorder characterized by autoimmunity, systemic inflammation, vascular injury, and tissue fibrosis (1). Hippocrates provided the first description of their "thickened" skin texture around 400 BCE followed by labeling of the skin as "wood-like" by Curzio (2). In 1836, Fantonetti applied the term "scleroderma," derived from the Greek words skleros (hard or indurated) and derma (skin), to describe the human skin and joint disease presenting with tightened dark leathered skin leading to impaired joint mobility (2).

Classification of patients with SSc is based on the extent of skin involvement- diffuse cutaneous sclerosis (dcSSc) or limited cutaneous sclerosis (lcSSc), the latter characterized by skin sclerosis restricted to the hands, face, neck and distal extremities (3). Although SSc mainly affects the skin, pulmonary manifestations have an unpredictable course and remain the main cause of morbidity and mortality (4).

EPIDEMIOLOGY

The overall incidence rate of SSc in the adult population of the United States is approximately 20 per million per year (5) and approximately one in 10,000 individuals worldwide (1). Incidence and prevalence rates are fairly similar for Europe, the United States, Australia, and Argentina suggesting a prevalence of 150–300 cases per million; Scandinavia, Japan, the UK, Taiwan, and India report lower prevalence (6). The European League Against Rheumatism (EULAR) study showed a median disease duration of 7.1 years for patients with dcSSc and 15.0 years for lcSSc (7). The ratio of women to men developing SSc is 4:1 with an age of 45–55 at presentation (8). Cigarette smoking contributes to disease severity, but is not associated with risk of developing SSc-ILD (9).

In a review of patients with SSc-ILD, pulmonary fibrosis accounted for 19% of deaths and pulmonary hypertension (PH) in 14% (4). In an Italian cohort, the survival of SSc-ILD patients was reported to be 29–69% at 10 years from diagnosis with a female to male ratio of 9.7:1 (10).

African-American scleroderma patients have an earlier onset and more severe pulmonary disease. However, African American race is not a significant risk factor for mortality after adjustment for socioeconomic factors (11). Al-Sheikh reported that European-descent white subjects (55%, 95% CI 51–60) have poorer survival compared to Hispanic subjects (81.3%, 95% CI 63–100). East Asians have the longest median survival time (43.3 years) and Arabs the shortest median survival time (15 years) (12). Independent of race, lower median household income predicted increased mortality (11).

MECHANISM OF FIBROSIS IN SSC-ILD

Similar to other fibrotic lung diseases, injury to epithelial cells, activation of innate and adaptive immunity, and fibroblast recruitment and activation may lead to excessive extracellular matrix production and scarring in SSc-ILD (13). The factors that promote the activation and increased matrix production of fibrogenic fibroblasts in SSc-ILD are not well studied. However, recent data suggest that myofibroblast differentiation and proliferation are key pathological mechanisms driving fibrosis in SSc-ILD (14).

In bronchoalveolar lavage (BAL) fluid from patients with SSc-ILD, the pro- inflammatory cytokines interleukin (IL)-8, tumor necrosis factor-a (TNF), and macrophage inflammatory protein—1a are increased (15). Lung biopsies from patients with SSc-ILD demonstrate increased expression of Toll-like receptor (TLR) 4 in fibroblasts (11, 16). TLR4 is widely recognized as central to the innate response to gram-negative bacteria, but it can also be activated by endogenous ligands generated by cellular injury, autoimmune response, and oxidative stress. TLR4 activation potentiates TGF–β signaling and suppresses antifibrotic microRNAs (miR-101, miR 18a5p, miR-1343, miR-153, miR-326, miR-27b, miR-489, miR26a) (11, 17). TGF-β, through indirect influence on cytokines, primarily platelet derived growth factor (PDGF), promotes fibrogenesis (18). Elevated levels of IL-33 have been correlated with the severity of skin and lung fibrosis (19).

OTHER PULMONARY MANIFESTIONS IN SSC

Lung involvement including ILD, PH, or a combination of ILD and PH, occurs in more than 70% of patients with SSc. Pulmonary vascular disease, primarily pulmonary arterial hypertension, occurs in 10–40% of patients with SSc. Recently, coexisting PH was reported in a large SSc-ILD cohort often occurring early after diagnosis of SSc-ILD (20).

CLINICAL DIAGNOSIS OF SSC-ILD

The diagnosis of SSc-ILD is based on finding ILD on HRCT of the chest in a patient with known SSc accompanied by normal or abnormal pulmonary function tests showing restriction. Approximately one third of patients with SSc have positive anti-topoisomerase (Scl-70) antibodies; these patients have a greater likelihood of developing ILD, compared to those with lcSSc or those with positive anti-centromere antibodies (21). In the EULAR analysis, 53% of cases with dcSSc and 35% of cases with lcSSc had SSc-ILD (22). Historically, African American ethnicity, higher Rodman skin score (a measure of skin thickness), high creatinine and serum CPK levels, hypothyroidism, and cardiac involvement are associated with increased risk for the development of ILD (23, 24). Current risk factors for progression include diffuse vs. limited disease, a disease duration of >5 years, extent of parenchymal disease on HRCT of >20%, a forced vital capacity (FVC) of <70%, and the detection of anti-topoisomerase antibody (25).

DIAGNOSIS OF SSC-ILD

The most common symptoms of SSc-ILD are dyspnea, fatigue, and non-productive cough (26). Early ILD is frequently asymptomatic. As part of the diagnostic evaluation for a patient with SSc-ILD, auscultation of bibasilar fine inspiratory crackles at the lung bases should warrant a HRCT of the chest (27). The most common radiological finding is a non-specific interstitial pneumonia pattern with peripheral, bibasilar distribution of ground glass opacities (28, 29) (**Figure 2**). A pattern of usual interstitial pneumonia, characterized by honeycomb cysts and traction bronchiectasis may also be seen in up to a third of patients with SSc-ILD (29). The presence of ground glass opacities may herald the development of pulmonary fibrosis (30).

The most common histopathologic finding on lung biopsy is fibrotic NSIP (31) (**Figure 3**). A usual interstitial pneumonia (UIP) pattern can also be seen. When compared to lung biopsies of patients with idiopathic pulmonary fibrosis, SSc-ILD patients have more germinal centers and fewer fibroblast foci (32).

Almost all patients with SSc-ILD have positive antinuclear antibodies; this can be accompanied by anti-topoisomerase I (anti-Scl-70), anti- Th/To, anti-U3 ribonucleoprotein (RNP), anti- U11/U12 RNP, and rarely anti-centromere antibodies (33). The sensitivity and specificity of these autoantibodies varies in SSc depending on ethnicity, geographic region of origin, and method of detection (34).

Pulmonary function tests may be normal at presentation, but can be helpful in the follow up of SSc-ILD (35). Forced vital capacity below 80%, low diffusing capacity of the lungs for carbon monoxide (DLCO), and older age are predictors for mortality in SSc-ILD (15, 36). A rapid decline in DLCO may be the single most significant predictor of poor outcome and extent of ILD (37–39).

Analysis of BAL from patients with SSc-ILD typically shows increased number of granulocytes, especially neutrophils and eosinophils, and sometimes an increased level of lymphocytes and mast cells (40). In a series of 156 patients with SSc-ILD, a high percentage of neutrophils in BAL was associated with a 30% increase in risk of mortality (41).

The diagnosis of SSc-ILD is based on finding ILD on the HRCT of the chest in a patient with known SSc, and with exclusion of other etiologies of pulmonary parenchymal disease such as drug induced lung toxicity, heart failure, or recurrent aspiration. A lung biopsy may be considered if there is suspicion for malignancy or granulomatous disease (40).

BIOMARKERS IN THE DIAGNOSIS OF SSC-ILD

There are no biomarkers that are part of a standard of care diagnostic work-up. In two study cohorts that included 427 individuals with SSc, lung-epithelial-derived surfactant protein (SP-D) was identified as a potential biomarker of SSc-ILD. It is suggested that elevated serum levels of SP-D would increase the risk of finding pulmonary fibrosis on chest images 3-fold (OR: 3.15 [1.81–5.48], $p < 0.001$) (42). Chemokine (C-C motif) ligand 18 (CCL18) is another biomarker that may predict the progression of ILD. The CCL18 is a pro-fibrotic factor and is found elevated in serum, BAL and lung tissue from patients with IPF or SSc-ILD (43). CCL18 is secreted predominantly by alveolar macrophages and is reflective of active lung injury (44).

The levels of Krebs von den Lungen-6 (KL-6), a glycoprotein found predominantly on type II pneumocytes and alveolar macrophages, are elevated in the serum of patients with SSc-ILD and may correlate with the presence of pneumonitis and the radiological fibrosis score in patients with SSc (45). KL-6 has been used as a marker for acuteness of lung fibrosis and the presence of pneumonitis (42). In a study of lung biopsies from 112 patients, the KL-6 level was significantly higher in patients with clinically

active pneumonitis (1,497 +/- 560 U/ml) compared with inactive pneumonitis (441 ± 276 U/ml ($p < 0.001$) (46).

CLINICAL MANAGEMENT OF PATIENTS WITH SSC-ILD

The importance of a decline in lung function and survival in patients with SSc was noted by Ferri (47). SSc-ILD is classified as limited or extensive based on the findings of high-resolution computed tomography (HRCT) and lung function FVC (15). Patients with >20% HRCT abnormalities are considered to have extensive lung disease and those with <20% HRCT changes as limited disease. If the FVC is <70%, patients have extensive lung disease, and if the FVC is >70%, patients have limited disease (15). Patients with extensive disease have higher mortality and risk of lung function deterioration (15).

The treatment for SSc-ILD has focused on immunosuppressive therapies, particularly cyclophosphamide (CYC) and mycophenylate mofetil (MMF) based on the results of two pivotal clinical trials. Results from the Scleroderma Lung Study 1 showed a 1% change in FVC in the placebo group compared to a 2.6% change in FVC in the treated SSc subjects at 12 and 18 months (31). After 24 months, there were no differences between groups (48, 49). The results of the Scleroderma Lung Study I supported CYC as a standard of care until smaller studies reported beneficial effects of MMF in SSc-ILD. This led to the Scleroderma Lung Study II comparing

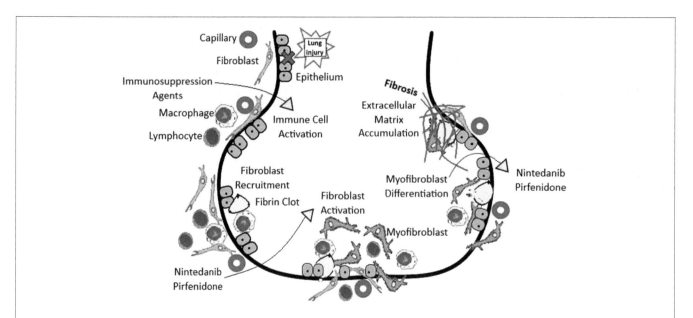

FIGURE 1 | The pathogenesis of SSc-ILD involves vascular, immunological, and fibrotic processes. The initial injury begins with endothelial and alveolar cell injury, which upregulates adhesion molecules and chemokines to attract leukocytes, which enable both innate and adaptive immune responses. Anti-topoisomerase 1 antibodies form immune complexes, and are taken up via Fc receptors, and activate endosomal Toll-like receptors in immune cells, which leads to type I interferon production. IFN release can induce TLR 3 expression on the surface of fibroblasts, causing pro-collagen production. Ligands for Toll-like receptors (TLRs) stimulate dendritic cells to produce IFN-α and interleukin (IL)-6, which in turn activate Th2 cells, produce IL-4 and IL-13, and stimulate pro-fibrotic macrophages. Macrophages produce multiple profibrotic factors including: TGFβ, connective tissue growth factor (CTGF), and PDGF, which promote fibroblast recruitment, invasion and proliferation. Fibroblast activation then occurs, and differentiation to a contractile myofibroblast phenotype result in overproduction and accumulation of extracellular matrix, resulting in progressive fibrosis. *Immunosuppression agents: mycophenolate mofetil, cyclophosphamide, tacrolimus, cyclosporine, tocilizumab, rituximab.

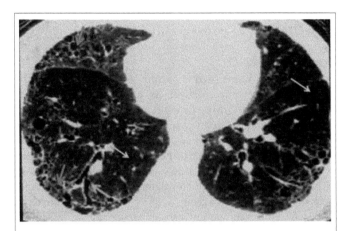

FIGURE 2 | HRCT of a usual interstitial pneumonia (UIP) pattern, characterized by honeycombing (red arrows), and traction bronchiectasis (blue arrow). Normal lung tissue is signaled with green arrows.

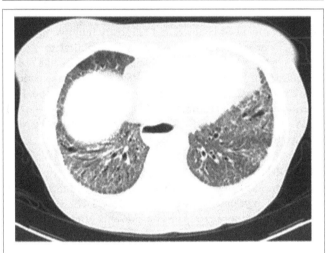

FIGURE 3 | Fibrotic nonspecific interstitial pneumonia (NSIP).

CYC vs. MMF showing that MMF was as effective and safer than CYC over a 24-month time period (54). Although this trial had a large dropout rate and lacked a placebo arm, MMF fell into a standard of care for SSc-ILD (54). Goldin et al. recently reported that changes in quantitative fibrosis scoring of the HRCT in SLS II correlated with FVC and the transition dyspnea index (50).Despite a previously negative trial with a tyrosine kinase inhibitor, imatinib (51), the recently completed SENSCIS trial in which 50% of the subjects were on a stable dose of MMF demonstrated an improvement in FVC with the addition of nintedanib (52). Of note, 50% had diffuse SSc and 60% of the participants were anti-topoisomerase positive.

The optimal treatment of SSc-ILD is not known. Developing treatments that would prevent SSc-ILD disease progression rather than disease regression is a research goal (39). Current management includes initiation of immunosuppressive treatment for SSc-ILD with ongoing evidence of disease progression based on PFT decline or radiographic deterioration. Initial therapy does not include steroids in light of the risk of renal crisis especially in dsSSc patients. Patients are more likely to benefit from immunosuppressant therapy during the early course of the disease, before substantial loss of lung function occurs (53). The most rapid decline in FVC occurs within the initial 3 years of disease onset (54). When therapy is initiated, exercise tolerance and PFTs should be monitored at 6-month intervals (55). Frequent HRCT images are not recommended and can be repeated when a change in clinical symptoms occur. (56) Most physicians seem to treat patients with extensive lung disease (presentation in HRCT and lung biopsy with UIP pattern, and evidence of ground glass opacities occupying more than 10% of lungs (Figures 1, 2). With the completion of more randomized clinical trials, newer treatments with or without the adopted immunosuppressive agents may demonstrate efficacy in SSc-ILD.

Mycophenolate Mofetil (MMF)

Mycophenolate mofetil (MMF)is an inhibitor of lymphocyte proliferation and is often used as first line treatment in patients with SSc-ILD who are at risk for progressive ILD (57). The role of MMF in SSc-ILD was studied in the Scleroderma Lung Study II that evaluated 142 patients with SSc-ILD with FVC of <80%, and ground glass opacities on HRCT. Participants were given either 1,500 mg MMF twice daily for 24 months or oral cyclophosphamide (CYC) titrated up to a maximum dose of 1.8–2.3 mg/kg for 12 months. MMF was better tolerated than CYC and had a lower incidence of leukopenia and thrombocytopenia (57). Bone marrow suppression and gastrointestinal (GI) symptoms were the most commonly observed adverse effects of MMF. A complete blood count should be performed before starting therapy and during treatment. The target dose of MMF is generally between 1.5 and 3 g daily usually in two divided doses to avoid GI side effects.

In an observational study, 13 patients received anti-thymocyte globulin plus prednisolone for 5 days, followed by MMF maintenance therapy for 12 months. Long-term MMF was well tolerated, but there was no change in mean FVC or diffusion capacity after receiving this combined therapy (58).

Cyclophosphamide (CYC)

Cyclophosphamide (CYC) is considered an alternative to MMF based on the results of the Scleroderma Lung Study II. The unfavorable adverse effect profile includes infertility, opportunistic infections, hemorrhagic cystitis, bladder cancer, and neutropenia (59). Monthly intravenous administration of CYC is preferred over oral administration, due to a lower cumulative dose effect, less frequent adverse effects, and the ability to ensure adequate hydration before administration (28). Six CYC monthly intravenous infusions are recommended (60), with monthly monitoring of white blood cell count, renal function, and urinalysis. Corticosteroid pulses have been used with CYC with favorable results, but not as monotherapy (61). After completing a course of CYC, the treatment is commonly switched to a less toxic maintenance agent such as MMF or Azathioprine. Improvement in lung function after CYC treatment tends to decrease after discontinuation (62). For this reason, maintenance therapy is recommended, preferably with MMF (57).

Azathioprine

Azathioprine is a less efficacious initial therapy for SSc-ILD than CYC. In a randomized, double-blind trial, 60 patients with early SSc-ILD received either Azathioprine or CYC. During the first 6 months of therapy, patients also received prednisone, which was tapered subsequently. After 18 months FVC ($-11.1 \pm 1\%$), and DLCO ($-11.6 \pm 1.3\%$) were significantly worse ($p < 0.001$) in the Azathioprine group. In the CYC group, DLCO and FVC remained unchanged (63).

Cyclosporine and Tacrolimus

Cyclosporine and tacrolimus selectively inhibit calcineurin, thereby impairing the transcription of IL-2 and several other cytokines in T lymphocytes. Cyclosporine is an immunosuppressive agent mainly used to treat organ rejection post- transplant. Cyclosporine is a highly nephrotoxic agent that causes a decrease in the glomerular filtration rate (GFR) and a decrease in creatinine clearance (64). In a retrospective, observational study, tacrolimus may have some benefits for SSc-ILD. Twenty patients with SSc-ILD treated with CYC were divided into two groups: one treated with tacrolimus and low-dose corticosteroids following CYC and the other treated with low-dose corticosteroids after CYC. No difference was observed in PFTs at baseline in each group (%VC: $79.5 \pm 16.1\%$ vs. $87.4 \pm 18.8\%$, %DLCO: $59.5 \pm 11.5\%$ vs. $63.7 \pm 14.6\%$). In 3 years follow up; subjects treated with tacrolimus did not demonstrate disease progression (65). Neither CYC or tacrolimus is considered standard of care management for SSc-ILD.

Bosentan

Bosentan, is a nonselective endothelin receptor antagonist, used in the treatment of pulmonary hypertension. It is known that the endothelin system participates in the pathogenesis of SSc, and that it could delay the progression of SSc-ILD. A prospective, double-blind, randomized, placebo-controlled, parallel group study was conducted to evaluate changes in 6 min walk test distance, FVC and DLCO changes. 163 patients were enrolled, 77 were randomized to receive Bosentan, and 86 were randomized to receive placebo for 12 months. No significant difference between treatment groups was observed for change in the 6-min walk distance. No deaths occurred in this study group. FVC and DLCO remained stable. In Conclusion, these data do not support the use of endothelin receptor antagonists as therapy for SSc-ILD (66).

BIOLOGICAL IMMUNOTHERAPIES

Rituximab

Rituximab, a monoclonal antibody that targets CD20 positive B-lymphocytes, is suggested for patients with refractory SSC-ILD (67). In a pilot study, rituximab plus standard therapy (prednisone, CYC, and/or MMF) compared to standard therapy alone showed that the 8 patients in the rituximab group had a significantly better FVC, and DLCO (median percentage of improvement of 10.25 and 19.46%, respectively) at 1 year, than the other 6 patients receiving standard therapy alone (68).

Further studies are need to assess the efficacy of rituximab in SSc-ILD (69).

Tocilizumab

Tocilizumab, a humanized monoclonal antibody against the human IL-6 receptor a chain, is approved for treatment of rheumatoid arthritis, juvenile idiopathic arthritis, and Castleman's disease (70). In patients with SSc-ILD, higher levels of serum IL-6 appear to be predictive of early disease progression in patients with mild ILD, this could be used to target treatment in this group of patients (71). In a randomized 48-week trial of 87 patients with dcSSc, FVC was significantly improved after 24 weeks in the Tocilizumab group (-34 vs. -171 ml respectively, $p = 0.0368$). However, no significant difference in FVC was found between the treated and control groups at 48 weeks (72).

Pomalidomide (POM)

Pomalidomide (POM), is an immunomodulator with antiangiogenic properties, and cytotoxic activity. Approved for the treatment of relapsed and refractory multiple myeloma (73). A 52 week randomized, double blind clinical trial of 23 patients with SSc-ILD was conducted to evaluate the safety and efficacy of POM on FVC and mRSS. Twenty-three patients were enrolled and randomized to receive POM or placebo. FVC deteriorated in both treatments (POM -5.2%, placebo -2.7%), mRSS (POM -2.7, placebo -3.7). Since very few subjects were enrolled the results were inconclusive (74).

Bortezomib

Bortezomib, is a FDA approved medication for the treatment of multiple myeloma. Bortezomib inhibits TGF- signaling *in vitro*, promotes normal repair and prevents lung fibrosis. The objective of the trial is to establish the safety and tolerability of bortezomib in SSc patients as well as exploratory effects on FVC. Participants receive MMF (1.5 g twice a day orally) and Bortezomib(1.3 mg/m²) subcutaneously once per week for the first 2 weeks vs. MMF plus placebo (normal saline) for 24 weeks. The trial is planned for completion in June 2019.

ANTI-FIBROTIC AGENTS

Nintedanib and pirfenidone have anti-fibrotic effects and are approved for use in patients with idiopathic pulmonary fibrosis (IPF). In a case series of five patients with SSc-ILD, pirfenidone (1,200–1,800 mg/day) was associated with a reduction in dyspnea and an increase in VC (10%) from baseline (75). LOTUSS, a 16-week open label phase II trial of the safety and tolerability of pirfenidone on patients with SSc-ILD, pirfenidone was generally well tolerated, but there were no significant changes in FVC (76). SLS III, a double-blind, parallel group, randomized and placebo-controlled clinical trial is currently being conducted in patients with SSc-ILD. Participants must be treatment naive. The objective of this study is to determine the efficacy and safety of the combination of MMF with Pirfenidone. Subjects will be randomized 1:1 to receive MMF plus Pirfenidone or MMF plus placebo. The trial is scheduled for completion on May 2021.

Nintedanib, is a tyrosine kinase inhibitor (77) for vascular endothelial growth factor (VEGF), fibroblast growth factor (FGF), and platelet-derived growth factor (PDGF), and colony stimulating factor 1 receptor (CSF1R) (78), slows disease progression and improves survival in patients with IPF. The SENCSIS trial, a double blind, randomized, placebo-controlled trial evaluated the efficacy and safety of oral nintenadib (150 mg bid) treatment for at least 52 weeks in patients with SSc-ILD (79). In the SENSCIS trial, 50% of the subjects had dsSSc and were on a stable dose of MMF. Subjects had a diagnosis of SSc with an onset of the first non-Raynaud's symptom within the past 7 years before entry and a HRCT that showed fibrosis affecting at least 10% of the lungs. The primary end point was the annual rate of decline in FVC. Key secondary end points were absolute changes from baseline in the modified Rodnan skin score (MRSS) and in the total score on the St. George's Respiratory Questionnaire (SGRQ). Neither of the two secondary endpoints achieved statistical significance highlighting the variability and poor reproducibility of the MRSS and the questionable applicability of the SGRQ for understanding dyspnea in SSc-ILD. The adjusted annual rate of change in FVC was -52.4 ml per year in the nintedanib group and -93.3 ml per year in the placebo group (difference, 41.0 ml per year; 95% [CI], 2.9–79.0; $P = 0.04$). Patients on a stable MMF dose did not elicit further improvement with add-on therapy with nintenadib.

Diarrhea, the most common adverse event, was reported in 75.7% of the patients in the nintedanib group and in 31.6% of those in the placebo group (52). An extension trial, SENSCIS-ON will assess long-term safety of treatment with oral Nintedanib in 450 subjects who completed the SENSCIS trial. This trial should be completed by July 2021.

OTHER TREATMENT MODALITIES

Lung Transplantation

Lung transplantation should be considered in the early stage of respiratory failure for all patients with chronic lung disease. However, gastrointestinal comorbidities that are often seen in patients with SSc-ILD may complicate the transplant evaluation (80). A systematic review by Khan et al. was performed to identify studies of the survival outcome post lung transplantation between patients with SSc vs. patients with no Ssc (ILD patients requiring lung transplantation) (81). SSc post-transplantation survival ranged 69–91% at 30-days, 69–85% at 6-months, 59–93% at 1-year, 49–80% at 2-years, and 46–79% at 3-years (82–85). The short-term and intermediate-term survival post-lung transplantation are similar to ILD patients requiring lung transplantation.

TABLE 1 | Completed clinical trials for patients with SSc-ILD.

Drug and study design	Name of study	Indications	Adverse effects
Mycophenolate mofetil (MMF). 2-year randomized, double-blind, active comparator/placebo-controlled trial	SLSII (57) NCT00883129	-First line treatment in patients who are at risk of progressive ILD. -Maintenance therapy	-Bone marrow suppression -Gastrointestinal (nausea, diarrhea, abdominal cramping) -Pancytopenia -Hypertension -Hyperglycemia
Cyclophosphamide (CYC) 1-year, randomized, double-blind, placebo-controlled trial plus 1 additional year of follow-up without study medication	SLS I (28, 59) NCT00004563	Second line treatment	-Infertility -Opportunistic infections -Hemorrhagic cystitis -Bladder cancer -Leukopenia -Thrombocytopenia
Bosentan 12-month randomized, double-blind, placebo-controlled trial	BUILD-2 (66) NCT00070590	Investigational approach	-Gastrointestinal (weight gain, nausea, vomiting) -Fatigue, Dizziness -Edema
Pirfenidone 16-week randomized, open-label comparison of two titration schedules	LOTUSS (76) NCT01933334	Investigational approach	-Gastrointestinal -Skin(sun sensitivity and rash) - Elevated liver enzymes
Pomalidomide 52 week randomized, double-blind, placebo-controlled, parallel-group study	CC-4047 (1, 74) NCT01559129	Investigational approach	-Gastrointestinal -Leuokopenia
Nintedanib 52 week, double blind, randomized, placebo-controlled trial evaluating FVC changes, efficacy and safety	SENCSIS trial (52, 79) NCT02597933	Investigational approach	-Gastrointestinal, mainly diarrhea -High blood pressure
Hematopoietic bone marrow stem cell transplant Randomized, open-label, phase II multicenter study of high-dose immunosuppressive Therapy	Scleroderma: cyclophosphamide or transplantation (SCOT) NCT00114530	Investigational approach	-Immunosuppression

TABLE 2 | Ongoing clinical trials for SSc-ILD patients.

TABLE 2 | Ongoing clinical trials for SSc-ILD patients.

Drug and study design	Name of study	Clinical trial identifier	Phase trial
Nintedanib An open-label extension trial of the long term safety of Nintedanib.	SENCSIS trial	NCT03313180	III
Bortezomib	Comparing and combining Bortezomib and Mycophenolate in SSc pulmonary fibrosis	NCT02370693	II, recruiting
Pirfenidone plus MMF vs. MMF plus placebo.	Scleroderma Lung Study III	NCT03221257	II, recruiting

Autologous Hematopoietic Stem Cell Transplantation (AHSCT)

Autologous hematopoietic stem cell transplantation (AHSCT) has been proposed as a potential therapy for severe SSc disease (86). In a meta-analysis study including patients with SSc-ILD on cyclophosphamide who underwent AHSCT, AHSCT reduced all-cause mortality (risk ratio [RR], 0.5 [95% confidence interval, 0.33–0.75]) and improved FVC (mean difference [M] 9.58% [95% CI, 3.89–15.18]), total lung capacity (M, 6.36% [95% CI, 1.23–11.49]), and assessment of quality of life (QOL) using a Short Form Health Survey showed improvement (M, 6.99% [95% CI, 2.79–11.18]) (87). Treatment-related mortality considerably varied between trials, but was overall higher with AHSCT (RR, 9.00 [95% CI, 1.57–51.69]). In the ASSIST trial, HSCT and antithymocyte globulin therapy preceded by CYC and filgrastim was superior to CYC with regards to skin score and lung volumes, although no difference was observed in DLco No deaths occurred in either group over 24 months of follow up (88). Recently, the SCOT (Scleroderma: CYC or transplantation) trial in patients with severe dcSSc with renal or pulmonary involvement, which goal was to determine the safety and effectiveness of high dose immunosuppressive therapy followed by AHSCT compared to CYC alone. The study demonstrated that myeloablative CD34+ selected AHSCT promoted greater event-free survival (survival without significant organ damage or death) than 12 months of CYC. The survival benefit was also noted at 54 months (79 vs. 50%) and at 72 months (74 vs. 47%) (89). **Tables 1, 2** show a summary of ongoing and completed clinical trials on Ssc-ILD treatment.

CONCLUSIONS

Although there is no consensus statement that defines the criteria for SSc-ILD, HRCT, and PFTs serve as the primary diagnostic and staging parameters for establishing a diagnosis. Although MMF has been the initial treatment choice for SSc-ILD due to safer toxicity profiles and outcomes, more recent trials raise the option of antifibrotics or combination immunomodulatory/antifibrotic therapy as potential new treatments for patients with SSc-ILD. Lung transplant should be considered as an option, but the significant comorbidities associated with SSc including GI comorbidities should be addressed with medical and surgical evaluations prior to referring for transplant.

Many questions remain unanswered. When should treatment be initiated for SSc-ILD? What treatment regimen is most efficacious? How long should the patient be treated with SSc-ILD? With the development of more sophisticated classification criteria and assessment of HRCT, availability of reliable and reproducible biomarkers and molecular profiling, answers for these questions will impact treatment strategies for patients with SSc-ILD.

AUTHOR CONTRIBUTIONS

PB conducted literature review, conducted exploratory analysis, and helped to develop the first draft of the manuscript. MG helped in developing the first draft of the manuscript. MM conducted literature review, conducted exploratory analysis, and developed the final version of the manuscript.

ACKNOWLEDGMENTS

We thank Dr. Aryeh Fischer who contributed HRCT images for this review.

REFERENCES

1. Meyer KC. Scleroderma with fibrosing interstitial lung disease: where do we stand? *Ann Am Thorac Soc.* (2018) 15:1273–5. doi: 10.1513/AnnalsATS.201808-544ED

2. Armando Laborde H, Young P. History of systemic sclerosis. *Gac Med Mex.* (2012) 148:201–8.

3. Gabrielli A, Avvedimento EV, Krieg T. Scleroderma. *N Engl J Med.* (2009) 360:1989–2003. doi: 10.1056/NEJMra0806188

4. Solomon JJ, et al. Scleroderma lung disease. *Eur Respir Rev.* (2013) 22:6–19. doi: 10.1183/09059180.00005512

5. Mayes MD. Scleroderma epidemiology. *Rheum Dis Clin North Am.* (2003) 29:239–54. doi: 10.1016/S0889-857X(03)00022-X

6. Barnes J, Mayes MD. Epidemiology of systemic sclerosis: incidence, prevalence, survival, risk factors, malignancy, and environmental triggers. *Curr Opin Rheumatol.* (2012) 24:165–70. doi: 10.1097/BOR.0b013e32834ff2e8

7. Tyndall AJ, Bannert B, Vonk M, Airò P, Cozzi F, Carreira PE, et al. Causes and risk factors for death in systemic sclerosis: a study from the EULAR Scleroderma Trials and Research (EUSTAR) database. *Ann Rheum Dis.* (2010) 69:1809–15. doi: 10.1136/ard.2009.114264

8. Singh D, Parihar AK, Patel S, Srivastava S, Diwan P, Singh MR. Scleroderma: an insight into causes, pathogenesis and treatment strategies. *Pathophysiology.* (2019) 26:103–14. doi: 10.1016/j.pathophys.2019.05.003

9. Chaudhary P, Chen X, Assassi S, Gorlova O, Draeger H, Harper BE, et al. Cigarette smoking is not a risk factor for systemic sclerosis. *Arthritis Rheumatol.* (2011) 63:3098–102. doi: 10.1002/art.30492

10. Lo Monaco A, Bruschi M, La Corte R, Volpinari S, Trotta F. Epidemiology of systemic sclerosis in a district of Northern Italy. *Clin Exp Rheumatol.* (2011) 29(2 suppl. 65):S10–4.

11. Bhattacharyya S, Kelley K, Melichian DS, Tamaki Z, Fang F, Su Y, et al. Toll-like receptor 4 signaling augments transforming growth factor-beta responses: a novel mechanism for maintaining and amplifying fibrosis in scleroderma. *Am J Pathol.* (2013) 182:192–205. doi: 10.1016/j.ajpath.2012.09.007

12. Al-Sheikh H, Ahmad Z, Johnson SR. Ethnic variations in systemic sclerosis disease manifestations, internal organ involvement, and mortality. *J Rheumatol*. (2019) 46:1103–8. doi: 10.3899/jrheum.180042

13. Tamby MC, Chanseaud Y, Guillevin L, Mouthon L. New insights into the pathogenesis of systemic sclerosis. *Autoimmun Rev*. (2003) 2:152–7. doi: 10.1016/S1568-9972(03)00004-1

14. Valenzi E, Bulik M, Tabib T, Morse C, Sembrat J, Trejo Bittar H, et al. Single-cell analysis reveals fibroblast heterogeneity and myofibroblasts in systemic sclerosis-associated interstitial lung disease. *Ann Rheum Dis*. (2019) 78:1379–87. doi: 10.1136/annrheumdis-2018-214865

15. Goh NS, Desai SR, Veeraraghavan S, Hansell DM, Copley SJ, Maher TM, et al. Interstitial lung disease in systemic sclerosis: a simple staging system. *Am J Respir Crit Care Med*. (2008) 177:1248–54. doi: 10.1164/rccm.200706-877OC

16. Bhattacharyya S, Midwood KS, Yin H, Varga J. Toll-like receptor-4 signaling drives persistent fibroblast activation and prevents fibrosis resolution in scleroderma. *Adv Wound Care*. (2017) 6:356–69. doi: 10.1089/wound.2017.0732

17. Kang H. Role of microRNAs in TGF-β signaling pathway-mediated pulmonary fibrosis. *Int J Mol Sci*. (2017) 18:E2527. doi: 10.3390/ijms18122527

18. Yamakage A, Kikuchi K, Smith EA, LeRoy EC, Trojanowska M. Selective upregulation of platelet-derived growth factor alpha receptors by transforming growth factor beta in scleroderma fibroblasts. *J Exp Med*. (1992) 175:1227–34. doi: 10.1084/jem.175.5.1227

19. Yanaba K, Yoshizaki A, Asano Y, Kadono T, Sato S. Serum IL-33 levels are raised in patients with systemic sclerosis: association with extent of skin sclerosis and severity of pulmonary fibrosis. *Clin Rheumatol*. (2011) 30:825–30. doi: 10.1007/s10067-011-1686-5

20. Young A, Vummidi D, Visovatti S, Homer K, Wilhalme H, White ES, et al. Prevalence, treatment and outcomes of coexistent pulmonary hypertension and interstitial lung disease in systemic sclerosis. *Arthritis Rheumatol*. (2019) 71:1339–49. doi: 10.1002/art.40862

21. Fischer A, Swigris JJ, Groshong SD, Cool CD, Sahin H, Lynch DA, et al. Clinically significant interstitial lung disease in limited scleroderma: histopathology, clinical features, and survival. *Chest*. (2008) 134:601–5. doi: 10.1378/chest.08-0053

22. Walker UA, Tyndall A, Czirják L, Denton C, Farge-Bancel D, Kowal-Bielecka O, et al. Clinical risk assessment of organ manifestations in systemic sclerosis: a report from the EULAR Scleroderma Trials And Research group database. *Ann Rheum Dis*. (2007) 66:754–63. doi: 10.1136/ard.2006.062901

23. McNearney TA, Reveille JD, Fischbach M, Friedman AW, Lisse JR, Goel N, et al. Pulmonary involvement in systemic sclerosis: associations with genetic, serologic, sociodemographic, and behavioral factors. *Arthritis Rheumatol*. (2007) 57:318–26. doi: 10.1002/art.22532

24. Greidinger EL, Flaherty KT, White B, Rosen A, Wigley FM, Wise RA. African-American race and antibodies to topoisomerase I are associated with increased severity of scleroderma lung disease. *Chest*. (1998) 114:801–7. doi: 10.1378/chest.114.3.801

25. Goh NS, Hoyles RK, Denton CP, Hansell DM, Renzoni EA, Maher TM, et al. Short-term pulmonary function trends are predictive of mortality in interstitial lung disease associated with systemic sclerosis. *Arthritis Rheumatol*. (2017) 69:1670–8. doi: 10.1002/art.40130

26. Cappelli S, Bellando Randone S, Camiciottoli G, De Paulis A, Guiducci S, Matucci-Cerinic M. Interstitial lung disease in systemic sclerosis: where do we stand? *Eur Respir Rev*. (2015) 24:411–9. doi: 10.1183/16000617.00002915

27. King TE Jr. Smoking and subclinical interstitial lung disease. *N Engl J Med*. (2011) 364:968–70. doi: 10.1056/NEJMe1013966

28. Tashkin DP, Elashoff R, Clements PJ, Goldin J, Roth MD, Furst DE, et al. Cyclophosphamide versus placebo in scleroderma lung disease. *N Engl J Med*. (2006) 354:2655–66. doi: 10.1056/NEJMoa055120

29. Goldin JG, Lynch DA, Strollo DC, Suh RD, Schraufnagel DE, Clements PJ, et al. High-resolution CT scan findings in patients with symptomatic scleroderma-related interstitial lung disease. *Chest*. (2008) 134:358–67. doi: 10.1378/chest.07-2444

30. Remy-Jardin M, Remy J, Wallaert B, Bataille D, Hatron PY. Pulmonary involvement in progressive systemic sclerosis: sequential evaluation with CT, pulmonary function tests, and bronchoalveolar lavage. *Radiology*. (1993) 188:499–506. doi: 10.1148/radiology.188.2.8327704

31. Fujita J, Yoshinouchi T, Ohtsuki Y, Tokuda M, Yang Y, Yamadori I, et al. Non-specific interstitial pneumonia as pulmonary involvement of systemic sclerosis. *Ann Rheum Dis*. (2001) 60:281–3. doi: 10.1136/ard.60.3.281

32. Song JW, Do KH, Kim MY, Jang SJ, Colby TV, Kim DS. Pathologic and radiologic differences between idiopathic and collagen vascular disease-related usual interstitial pneumonia. *Chest*. (2009) 136:23–30. doi: 10.1378/chest.08-2572

33. Hamaguchi Y. Autoantibody profiles in systemic sclerosis: predictive value for clinical evaluation and prognosis. *J Dermatol*. (2010) 37:42–53. doi: 10.1111/j.1346-8138.2009.00762.x

34. Mehra S, Walker J, Patterson K, Fritzler MJ. Autoantibodies in systemic sclerosis. *Autoimmun Rev*. (2013) 12:340–54. doi: 10.1016/j.autrev.2012.05.011

35. Schoenfeld SR, Castelino FV. Interstitial lung disease in scleroderma. *Rheum Dis Clin North Am*. (2015) 41:237–48. doi: 10.1016/j.rdc.2014.12.005

36. Winstone TA, Assayag D, Wilcox PG, Dunne JV, Hague CJ, Leipsic J, et al. Predictors of mortality and progression in scleroderma-associated interstitial lung disease: a systematic review. *Chest*. (2014) 146:422–36. doi: 10.1378/chest.13-2626

37. Plastiras SC, Karadimitrakis SP, Ziakas PD, Vlachoyiannopoulos PG, Moutsopoulos HM, Tzelepis GE. Scleroderma lung: initial forced vital capacity as predictor of pulmonary function decline. *Arthritis Rheumatol*. (2006) 55:598–602. doi: 10.1002/art.22099

38. Guler SA, Winstone TA, Murphy D, Hague C, Soon J, Sulaiman N, et al. Does systemic sclerosis-associated interstitial lung disease burn out? Specific phenotypes of disease progression. *Ann Am Thorac Soc*. (2018) 15:1427–33. doi: 10.1513/AnnalsATS.201806-362OC

39. Bouros D, Wells AU, Nicholson AG, Colby TV, Polychronopoulos V, Pantelidis P, et al. Histopathologic subsets of fibrosing alveolitis in patients with systemic sclerosis and their relationship to outcome. *Am J Respir Crit Care Med*. (2002) 165:1581–6. doi: 10.1164/rccm.2106012

40. Kowal-Bielecka O, Kowal K, Highland KB, Silver RM. Bronchoalveolar lavage fluid in scleroderma interstitial lung disease: technical aspects and clinical correlations: review of the literature. *Semin Arthritis Rheumatol*. (2010) 40:73–88. doi: 10.1016/j.semarthrit.2008.10.009

41. Kinder BW, Brown KK, Schwarz MI, Ix JH, Kervitsky A, King TE. Baseline BAL neutrophilia predicts early mortality in idiopathic pulmonary fibrosis. *Chest*. (2008) 133:226–32. doi: 10.1378/chest.07-1948

42. Elhai M, Hoffmann-Vold AM, Avouac J, Pezet S, Cauvet A, Leblond A, et al. Performance of candidate serum biomarkers for systemic sclerosis-associated interstitial lung disease. *Arthritis Rheumatol*. (2019) 71:972–82. doi: 10.1002/art.40815

43. Prasse A, Pechkovsky DV, Toews GB, Schäfer M, Eggeling S, Ludwig C, et al. CCL18 as an indicator of pulmonary fibrotic activity in idiopathic interstitial pneumonias and systemic sclerosis. *Arthritis Rheumatol*. (2007) 56:1685–93. doi: 10.1002/art.22559

44. Hant FN, Ludwicka-Bradley A, Wang HJ, Li N, Elashoff R, Tashkin DP, et al. Surfactant protein D and KL-6 as serum biomarkers of interstitial lung disease in patients with scleroderma. *J Rheumatol*. (2009) 36:773–80. doi: 10.3899/jrheum.080633

45. Oguz EO, Kucuksahin O, Turgay M, Yildizgoren MT, Ates A, Demir N, et al. Association of serum KL-6 levels with interstitial lung disease in patients with connective tissue disease: a cross-sectional study. *Clin Rheumatol*. (2016) 35:663–6. doi: 10.1007/s10067-015-3167-8

46. Kobayashi J, Kitamura S. KL-6: a serum marker for interstitial pneumonia. *Chest*. (1995) 108:311–5. doi: 10.1378/chest.108.2.311

47. Ferri C, Valentini G, Cozzi F, Sebastiani M, Michelassi C, La Montagna G, et al. Systemic sclerosis: demographic, clinical, and serologic features and survival in 1,012 Italian patients. *Medicine*. (2002) 81:139–53. doi: 10.1097/00005792-200203000-00004

48. Volkmann ER, Tashkin DP, Sim M, Li N, Khanna D, Roth MD, et al. Cyclophosphamide for systemic sclerosis-related interstitial lung disease: a

comparison of scleroderma lung study I and II. *J Rheumatol.* (2019) 46:1316–25. doi: 10.3899/jrheum.180441

49. Kafaja S, Clements PJ, Wilhalme H, Tseng CH, Furst DE, Kim GH, et al. Reliability and minimal clinically important differences of forced vital capacity: results from the scleroderma lung studies (SLS-I and SLS-II). *Am J Respir Crit Care Med.* (2018) 197:644–52. doi: 10.1164/rccm.201709-1845OC

50. Goldin JG, Kim GHJ, Tseng CH, Volkmann E, Furst D, Clements P, et al. Longitudinal changes in quantitative interstitial lung disease on computed tomography after immunosuppression in the scleroderma lung study II. *Ann Am Thorac Soc.* (2018) 15:1286–95. doi: 10.1513/AnnalsATS.201802-079OC

51. Fraticelli P, Gabrielli B, Pomponio G, Valentini G, Bosello S, Riboldi P, et al. Low-dose oral imatinib in the treatment of systemic sclerosis interstitial lung disease unresponsive to cyclophosphamide: a phase II pilot study. *Arthritis Res Ther.* (2014) 16:R144. doi: 10.1186/ar4606

52. Distler O, Highland KB, Gahlemann M, Azuma A, Fischer A, Mayes MD, et al. Nintedanib for systemic sclerosis-associated interstitial lung disease. *N Engl J Med.* (2019) 380:2518–28. doi: 10.1056/NEJMoa1903076

53. Moore OA, Goh N, Corte T, Rouse H, Hennessy O, Thakkar V, et al. Extent of disease on high-resolution computed tomography lung is a predictor of decline and mortality in systemic sclerosis-related interstitial lung disease. *Rheumatology.* (2013) 52:155–60. doi: 10.1093/rheumatology/kes289

54. Steen VD, Medsger TA Jr. Severe organ involvement in systemic sclerosis with diffuse scleroderma. *Arthritis Rheumatol.* (2000) 43:2437–44. doi: 10.1002/1529-0131(200011)43:11<2437::AID-ANR10>3.0.CO;2-U

55. Rizzi M, Sarzi-Puttini P, Airoldi A, Antivalle M, Battellino M, Atzeni F. Performance capacity evaluated using the 6-minute walk test: 5-year results in patients with diffuse systemic sclerosis and initial interstitial lung disease. *Clin Exp Rheumatol.* (2015) 33(4 suppl. 91):S142–7.

56. Katzen JB, Raparia K, Agrawal R, Patel JD, Rademaker A, Varga J, et al. Early stage lung cancer detection in systemic sclerosis does not portend survival benefit: a cross sectional study. *PLoS ONE.* (2015) 10:e0117829. doi: 10.1371/journal.pone.0117829

57. Tashkin DP, Roth MD, Clements PJ, Furst DE, Khanna D, Kleerup EC, et al. Mycophenolate mofetil versus oral cyclophosphamide in scleroderma-related interstitial lung disease (SLS II): a randomised controlled, double-blind, parallel group trial. *Lancet Respir Med.* (2016) 4:708–19. doi: 10.1016/S2213-2600(16)30152-7

58. Stratton RJ, Wilson H, Black CM. Pilot study of anti-thymocyte globulin plus mycophenolate mofetil in recent-onset diffuse scleroderma. *Rheumatology.* (2001) 40:84–8. doi: 10.1093/rheumatology/40.1.84

59. Furst DE, Tseng CH, Clements PJ, Strange C, Tashkin DP, Roth MD, et al. Adverse events during the Scleroderma Lung Study. *Am J Med.* (2011) 124:459–67. doi: 10.1016/j.amjmed.2010.12.009

60. Hoyles RK, Ellis RW, Wellsbury J, Lees B, Newlands P, Goh NS, et al. A multicenter, prospective, randomized, double-blind, placebo-controlled trial of corticosteroids and intravenous cyclophosphamide followed by oral azathioprine for the treatment of pulmonary fibrosis in scleroderma. *Arthritis Rheumatol.* (2006) 54:3962–70. doi: 10.1002/art.22204

61. Yiannopoulos G, Pastromas V, Antonopoulos I, Katsiberis G, Kalliolias G, Liossis SN, et al. Combination of intravenous pulses of cyclophosphamide and methylprednizolone in patients with systemic sclerosis and interstitial lung disease. *Rheumatol Int.* (2007) 27:357–61. doi: 10.1007/s00296-006-0217-1

62. Tashkin DP, Elashoff R, Clements PJ, Roth MD, Furst DE, Silver RM, et al. Effects of 1-year treatment with cyclophosphamide on outcomes at 2 years in scleroderma lung disease. *Am J Respir Crit Care Med.* (2007) 176:1026–34. doi: 10.1164/rccm.200702-326OC

63. Nadashkevich O, Davis P, Fritzler M, Kovalenko W. A randomized unblinded trial of cyclophosphamide versus azathioprine in the treatment of systemic sclerosis. *Clin Rheumatol.* (2006) 25:205–12. doi: 10.1007/s10067-005-1157-y

64. Tapia C, Basehore BM, Zito PM. *Cyclosporine, in StatPearls.* Treasure Island, FL: StatPearls Publishing (2019).

65. Tochimoto A, Kawaguchi Y, Hara M, Tateishi M, Fukasawa C, Takagi K, et al. Efficacy and safety of intravenous cyclophosphamide pulse therapy with oral prednisolone in the treatment of interstitial lung disease with systemic sclerosis: 4-year follow-up. *Mod Rheumatol.* (2011) 21:296–301. doi: 10.1007/s10165-010-0403-6

66. Seibold JR, Denton CP, Furst DE, Guillevin L, Rubin LJ, Wells A, et al. Randomized, prospective, placebo-controlled trial of bosentan in interstitial lung disease secondary to systemic sclerosis. *Arthritis Rheumatol.* (2010) 62:2101–8. doi: 10.1002/art.27466

67. Daoussis D, Liossis SN, Tsamandas AC, Kalogeropoulou C, Paliogianni F, Sirinian C, et al. Effect of long-term treatment with rituximab on pulmonary function and skin fibrosis in patients with diffuse systemic sclerosis. *Clin Exp Rheumatol.* (2012) 30(2 suppl. 71):S17–22.

68. Daoussis D, Liossis SN, Tsamandas AC, Kalogeropoulou C, Kazantzi A, Sirinian C, et al. Experience with rituximab in scleroderma: results from a 1-year, proof-of-principle study. *Rheumatology.* (2010) 49:271–80. doi: 10.1093/rheumatology/kep093

69. Jordan S, Distler JH, Maurer B, Huscher D, van Laar JM, Allanore Y, et al. Effects and safety of rituximab in systemic sclerosis: an analysis from the European Scleroderma Trial and Research (EUSTAR) group. *Ann Rheum Dis.* (2015) 74:1188–94. doi: 10.1136/annrheumdis-2013-204522

70. Nishimoto N, Kishimoto T. Interleukin 6: from bench to bedside. *Nat Clin Pract Rheumatol.* (2006) 2:619–26. doi: 10.1038/ncprheum0338

71. De Lauretis A, Sestini P, Pantelidis P, Hoyles R, Hansell DM, Goh NS, et al. Serum interleukin 6 is predictive of early functional decline and mortality in interstitial lung disease associated with systemic sclerosis. *J Rheumatol.* (2013) 40:435–46. doi: 10.3899/jrheum.120725

72. Khanna D, Denton CP, Jahreis A, van Laar JM, Frech TM, Anderson ME, et al. Safety and efficacy of subcutaneous tocilizumab in adults with systemic sclerosis (faSScinate): a phase 2, randomised, controlled trial. *Lancet.* (2016) 387:2630–40. doi: 10.1016/S0140-6736(16)00232-4

73. Lacy MQ, McCurdy AR. Pomalidomide. *Blood.* (2013) 122:2305–9. doi: 10.1182/blood-2013-05-484782

74. Hsu VM, Denton CP, Domsic RT, Furst DE, Rischmueller M, Stanislav M, et al. Pomalidomide in patients with interstitial lung disease due to systemic sclerosis: a phase II, multicenter, randomized, double-blind, placebo-controlled, parallel-group study. *J Rheumatol.* (2018) 45:405–10. doi: 10.3899/jrheum.161040

75. Miura Y, Saito T, Fujita K, Tsunoda Y, Tanaka T, Takoi H, et al. Clinical experience with pirfenidone in five patients with scleroderma-related interstitial lung disease. *Sarcoidosis Vasc Diffuse Lung Dis.* (2014) 31:235–8.

76. Khanna D, Albera C, Fischer A, Khalidi N, Raghu G, Chung L, et al. An open-label, phase II study of the safety and tolerability of pirfenidone in patients with scleroderma-associated interstitial lung disease: the LOTUSS trial. *J Rheumatol.* (2016) 43:1672–9. doi: 10.3899/jrheum.151322

77. Wollin L, Wex E, Pautsch A, Schnapp G, Hostettler KE, Stowasser S, et al. Mode of action of nintedanib in the treatment of idiopathic pulmonary fibrosis. *Eur Respir J.* (2015) 45:1434–45. doi: 10.1183/09031936.00174914

78. Richeldi L, Costabel U, Selman M, Kim DS, Hansell DM, Nicholson AG, et al. Efficacy of a tyrosine kinase inhibitor in idiopathic pulmonary fibrosis. *N Engl J Med.* (2011) 365:1079–87. doi: 10.1056/NEJMoa1103690

79. Distler O, Brown KK, Distler JHW, Assassi S, Maher TM, Cottin V, et al. Design of a randomised, placebo-controlled clinical trial of nintedanib in patients with systemic sclerosis-associated interstitial lung disease (SENSCIS). *Clin Exp Rheumatol.* (2017) 35 (suppl. 106):75–81.

80. Bernstein EJ, Peterson ER, Sell JL, D'Ovidio F, Arcasoy SM, Bathon JM, et al. Survival of adults with systemic sclerosis following lung transplantation: a nationwide cohort study. *Arthritis Rheumatol.* (2015) 67:1314–22. doi: 10.1002/art.39021

81. Khan IY, Singer LG, de Perrot M, Granton JT, Keshavjee S, Chau C, et al. Survival after lung transplantation in systemic sclerosis. A systematic review. *Respir Med.* (2013) 107:2081–7. doi: 10.1016/j.rmed.2013.09.015

82. Massad MG, Powell CR, Kpodonu J, Tshibaka C, Hanhan Z, Snow NJ, et al. Outcomes of lung transplantation in patients with scleroderma. *World J Surg.* (2005) 29:1510–5. doi: 10.1007/s00268-005-0017-x

83. Schachna L, Medsger TA, Dauber JH, Wigley FM, Braunstein NA, White B, et al. Lung transplantation in scleroderma compared with idiopathic pulmonary fibrosis and idiopathic pulmonary arterial hypertension. *Arthritis Rheumatol.* (2006) 54:3954–61. doi: 10.1002/art.22264

84. Shitrit D, Amital A, Peled N, Raviv Y, Medalion B, Saute M, et al. Lung transplantation in patients with scleroderma: case series, review of the literature, and criteria for transplantation. *Clin Transplant.* (2009) 23:178–83. doi: 10.1111/j.1399-0012.2009.00958.x

85. Saggar R, Khanna D, Furst DE, Belperio JA, Park GS, Weigt SS, et al. Systemic sclerosis and bilateral lung transplantation: a single centre

experience. *Eur Respir J.* (2010) 36:893–900. doi: 10.1183/09031936.001 39809

86. van Laar JM, Farge D, Sont JK, Naraghi K, Marjanovic Z, Larghero J, et al. Autologous hematopoietic stem cell transplantation vs intravenous pulse cyclophosphamide in diffuse cutaneous systemic sclerosis: a randomized clinical trial. *JAMA.* (2014) 311:2490–8. doi: 10.1001/jama.2014.6368

87. Shouval R, Furie N, Raanani P, Nagler A, Gafter-Gvili A. Autologous hematopoietic stem cell transplantation for systemic sclerosis: a systematic review and meta-analysis. *Biol Blood Marrow Transplant.* (2018) 24:937–44. doi: 10.1016/j.bbmt.2018.01.020

88. Burt RK, Shah SJ, Dill K, Grant T, Gheorghiade M, Schroeder J, et al. Autologous non-myeloablative haemopoietic stem-cell transplantation compared with pulse cyclophosphamide once per month for systemic sclerosis (ASSIST): an open-label, randomised phase 2 trial. *Lancet.* (2011) 378:498–506. doi: 10.1016/S0140-6736(11)60982-3

89. Sullivan KM, Goldmuntz EA, Keyes-Elstein L, McSweeney PA, Pinckney A, Welch B, et al. Myeloablative autologous stem-cell transplantation for severe scleroderma. *N Engl J Med.* (2018) 378:35–47. doi: 10.1056/NEJMoa1703327

7

Management of Acute Exacerbation of Idiopathic Pulmonary Fibrosis in Specialised and Non-specialised ILD Centres Around the World

Markus Polke[1], Yasuhiro Kondoh[2], Marlies Wijsenbeek[3], Vincent Cottin[4],
Simon L. F. Walsh[5], Harold R. Collard[6], Nazia Chaudhuri[7], Sergey Avdeev[8],
Jürgen Behr[9,10], Gregory Calligaro[11], Tamera J. Corte[12], Kevin Flaherty[13],
Manuela Funke-Chambour[14], Martin Kolb[15], Johannes Krisam[16], Toby M. Maher[17,18],
Maria Molina Molina[19,20], Antonio Morais[21], Catharina C. Moor[3], Julie Morisset[22],
Carlos Pereira[23], Silvia Quadrelli[24,25], Moises Selman[26], Argyrios Tzouvelekis[27],
Claudia Valenzuela[28], Carlo Vancheri[29], Vanesa Vicens-Zygmunt[30], Julia Wälscher[1,31],
Wim Wuyts[32], Elisabeth Bendstrup[33] and Michael Kreuter[1,10]*

[1] Center for Interstitial and Rare Lung Diseases, Pneumology, Thoraxklinik, University of Heidelberg, Heidelberg, Germany,
[2] Department of Respiratory Medicine and Allergy, Tosei General Hospital, Seto, Japan, [3] Department of Respiratory Medicine,
Centre for Interstitial Lung Diseases and Sarcoidosis, Erasmus University Medical Centre, Rotterdam, Netherlands, [4] National
Coordinating Reference Centre for Rare Pulmonary Diseases, Louis Pradel Hospital, Hospices Civils de Lyon, University
Claude Bernard Lyon 1, Lyon, France, [5] Imperial College, National Heart and Lung Institute, London, United Kingdom,
[6] Department of Medicine, University of California, San Francisco, San Francisco, CA, United States, [7] North West Interstitial
Lung Disease Unit, Manchester University NHS Foundation Trust, Wythenshawe, Manchester, United Kingdom, [8] Sechenov
First Moscow State Medical University, Moscow, Russia, [9] Medizinische Klinik und Poliklinik V, LMU Klinikum, University of
Munich, Munich, Germany, [10] German Center for Lung Research (DZL), Marburg, Germany, [11] Division of Pulmonology,
Department of Medicine, University of Cape Town, Cape Town, South Africa, [12] Royal Prince Alfred Hospital, University of
Sydney, Sydney, NSW, Australia, [13] Department of Medicine, University of Michigan, Ann Arbor, MI, United States,
[14] Department of Pulmonary Medicine, Inselspital, Bern University Hospital, University of Bern, Bern, Switzerland,
[15] Department of Medicine, Firestone Institute for Respiratory Health, Research Institute at St Joseph's Healthcare, McMaster
University, Hamilton, ON, Canada, [16] Institute of Medical Biometry and Informatics, University of Heidelberg, Heidelberg,
Germany, [17] Hastings Centre for Pulmonary Research and Division of Pulmonary, Critical Care, and Sleep Medicine, Keck
School of Medicine, University of Southern California, Los Angeles, CA, United States, [18] Interstitial Lung Disease Unit,
Imperial College London, National Heart and Lung Institute, Royal Brompton and Harefield NHS Foundation Trust, London,
United Kingdom, [19] Institut d'Investigació Biomèdica de Bellvitge (IDIBELL), University Hospital of Bellvitge, L'Hospitalet de
Llobregat, Barcelona, Spain, [20] Centro de Investigación Biomédica en Red Enfermedades Respiratorias (CIBERES), Madrid,
Spain, [21] Department of Pneumology, Faculdade de Medicina, Centro Hospitalar São João, Universidade do Porto, Porto,
Portugal, [22] Département de Médecine, Centre Hospitalier de l'Université de Montréal, Montréal, QC, Canada, [23] Lung
Disease Department, Paulista School of Medicine, Federal University of São Paulo, São Paulo, Brazil, [24] Hospital Británico,
Buenos Aires, Argentina, [25] Sanatorio Güemes, Buenos Aires, Argentina, [26] Instituto Nacional de Enfermedades Respiratorias
Ismael Cosío Villegas, Mexico City, Mexico, [27] Department of First Academic Respiratory, Sotiria General Hospital for Thoracic
Diseases, University of Athens, Athens, Greece, [28] ILD Unit, Pulmonology Department Hospital Universitario de La Princesa,
Universidad Autonoma de Madrid, Madrid, Spain, [29] Regional Referral Centre for Rare Lung Diseases, A.O.U.
Policlinico-Vittorio Emanuele, University of Catania, Catania, Italy, [30] Unit of Interstitial Lung Diseases, Department of
Pneumology, Pneumology Research Group, IDIBELL, L'Hospitalet de Llobregat, University Hospital of Bellvitge, Barcelona,
Spain, [31] Department of Pulmonary Medicine, Centre for Interstitial and Rare Lung Diseases, Ruhrlandklinik University Hospital
Essen, Essen, Germany, [32] Unit for Interstitial Lung Diseases, Department of Respiratory Diseases, University Hospitals
Leuven, Leuven, Belgium, [33] Department of Respiratory Diseases and Allergy, Aarhus University Hospital, Aarhus C, Denmark

*Correspondence:
Michael Kreuter
kreuter@uni-heidelberg.de

Background: Acute exacerbation of idiopathic pulmonary fibrosis (AE-IPF) is a severe complication associated with a high mortality. However, evidence and guidance on management is sparse. The aim of this international survey was to assess differences in prevention, diagnostic and treatment strategies for AE-IPF in specialised and non-specialised ILD centres worldwide.

Material and Methods: Pulmonologists working in specialised and non-specialised ILD centres were invited to participate in a survey designed by an international expert panel. Responses were evaluated in respect to the physicians' institutions.

Results: Three hundred and two (65%) of the respondents worked in a specialised ILD centre, 134 (29%) in a non-specialised pulmonology centre. Similarities were frequent with regards to diagnostic methods including radiology and screening for infection, treatment with corticosteroids, use of high-flow oxygen and non-invasive ventilation in critical ill patients and palliative strategies. However, differences were significant in terms of the use of KL-6 and pathogen testing in urine, treatments with cyclosporine and recombinant thrombomodulin, extracorporeal membrane oxygenation in critical ill patients as well as antacid medication and anaesthesia measures as preventive methods.

Conclusion: Despite the absence of recommendations, approaches to the prevention, diagnosis and treatment of AE-IPF are comparable in specialised and non-specialised ILD centres, yet certain differences in the managements of AE-IPF exist. Clinical trials and guidelines are needed to improve patient care and prognosis in AE-IPF.

Keywords: idiopathic pulmonary fibrosis, acute exacerbation, questionnaire, pulmonologists, specialised ILD centres, non-specialised ILD centres

INTRODUCTION

Idiopathic pulmonary fibrosis (IPF) is a chronic and progressive fibrosing interstitial lung disease associated with a poor prognosis with a five-year survival rate of 20–40% and a median survival time of 2–5 years (1, 2). An acute exacerbation of IPF contributes to the dismal prognosis and disease progression and is defined as an acute, clinically significant respiratory deterioration characterised by evidence of new widespread alveolar abnormality in patients with IPF and after the exclusion of cardiac failure or fluid overload (3). The annual incidence is up to 20%, depending on the population analysed (4, 5). AE-IPF is associated with a median survival of ~3–4 months (6, 7) and may account for more than 40% of all death in patients with IPF (8). The aetiology is still obscure, but AE-IPF might be triggered e.g. by infection or procedures/operation, or may occur idiopathic (6). Evidence on prevention, diagnosis and therapy of AE-IPF is sparse and no international guidelines exist (3, 9). Accordingly, there is a huge variability with regards to preventive, diagnostic and therapeutic approaches worldwide (10). It is unknown whether these different strategies are partially explainable by differences between specialised and non-specialised ILD centres. Therefore, this study aimed to compare preventive, diagnostic and therapeutic strategies for AE-IPF between specialised and non-specialised ILD centres.

MATERIALS AND METHODS
Questionnaire and Participating Physicians

As described previously (10), as a first step we conducted a literature research on diagnostics, therapy, prevention and management of AE-IPF to identify items to be included in this survey. Then, an expert panel was created, comprising pulmonologists with expertise in the diagnosis and management of ILD working in specialist ILD centres and a track record of publication in this field, to participate in an email-based interview to structure the survey. The final questionnaire consisted of 20 questions regarding diagnosis, treatment and prevention of AE-IPF and suggested future perspectives in AE-IPF research (10). To identify working place (specialised and non-specialised ILD centres), country of origin, number of patients with IPF under care, and estimated number of AE-IPF seen, additional questions were included into this survey. From July 1 2017 to November 30 2017 pulmonologists worldwide with interest in ILD were identified, including the European Respiratory Society assembly on Diffuse Parenchymal Lung Disease, the American Thoracic Society assembly on Clinical Problems, the Japanese Respiratory Society assembly on Diffuse Parenchymal Lung Disease and participants of the IPF Project Consortium (www.theipfproject.com) (11). Nationality, academic status (working at a university hospital or not) or subspecialist interests within respiratory medicine did not influence inclusion eligibility. The questionnaire was provided by the online survey tool SurveyMonkey® from December 2017 to April 2018.

Statistical Analysis

For questions with categorical answers, absolute and relative frequencies were calculated and chi-squared tests were used to assess differences between specialised and non-specialised ILD centres. For questions with answers on a continuous scale, median, first and third quartile, minimum and maximum were determined and differences between continents were assessed using Kruskal–Wallis tests. Due to the exploratory nature of this survey, all resulting *p*-values are solely to be interpreted descriptively and no adjustment for multiple testing was conducted. *p*-values smaller than 0.05 were regarded as statistically significant. All analyses were conducted using R v.3.4.2 (http://r-project.org).

RESULTS

Participants

Overall, 509 pulmonologists from 66 countries responded. Three hundred and thirty four (65.9%) of the participants worked in a specialised ILD centre, 142 (28.0%) in non-specialised ILD centres i.e. in a general pulmonology department, 4 (0.8%) on an intensive care unit and 27 (5.3%) did not indicate their institution. Physicians working on an intensive care unit or who did not indicate their institution were excluded from the analysis. A total of 436 pulmonologists working in a specialised or non-specialised ILD centre were included in this analysis. On average 331 cases of AE-IPF were seen in specialised ILD centres and 139 in non-specialised ILD centres. **Figure 1** shows the place of work (continent) of the respondents in specialised and non-specialised ILD centres.

Diagnostic Procedures for AE-IPF

Most diagnostic tools, including multi-slice thin-section computer tomography without contrast media (HRCT), CT with contrast media in the absence of clinical suspicion of pulmonary embolism, bronchoalveolar lavage (BAL), echocardiography, assessment for pathogens, NT-proBNP/BNP, D-Dimer and troponins were used similarly between specialised and non-specialised ILD centres. The main difference was the sampling of sputum for microbiology (induced sputum) which was

more frequent in non-specialised ILD centres (22 vs. 12%, *p* = 0.0106). Conversely, pathogen testing in urine was performed significantly more often in specialised ILD centres than in non-specialised ILD centres (42 vs. 28%, *p* = 0.0068). 50% of specialised ILD centres screened for RSV (respiratory syncytial virus), compared to only 33% in non-specialised ILD centres (*p* = 0.0024). The use of biomarker KL-6 was higher in non-specialised ILD centres than in specialised ILD centres (24 vs. 15%, *p* = 0.0313). The most relevant diagnostic procedures applied for AE-IPF are shown in **Figure 2**. Other diagnostic procedures such as laboratory parameters or specific pathogens are shown in **Supplementary 1**.

Treatment Approaches for AE-IPF

The majority of participating pulmonologists treated AE-IPF with methylprednisolone or equivalent with a dosage of 500–1,000 mg per day for 3 days followed by a slow tapering similarly in both types of institutions (63 vs. 66%).

Other immunosuppressive therapies such as cyclosporine, cyclophosphamide (i.v. bolus), tacrolimus and rituximab were rarely used in both specialised and non-specialised ILD centres, but cyclosporine was significantly more frequently used in non-specialised ILD centres (13 vs. 6%, *p* = 0.0288).

Other therapies such as polymyxin B hemoperfusion (7 vs. 10%), and plasmapheresis/plasma exchange (4 vs. 5%) were also less commonly used in specialised and non-specialised ILD centres. However, significantly more pulmonologists treated their patients with recombinant thrombomodulin in non-specialised ILD centres than in specialised ILD centres (15 vs. 8%, *p* = 0.0342).

Differences between institutions in the use of treatment strategies are shown in **Figure 3**. *See also* **Supplementary 1**.

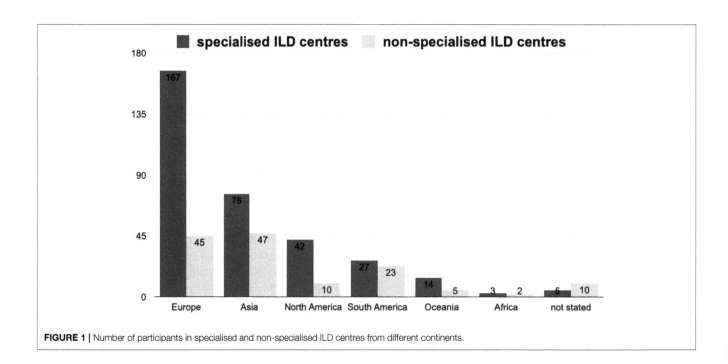

FIGURE 1 | Number of participants in specialised and non-specialised ILD centres from different continents.

Antifibrotic Therapy Management During AE-IPF

In patients without antifibrotic therapy, the majority of the survey participants see a reason to initiate an antifibrotic therapy in the event of an AE-IPF in specialised and non-specialised ILD centres (66 vs. 69%).

The choice of the antifibrotic drug did also not differ significantly between specialised and non-specialised centres (nintedanib 20 vs. 20%, pirfenidone 11 vs. 19%, no preference for specific anti-fibrotic drug 35 vs. 28%).

For patients already on antifibrotic therapy at the time of AE-IPF, there was no significant difference in the approach: 80% of respondents in specialised ILD centres would continue and 5% would discontinue antifibrotic therapy, compared to 70% continuing ($p = 0.0513$) and 7% discontinuing therapy ($p = 0.5491$) in non-specialised ILD centres. The dose was reduced by 1 % in specialised ILD centres compared to 5% in non-specialised ILD centres ($p = 0.0301$), 9% would switch to the alternative antifibrotic therapy in specialist ILD centres and similarly 10% would switch in non-specialised ILD centres ($p = 0.999$).

Different strategies in this situation are also shown in **Figure 4**. For further strategies *see* **Supplementary 1**.

Management of Pulmonary Hypertension (PH) During AE-IPF

In the case of suspected PH on clinical investigations (e.g. echocardiography, BNP, clinical signs) during an AE-IPF,

significantly more physicians in specialised ILD centres would start diuretic therapy than in non-specialised ILD centre (54 vs. 41%, $p = 0.0210$). Only a minority in both institutions would perform right heart catheterization in AE-IPF in suspected PH (6 vs. 7%). Seven percentage would start a PH specific treatment after an established PH diagnosis in a specialised ILD centre, significantly more (14%) would do so in a non-specialised ILD centre ($p = 0.0494$). Only 3% of physicians in a specialised ILD centre and 1% in a non-specialised centre would start a PH specific treatment without a confident diagnosis. After stabilisation of AE-IPF, more than 50% of physicians would evaluate a PH specific treatment by subsequently performing right heart catheterization (56 vs. 55%). A quarter of all participating pulmonologists in specialised and non-specialised ILD centres saw no indication for a PH treatment during or after AE-IPF (**Supplementary 1**).

Intensive Care Unit (ICU) and Palliative Care in AE-IPF

With regards to the care for critically ill patients with AE, there were no differences in specialised and non-specialised ILD centres for the use of high-flow oxygen (84 vs. 78%) and non-invasive ventilation (NIV) (72 vs. 77%). 9% of specialised and 11% of non-specialised ILD centres use invasive ventilation for all critical ill patients, whereas 48 vs. 39% respectively would only use invasive ventilation in patients suitable for lung transplantation (LTX) as a bridge to LTX or in very selected cases.

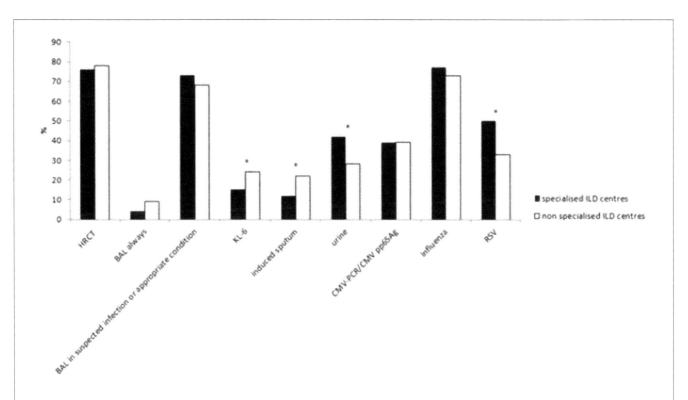

FIGURE 2 | The main diagnostic procedures applied for AE-IPF in specialised and non-specialised ILD centres. Statistically significant differences are labelled with a * (p-value = <0.05).

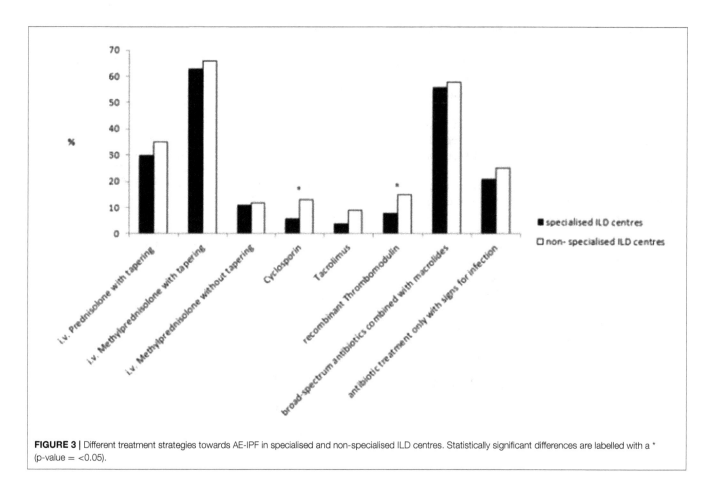

FIGURE 3 | Different treatment strategies towards AE-IPF in specialised and non-specialised ILD centres. Statistically significant differences are labelled with a *
(p-value = <0.05).

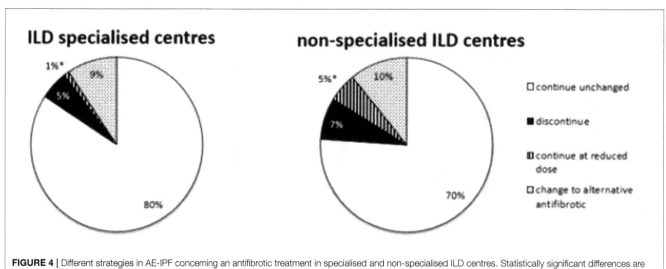

FIGURE 4 | Different strategies in AE-IPF concerning an antifibrotic treatment in specialised and non-specialised ILD centres. Statistically significant differences are
labelled with a * (p-value = <0.05).

Significantly more physicians in specialised ILD centres offered extracorporeal membrane oxygenation (ECMO) to patients suitable for LTX as a bridge to LTX than in non-specialised ILD centres (49 vs. 36%, $p = 0.0287$).

Palliative care was considered similarly in both types of institutions (65 vs. 62%).

Institutional differences in these approaches are shown in **Figure 5** (**Supplementary 1**).

Preventive Strategies for AE-IPF

Measures aimed at preventing the occurrence of AE-IPF was equal amongst specialised and non-specialised ILD centres

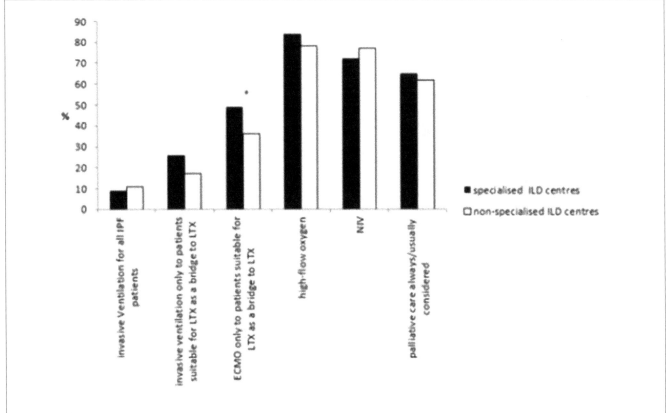

FIGURE 5 | Different management strategies in critically ill patients with AE-IPF in specialised and non-specialised ILD centres. Statistically significant differences are labelled with a * (p-value = <0.05).

and included vaccinations, antifibrotic therapy and pulmonary rehabilitation or other forms of structured exercise therapy. Antacid drugs were prescribed significantly more in non-specialised ILD centres than in specialised ILD centres (61 vs. 50%, $p = 0.0438$) in all IPF patients. Long-term azithromycin, low dose steroids ($\leq$10 mg) and anticoagulation (to prevent AE-IPF) were only used by a minority in both types of institutions.

In terms of planned surgical procedures, significantly more physicians in specialised ILD centres favoured preventive anaesthetic measures such as low tidal volume and avoidance of hyperoxygenation compared to physicians in non-specialised ILD centres (72 vs. 61%, p=0.0368).

Institutional differences in preventive strategies are shown in **Figure 6**. *See also* **Supplementary 1**.

Unmet Needs in AE-IPF

Pulmonologists in both specialised and non-specialised ILD centres advocate more intensive collaboration between different ILD specialists; improved education and training of physicians; education of patients and caregivers as well as enhanced research to improve the understanding of the pathophysiology, diagnosis and management of AE-IPF. Physicians working in specialised ILD centres saw a stronger need for intensified research and projects on the treatment of AE-IPF (90 vs. 80%, $p = 0.0101$). There were more pulmonologists in non-specialised ILD centres

who saw a need of improvement in multidisciplinary strategies for diagnosing and discussions than in specialised ILD centres (67 vs. 53%, $p = 0.0088$).

DISCUSSION

Despite the fact that AE-IPF is one of the most common causes of death in IPF (3), evidence on prevention, additional diagnostic approaches besides HRCT and treatment of this complication is sparse and differs significantly worldwide (10). No particular evidence-based guidance exists. Here we report analyses on similarities and differences in the management of AE-IPF in specialised vs. non-specialised ILD centres. The strength of our report was the significant number of physicians who replied to our survey representing both specialised and non-specialised ILD centres.

Diagnostic procedures were almost identical in both specialised and non-specialised ILD centres, including radiology and screening for infections. Molyneaux et al. have showed that there is an increased bacterial load in the BAL of IPF patients with AE-IPF compared to stable IPF patients (12) suggesting a potential causative role in AE-IPF. There is evidence for the contribution of lung microbiota in disease progression and in acute exacerbation (13, 14). Microbiological confirmation may therefore play an important role in the diagnostic process and may be useful for future therapeutic and preventive strategies.

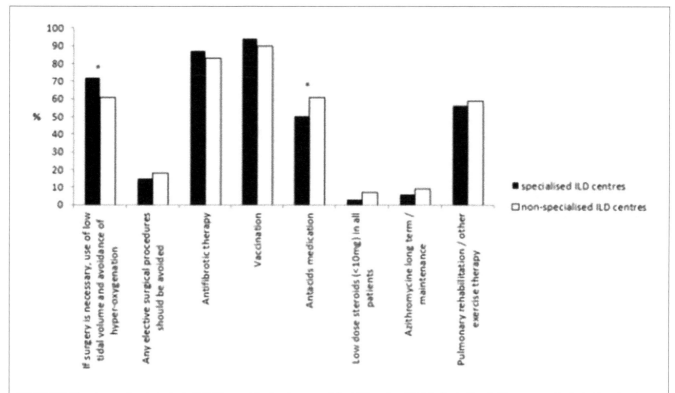

FIGURE 6 | Different preventive strategies in AE-IPF in specialised and non-specialised ILD centres. Statistically significant differences are labelled with a * (p-value = <0.05).

The majority of physicians in specialised and non-specialised ILD centres screen for pathogens in sputum, deemed a safer method to screen for pathogens compared to bronchoscopy. A recent study supports this approach as a positive bronchoscopy only affected management in 13% of patients and resulted in a change of treatment in <5% (15). Furthermore, in the same study, a significant number of patients required intubation and transfer to the ICU with poor extubation success post bronchoscopy (15). Conversely, a study has demonstrated the feasibility and safety of performing BAL aided by NIV as a useful tool for differentiating or confirming triggered AE (16).

Furthermore, there is a similarity in therapeutic approaches. The majority of pulmonologists in specialised and non-specialised ILD centres use antibiotic therapy, namely broad-spectrum antibiotic combined with macrolide. High dose steroids are widely administered in non-specialised and specialised ILD centres in AE-IPF. High dose long-term steroid use was associated with an increased mortality in the PANTHER trial (17) and a history of previous immunosuppression before AE-IPF has a negative impact on mortality (18). Recently, a retrospective study with 82 AE-IPF patients showed that subjects receiving corticosteroids were more likely to require ICU level care and mechanical ventilation and therefore did not benefit from treatment with corticosteroids (19). However, future studies with larger cohorts are necessary to prove the deleterious effects of steroid therapy.

Other immunosuppressants and strategies are used less frequently. Very few pulmonologists never use immunosuppression for AE-IPF. Although there is only low evidence base for the use of more potent anti-inflammatory treatment approaches such as cyclosporine A, intravenous cyclophosphamide or tacrolimus (20–24), they are used by some pulmonologists in non-specialised and specialised ILD centres. A randomised, double-blinded clinical trial of cyclophosphamide in AE-IPF with 120 patients was completed and results are eagerly awaited (https://clinicaltrials.gov/ct2/show/NCT02460588).

The international guidelines recommend avoiding ICU in patients with AE-IPF (weak recommendation) (25) because the mortality of patients with AE-IPF admitted to ICU, particularly in ventilated patients, is high (26). Some patients who do not respond to conventional oxygen therapy benefit from high flow oxygen (27). NIV may be a reasonable option for some critically ill patients (28). Trudzinski et al. showed that ECMO is only an option for patients who are suitable for LTX, as it conferred limited impact on the poor prognosis for those who were not LTX candidates (29). This might be a reason for pulmonologists in no matter what kind of institution to prefer NIV and high-flow oxygen in patients with AE-IPF. Data on this is however limited.

In non-specialised and specialised ILD centres prevention strategies towards AE-IPF were performed to the same extent. Vaccinations were most frequently used; although their use is recommended by the international guideline, there is a lack of evidence to support this recommendation (30).

The approach by physicians to utilise antifibrotic drugs as a form of preventive strategy is supported by recent data of controlled trials that suggest nintedanib may prolong the time to the first AE-IPF (31) and reduces mortality after AE-IPF (32). Pirfenidone reduces the risk for respiratory related hospitalisation in *post-hoc* analyses (33). Data proving a reduced frequency of AE-IPF with pirfenidone is sparse: In a Phase 2 trial of 107 patients Azuma et al. found a significant reduction of AE-IPF in patients using pirfenidone (34). A larger trial could not prove this (35).

While a Japanese study suggested a role for anticoagulants to prevent AE-IPF (Kubo et al.), a more recent study did not support this (36). This is in line with the results shown here: only a minority use anticoagulants to prevent AE-IPF. This is further supported by data suggesting a negative impact of anticoagulants on survival in IPF in general (37, 38).

Besides many similarities in the approach towards AE-IPF, there are also some differences in ILD specialised and non-specialised ILD centres.

PH is common in patients with IPF (39). Its prevalence at baseline means a higher risk for a subsequent AE-IPF, it is associated with a poorer overall survival but until now no specific PH treatment could show a benefit for IPF patients (40, 41). Significantly more pulmonologists in specialised ILD centres start diuretics compared to non-specialised ILD centres, and in line with the lack of benefits for specific PH treatment, most physicians do not use a specific PH treatment.

Many physicians use antacid drugs as a preventive strategy for AE-IPF, significantly more in non-specialised ILD centres. Lee et al. reported a higher pepsin level in the BAL of patients with AE-IPF compared to patients with stable disease (42) and a retrospective analysis showed a positive impact of antacid drugs on the course of IPF (43, 44). Other studies could not repeat this effect and suggested potentially higher rates of respiratory infections (45) and AE-IPF (46). The reason for the difference in the use of anti-acid drugs remains unclear, maybe because specialised ILD centres treat patients who are more ill or receive palliative treatment. Also different prescription rules in different countries or the fact that an old statement published by international societies from 2011 recommended their use (9) may be responsible.

Only a few pulmonologists use low dose steroids as a preventive strategy for AE-IPF, most of them in non-specialised ILD centres. This approach is in line with the international guideline where it is not recommended to use steroids beyond AE-IPF (17, 25). Furthermore, the use of corticosteroids has a negative effect on the outcome of IPF patients who received nintedanib (47).

Both pulmonologists in specialised and non-specialised ILD centres saw a high requirement for improved research strategies for AE-IPF. Significantly more non-specialised ILD centres saw the need for improvement in multidisciplinary strategies for diagnosing and discussion compared to pulmonologists in specialised ILD centres. Multidisciplinary team (MTD) meetings are widely used in the process of diagnostic and patient management (48) and they improve confidence in ILD diagnostics (49). MTD meetings are officially recommended (50). Arguably, MTD are more available in specialised ILD centres.

Many of the differences observed underscore the high and still unmet need for intensive research in AE-IPF. However, others might be associated with strategies applied outside current evidence. This demonstrates how important education in rare diseases and their complications is.

Our survey has some limitations: The survey was not designed for a data driven assessment of management practises but mainly to evaluate attitudes towards different aspects of AE-IPF. Participation was voluntarily and biased by involvement i.e. non-participating centres may have answered differently. Additionally, there was an imbalance between the number of specialised and non-specialised ILD institutions. Moreover, the number of ILD centres and patient numbers and thus experiences of diagnosis and management of AE-IPF may vary from country to country. Arguably, the number of IPF patients and cases of AE-IPF are higher in Japan as an example, than in other countries (51). Therefore, non-specialised ILD centres in Japan may have a higher number of patients to treat and thus greater experience than other non-specialised ILD centres elsewhere. More experienced physicians in the field of AE-IPF might have influenced the results of this questionnaire. Furthermore, the availability of treatments differs clearly between countries/continents, e.g., recombinant thrombomodelin is used almost exclusively in Asia and here by a quarter of all physicians (10). This might explain the fact that thrombomodulin is used more often in non-specialised ILD centres. The same applies for the use of KL-6 in the diagnostic process of AE-IPF. Finally, not all aspects of approaches to AE-IPF could be addressed in the questionnaire. The current COVID-19 pandemic was not part of the questionnaire because it was sent out before. This situation might have a huge impact on how AE-IPF is managed and this was not assed in the survey.

In conclusion, specialised and non-specialised ILD centres throughout the world do only differ in some aspects in the management of AE-IPF. Due to scant evidence and missing focused guidelines basic research and clinical trials have to be performed to establish optimal approaches to this deadly complication.

ETHICS STATEMENT

Ethical review and approval was not required for the study on human participants in accordance with the local legislation and institutional requirements. Written informed consent from the participants was not required to participate in this study in accordance with the national legislation and the institutional requirements.

AUTHOR CONTRIBUTIONS

MP and MK contributed mainly to the conception and design

of the study. MP wrote the first draft of the manuscript. JK performed the statistical analysis. All authors contributed to manuscript revision, read, and approved the submitted version.

ACKNOWLEDGMENTS

We would like to thank all participants who generously agreed to participate in this study.

REFERENCES

1. Ley B, Collard HR, King TE Jr. Clinical course and prediction of survival in idiopathic pulmonary fibrosis. *Am J Respir Crit Care Med.* (2011) 183:431–40. doi: 10.1164/rccm.201006-0894CI

2. Kreuter M, Koegler H, Trampisch M, Geier S, Richeldi L. Differing severities of acute exacerbations of idiopathic pulmonary fibrosis (IPF): insights from the INPULSIS® trials. *Respir Res.* (2019) 20:71. doi: 10.1186/s12931-019-1037-7

3. Collard HR, Ryerson CJ, Corte TJ, Jenkins G, Kondoh Y, Lederer DJ, et al. Acute exacerbation of idiopathic pulmonary fibrosis. an international working group report. *Am J Respir Crit Care Med.* (2016) 194:265–75. doi: 10.1164/rccm.201604-0801CI

4. Song JW, Hong SB, Lim CM, Koh Y, Kim DS. Acute exacerbation of idiopathic pulmonary fibrosis: incidence, risk factors and outcome. *Eur Respir J.* (2011) 37:356–63. doi: 10.1183/09031936.00159709

5. Idiopathic Pulmonary Fibrosis Clinical Research Network, Zisman DA, Schwarz M, Anstrom KJ, Collard HR, Flaherty KR, et al. A controlled trial of sildenafil in advanced idiopathic pulmonary fibrosis. *N Engl J Med.* (2010) 363:620–8. doi: 10.1056/NEJMoa1002110

6. Simon-Blancal V, Freynet O, Nunes H, Bouvry D, Naggara N, Brillet PY, et al. Acute exacerbation of idiopathic pulmonary fibrosis: outcome and prognostic factors. *Respiration.* (2012) 83:28–35. doi: 10.1159/000329891

7. Collard HR, Yow E, Richeldi L, Anstrom KJ, Glazer C. IPFnet investigators. Suspected acute exacerbation of idiopathic pulmonary fibrosis as an outcome measure in clinical trials. *Respir Res.* (2013) 14:73. doi: 10.1186/1465-9921-14-73

8. Natsuizaka M, Chiba H, Kuronuma K, Otsuka M, Kudo K, Mori M, et al. Epidemiologic survey of Japanese patients with idiopathic pulmonary fibrosis and investigation of ethnic differences. *Am J Respir Crit Care Med.* (2014) 190:773–9. doi: 10.1164/rccm.201403-0566OC

9. Raghu G, Collard HR, Egan JJ, Martinez FJ, Behr J, Brown KK, et al. An official ATS/ERS/JRS/ALAT statement: idiopathic pulmonary fibrosis: evidence-based guidelines for diagnosis and management. *Am J Respir Crit Care Med.* (2011) 183:788–824. doi: 10.1164/rccm.2009-040GL

10. Kreuter M, Polke M, Walsh SLF, Krisam J, Collard HR, Chaudhuri N, et al. Acute exacerbation of idiopathic pulmonary fibrosis: international survey and call for harmonisation. *Eur Respir J.* (2020) 55:1901760. doi: 10.1183/13993003.01760-2019

11. Walsh SLF, Maher TM, Kolb M, Poletti V, Nusser R, Richeldi L, et al. Diagnostic accuracy of a clinical diagnosis of idiopathic pulmonary fibrosis: an international case-cohort study. *Eur Respir J.* (2017) 50:1700936. doi: 10.1183/13993003.00936-2017

12. Molyneaux PL, Cox MJ, Wells AU, Kim HC, Ji W, Cookson WO, et al. Changes in the respiratory microbiome during acute exacerbations of idiopathic pulmonary fibrosis. *Respir Res.* (2017) 18:29. doi: 10.1186/s12931-017-0511-3

13. O'Dwyer DN, Ashley SL, Gurczynski SJ, Xia M, Wilke C, Falkowski NR, et al. Lung microbiota contribute to pulmonary inflammation and disease progression in pulmonary fibrosis. *Am J Respir Crit Care Med.* (2019) 199:1127–38. doi: 10.1164/rccm.201809-1650OC

14. D'Alessandro-Gabazza CN, Kobayashi T, Yasuma T, Toda M, Kim H, Fujimoto H, et al. A Staphylococcus pro-apoptotic peptide induces acute exacerbation of pulmonary fibrosis. *Nat Commun.* (2020) 11:1539. doi: 10.1038/s41467-020-15344-3

15. Arcadu A, Moua T. Bronchoscopy assessment of acute respiratory failure in interstitial lung disease. *Respirology.* (2017) 22:352–9. doi: 10.1111/resp.12909

16. Teramachi R, Kondoh Y, Kataoka K, Taniguchi H, Matsuda T, Kimura T, et al. Outcomes with newly proposed classification of acute respiratory deterioration in idiopathic pulmonary fibrosis. *Respir Med.* (2018) 143:147–52. doi: 10.1016/j.rmed.2018.09.011

17. Idiopathic Pulmonary Fibrosis Clinical Research Network, Raghu G, Anstrom KJ, King TE Jr, Lasky JA, Martinez FJ. Prednisone, azathioprine, and N-acetylcysteine for pulmonary fibrosis. *N Engl J Med.* (2012) 366:1968–77. doi: 10.1056/NEJMoa1113354

18. Papiris SA, Kagouridis K, Kolilekas L, Papaioannou AI, Roussou A, Triantafillidou C, et al. Survival in Idiopathic pulmonary fibrosis acute exacerbations: the non-steroid approach. *BMC Pulm Med.* (2015) 15:162. doi: 10.1186/s12890-015-0146-4

19. Farrand E, Vittinghoff E, Ley B, Butte AJ, Collard HR. Corticosteroid use is not associated with improved outcomes in acute exacerbation of IPF. *Respirology.* (2020) 25:629–35. doi: 10.1111/resp.13753

20. Sakamoto S, Homma S, Miyamoto A, Kurosaki A, Fujii T, Yoshimura K. Cyclosporin A in the treatment of acute exacerbation of idiopathic pulmonary fibrosis. *Intern Med.* (2010) 49:109–15. doi: 10.2169/internalmedicine.49.2359

21. Novelli L, Ruggiero R, De Giacomi F, Biffi A, Faverio P, Bilucaglia L, et al. Corticosteroid and cyclophosphamide in acute exacerbation of idiopathic pulmonary fibrosis: a single center experience and literature review. *Sarcoidosis Vasc Diffuse Lung Dis.* (2016) 33:385–91.

22. Horita N, Akahane M, Okada Y, Kobayashi Y, Arai T, Amano I, et al. Tacrolimus and steroid treatment for acute exacerbation of idiopathic pulmonary fibrosis. *Intern Med.* (2011) 50:189–95. doi: 10.2169/internalmedicine.50.4327

23. Donahoe M, Valentine VG, Chien N, Gibson KF, Raval JS, Saul M, et al. Autoantibody-targeted treatments for acute exacerbations of idiopathic pulmonary fibrosis. *PLoS ONE.* (2015) 10:e0127771. doi: 10.1371/journal.pone.0127771

24. Kolb M, Kirschner J, Riedel W, Wirtz H, Schmidt M. Cyclophosphamide pulse therapy in idiopathic pulmonary fibrosis. *Eur Respir J.* (1998) 12:1409–14. doi: 10.1183/09031936.98.12061409

25. Raghu G, Rochwerg B, Zhang Y, Garcia CA, Azuma A, Behr J, et al. An official ATS/ERS/JRS/ALAT clinical practice guideline: treatment of idiopathic pulmonary fibrosis. An update of the 2011 clinical practice guideline. *Am J Respir Crit Care Med.* (2015) 192:e3–19. doi: 10.1164/rccm.201506-1063ST

26. Rangappa P, Moran JL. Outcomes of patients admitted to the intensive care unit with idiopathic pulmonary fibrosis. *Crit Care Resusc.* (2009) 11:102–9.

27. Vianello A, Arcaro G, Molena B, Turato C, Braccioni F, Paladini L, et al. High-flow nasal cannula oxygen therapy to treat acute respiratory failure in patients with acute exacerbation of idiopathic pulmonary fibrosis. *Ther Adv Respir Dis.* (2019) 13:1753466619847130. doi: 10.1177/1753466619847130

28. Yokoyama T, Kondoh Y, Taniguchi H, Kataoka K, Kato K, Nishiyama O, et al. Noninvasive ventilation in acute exacerbation of idiopathic pulmonary fibrosis. *Intern Med.* (2010) 49:1509–14. doi: 10.2169/internalmedicine.49.3222

29. Trudzinski FC, Kaestner F, Schäfers HJ, Fähndrich S, Seiler F, Böhmer P, et al. Outcome of patients with interstitial lung disease treated with extracorporeal membrane oxygenation for acute respiratory failure. *Am J Respir Crit Care Med.* (2016) 193:527–33. doi: 10.1164/rccm.201508-1701OC

30. Cottin V, Crestani B, Valeyre D, Wallaert B, Cadranel J, Dalphin JC, et al. Diagnosis and management of idiopathic pulmonary fibrosis: French practical guidelines. *Eur Respir Rev.* (2014) 23:193–214. doi: 10.1183/09059180.00001814

31. Richeldi L, du Bois RM, Raghu G, Azuma A, Brown KK, Costabel U, et al. Efficacy and safety of nintedanib in idiopathic pulmonary fibrosis. *N Engl J Med.* (2014) 370:2071–82. doi: 10.1056/NEJMoa1402584

32. Collard HR, Richeldi L, Kim DS, Taniguchi H, Tschoepe I, Luisetti M, et al. Acute exacerbations in the INPULSIS trials of nintedanib in idiopathic pulmonary fibrosis. *Eur Respir J.* (2017) 49:1601339. doi: 10.1183/13993003.01339-2016

33. Ley B, Swigris J, Day BM, Stauffer JL, Raimundo K, Chou W, et al. Pirfenidone reduces respiratory-related hospitalizations in idiopathic pulmonary fibrosis. *Am J Respir Crit Care Med.* (2017) 196:756–61. doi: 10.1164/rccm.201701-0091OC

34. Azuma A, Nukiwa T, Tsuboi E, Suga M, Abe S, Nakata K, et al. Double-blind, placebo-controlled trial of pirfenidone in patients with

idiopathic pulmonary fibrosis. *Am J Respir Crit Care Med.* (2005) 171:1040–7. doi: 10.1164/rccm.200404-571OC

35. Taniguchi H, Ebina M, Kondoh Y, Ogura T, Azuma A, Suga M, et al. Pirfenidone in idiopathic pulmonary fibrosis. *Eur Respir J.* (2010) 35:821–9. doi: 10.1183/09031936.00005209

36. Kreuter M, Wijsenbeek MS, Vasakova M, Spagnolo P, Kolb M, Costabel U, et al. Unfavourable effects of medically indicated oral anticoagulants on survival in idiopathic pulmonary fibrosis: methodological concerns. *Eur Respir J.* (2016) 48:1524–6. doi: 10.1183/13993003.01482-2016

37. Noth I, Anstrom KJ, Calvert SB, de Andrade J, Flaherty KR, Glazer C, et al. A placebo-controlled randomized trial of warfarin in idiopathic pulmonary fibrosis. *Am J Respir Crit Care Med.* (2012) 186:88–95. doi: 10.1164/rccm.201202-0314OC

38. King CS, Freiheit E, Brown AW, Shlobin OA, Aryal S, Ahmad K, et al. Association between anticoagulation and survival in interstitial lung disease: an analysis of the pulmonary fibrosis foundation patient registry. *Chest.* (2020) 3692:34911–4. doi: 10.1016/j.chest.2020.10.019

39. Nathan SD, Shlobin OA, Ahmad S, Urbanek S, Barnett SD. Pulmonary hypertension and pulmonary function testing in idiopathic pulmonary fibrosis. *Chest.* (2007) 131:657–63. doi: 10.1378/chest.06-2485

40. Judge EP, Fabre A, Adamali HI, Egan JJ. Acute exacerbations and pulmonary hypertension in advanced idiopathic pulmonary fibrosis. *Eur Respir J.* (2012) 40:93–100. doi: 10.1183/09031936.00115511

41. Cano-Jiménez E, Hernández González F, Peloche GB. Comorbidities and Complications in Idiopathic Pulmonary Fibrosis. *Med Sci (Basel).* (2018) 6:71. doi: 10.3390/medsci6030071

42. Lee JS, Song JW, Wolters PJ, Elicker BM, King TE Jr, Kim DS, et al. Bronchoalveolar lavage pepsin in acute exacerbation of idiopathic pulmonary fibrosis. *Eur Respir J.* (2012) 39:352–8. doi: 10.1183/09031936.00050911

43. Lee JS Ryu JH, Elicker BM, Lydell CP, Jones KD, Wolters PJ, et al. Gastroesophageal reflux therapy is associated with longer survival in patients with idiopathic pulmonary fibrosis. *Am J Respir Crit Care Med.* (2011) 184:1390–4. doi: 10.1164/rccm.201101-0138OC

44. Lee JS, Collard HR, Anstrom KJ, Martinez FJ, Noth I, Roberts RS, et al. Anti-acid treatment and disease progression in idiopathic pulmonary fibrosis: an analysis of data from three randomised controlled trials. *Lancet Respir Med.* (2013) 1:369–76. doi: 10.1016/S2213-2600(13)70105-X

45. Kreuter M, Wuyts W, Renzoni E, Koschel D, Maher TM, Kolb M, et al. Antacid therapy and disease outcomes in idiopathic pulmonary fibrosis: a pooled analysis. *Lancet Respir Med.* (2016) 4:381–9. doi: 10.1016/S2213-2600(16)00067-9

46. Costabel U, Behr J, Crestani B, Stansen W, Schlenker-Herceg R, Stowasser S, et al. Anti-acid therapy in idiopathic pulmonary fibrosis: insights from the INPULSIS® trials. *Respir Res.* (2018) 19:167. doi: 10.1186/s12931-018-0866-0

47. Cottin V LH, Luppi F, Le Maulf F, Schlenker-Herceg R, Stowasser S, Du Bois RM. Effect of baseline corticosteroid medication on reduction in FVC decline with nintedanib. *Eur Respir J.* (2015) 46:OA4498. doi: 10.1183/13993003.congress-2015.OA4498

48. Richeldi L, Launders N, Martinez F, Walsh SLF, Myers J, Wang B, et al. The characterisation of interstitial lung disease multidisciplinary team meetings: a global study. *ERJ Open Res.* (2019) 5:00209-2018. doi: 10.1183/23120541.00209-2018

49. Walsh SLF, Wells AU, Desai SR, Poletti V, Piciucchi S, Dubini A, et al. Multicentre evaluation of multidisciplinary team meeting agreement on diagnosis in diffuse parenchymal lung disease: a case-cohort study. *Lancet Respir Med.* (2016) 4:557–65. doi: 10.1016/S2213-2600(16)30033-9

50. Raghu G, Remy-Jardin M, Myers JL, Richeldi L, Ryerson CJ, Lederer DJ, et al. Diagnosis of idiopathic pulmonary fibrosis. An official ATS/ERS/JRS/ALAT clinical practice guideline. *Am J Respir Crit Care Med.* (2018) 198:e44–e68. doi: 10.1164/rccm.201807-1255ST

51. Saito S, Lasky JA, Hagiwara K, Kondoh Y. Ethnic differences in idiopathic pulmonary fibrosis: The Japanese perspective. *Respir Investig.* (2018) 56:375–83. doi: 10.1016/j.resinv.2018.06.002

8

The Role of the Multidisciplinary Evaluation of Interstitial Lung Diseases

Federica Furini [1]*, Aldo Carnevale [2], Gian Luca Casoni [3], Giulio Guerrini [1],
Lorenzo Cavagna [4], Marcello Govoni [1] and Carlo Alberto Sciré [1]

[1] Section of Rheumatology, Department of Medical Sciences, University of Ferrara and Azienda Ospedaliero-Universitaria
Sant'Anna di Ferrara, Cona, Italy, [2] Department of Radiology, Azienda Ospedaliero-Universitaria Sant'Anna di Ferrara, Cona,
Italy, [3] Department of Medical Sciences, Research Centre on Asthma and COPD, University of Ferrara, Ferrara, Italy, [4] Division
of Rheumatology, University and IRCCS Policlinico S. Matteo Foundation, Pavia, Italy

*Correspondence:
Federica Furini
fefe.furini@gmail.com

The opportunity of a multidisciplinary evaluation for the diagnosis of interstitial pneumonias highlighted a major change in the diagnostic approach to diffuse lung disease. The new American Thoracic Society, European Respiratory Society, Japanese Respiratory Society, and Latin American Thoracic Society guidelines for the diagnosis of idiopathic pulmonary fibrosis have reinforced this assumption and have underlined that the exclusion of connective tissue disease related lung involvement is mandatory, with obvious clinical and therapeutic impact. The multidisciplinary team discussion consists in a moment of interaction among the radiologist, pathologist and pulmonologist, also including the rheumatologist when considered necessary, to improve diagnostic agreement and optimize the definition of those cases in which pulmonary involvement may represent the first or prominent manifestation of an autoimmune systemic disease. Moreover, the proposal of classification criteria for interstitial lung disease with autoimmune features (IPAF) represents an effort to define lung involvement in clinically undefined autoimmune conditions. The complexity of autoimmune diseases, and in particular the lack of classification criteria defined for pathologies such as anti-synthetase syndrome, makes the involvement of the rheumatologist essential for the correct interpretation of the autoimmune element and for the application of classification criteria, that could replace clinical pictures initially interpreted as IPAF in defined autoimmune disease, minimizing the risk of misdiagnosis. The aim of this review was to evaluate the available evidence about the efficiency and efficacy of different multidisciplinary team approaches, in order to standardize the professional figures and the core set procedures that should be necessary for a correct approach in diagnosing patients with interstitial lung disease.

Keywords: interstitial lung disease (ILD), connective tissue disease (CTD), multidisciplinary team (MDT), rheumatologist, interstitial pneumonia with autoimmune features (IPAF)

INTRODUCTION

Multidisciplinary discussion (MDD) is currently recommended during the diagnostic process of interstitial lung diseases (ILD) in particular when idiopathic pulmonary fibrosis (IPF) is suspected (1, 2). IPF has the worst prognosis among the different forms of ILD, with a median survival of 3–5 years from the diagnosis. It can generally be suspected in male subjects over the age of 60 who present an usual interstitial pneumonia pattern (UIP) at radiology and histology. In subjects with a radiological pattern compatible with UIP and in the absence of a detectable etiology, surgical lung biopsy (SLB) is not necessary, whereas it should be considered in patients with probable or indeterminate radiological patterns for UIP especially when an alternative diagnosis is not achievable (1). MDD is currently replacing the histological evaluation, due to its limited reliability and intrinsic risks particularly in elderly or highly comorbid patients (3). Given the poor prognosis of IPF and the availability of new anti-fibrotic drugs such as pirfenidone and nintedanib, the diagnosis formulated via MDD is currently considered the gold standard (4–6). Despite this guideline for IPF diagnosis, there are no available studies that clearly assess the impact of multidisciplinary team (MDT) in the approach to patients with ILD and we do not know if the evaluation by experts can actually be better than MDD. Nonetheless, the participation by clinicians, radiologists, and when applicable histopathologists, could be considered useful to share clinical cases between physicians with different points of view in order to establish a "common language" and improve the knowledge of the singles (7).

Applying the guidelines of the American Thoracic Society, European Respiratory Society, Japanese Respiratory Society and Latin American Thoracic Association (ATS/ERS/JRS/ALAT), the recommended MDT is generally composed by a clinician (often a pulmonologist), a thoracic radiologist and pathologist with experience in ILD. Other physicians as rheumatologist should be considered only in selected cases (8). Current clinical practice guidelines for IPF recommend to perform a battery of serological test as C-reactive protein (CRP), erythrocyte sedimentation rate (ESR), antinuclear antibodies (ANA) by immunofluorescence, rheumatoid factor (RF), myositis panel, and anti–cyclic citrullinated peptide (ACPA) without a previous consultation with rheumatologist, reserving this possibility in case of positivity of serological tests or presence of clinical manifestations suggesting an underling rheumatological disease (especially in women <60 years old) (8).

Hence ILD could be related to rheumatoid arthritis (RA), systemic vasculitis (especially antineutrophil Cytoplasmic Antibodies (ANCA)-associated Vasculitis) (9) and different connective tissue disease (CTD) especially systemic sclerosis (SSc), myositis spectrum disorders comprising overlap myositis and antisynthetase syndrome (ASSD) but also systemic lupus erythematosus, primary Sjögren's syndrome, and mixed CTD (10, 11). Specific classification criteria are available for most CTDs, while classification criteria currently lack for diseases such as ASSD, making the correct diagnosis very challenging (12).

The recent introduction of criteria defining interstitial pneumonias with autoimmune features (IPAF) has allowed to reclassify those ILD that did not meet any CTD criteria, creating a growing interest in research concerning these new entities, especially on their possible evolution in CTD and overall prognosis (13).

The primary objective of this study was to perform a systematic review of literature to explore the evidence on the organization and outcome of MDT for the diagnosis and management of ILD, and to evaluate the role of rheumatologist. A secondary objective is to elaborate a definite proposal of ILD multidisciplinary evaluation.

MATERIALS AND METHODS

A systematic literature review was performed using electronic databases Pubmed (1999–2019) and Embase (1999–2019). The search strategy was elaborated to include the greatest number of references dealing with the populations and the interventions object of the study by using the following keywords in combination with the Boolean operators OR and AND: "interstitial," "pneumonia," "multidisciplinary," "lung disease, interstitial," "pulmonary fibrosis," "interstitial pneumonias," "multidisciplinary team," and "multidisciplinary approach." Three reviewers (FF, GG, and AC) independently screened the titles and abstracts of all retrieved papers and selected the studies to be included in this review, after removing duplicates. All the articles selected by at least one of the reviewers were retrieved for full text evaluation. Article were selected according *a priori* inclusion criteria according to PICO methodology: (a) population: subjects aged >18 years with a suspected or established diagnosis of ILD; (b) intervention: multidisciplinary approach involving at least two different physicians of two different specialties; (c) type of study: metanalysis, randomized controlled trial (RCT), cohort, case control and case series (>5 patients) in English language. Other languages and other study designs (narrative review, case reports and meeting abstracts) were excluded. In case of disagreement between the reviewers, a further author (CS) was consulted to achieve a consensus. Primary outcome of this systematic review was the definition of the organization and physicians involved in the MDT with particular attention to clinical data collected and instrumental exams performed. A secondary objective was to evaluate the outcome of multidisciplinary approach (e.g., diagnosis or management) and to evaluate the role of rheumatologist. Selected articles were reviewed independently by three reviewers (FF, GG, and AC) and all data were extracted using an extraction form designed to respond to primary and secondary objectives of the review. The following data were extracted: authors, journal, year of publication, study design, inclusion and exclusion criteria, number of participants, population (ILD onset or established ILD, IPF, CTD related ILD, or both), interventions (physicians involved, instrumental examinations considered during the MDD) and outcomes evaluated (diagnosis, prognosis, efficacy of a treatment and other).

RESULTS

The search provided a total number of 333 citations from Pubmed and 955 from Embase. After excluding duplicates, a total

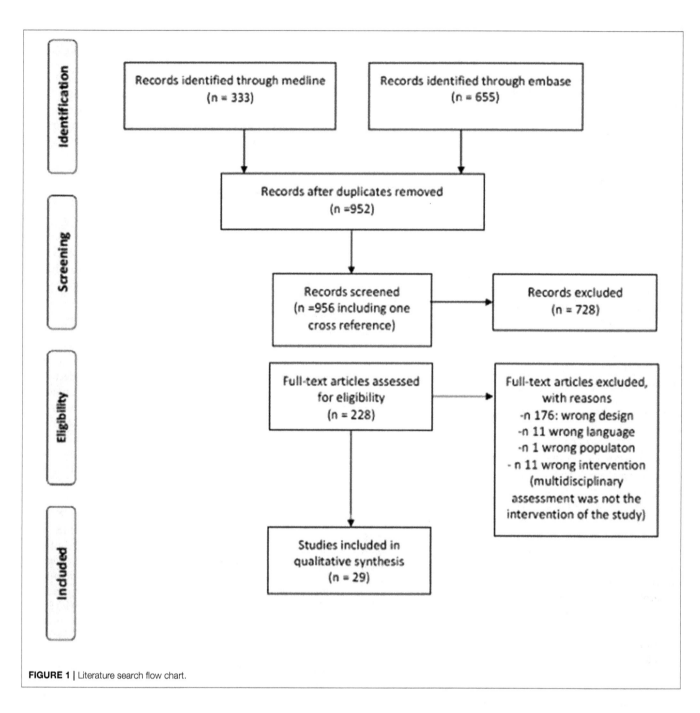

FIGURE 1 | Literature search flow chart.

of 952 references were screened for title and abstract and a total of 228 (including one cross reference) for full text analysis. A total of 29 papers were finally included for data extraction. **Figure 1** summarizes the number of papers excluded and the reason for exclusion. **Table 1** summarizes the main characteristics of the included studies.

Physician Involved in the MDT

In the included studies, the professional figures most frequently involved in MDT were: pulmonologist (29/29), thoracic radiologist (26/29), and thoracic pathologist (23/29). The rheumatologist role was described in 7 studies. Other professional figures were reported in 7 studies, including: clinical nurse specialist, cardiothoracic surgeon and lung transplantation team, occupational therapists, cardiologist, immunologist, palliative care expert, respiratory therapist, physiotherapist, and dietitian.

Some studies compared different compositions of MDT. Lok performed a comparison between a general respiratory clinic composed only by a pneumologist and a nurse (84 patients) and an ILD clinic setting including a specialist with interest in ILD with the support of radiologist, pathologist, and access to transplant and cardiothoracic program (54 patients). A multidisciplinary approach-based follow-up seemed

TABLE 1 | Characteristics and results of selected studies.

References	Study design	Population	Number of participants	Mean age(years) mean ± SD or (IQR)	Female %	Mean follow-up (months)
Burge et al. (14)	Retrospective cohort	ILD onset	71	/	/	/
Chartrand et al. (15)	Retrospective cohort	ILD established, myositis spectrum of disease, and/or SynS	33	55	22 (66.7%)	/
Castelino et al. (16)	Retrospective cohort	ILD onset	50	64 (32–80)	27 (54%)	12
De Sadeleer et al. (17)	Retrospective cohort	ILD onset	938	60.8 (14–90)	34.8%	
Ferri et al. (18)	Retrospective case-control	UCTD, IPAF, U-ILD	52 UCTD vs. 50 (35 IPAF-15 U-ILD)	UCTD 55 ± 13, IPAF 63 ± 12, U-ILD 68 ± 8.9	UCTD 44 (86%) IPAF 24(69%) U-ILD 9(60%)	/
Flaherty et al. (19)	Retrospective cohort	ILD onset (CTD excluded)	58	/	/	/
Fujisawa et al. (20)	Retrospective cohort	ILD onset (subjected to Surgical Lung Biopsy)	465	65	35%	7
Han et al. (21)	Retrospective cohort	Idiopathic ILD	56	56.9 ± 12.6	32 (57.1%)	7
Jeong et al. (22)	Prospective cohort	ILD related to CTD Idiopathic ILD	44 (23 CTD-ILD vs. 21 IPF)	CTD-ILD: 58.5, Idiopathic ILD: 70	CTD-ILD: 69.6%, Idiopathic ILD: 23.8%	
Jo et al. (23)	Retrospective cohort	Idiopathic ILD	417		31	26.16
Jo et al. (24)	Retrospective cohort	Idiopathic ILD, ILD related to CTD, unclassifiable ILD	90	67 ± 11	36 (40%)	/
Kalluri et al. (25)	Retrospective case-control/retrospective cohort	Idiopathic ILD	32	MDC group: 22, no MDC group: 10	MDC group: 36%, no MDC group: 40%	No MDC group: 17.4; MDC group: 14.4
Kohashi et al. (26)	Retrospective cohort	Idiopathic ILD that underwent to SLB	47	62 (56–67)	14 (29.8%)	1,582 (1,213–1,935) days
Kondoh et al. (27)	Retrospective cohort	Idiopathic ILD, Unclassifiable ILD, NSIP, hypersensitivity Pneumonia, ILD related to CTD	179	65 (60–70)	56 (31.3%)	/
Levi et al. (28)	Prospective cohort	New onset: ILD related CTD, Idiopathic ILD, IPAF	60	67.3 ± 12	27(45%)	/
Lok (29)	Retrospective cohort	/	138	General respiratory clinic: 64.6 vs. Patients of ILD clinic: 55.9	General respiratory clinic 31 (37%) ILD clinic: 28 (52%)	General respiratory clinic 31.9 vs. ILD clinic 22.3
Chaudhuri et al. (30)	Retrospective cohort	ILD established: ILD related to CTD, Idiopathic ILD	318	/	/	/
Nakamura et al. (31)	Retrospective cohort	U-ILD	33	64.4 ± 8.8	17(51.5%)	60.5
Newton et al. (32)	Retrospective cohort	familial pulmonary fibrosis	115	58 ± 10	57 (49.6%)	180
Patterson et al. (3)	Case control study	ILD onset	327 (80 of age>70)	54 ± 12 non-elderly vs. 76 ± 4 elderly	115(47%) non-elderly, 54 (68%) elderly	/
Pezzuto et al. (33)	Retrospective cohort	ILD onset	124	69 ± 7.9	37 (29.8%)	/

(Continued)

TABLE 1 | Continued

References	Study design	Population	Number of participants	Mean age(years) mean ± SD or (IQR)	Female %	Mean follow-up (months)
Tanizawa et al. (34)	Retrospective cohort	ILD established (UIP pattern at histology) CTD-ILD related are excluded	252.215 IPF, 19 U-ILD, 13 hypersensitivity pneumonitis	68.1 (62.1–72.6) with BCF vs. 67.7 (62.5–73.8) without BCF	32 (33.3%) in with BCF vs. 43(27.6%) without BCF	/
Thomeer et al. (35)	RCT	ILD established	182	18–75	NA	12
Tomassetti et al. (36)	Cross sectional	ILD established (without define UIP pattern on HRCT)	117 (59 BLC vs. 59 SLB)	59 (29–77) BLC vs. 59 (34–74) SLB	31 (53.4%) in BLC vs. 31 (52.5%) in SLB	/
Tominaga et al. (37)	Retrospective cohort	Idiopathic ILD	95	63 (40–79)	17 (10.7%)	/
Oltmanns et al. (38)	Retrospective cohort	ILD established	63	68 ± 7	16. (25%)	11±7
Ussavarungsi et al. (39)	Retrospective cohort	U-ILD	74	63 (20–89)	33(45%)	/
Walsh et al. (40)	Retrospective cohort	ILD onset	70	60.9 ± 15.5	46(66%)	67
Yamauchi et al. (41)	Prospective cohort	Idiopathic ILD	30	64.5 ± 6.3	8(26.7%)	/

SD, standard deviation; IQR, interquartile range; MDT, multidisciplinary team; ILD, interstitial lung disease; HRCT, high resolution computer tomography; PFT, pulmonary function test; CT, computed tomography; ASSD/Syns, antisynthetase; UCTD, undifferentiated connective tissue disease; IPAF, Interstitial pneumonia with autoimmune features; U-ILD, undifferentiated connective tissue disease; CTD, connective tissue diseases; CTD-ILD, interstitial lung disease related to connective tissue diseases; MDC, multidisciplinary collaborative; SLB, surgical lung biopsy; NSIP, nonspecific interstitial pneumonia; UIP, usual interstitial pneumonia; BLC, bronchoscopic lung biopsy; I, not reported.

to give an advantage in terms of survival in patients aged <60 years, being age an important negative prognostic factors in this population (29). In the study by Burge et al., the MDT was composed by a clinical nurse specialist as well as the classical organization which included specialist radiologist, histopathologist, and clinician. The authors highlighted the importance of MDD in the diagnosis of ILD compared to histology. The 71 patients in the study had in fact undergone video-assisted thoracoscopic surgery (VATS), and a retrospective analysis by MDT of the histological, clinical and radiological data was performed. In 30% of cases after MDD the diagnosis differed significantly from the histology report, and in a further 12% MDD changed the diagnosis from probable to confident (14).

Not all cases must necessarily be submitted to MDD. Chaudhuri et al. applied the MDD in the retrospective evaluation of 318 patients. The MDT of this study met weekly, and only patients sent by ILD expert clinicians were evaluated. The authors emphasized that after the multidisciplinary analysis the diagnosis could change, and that in doubtful cases, where biopsy was not possible due to comorbidities, the diagnosis could be reconsidered and reviewed over time based on the evolution and any response to therapy (30). Flaherty et al. highlighted how in the evaluation of patients with suspected IPF the review of the case by the radiologist, pathologist and clinician is fundamental, and that the sharing of clinical, radiological and possibly histopathological information can modify the diagnosis and/or increase diagnostics confidence and interobserver agreement. The diagnostic process described in this study was in fact organized through 4 different steps during which more information were progressively shared and the progressive interaction between the MDT members was permitted. The agreement between clinicians and radiologists was thus increased from the beginning to the end of the diagnostic process (0.39 vs. 0.88) (19).

The multidisciplinary approach, while representing the gold standard in the diagnosis of ILD, is not always practicable in normal clinical routine since local structures may not have experts in this field or meetings may be difficult to organize due to the geographical distance between the participants or time-related limits. A solution to overcome these limits could be provided by digital platforms. Fujisawa et al. validated a digital platform for the organization of MDD. The clinical data and radiological and histological images of 465 patients with suspected ILD (all therefore subjected to SLB) were included in an electronic database accessible via the web. Each patient was given a numerical identification code. The members of the MDT (clinicians, radiologists, and pathologists) could then separately access the various information and then a web conference to discuss with the other two members of the MDT. Also in this study, the MDD made possible to reformulate the initial diagnosis in a conspicuous number of cases (49%), and from the analysis of the survival curves it was shown that also this MDD modality is able to identify those diagnoses with the worse prognosis (like IPF) [(20); **Table 2**].

TABLE 2 | Physicians involved in the MDT.

References	Pulmonologist	Radiologist	Pathologist	Rheumatologist
Burge et al. (14)	1	1	1	0
Chartrand et al. (15)	1	1	1	1
De Sadeleer et al. (17)	1	1	1	1
Ferri et al. (18)	1	1	1	1
Kondoh et al. (27)	1	1	1	0
Levi et al. (28)	1	1	1	1
Jo et al. (24) 10/1/2019 9:37:00 p.m.	1	1	1	1
Flaherty et al. (19)	1	1	1	0
Fujisawa et al. (20)	1	1	1	0
Han et al. (21)	1	1	1	0
Jo et al. (42)	1	1	1	0
Kohashi et al. (26)	1	1	1	0
Lok (29)	1	1	1	0
Chaudhuri et al. (30)	1	1	1	0
Nakamura et al. (31)	1	1	1	0
Patterson et al. (3)	1	1	1	0
Pezzuto et al. (33)	1	1	1	0
Tanizawa et al. (34)	1	1	1	0
Thomeer et al. (35)	1	1	1	0
Tomassetti et al. (36)	1	1	1	0
Tominaga et al. (37)	1	1	1	0
Oltmanns et al. (38)	1	1	1	0
Walsh et al. (40)	1	1	1	0
Yamauchi et al. (41)	1	1	1	0
Jeong et al. (22)	1	1	0	1
Newton et al. (32)	1	1	0	0
Ussavarungsi et al. (39)	1	1	0	0
Castelino et al. (16)	1	0	0	1
Kalluri et al. (25)	1	0	0	0

Variables Evaluated During MDD

Clinical history assessment is reported in 24 of the 29 included studies. In addition to demographics (age and sex), the most frequently collected data concerned smoke (17/29) and environmental exposure (11/29). The evaluation of symptoms related to the possible presence of CTD and physical examination were reported in 7 studies.

High resolution computed tomography (HRCT) was evaluated in all studies except two: one dealing with a multidisciplinary approach not for the diagnosis, but for palliative care of ILD patients (25), and one focused on transbronchial lung cryobiopsy (39). HRCT was usually acquired only at baseline during the diagnostic process (24/27 studies). In 3 studies including longitudinal information, HRCT was repeated after 3–6 months in two studies (22, 31), and not specified in one study (35). Baseline chest X-ray was described in only one study (37).

Pulmonary function tests (PFT) were part of the core set of parameters analyzed during multidisciplinary evaluation in almost all studies (27/29). PFT were not performed in the same two previously described studies, in which even HRCT was not performed (25, 39). In 21 studies, PFTs were performed only at the baseline while in 6 studies repetition was described during follow-up with different timing: 1–3 months (38), 3 months (22), 3–6 months (31), annually (27), and not specified (32). The parameters considered were in most cases the forced vital capacity (FVC), the ability to spread carbon monoxide (DLCO) and forced expiratory volume in the 1st second (FEV1); less frequently, total lung capacity (TLC); and residual volume (RV).

Pulmonary histology was evaluated in 21 studies. The role in the MDD of biopsy and especially of two different techniques (namely surgical lung biopsy SLB, and bronchoscopic lung biopsy BLC) was evaluated in a cross-sectional study involving 171 patients (58 BLC vs. 59 SLB). Both the modalities of biopsy increased the diagnostic accuracy of IPF (36). Ussavarungsi evaluated the role of Transbronchial Cryobiopsy (TBC) in the MDD; in this series of 74 patients, TBC failed to obtain histological samples demonstrating a specific UIP or NSIP pattern (39). In a retrospective cohort of 124 patients with suspected IPF, authors suggested to perform HRCT at baseline together with PFT (FVC, TLC; RV and DLCO), laboratory test for CTD and vasculitis, and bronchoalveolar lavage (BAL) for cytological and microbiological tests. HRCT results were then reviewed by MDT and classified according to the ATS/ERS/JRS/ALAT guidelines in UIP pattern, probable UIP and inconsistent with UIP patterns. Only in the last two and in presence of clinical, immunological, microbiological, and cytological abnormalities suggestive for IPF, the authors recommended biopsy. 15/124 patients could not be classified in neither of proposed definitions of HRCT patterns, but they were subsequently diagnosed with IPF after MDD and biopsy (33).

Serological data were reported in 17/29 studies, and 14 included autoantibody profile tests, especially RF, ACPA, ANA, antibodies against extractable nuclear antigens (ENA), myositis specific antibodies (including anti-synthetase) and myositis associated. Two studies reported genetic evaluation. Newton correlated traditional parameters evaluated during MDD (demographic data, physical examination, PFT, and HRCT) with four telomere-related genes mutations (TERT, TERC, RTEL1, and PARN). These genetic investigations were not usually performed during the traditional MDD for ILD, but this study focused on the evaluation of hereditary forms of pulmonary fibrosis (32). Another genetic test relating the MUC5B gene (rs35705950), associated with susceptibility to IPF, was obtained in a study cohort involving 252 ILD patients considered through MDD for diagnosis. In this study, the presence of bronchiolocentric fibrosis seemed not to correlated with MUC5B gene, telomere length, and IPF diagnosis formulated through MDD (34).

Further instrumental investigations evaluated during MDD were described in 15 studies, including BAL, doppler echocardiography, and 6-min walking test (**Table 3**).

Outcome Evaluated by MDT

Fifteen studies had as outcome a reference standard diagnosis, 7 prognostic evaluation, 5 both diagnosis and prognosis, 1 evaluated efficacy of pirfenidone treatment, and 1 the effect of multidisciplinary approach on patient perception of the disease.

Evaluating in detail the studies in which the outcome was the diagnosis, after the assessment by the MDT of a large cohort of 417 patients collected in the Australian IPF Registry (AIPFR), it was shown that in 23% of cases the guidelines for IPF were not applied by referring physicians (42). Despite this observation, in another study by the same authors the MDD showed to be relevant not only for the diagnosis, but also for the investigations prescribed and therapeutic behavior. After multidisciplinary evaluation of 93 patients, in fact, ILD diagnosis was changed in 53% of patients referred, and 71% of unclassifiable disease were re-classified under a specific diagnosis with obvious implication on therapeutic approach including an increased recommendation for anti-fibrotic therapy and referral for clinical trials (24). In a larger study by De Sadeleer involving 938 patients sent for multidisciplinary evaluation, the diagnosis was reached in 79.5% and modified in 41.9% of cases after MDD, while a diagnostic conclusion was not achieved only in 19.5% of the patients; however, in this case further investigations (16% of the total court) were at least suggested. This study demonstrated that a correct diagnosis also correlated with better prognosis, and that MDT could be helpful for the identification

of those patients with worse prognosis. Indeed patients who were diagnosed as IPF demonstrated a worse prognosis than those classified as not-IPF after MDD [Hazard ratio (HR) 4.31, $p <0.001$], while patients initially classified as IPF who reported a change in their diagnosis after MDD showed a better prognosis compared to patients definitely diagnosed with IPF (HR 0.37, $p = 0.094$) (17). In another study of 33 patients with previous diagnosis of unclassifiable-ILD (U-ILD), clinical, radiological and histological data were retrospectively evaluated by MDT. After MDD, the initial diagnosis was confirmed in 18 (54.5%) patients, but changed to collagen vascular disease-related interstitial pneumonia in 9 (27.3%), to chronic hypersensitivity pneumonitis in 3 (9.1%), to idiopathic pleuro-parenchymal fibroelastosis in 2 (6.1%), and IPF with emphysema in 1 (3.0%) patient (31).

The importance of cooperation between clinicians, radiologists and pathologists was reinforced by the analysis of patients enrolled in the IFIGENIA trial, a randomized placebo-controlled trial conducted on patients with IPF in which N-Acetylcysteine was associated referred to standard therapy (azathioprine plus steroid). Patients diagnosed as IPF by the clinician were subjected to a commission of thoracic radiology experts who evaluated chest HRCT images and by expert pathologists who evaluated the results of biopsies if performed. The diagnosis of IPF was rejected in 12.8% of cases formulated by the expert clinician after reviewing the histology and HRCT images thus demonstrating the importance of the multidisciplinary collaboration between clinicians, expert radiologists, and pathologists for a correct diagnosis of IPF (35). The reliability of MDD composed by these professional figures was also assessed. Seven different MDTs assessed 70 cases, for a total of 490 diagnoses [CTD-related ILD ($n = 146$), IPF ($n = 88$), idiopathic NSIP ($n = 50$), hypersensitivity pneumonitis ($n = 46$), and others ($n = 160$)]. Inter-MDT agreement for a first-choice diagnosis of IPF was good ($κ = 0.60$), good for CTD-related ILD ($κ = 0.64$), but fair for idiopathic NSIP ($κ = 0.25$), and hypersensitivity pneumonitis ($κ = 0.24$). The authors therefore recognized the excellent performance of the MDT in diagnosing IPF for which better defined classification criteria are available than for other conditions, i.e., hypersensitivity pneumonitis. Furthermore, the highest frequency of CTD-ILD, demonstrated the importance of including a rheumatologist in the multidisciplinary evaluation of ILD (40).

Besides the diagnostic process, MDD could be performed to evaluate the prognosis of particular populations of ILD patients. In a prospective cohort study involving 327 subjects, multidisciplinary approach was employed to evaluate the role of age onset to determine both diagnosis and prognosis of ILD patients (3). MDT can also be used not only in the diagnosis of IPF but also to identify sub-populations of patients with a worse prognosis. In a study conducted on 47 patients with IPF confirmed after SLB and MDD, the multidisciplinary evaluation allowed to identify the presence of emphysema and its extent as negative prognostic factors for survival (26). In the evaluation of the patient's suitability for starting pirfenidone therapy, the multidisciplinary meeting, where clinicians, radiologists and pathologists discussed clinical and instrumental data, was essential to identify IPF patients (38).

TABLE 3 | Variables evaluated during MDD.

References	Clinical evaluation	HRCT	PFT	Lung biopsy	Laboratory test	Other
Burge et al. (14)	History (brief clinical history, the duration of breathlessness, exposure, and smoking histories) Physical examination (crackles and clubbing)	Yes, pre-operative lung CT	Full lung function tests before biopsy (not described)	Yes	Immunological tests to identify collagen-vascular diseases, antibodies associated with hypersensitivity pneumonitis, and angiotensin converting enzyme levels	/
Chartrand et al. (15)	History (smoke, family history) BMI	Yes at baseline	Yes, FVC, DLCO	No	5 myositis-specific (Jo1, PL12, PL7, OJ, EJ, Mi2, SRP) and myositis-associated antibodies (Ro52, Ku, PM-Scl) antibodies (Jo1, PL-7, PL-12, EJ, OJ), 2 other myositis-specific antibodies (Mi-2, SRP), and 3 myositis-associated antibodies (Ku, PM-Scl, Ro-52)	/
Castelino et al. (16)	History (occupational and environmental exposures, medication history, family history) Physical examination (skin, mucus membranes, musculoskeletal, oropharyngeal, and gastrointestinal system)	Yes at baseline	Yes, FVC, DLCO	Yes	Anti-nuclear antibody (performed using HEp2 cell lines at BWH), ENAs, RF, inflammatory markers (ESR and CRP)	-Nailfold capillaroscopy -Echocardiography -Esophageal testing for pH or manometric studies
De Sadeleer et al. (17)	History (familial history, exposures, comorbidities, and medication use) -Physical examination	Yes at baseline	Yes not specified	Yes	Serological data (not specified)	BAL
Ferri et al. (18)	- History (demographic, occupational, smoking, medication, environmental, occupational, autoimmune manifestation)	Yes at baseline	Yes, including DLCO	Surgical lung biopsy Skin biopsy	ANA, anti-ENA, ESR, CRP, routine blood chemistry, urinalysis, infections, RF (first line), antiCCP, complement, ASMA, AMA, ANCA, antiphospholipid, organ specific antibodies, 24 h proteinuria (second line)	Doppler echocardiography, Joint echography, Nailfold capillaroscopy, Schirmer's test, Salivary gland echography, Minor salivary gland biopsy, Muscle biopsy, Electromyography
Flaherty et al. (19)	History (symptoms, environmental exposures, comorbid illnesses, medication use, smoking history, family history) -Physical examination findings	Yes at baseline	Yes, lung volumes and DLCO	No	Serological data (not specified)	/
Fujisawa et al. (20)	History (symptoms, environmental exposures, smoking history, family history, comorbid illnesses) -Physical examination	Yes, within 3 months from SLB	Yes, FVC, FEV1, DLCO	Yes	Blood test results, arterial blood gas analysis (or SpO2)	6-MWT, bronchoscopy, including bronchoalveolar lavage
Han et al. (21)	- History (smoking history; environmental, occupational and drug exposure; history of established connective tissue disease (CTD)]	Yes at baseline	Yes not specified	Yes	No	/

(Continued)

TABLE 3 | Continued

References	Clinical evaluation	HRCT	PFT	Lung biopsy	Laboratory test	Other
Jeong et al. (22)	- History (exercise status, Educational status, underlying rheumatic diseases)	Yes, repeat at 6 months	Yes, lung volumes, and DLCO, repeat at 3 months	No	No	The Brief Illness Perception Questionnaire (IPQ), Beliefs about Medicines Questionnaire (BMQ), Patient Health Questionnaire-2 (PHQ-2), Adherence measures
Jo et al. (42)	History (smoke, presence of underlying rheumatic diseases) -Physical examination(BMI)	Yes at baseline	Yes, FVC, FEV1/FVC, and DLCO	Yes	No	/
Jo et al. (24)	-History smokers (pack/years)	Yes at baseline	Yes, FVC, TLC, DLCO	Yes	Extended myositis screen and hypersensitivity precipitins and BNP	6-MWT, Resting SpO2, Nadir SpO2, Transthoracic echocardiogram, right heart catheterization
Kalluri et al. (25)	-Charlson Comorbidity Index -Pharmacotherapy (anti fibrotics, PPI, opioids, benzodiazepines)	No	Yes, FVC, DLCO	No	No	/
Kohashi et al. (26)	-History (smoke) - BMI	Yes at baseline	Yes, FVC, FEV1, FEV1/FVC, DLCO	No	BNP, LDH, KL-6, SP-D, ANA, RF, other autoantibodies	echocardiography
Kondoh et al. (27)	-History (smoke)	Yes at baseline	Yes, FVC, DLCO, FEV1/FVC repeated every year	Yes	No	BAL, PaO2
Levi et al. (28)	-History (smoke, family history of ILD, medications and environmental risk factors)	Yes at baseline	Yes, FVC%, DLCO%, and TLC%	Yes	Complete blood count, chemistry, renal and liver function tests, antinuclear antibody, rheumatoid factor (RF), C-reactive protein (CRP), anti-dsDNA, Scl70, anti-SSA, and anti-SSB were done. A cyclic citrullinated peptide (CCP) antibodies test was done in the case of a positive RF result, anti-Jo1, anti-RNP, anti-Smith, anticentromere, antimyeloperoxidase, antiproteinase–3, and anticardiolipin antibodies, erythrocyte sedimentation rate, various IgG subclasses including IgG4, and vitamin D (level)	Echocardiogram (Pulmonary hypertension, right heart failure), O2 saturation, Bronchoscopy (BAL only, TBB, Cryobiopsy, EBUS), 6-min walking distance (6MWD) test,
Lok (29)	-Evaluation of ongoing pharmacologic therapy	Yes at baseline	Yes, FEV1,FVC,TLC, DLCO	Yes	No	/
Chaudhuri et al. (30)	No	Yes at baseline	Yes, lung volumes, and DLCO	No	No	/
Nakamura et al. (31)	-Evaluation of Smoking index -GAP (Gender, Age, and Physiology) score	Yes, every 3–6 months	Yes, FVC, FEV1, DLCO, DLCO/VA every 3–6 months	Yes	Krebs von der Lungen-6, surfactant protein D, antinuclear antibody, auto-antibodies related to connective tissue diseases	Echocardiography

(Continued)

TABLE 3 | Continued

References	Clinical evaluation	HRCT	PFT	Lung biopsy	Laboratory test	Other
Newton et al. (32)	History (ethnicity, clinical manifestations: dyspnea, cough, smoking status) -Physical examination (crackles, clubbing)	Yes at baseline	Yes, FVC DLCO at baseline and during follow up without a established timing	No	No	/
Patterson et al. (3)	-History (race, smoking habits, clinical features of sarcoidosis, hypersensitivity pneumonitis, and CTD related ILD)	Yes at baseline	Yes, FVC, and DLCO at baseline and yearly	Yes	No	Walking distance, Hypoxemia
Pezzuto et al. (33)	No	Yes at baseline	Yes, at the time of evaluation FVC, TV, TLC, DLCO	Yes	For exclusion of CTD and vasculitis but not specified	BAL
Tanizawa et al. (34)	-History (ethnicity/race, smoking status, selected comorbidities) (asthma; congestive heart failure; gastroesophageal reflux; sleep apnea; diabetes), exposure history	Yes closed to biopsy. Categorized as definite UIP, possible UIP, or inconsistent with UIP pattern	Yes, close to biopsy FVC, FEV1, TLC, DLCO	Yes	No	MUC5B genotyping and telomere length measurement
Thomeer et al. (35)	No	Yes within 12 months before biopsy and during follow up	No	Yes	No	/
Tomassetti et al. (36)	-History: onset, symptoms, detailed history of exposure, family history, past medical history, and medications	Yes at baseline	Yes, at the time of evaluation FVC, RV, TLC, DLCO	No	Blood cell count, LDH, CRP, ESR, liver and kidney function profile, autoimmunity—ANA ENA ANCA	/
Tominaga et al. (37)	-History: onset, symptoms, detailed history of exposure, family history, past medical history, and medications	Yes, baseline	Yes VC, DLCO	Yes	Rheumatoid arthritis test, rheumatoid arthritis particle agglutination (RAPA) and ANA, serum biomarkers (Krebs von der Lungen-6 and surfactant protein-D)	/
Oltmanns et al. (38)	-History (comorbidities; smoking history)	Yes at baseline	/	Yes	Blood gas analysis, liver function test	/
Ussavarungsi et al. (39)	No	No	/	Yes	No	/
Walsh et al. (40)	-History (smoking habits, rheumatological disease, and rheumatological manifestation)	Yes at baseline	/	Yes	Autoantibodies	/
Yamauchi et al. (41)	-History (smoke)	Yes at baseline	/	No	KL-6, SP-D	/

CT, computer tomography; BMI, body mass index; FVC, forced vital capacity; DLCO, the ability to spread carbon monoxide; FEV1, forced expiratory volume in the 1st second; less frequently, TLC, total lung capacity; CRP, C-reactive protein; ESR, erythrocyte sedimentation rate; ANA, antinuclear antibodies; RF, rheumatoid factor; ACPA, anti-cyclic citrullinated peptide; ENA antibodies against extractable nuclear antigens; BAL, bronchoalveolar lavage; ASMA, antibodies against smooth muscle; ANCAs, anti-neutrophil cytoplasmic antibodies; CTD, connective tissue disease; SLB, surgical lung biopsy; ILD-CTD, interstitial lung disease related to connective tissue disease; IPF, idiopathic pulmonary fibrosis; SpO2, saturation of peripheral oxygen; BNP, natriuretic peptide B; LDH, lactic dehydrogenase; KL-6, Krebs von den Lungen 6; SP-D, surfactant protein-D; NSIP, idiopathic non-specific interstitial pneumonia; IPAF, interstitial pneumonia with autoimmune features; TBB, transbronchial biopsy; Scl70, anti-topoisomerase1; EBUS, endobronchial ultrasound; PaO2, Partial Pressure of Oxygen in Arterial Blood; U-ILD, undifferentiated interstitial lung disease; BCF, bronchiolocentric fibrosis; MUC5B, mucin 5B; /, not reported.

Possible applications of MDD could encompass the management of ILD patients. In a study by Kalluri, subjects with ILD secondary to rheumatic diseases referred to the MDT (composed of pneumologist and rheumatologist), were compared with patients suffering from IPF followed according to a normal care setting. While the disease progression assessed through the worsening of the HRCT and PFT parameters was comparable, patients evaluated by MDD experienced greater satisfaction and more participation in their care path (22). A multidisciplinary approach in palliative care involving the participation of ILD experts, a palliative respiratory care expert, nurse, respiratory therapist, physiotherapist, and a dietitian, compared to the standard approach (namely ILD experts and a nurse) proved efficacy in improving the management of a small series of 32 patient, in terms of reduced number of emergency visits and hospital admissions (25).

There is little evidence concerning the role of MDT activity in the follow up. The diagnosis of ILD can change over time in light of new clinical or serological elements that may emerge in the course of the disease, as well as the progress and response to therapy. In a retrospective study of 56 patients evaluated during a 7-month average follow-up, it was shown how the re-evaluation of new clinical elements and a second HRCT by the pulmonologist and radiologist can modify the diagnosis of a first multidisciplinary discussion (10.7%), as well as the level of agreement (25% of cases). The multidisciplinary evaluation should therefore be a dynamic process not limited to the initial phase of the diagnostic process but also considered during the follow up (21). In a retrospective cohort study, 30 patients with a probable UIP pattern on HRCT and histology compatible or probable for UIP were identified by MDD. The evolution of the radiological data and the prognostic implications of patients who evolved radiologically were therefore evaluated against a specific HRCT pattern. In this case, the MDT and in particular the interaction between the radiologist and pathologist was fundamental to identify the target population of this study (41).

Role of Rheumatologist

The rheumatologist was included in MDT in 7 studies. The retrospective study by Chartrand highlighted the role of the rheumatologist in the MDT while evaluating patients with ILD. From the National Jewish Health Metical database, the authors identified patients initially referred as IPF. After the multidisciplinary evaluation, the diagnosis was modified in 33 patients in ASSD (27/33) or a myositis spectrum disease (6/33). In these patients the identification of specific myositis antibodies (in particular anti-synthetase) or myositis associated were fundamental. The authors underlined that about a third of the patients was ANA negative, and so the research of the autoimmune profile should be extended to these antibodies that often recognize cytoplasmic antigens. Moreover, in 85% of cases at least one manifestation attributable to CTD was present, such as Raynaud's phenomenon, mechanic's hand, Gottron's papules, capillaroscopic alterations. Among these, the muscular manifestations were present only in a third of patients (15). A retrospective observational study of 50 patients, the MDD led to a final diagnosis of CTD-ILD in 25 patients, IPF in 15

and other forms of ILD in 10. In particular, in 7 of the 25 patients with CTD-ILD the pre-MDD diagnosis was IPF with completely different prognostic and therapeutic implications. Therapy therefore changed in 20 of 25 patients with CTD-ILD and in 4 of 15 patients with IPF after MDT evaluation (16). In the study by Ferri et al., the MDD was performed by a rheumatologist and a pneumologist. Other professional figures such as the thoracic radiologist, surgeon and pathologist were considered only in selected cases. Given the type of setting, the authors described a more detailed clinical and laboratory assessment set with particular attention to the evaluation of autoimmune clinical manifestations and serological investigations. In the evaluation of the patient, specific instrumental investigations were also included, such as nailfold capillaroscopy, joint and salivary glands ultrasound, suggesting an application based on clinical suspicion (18). In a prospective study of 60 patients the role of the rheumatologist in the classification of patients with ILD at the onset is again emphasized. The diagnostic process was divided into three phases: a first phase in which the traditional MDT was involved, consisting of pulmonologist, radiologist and pathologist, and a second one where a rheumatologist evaluated the cases independently. In the course of traditional MDT clinical information, PFT, HRCT, biopsy, and BAL when available were evaluated. Serological investigations routinely performed included ANA, anti-dsDNA, anti-topoisomerase-1(Scl70), anti-SSA, and anti-SSB, ACPA (done in the case of a positive RF result). To these tests, the following could be added after the rheumatologic evaluation: anti-Jo1, anti-RNP, anti-Smith, anticentromere, ANCA, and anticardiolipin antibodies, various IgG subclasses including IgG4. Also anti-synthetase antibodies were tested if deemed necessary by the rheumatologist. Finally, there was a third phase of comparison between MDT and rheumatologist, in which some diagnoses formulated by the MDT were modified. In particular 21.9% of IPF cases and 28.5% of hypersensitivity pneumonia cases (HP) the diagnosis was modified in favor of pathologies of rheumatological interest such as Sjogren's syndrome, associated ANCA-associated vasculitis, RA, ASSD, SSc, and related IgG4 pathology. The authors also argued that the rheumatological evaluation could have avoided 7 bronchoscopies and 1 lung biopsy (28).

DISCUSSION

Before the publication of the 2002 ATS guidelines, the diagnosis of ILD was based on histopathology. However, the interobserver agreement between expert histopathologists was reported low, especially in the presence of non-specific interstitial pneumonia (NSIP) pattern (43). The level of diagnostic accuracy and interobserver agreement between radiologists was better than between pathologists, and HRCT is currently the most used diagnostic tool in the evaluation of patients with ILD, being less invasive than lung biopsy. Furthermore, different histopathological findings may be present in different lobes of the same patient. Already before the publication of ATS/ERS/JRS/ALAT guidelines, the importance of a multidisciplinary evaluation of IPF patients was proposed

(29). Current clinical practice guidelines suggest that in patients with suspected IPF a definite UIP pattern at HRCT could be considered a sufficient criterion for making the diagnosis. About half of the patients, however, presents a probable or inconsistent UIP pattern. In this group of patients the MDT is fundamental (44), especially for the identification of IPF which is the form of ILD with the worst prognosis with an average survival of 2–3 years from diagnosis. Given the current availability of effective anti-fibrotic drugs such as nintedanib and pirfenidone, a correct and early diagnosis of IPF is crucial (5).

SLB is generally considered in cases where imaging is inconsistent with UIP and in case of conflicting clinical data. Nevertheless, an UIP patter at histology is not necessarily indicative of IPF as demonstrated in the study by Tominaga, where the clinical information and HRCT images of 95 patients diagnosed as IPF and confirmed by a histological pattern compatible with UIP, were first re-evaluated separately and later on the course of MDD by a group of radiologists and pulmonologists. The two groups were progressively provided with more clinical data and radiological images. With the increase of clinical and radiological information, the degree of certainty in the diagnosis was reduced to a low or to an intermediate level in 41% of cases (37).

Multidisciplinary evaluation is essential in patients who do not have a definite UIP pattern at HRCT. Especially for probable UIP pattern, different studies have reported a variable frequency of IPF from 90 to 60%. Given the prognostic importance of a correct diagnosis, integration of imaging with clinical and histological data is fundamental, as demonstrated in a cohort of 179 patients with probable UIP pattern at HRCT in which the 50% of cases were diagnosed by MDD as IPF presenting worse prognosis compared to patients without IPF (27).

MDT classically include a pulmonologist, a radiologist and pathologist expert in ILD, but other professional figures including specialists in rheumatology, thoracic surgery, lung transplantation, and occupational medicine are often involved on demand (17). Despite the importance of MDD and available recommendations, there are no indications on the optimal composition of the MDT, on the timing or how to organize these meetings. Although in most cases the MDD aims to make an accurate diagnosis of ILD, the multidisciplinary approach can be used in patient care or for follow-up. Depending on the aims and degree of experience of the MDT itself, the organization may be different. For example, members of a recently established MDT could meet more frequently while in the case of clinicians with more experience in multidisciplinary discussion, the assessment could only be performed in selected cases. Depending on the purpose of the MDD, the members could be different, for example in the diagnostic evaluation the thoracic surgeon might not be useful (44).

Despite the recommendations and the available studies, it is currently not known whether the multidisciplinary approach is better than the single expert's clinical judgment in the diagnosis of patients with ILD. Moreover, the strict application of the guidelines for IPF is not always feasible; for example it is not always possible to perform SLB for safety reasons, and in the definition of the UIP pattern (both radiological and pathological)

often the agreement between the observers is only moderate. Finally, the guidelines do not indicate how some clinical aspects, which may help to increase diagnostic confidence, should be included in MDD. This means that the multidisciplinary approach is not always applicable, and often the diagnosis is left to the opinion of the expert. The concept of "working diagnosis" recently proposed by the Fleischner Society allows to justify a disease-specific therapy despite a non-definite diagnosis (45). The lack of a standardized ontological framework can also determine heterogeneity in diagnosis for patients with ILD. Ryerson et al. made a proposal to standardize the terminology, by subdividing according to the degree of diagnostic confidence (> 90%, between 89 and 50% and <50%) the wording in the diagnosis of ILD in "confident," "provisional," and "unclassifiable ILD" (46). An international study involving 404 physicians that evaluated 60 cases of suspected IPF employed these standardized definitions to evaluate the impact of diagnostic likelihood on physician's decision to performed biopsy and on which treatment prescribe. This study showed that in presence of a provisional high confidence IPF diagnosis only a minority of patients (29.6%) would be addressed to SLB. Furthermore, most physicians prescribed anti-fibrotic therapy without performing histological evaluation in 63% of patients with a diagnostic likelihood of 70%, and in 63.0 and 41.5% of provisional high confidence and low confidence IPF diagnoses, respectively. The behavior of experts participating to this study was in most cases different from the guidelines; for instance, especially university hospital physicians tended not to require biopsy and to choose therapy according to a "working diagnosis" instead of a certain diagnosis as defined by the current guidelines. Therefore, the MDD would have a role in training physicians especially when they work in isolation (47).

The ATS guidelines emphasize the need to exclude the presence of a CTD during the evaluation of a patient with ILD. Despite this recommendation, rheumatologists are not considered mandatory among professional figures involved in the MDD, reserving the rheumatological evaluation only to patients with positive autoantibody serology, suspicious clinical manifestations for CTD and other rheumatological diseases, or in case with demographic characteristics atypical for IPF (e.g., female, age younger than 60 years, not smokers). The presence of a rheumatologist could therefore be fundamental in identifying specific non-pulmonary clinical manifestations that could not be easily recognized by traditional members of MDT, especially in patients with demographic, clinical and histopathological features inconsistent with IPF (15). For example, in female patients younger than 50 years, a diagnosis of IPF is unlikely compared to a male smoker over 60. Furthermore, some radiological patterns such as NSIP or organizing pneumonia (OP) are more characteristic of ILD associated with CTD. The presence of a definite UIP pattern, however, does not exclude the presence of an underlying autoimmune disease especially RA and some cases of SSc (48). Histological UIP pattern is indistinguishable between IPF and CTD-ILD, but some characteristics such as increased expression of lymphoid hyperplasia with germinal centers, more plasmatic infiltration, and less severe honeycombing are typical for CTD.

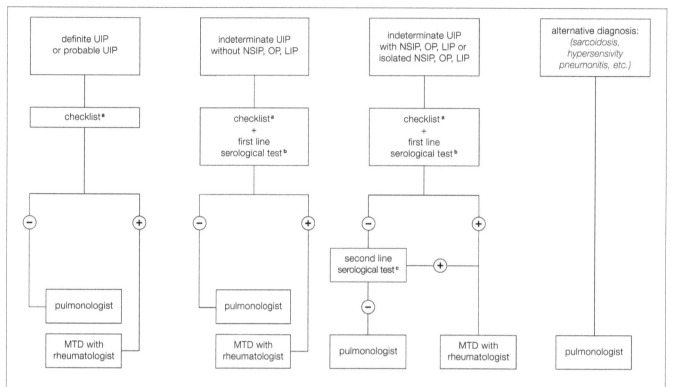

FIGURE 2 | Proposal for a multidisciplinary team (MDT) involving the rheumatologist. (a) Checklist regarding signs and symptoms compatible with CTD or arthritis. (b) First line serological test: RF, ACPA, ANA, CPK. (c) Second line serological test: Anti-ds DNA, Anti-Ro (SS-A), Anti-La (SS-B), Anti-ribonucleoprotein, Anti-topoisomerase (Scl-70) Anti-tRNA synthetase, Anti-PM-Scl, Anti-MDA5.

ILD can be a manifestation developed during an established CTD, so the diagnostic approach, therapy, and follow-up are better defined, and the rheumatologist is naturally involved in patient management. In other contexts, ILD may be the first manifestation at the onset of a not recognized CTD and the other typical clinical features may appear after the pulmonary involvement. This is known for example, especially in myositis spectrum disorders where in 10–30% of cases ILD may be the predominant manifestation (10), in particular in case of ASSD where the classical triad arthritis, myositis and ILD may develop during the follow up (49). The lack of specific classification criteria for ASSD makes the correct diagnosis for these patients more difficult, and an expert rheumatologist would be essential during the evaluation of these patients (12). Moreover, very few patients affected by SSc or RA may present as ILD at the onset, so in these cases the diagnostic process could be very challenging. In these pathological contexts the rheumatologist is crucial to identify the signs and symptoms more nuanced and less clear that cannot be recognized by other professional figures traditionally involved in the MDT.

The evaluation of the patient with ILD cannot be independent of the execution of blood tests, in particular autoimmunity, and different guidelines have proposed the execution of different biochemical test. The French guidelines recommends to evaluate complete blood cell count, CRP, serum creatinine, transaminases, γ-glutamyltransferase, and alkaline phosphatases, ANA, ACPA, and RF, reserving the search of other more

specific antibodies (anti-SSA, anti-SSB, anti-centromeres, Scl70, anti-U3RNP, anti-synthetase antibodies, anti-thyroid antibodies) in case of positivity of first line antibodies or in presence of clinical manifestation compatible with CTD (50). The ATS/ERS/JRS/ALAT guideline recommends CRP, ESR, ANA (by immunofluorescence), RF, myositis panel and ACPA performing other test according to symptoms and signs (8). In the last few years, the diffusion of laboratory kits able to identify specific and associated myositis antibodies has made possible to reclassify patients with doubtful clinical pictures especially in the presence of negative ANA or with cytoplasmatic patterns. In particular antibodies such as MDA-5 and specific anti-synthetase antibodies such as PL2 and PL7 identify myositis with prevalent pulmonary expression that could be the first clinical manifestation up to 10–30% of cases of myositis spectrum disease (10).

The studies included in this review show that there is not a common behavior in serological evaluation, and only in 17 studies biochemical tests were evaluated during MDD. Fourteen studies reported the evaluation of autoantibodies without a clear suggestion of which test should be performed, and in 5 studies is not reported which serological test was chosen.

Another diagnostic challenge is represented by IPAF, a clinical entity of more recent characterization and of which classification criteria have been formulated (13). IPAF could be considered an ILD in which clinical or serological abnormalities typical of CTD are present but insufficient to satisfy classification criteria of a defined autoimmune disease. These classification criteria share many characteristics with undifferentiated connective tissues and allow to identify as IPAF very different clinical entities including patients with very early SSc or other CTD such as myositis spectrum diseases with a predominant pulmonary manifestation at onset. This could result in a mis-classification of patients especially without a rheumatologic evaluation (51).

Despite these considerations, no clear indications are available about the rheumatologist involvement in MDT. Only 7/29 studies included in this review described a rheumatological evaluation during MDD paying attention to the correct re-classification of patients who were initially classified as IPF (15, 16), and to the possibility of avoiding not necessary diagnostic procedures (28). From the available studies it is not possible to identify a univocal attitude on the modalities and timing of involvement of the rheumatologist in such a context.

For these reasons we have formulated a proposal for the organization of the MDT that provides different scenarios to suggest when and how the rheumatologist should be included in MDD, especially to help to identify CTD-ILD and IPAF (**Figure 2**). A first scenario includes ILD patients with HRCT pattern typical for UIP which is less frequent in cases of ILD associated with autoimmune diseases and more typical of IPF. However, it is still possible that a UIP pattern could be found, even if less frequently, in course of rheumatological disorders, especially RA and SSc. We have therefore proposed that the pulmonologist participating to MDT should be trained to identify clinical manifestations compatible with CTD or RA belonging to the checklist reported in **Table 4**. This core set includes main signs and symptoms typical of rheumatologic diseases that can be more frequently complicated with ILD: SSc, RA, Sjogren syndrome, and myositis spectrum disorder. For joint involvement, we have decided to include patients presenting at least one swollen or tender joint on examination excluding distal interphalangeal joints, first carpometacarpal joints, and first metatarsophalangeal in agreement with the definition reported in 2010 classification criteria for RA (54). For myositis spectrum disorders we have included the search for weakness of proximal musculature of the upper and lower limbs and for the presence of typical cutaneous manifestations (Gottron's papules and sign) described in the classification criteria of 2017 for idiopathic inflammatory myopathies (53). To identify patients affected by ASSD, fever, mechanic's hands, Raynaud's phenomenon and dysphagia have been included in the checklist. In particular, the last two manifestations together with puffy fingers, sclerodactyly, and telangiectasias, belong to scleroderma spectrum manifestations and so they should be considered as part of the coreset of clinical manifestations to be evaluated during diagnostic approach of patients with ILD. Finally, the sicca syndrome has been described according to the 2002 classification criteria for Sjogren's syndrome as a sensation of daily dryness, ocular or oral duration longer than 3 months (52). In case of positivity of at least one of these clinical criteria, we have proposed to involve the rheumatologist for a second evaluation in order to confirm the first clinical impression and therefore to perform further instrumental examinations, such as biochemical tests (including

TABLE 4 | Signs and symptoms to be assessed in the suspicion of a rheumatological disease.

Clinical manifestation of autoimmune disease	Description
Joint involvement	Any swollen or tender joint on examination excluding distal interphalangeal joints, first carpometacarpal joints, and first metatarsophalangeal joints are excluded from assessment. Synovitis could be confirmed by imaging (Definition according 2010 Rheumatoid Arthritis Classification Criteria)
Raynaud syndrome	A vascular disorder especially of the fingers and toes, that is characterized by pallor, cyanosis, and redness in succession usually upon exposure to cold
Puffy fingers or sclerodactyly	Swelling or thickening of fingers
Distal digital tip ulceration	Loss of epithelialization and tissues involving, in different degrees, the epidermis, the dermis, the subcutaneous tissue, and sometimes also involving the bone
Telangiectasia	Small dilated-blood vessels near the surface of the skin or mucous membranes, measuring between 0.5 and 1 ml in diameter, especially localized on finger or face
Mechanics hand	Rough, cracked, hyperkeratotic, aspect of palmar areas of the fingers with fissures of the skin
Sicca syndrome	Sensation of dryness of eyes and/or mouth daily and persistent for 3 months (52)
Gottron signs	Fixed rash or patches on the extensor surfaces of the joints (especially elbows and/or knees)
Gottron papules	Erythematous to violaceous papules and plaques over the extensor surfaces of the metacarpophalangeal and interphalangeal joints
Eliotrophic rash	Violaceous erythema of the upper eyelids often with associated edema and telangiectasia
Fever	Unexplained by other causes
Muscle weakness	Weakness of proximal upper and lower extremities as Distal muscles are less involved. Weakness of neck flexors is usually more severe than of neck extensors (53)
Dysphagia	Difficulty in swallowing

autoantibodies), capillaroscopy or echography suggested by the rheumatologist based on his clinical suspicion, thus avoiding useless and expensive investigations. Furthermore, this approach makes it possible to identify IPAF. According to the ATS classification criteria, in fact, being absent the morphological domain [HRCT pattern compatible with NSIP, OP or LIP (lymphoid interstitial pneumonia)], both the serological and the clinical domain are required. Therefore, our checklist including all the manifestations present in the clinical domain of these criteria, allows to identify patients with suspected IPAF and to confirm the suspicion after performing serological investigations.

Another scenario includes ILD patients with probable UIP pattern, indeterminate UIP pattern on HRCT. In this case, patterns frequently observed during CTD as NSIP, OP, and LIP would be included so the probability to observe an ILD secondary to an autoimmune disease is greater than in case of typical UIP pattern. For this reason, we have added to the clinical domain a biochemical screening test including ANA, RF, ACPA, and creatine phosphokinase (CPK). In case of negativity of both clinical and serological domain, patients presenting NSIP, OP, or LIP pattern are subjected to further serological evaluation in order to exclude IPAF or myositis spectrum disorders, and evaluated by a rheumatologist. In case of positivity of at least one of clinical or serological parameters during the screening, patients would be referred to rheumatologist that would suggest to perform further instrumental investigations such as biochemical tests (including autoantibodies), capillaroscopy, or echography based on clinical suspicion in order to avoid unnecessary investigations and to accurately diagnose patients with CTD-ILD (**Figure 2**).

CONCLUSION

The role of the rheumatologist in MDD for the evaluation of patients with ILD is still not defined but could be fundamental

for the correct diagnosis of CTD-ILD and IPAF. From the literature review, it emerges that in most cases the MDT is composed by the pulmonologist, radiologist and pathologist. The first being an essential member of the MDT, could be trained to be able to identify patients with suspected CTD-ILD and IPAF in order to select them for rheumatological evaluation. This organization could simplify the multidisciplinary meeting, reducing the times in which all professions are required for MDD. Our proposal for the organization of the MDT also provides a minimum core set of blood tests for screening, reserving the execution of second-level investigations only after a rheumatological indication and targeted according to the clinical suspicion, thus avoiding unnecessary and confounding tests.

AUTHOR CONTRIBUTIONS

FF and CS formulated the concept and design the paper. FF, GG, and AC performed SRL. FF wrote the manuscript. CS, GC, LC, and MG revised the manuscript critically, approved the final manuscript, and agreed to be accountable for all aspects of the manuscript.

REFERENCES

1. Travis WD, Costabel U, Hansell DM, King TEJ, Lynch DA, Nicholson AG, et al. An official American Thoracic Society/European Respiratory Society statement: update of the international multidisciplinary classification of the idiopathic interstitial pneumonias. *Am J Respir Crit Care Med.* (2013) 188:733–48. doi: 10.1164/rccm.201308-1483ST
2. Wells AU, Hirani N, on behalf of the BTS Interstitial Lung Disease Guideline Group, a subgroup of the British Thoracic Society Standards of Care Committee, in collaboration with the Thoracic Society of Australia and New Zealand and the Irish Thoracic Society. Interstitial lung disease guideline. *Thorax.* (2008) 63:v1–58. doi: 10.1136/thx.2008.101691
3. Patterson KC, Shah RJ, Porteous MK, Christie JD, D'Errico CA, Chadwick M, et al. Interstitial lung disease in the elderly. *Chest.* (2017) 151:838–44. doi: 10.1016/j.chest.2016.11.003
4. Sontake V, Gajjala PR, Kasam RK, Madala SK. New therapeutics based on emerging concepts in pulmonary fibrosis. *Expert Opin Ther Targets.* (2019) 23:69–81. doi: 10.1080/14728222.2019.1552262
5. Ahmad K, Nathan SD. Novel management strategies for idiopathic pulmonary fibrosis. *Expert Rev Respir Med.* (2018) 12:831–42. doi: 10.1080/17476348.2018.1513332
6. Distler O, Brown KK, Distler JHW, Assassi S, Maher TM, Cottin V, et al. Design of a randomised, placebo-controlled clinical trial of nintedanib in patients with systemic sclerosis-associated interstitial lung disease (SENSCIS™). *Clin Exp Rheumatol.* (2017) 35(Suppl. 106):75–81.
7. Cottin V, Castillo D, Poletti V, Kreuter M, Corte TJ, Spagnolo P. Should patients with interstitial lung disease be seen by experts? *Chest.* (2018) 154:713–4. doi: 10.1016/j.chest.2018.05.044
8. Raghu G, Remy-Jardin M, Myers JL, Richeldi L, Ryerson CJ, Lederer DJ, et al. Diagnosis of idiopathic pulmonary fibrosis. An official ATS/ERS/JRS/ALAT clinical practice guideline. *Am J Respir Crit Care Med.* (2018) 198:e44–68. doi: 10.1164/rccm.201807-1255ST
9. Mohammad AJ, Mortensen KH, Babar J, Smith R, Jones RB, Nakagomi D, et al. Pulmonary involvement in antineutrophil cytoplasmic antibodies (ANCA)-associated vasculitis: the influence of ANCA subtype. *J Rheumatol.* (2017) 44:1458–67. doi: 10.3899/jrheum.161224
10. Cottin V. Idiopathic interstitial pneumonias with connective tissue diseases features: a review. *Respirology.* (2016) 21:245–58. doi: 10.1111/resp.12588
11. Narula N, Narula T, Mira-Avendano I, Wang B, Abril A. Interstitial lung disease in patients with mixed connective tissue disease: pilot study on predictors of lung involvement. *Clin Exp Rheumatol.* (2018) 36:648–51.

12. Castañeda S, Cavagna L, González-Gay MA. New criteria needed for antisynthetase syndrome. *JAMA Neurol.* (2018) 75:258–59. doi: 10.1001/jamaneurol.2017.3872
13. Fischer A, Antoniou KM, Brown KK, Cadranel J, Corte TJ, du Bois RM, et al. An official European Respiratory Society/American Thoracic Society research statement: interstitial pneumonia with autoimmune features. *Eur Respir J.* (2015) 46:976–87. doi: 10.1183/13993003.00150-2015
14. Burge PS, Reynolds J, Trotter S, Burge GA, Walters G. Histologist's original opinion compared with multidisciplinary team in determining diagnosis in interstitial lung disease. *Thorax* 72:280–1. (2017). doi: 10.1136/thoraxjnl-2016-208776
15. Chartrand S, Swigris JJ, Peykova L, Chung J, Fischer A. A Multidisciplinary evaluation helps identify the antisynthetase syndrome in patients presenting as idiopathic interstitial pneumonia. *J Rheumatol.* (2016) 43:887–92. doi: 10.3899/jrheum.150966
16. Castelino FV, Goldberg H, Dellaripa PF. The impact of rheumatological evaluation in the management of patients with interstitial lung disease. *Rheumatology.* (2011) 50:489–93. doi: 10.1093/rheumatology/keq233
17. De Sadeleer LJ, Meert C, Yserbyt J, Slabbynck H, Verschakelen JA, Verbeken EK, et al. Diagnostic ability of a dynamic multidisciplinary discussion in interstitial lung diseases: a retrospective observational study of 938 cases. *Chest.* (2018) 153:1416–23. doi: 10.1016/j.chest.2018.03.026
18. Ferri C, Manfredi A, Sebastiani M, Colaci M, Giuggioli D, Vacchi C, et al. Interstitial pneumonia with autoimmune features and undifferentiated connective tissue disease: Our interdisciplinary rheumatology-pneumology experience, and review of the literature. *Autoimm Rev.* (2016) 15:61–70. doi: 10.1016/j.autrev.2015.09.003
19. Flaherty KR, King TEJ, Raghu G, Lynch J, Colby TV, Travis WD, et al. Idiopathic interstitial pneumonia: what is the effect of a multidisciplinary approach to diagnosis? *Am J Respir Crit Care Med.* (2004) 170:904–10. doi: 10.1164/rccm.200402-147OC
20. Fujisawa T, Mori K, Mikamo M, Ohno T, Kataoka K, Sugimoto C, et al. Nationwide cloud-based integrated database of idiopathic interstitial pneumonias for multidisciplinary discussion. *Eur Respir J.* (2019) 53:1802243. doi: 10.1183/13993003.02243-2018
21. Han Q, Wang H-Y, Zhang X-X, Wu L-L, Wang L-L, Jiang Y, et al. The role of follow-up evaluation in the diagnostic algorithm of idiopathic interstitial pneumonia: a retrospective study. *Sci. Rep.* (2019) 9:6452. doi: 10.1038/s41598-019-42813-7

22. Jeong SO, Uh S-T, Park S, Kim H-S. Effects of patient satisfaction and confidence on the success of treatment of combined rheumatic disease and interstitial lung disease in a multidisciplinary outpatient clinic. *Int J Rheum Dis.* (2018) 21:1600–8. doi: 10.1111/1756-185X. 13331

23. Jo HE, Prasad JD, Troy LK, Mahar A, Bleasel J, Ellis SJ, et al. Diagnosis and management of idiopathic pulmonary fibrosis: thoracic society of Australia and New Zealand and Lung Foundation Australia position statements summary. *Med J Aust.* (2018) 208:82–8. doi: 10.5694/mja17. 00799

24. Jo HE, Glaspole IN, Levin KC, McCormack SR, Mahar AM, Cooper WA, et al. Clinical impact of the interstitial lung disease multidisciplinary service. *Respirology.* (2016) 21:1438–44. doi: 10.1111/resp.12850

25. Kalluri M, Claveria F, Ainsley E, Haggag M, Armijo-Olivo S, Richman-Eisenstat J. Beyond Idiopathic pulmonary fibrosis diagnosis: multidisciplinary care with an early integrated palliative approach is associated with a decrease in acute care utilization and hospital deaths. *J Pain Symptom Manage.* (2018) 55:420–6. doi: 10.1016/j.jpainsymman.2017. 10.016

26. Kohashi Y, Arai T, Sugimoto C, Tachibana K, Akira M, Kitaichi M, et al. Clinical impact of emphysema evaluated by high-resolution computed tomography on idiopathic pulmonary fibrosis diagnosed by surgical lung biopsy. *Respir Int Rev Thor Dis.* (2016) 92:220–8. doi: 10.1159/000448118

27. Kondoh Y, Taniguchi H, Kataoka K, Furukawa T, Shintani A, Fujisawa T, et al. Clinical spectrum and prognostic factors of possible UIP pattern on high-resolution CT in patients who underwent surgical lung biopsy. *PLoS ONE.* (2018) 13:e0193608. doi: 10.1371/journal.pone.0193608

28. Levi Y, Israeli-Shani L, Kuchuk M, Epstein Shochet G, Koslow M, Shitrit D. Rheumatological assessment is important for interstitial lung disease diagnosis. *J Rheumatol.* (2018) 45:1509–14. doi: 10.3899/jrheum. 171314

29. Lok SS. Interstitial lung disease clinics for the management of idiopathic pulmonary fibrosis: a potential advantage to patients. Greater Manchester Lung Fibrosis Consortium. *J Heart Lung Transpl.* (1999) 18:884–90.

30. Chaudhuri N, Spencer L, Greaves M, Bishop P, Chaturvedi A, Leonard C, et al. A review of the multidisciplinary diagnosis of interstitial lung diseases: a retrospective analysis in a single UK specialist centre. *J Clin Med.* (2016) 5:E66. doi: 10.3390/jcm5080066

31. Nakamura Y, Sugino K, Kitani M, Hebisawa A, Tochigi N, Homma S. Clinico-radio-pathological characteristics of unclassifiable idiopathic interstitial pneumonias. *Respir Investig.* (2018) 56:40–7. doi: 10.1016/j.resinv.2017. 09.001

32. Newton CA, Batra K, Torrealba J, Kozlitina J, Glazer CS, Aravena C, et al. Telomere-related lung fibrosis is diagnostically heterogeneous but uniformly progressive. *Eur Respir J.* (2016) 48:1710–20. doi: 10.1183/13993003.00308-2016

33. Pezzuto G, Claroni G, Puxeddu E, Fusco A, Cavalli F, Altobelli S, et al. Structured multidisciplinary discussion of HRCT scans for IPF/UIP diagnosis may result in indefinite outcomes. *Sarcoid Vascul Diffuse Lung Dis.* (2015) 32:32–36.

34. Tanizawa K, Ley B, Vittinghoff E, Elicker BM, Henry TS, Wolters PJ, et al. Significance of bronchiolocentric fibrosis in patients with histopathological usual interstitial pneumonia. *Histopathology.* (2019) 74:1088–97. doi: 10.1111/his.13840

35. Thomeer M, Demedts M, Behr J, Buhl R, Costabel U, Flower CDR, et al. Multidisciplinary interobserver agreement in the diagnosis of idiopathic pulmonary fibrosis. *Eur Respir J.* (2008) 31:585–91. doi: 10.1183/09031936.00063706

36. Tomassetti S, Wells AU, Costabel U, Cavazza A, Colby TV, Rossi G, et al. Bronchoscopic lung cryobiopsy increases diagnostic confidence in the multidisciplinary diagnosis of idiopathic pulmonary fibrosis. *Am J Respir Critic Care Med.* (2016) 193:745–2. doi: 10.1164/rccm.201504-0711OC

37. Tominaga J, Sakai F, Johkoh T, Noma S, Akira M, Fujimoto K, et al. Diagnostic certainty of idiopathic pulmonary fibrosis/usual interstitial pneumonia: The effect of the integrated clinico-radiological assessment. *Eur J Radiol.* (2015) 84:1088–95. doi: 10.1016/j.ejrad.2015.08.016

38. Oltmanns U, Kahn N, Palmowski K, Träger A, Wenz H, Heussel CP, et al. Pirfenidone in idiopathic pulmonary fibrosis-experience from a german tertiary referral centre for interstitial lung diseases. *Am J Respir Crit Care Med.*

(2014) 189:199–207. doi: 10.1159/000363064

39. Ussavarungsi K, Kern RM, Roden AC, Ryu JH, Edell ES. Transbronchial cryobiopsy in diffuse parenchymal lung disease: retrospective analysis of 74 cases. *Chest.* (2017) 151:400–8. doi: 10.1016/j.chest.2016.09.002

40. Walsh SLF, Wells AU, Desai SR, Poletti V, Piciucchi S, Dubini A, et al. Multicentre evaluation of multidisciplinary team meeting agreement on diagnosis in diffuse parenchymal lung disease: a case-cohort study. *Lancet Respir Med.* (2016) 4:557–65. doi: 10.1016/S2213-2600(16) 30033-9

41. Yamauchi H, Bando M, Baba T, Kataoka K, Yamada Y, Yamamoto H, et al. Clinical course and changes in high-resolution computed tomography findings in patients with idiopathic pulmonary fibrosis without honeycombing. *PLoS ONE.* (2016) 11:e0166168. doi: 10.1371/journal.pone.0166168

42. Jo HE, Glaspole I, Goh N, Hopkins PMA, Moodley Y, Reynolds PN, et al. Implications of the diagnostic criteria of idiopathic pulmonary fibrosis in clinical practice: analysis from the Australian idiopathic pulmonary fibrosis registry. *Respirology.* (2019) 24:361–8. doi: 10.1111/resp.13427

43. Nicholson AG. Inter-observer variation between pathologists in diffuse parenchymal lung disease. *Thorax.* (2004) 59:500–5. doi: 10.1136/thx.2003.011734

44. Walsh SLF. Multidisciplinary evaluation of interstitial lung diseases: current insights: number 1 in the series "radiology" edited by Nicola Sverzellati and Sujal Desai. *Eur Respir Rev.* (2017) 26:170002. doi: 10.1183/16000617.0002-2017

45. Walsh SLF, Maher TM, Kolb M, Poletti V, Nusser R, Richeldi L, et al. Diagnostic accuracy of a clinical diagnosis of idiopathic pulmonary fibrosis: an international case-cohort study. *Eur Respir J.* (2017) 50:1700936. doi: 10.1183/13993003.00936-2017

46. Ryerson CJ, Corte TJ, Lee JS, Richeldi L, Walsh SLF, Myers JL, et al. A standardized diagnostic ontology for fibrotic interstitial lung disease. An international working group perspective. *Am J Respir Crit Care Med.* (2017) 196:1249–54. doi: 10.1164/rccm.201702-0400PP

47. Walsh SLF, Lederer DJ, Ryerson CJ, Kolb M, Maher TM, Nusser R, et al. Diagnostic likelihood thresholds that define a working diagnosis of idiopathic pulmonary fibrosis. *Am J Respir Crit Care Med.* (2019). doi: 10.1164/rccm.201903-0493OC. [Epub ahead of print]

48. Song JW, Do K-H, Kim M-Y, Jang SJ, Colby TV, Kim DS. Pathologic and radiologic differences between idiopathic and collagen vascular disease-related usual interstitial pneumonia. *Chest.* (2009) 136:23–30. doi: 10.1378/chest.08-2572

49. Bartoloni E, Gonzalez-Gay MA, Scirè C, Castaneda S, Gerli R, Lopez-Longo FJ, et al. Clinical follow-up predictors of disease pattern change in anti-Jo1 positive anti-synthetase syndrome: results from a multicenter, international and retrospective study. *Autoimmun Rev.* (2017) 16:253–7. doi: 10.1016/j.autrev.2017.01.008

50. Cottin V, Crestani B, Valeyre D, Wallaert B, Cadranel J, Dalphin J-C, et al. Diagnosis and management of idiopathic pulmonary fibrosis: French practical guidelines. *Eur Respir Rev.* (2014) 23:193–214. doi: 10.1183/09059180.00001814

51. Sambataro G, Sambataro D, Torrisi SE, Vancheri A, Pavone M, Rosso R, et al. State of the art in interstitial pneumonia with autoimmune features: a systematic review on retrospective studies and suggestions for further advances. *Eur Respir Rev.* (2018) 27:170139. doi: 10.1183/16000617. 0139-2017

52. Vitali C. Classification criteria for Sjogren's syndrome: a revised version of the European criteria proposed by the American-European Consensus Group. *Ann Rheum Dis.* (2002) 61:554–8. doi: 10.1136/ard.61. 6.554

53. Lundberg IE, Tjärnlund A, Bottai M, Werth VP, Pilkington C, de Visser M, et al. EULAR/ACR classification criteria for adult and juvenile idiopathic inflammatory myopathies and their major subgroups. *Ann Rheum Dis.* (2017) 76:1955–64. doi: 10.1136/annrheumdis-2017-211468

54. Aletaha D, Neogi T, Silman AJ, Funovits J, Felson DT, Bingham CO, et al. 2010 Rheumatoid arthritis classification criteria: an American College of Rheumatology/European League Against Rheumatism collaborative initiative. *Arthr Rheum.* (2010) 62:2569–81. doi: 10.1002/art.27584

9

Patient Reported Experiences and Delays During the Diagnostic Pathway for Pulmonary Fibrosis: A Multinational European Survey

Iris G. van der Sar[1†], Steve Jones[2†], Deborah L. Clarke[3], Francesco Bonella[4], Jean Michel Fourrier[5], Katarzyna Lewandowska[6], Guadalupe Bermudo[7], Alexander Simidchiev[8], Irina R. Strambu[9], Marlies S. Wijsenbeek[1] and Helen Parfrey[10*]

[1] Erasmus Medical Center, Rotterdam, Netherlands, [2] Action for Pulmonary Fibrosis, Lichfield, United Kingdom, [3] Galapagos NV, Mechelen, Belgium, [4] Ruhrlandklinik, University of Duisburg-Essen, Essen, Germany, [5] Association Pierre Enjalran Fibrose Pulmonaire Idiopathique, Meyzieu, France, [6] Department of Pulmonary Diseases, National Research Institute of Tuberculosis and Lung Diseases, Warsaw, Poland, [7] Hospital Universitari de Bellvitge, Barcelona, Spain, [8] Department of Functional Diagnostics, Medical Institute MVR, Sofia, Bulgaria, [9] Carol Davila University of Medicine and Pharmacy, Bucharest, Romania, [10] Royal Papworth Hospital, Cambridge, United Kingdom

*Correspondence:
Helen Parfrey
hp226@cam.ac.uk

[†] These authors share first authorship

Introduction: Pulmonary fibrosis includes a spectrum of diseases and is incurable. There is a variation in disease course, but it is often progressive leading to increased breathlessness, impaired quality of life, and decreased life expectancy. Detection of pulmonary fibrosis is challenging, which contributes to considerable delays in diagnosis and treatment. More knowledge about the diagnostic journey from patients' perspective is needed to improve the diagnostic pathway. The aims of this study were to evaluate the time to diagnosis of pulmonary fibrosis, identify potential reasons for delays, and document patients emotions.

Methods: Members of European patient organisations, with a self-reported diagnosis of pulmonary fibrosis, were invited to participate in an online survey. The survey assessed the diagnostic pathway retrospectively, focusing on four stages: (1) time from initial symptoms to first appointment in primary care; (2) time to hospital referral; (3) time to first hospital appointment; (4) time to final diagnosis. It comprised open-ended and closed questions focusing on time to diagnosis, factors contributing to delays, diagnostic tests, patient emotions, and information provision.

Results: Two hundred and seventy three participants (214 idiopathic pulmonary fibrosis, 28 sarcoidosis, 31 other) from 13 countries responded. Forty percent of individuals took ≥1 year to receive a final diagnosis. Greatest delays were reported in stage 1, with only 50.2% making an appointment within 3 months. For stage 2, 73.3% reported a hospital referral within three primary care visits. However, 9.9% reported six or more visits. After referral, 76.9% of patients were assessed by a specialist within 3 months (stage 3) and 62.6% received a final diagnosis within 3 months of their first hospital visit (stage 4). Emotions during the journey were overall negative. A major need for more information and support during and after the diagnostic process was identified.

Conclusion: The time to diagnose pulmonary fibrosis varies widely across Europe. Delays occur at each stage of the diagnostic pathway. Raising awareness about pulmonary fibrosis amongst the general population and healthcare workers is essential to shorten the time to diagnosis. Furthermore, there remains a need to provide patients with sufficient information and support at all stages of their diagnostic journey.

Keywords: pulmonary fibrosis, delayed diagnosis, diagnostic journey, survey, patient reported outcomes

INTRODUCTION

Interstitial lung disease (ILD) describes a relatively uncommon group of diseases characterised by inflammation and fibrosis of the lung interstitium. Pulmonary fibrosis is a chronic, and often progressive condition. There is, however, considerable variation amongst patients in terms of aetiology, treatment strategies, and disease course (1). Amongst all types of pulmonary fibrosis, idiopathic pulmonary fibrosis (IPF) is the most prevalent and accounts for about two-thirds of cases. It has the worst prognosis due to rapid disease progression with a mean survival of 4 years from diagnosis without anti-fibrotic therapy (2). Other types of progressive pulmonary fibrosis include chronic hypersensitivity pneumonitis, auto-immune disease related ILD, and occupational diseases such as asbestosis (1). Epidemiological data for all types of pulmonary fibrosis are limited as most registries and studies have focused on IPF or progressive phenotypes only (3). The reported prevalence (per 100,000 persons) of the ILDs that most often result in pulmonary fibrosis is 30.2 for sarcoidosis, 12.1 for ILD related to a connective tissue disease and 8.2 for IPF. Overall, the proportion of ILD patients who develop pulmonary fibrosis varies from 13 to 100% per individual disease (1).

The diagnostic journey usually starts with patients presenting to their primary care physicians with initial symptoms of cough or mild dyspnoea. These non-specific symptoms, combined with the heterogeneity, and rarity of pulmonary fibrosis, as well as requirement for multiple diagnostic investigations, results in a prolonged time to diagnosis with potential delays related to patient factors and healthcare systems (4). Reported time to diagnosis from the onset of initial symptoms varies in different studies but may be up to a median of 2.1 years (IQR 0.9–5.0) (5). Longer time to diagnosis is associated with worse outcomes in IPF (6, 7), causes delayed treatment, leads to more extensive fibrosis (8) and affects patients' well-being. Therefore, it is important to get better insights into patients' experiences during the diagnostic journey to identify reasons for potential delays. Understanding patients' experiences will also help healthcare workers guide and support patients during their diagnosis journey. However, to date, only a few studies have explored the reasons for diagnostic delays using data reported by pulmonary fibrosis patients (9–13). Most analyses are based on retrospective data obtained from healthcare records (5, 7, 8, 14–18).

In this paper, we present data obtained from a multinational patient survey regarding time to diagnosis and potential causes for diagnostic delays, together with patient experiences on the pathway to diagnosis. Based upon these findings, we provide general recommendations to improve the diagnostic process.

METHODS
Survey Design and Distribution

A survey was designed to collect quantitative and qualitative data from patients diagnosed with pulmonary fibrosis across Europe. This survey was developed based upon a market research survey on the IPF patient journey (unpublished data) carried out using a mixture of in-depth telephone interviews with 28 patients and 30 pulmonologists, and online interviews with 315 pulmonologists spanning USA, France, Germany, Italy, Spain, United Kingdom, Australia, Brazil, Canada, and Japan. The patient survey was developed jointly between Galapagos and two patient organisations: Action for Pulmonary Fibrosis (APF, based in the United Kingdom) and the European Idiopathic Pulmonary Fibrosis and Related Disorders Federation (EU-IPFF). Insights from this patient journey research resulted in a questionnaire incorporating both closed and open-ended questions, which focused on the following four stages of the patient journey to identify key points in the delay to diagnosis. The first stage was the time from first onset of symptoms at home, before seeking medical attention in a primary care setting; the second the amount of visits in primary care before being referred to a hospital specialist; the third the time taken to be seen in a hospital by a specialist; and the last the time taken to receive a diagnosis (**Figure 1A**). The survey also gathered data on the overall time from first onset of symptoms to diagnosis and information provided by healthcare workers. Patients were also asked about their feelings throughout the diagnostic journey and to provide advice for patients navigating this journey in the future. No personalised data were collected and all data were anonymised. The questionnaire was designed in English and translated into seven languages (Bulgarian, Dutch, French, German, Hungarian, Italian, and Spanish) by a certified translation agency. It was created using the Typeform® platform. Patients were invited to complete the questionnaire by an e-mail containing a link to the platform. The complete survey in English can be found in the **Supplementary Material 1**.

The survey was disseminated by the EU-IPFF through its member patient organisations in Europe; these organisations distributed the survey to members and other patients through email and social media. Patients with a self-reported diagnosis of pulmonary fibrosis, and who had an email address and

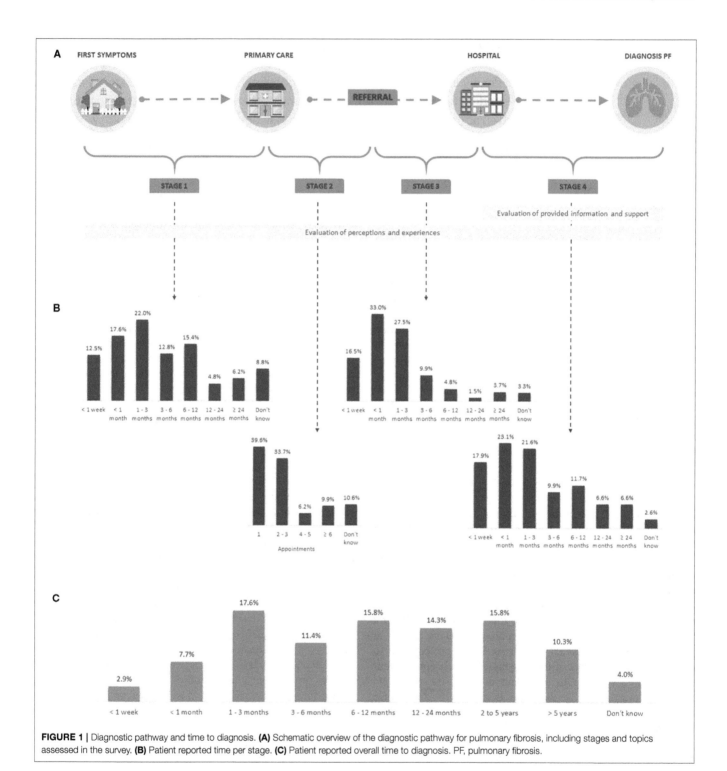

FIGURE 1 | Diagnostic pathway and time to diagnosis. **(A)** Schematic overview of the diagnostic pathway for pulmonary fibrosis, including stages and topics assessed in the survey. **(B)** Patient reported time per stage. **(C)** Patient reported overall time to diagnosis. PF, pulmonary fibrosis.

internet access were eligible to participate. The survey was sent out on 7th June 2020 with a reminder after 2 weeks. It closed on 1st July 2020. Ethical review was not required for this online questionnaire. Patients agreed with the use of their responses for further analysis without collection of personal data and were informed that all data was anonymised.

Data Analysis

Responses in languages other than English were translated into English by a certified translation agency. Open-ended questions were assessed qualitatively and coded or categorised for interpretation. Data were uploaded and calculations were performed in Excel (Microsoft, Redmond, WA, USA). R version 4.0.3 for Mac OS X GUI (PBC,

Boston, MA, USA) was used for creating a word cloud. All responses were included in the analysis, except for blank responses.

Literature Search

In addition to the survey, a literature search on diagnostic delays in ILD, with a focus on pulmonary fibrosis, was conducted in order to provide a complete overview of the available evidence from patient surveys, physician surveys, and medical file analysis.

The systematic literature search was performed in Embase, Medline, Web of science, Cochrane, and Google scholar databases. The following search terms were used: diagnostic delay, time to diagnosis, interstitial lung disease (including sarcoidosis, vasculitis, interstitial pneumonia). Full search and outcome can be found in the **Supplementary Material 2**. Animal studies, paediatric subjects and articles in languages other than English were excluded. The reference list was screened for relevance by title and abstract. Letters to the editor, abstracts, posters, and articles without available full text were excluded.

RESULTS

Respondent Characteristics

Two hundred and seventy three patients from thirteen different countries responded. The largest group of respondents were IPF patients ($n = 214$, 78.4%), followed by sarcoidosis ($n = 28$, 10.3%). Other types of pulmonary fibrosis diagnoses accounted for 31 respondents (11.4%) and included patients with autoimmune related disorders, chronic hypersensitivity pneumonitis, and other conditions. The majority of respondents received a diagnosis of pulmonary fibrosis in Spain (21.6%), Belgium (20.1%), United Kingdom (18.3%), Italy (17.2%), or Germany (10.6%). A smaller number of respondents were diagnosed in the Netherlands (3.3%), Bulgaria (2.6%), France (1.8%), Poland (1.8%), Austria (1.5%), Ireland (0.4%), Norway 0.4%), and Romania (0.4%). Shortness of breath, dry cough, and tiredness were the most common initial symptoms in all diagnosis groups (**Figure 2A**).

The total time from initial symptom onset to a final diagnosis of pulmonary fibrosis, varied greatly amongst patients (**Figure 1C**). Overall, nearly 30% received a diagnosis within 3 months, with 31.3% patients with IPF receiving a diagnosis within 3 months, compared to 14.3% for sarcoidosis and 19.4% for other types of pulmonary fibrosis. Moreover, 40.2% of all patients had to wait a year or more to be diagnosed, with the largest difference between the proportion of patient with IPF (36.4%) and other types of pulmonary fibrosis (58.1%).

Stages of the Diagnostic Process

Stage 1: From Initial Symptom Onset to First Primary Care Assessment

More than half of respondents made a first appointment with a primary care physician within 3 months of symptom onset (52.0%), but nearly 30% waited more than 6 months (**Figure 1B**, stage 1). A number of patients responded that they did not delay visiting their doctor (26.7%).

Of all patients with a delay in stage 1 of 6 months or less ($n = 177$), 65.0% reported a total time to diagnosis of 1 year or less. Where patients with a delay of more than 6 months ($n = 72$) in this stage, only 34.7% reported being diagnosed within a year.

There were a variety of reasons for delays (**Figure 2B**). In a large number of cases, patients delayed seeking medical advice because they were not concerned about their symptoms. Patients believed symptoms were related to other causes (e.g., cold, smoking, stress; 35.2%), related to age (25.6%), or due to another established disease (5.1%). The main reasons that triggered patients to make an appointment with their primary care physician were worries about their symptoms, including shortness of breath (45.1%), cough (31.9%), and fatigue (20.9%) (**Figure 2C**). For 18.7% of patients, it was the impact of symptoms on their daily activities, especially on physical activity (e.g., sports, climbing stairs, walking, household, gardening) and work-related activities that led them to consult their primary care physician. In addition, some patients were prompted to make an appointment following the suggestion from family members or friends (22.7%), or another physician (7%).

Stage 2: From Start of Primary Care Assessment to Referral to Pulmonologist

At the first primary care appointment, a variety of actions were taken by the treating physicians. Almost half of all patients were referred to a pulmonologist (**Figure 3**). Other reported physician's actions included additional tests (19.0%), treatment for another disease (16.5%), and referral to other specialists rather than a pulmonologist (10.3%). Overall, the majority (73.3%) of patients were referred to a pulmonologist within three primary care visits, but for 9.9% of patients it took six or more appointments (**Figure 1B**, stage 2).

Comparing the different diagnosis groups, 43.2% of IPF patients were referred to a pulmonologist after one primary care visit. This was lower for those with sarcoidosis (28.6%) and other types of pulmonary fibrosis (25.8%). Furthermore, 39.3% of sarcoidosis patients were referred after six or more primary care visits, compared to 6.6% of IPF and 6.7% of other fibrosis types in this cohort.

Stage 3: From Referral to First Hospital Appointment

Once patients were referred to a pulmonary specialist, 76.9% of all patients had their first visit within 3 months (**Figure 1B**, stage 3). This was lower for the subgroup of sarcoidosis patients (50.0%) compared to IPF (79.9%), and other types of pulmonary fibrosis (80.6%). Few IPF patients (2.3%) had a delay of more than a year from referral to first hospital appointment, in contrast to almost a third of the sarcoidosis patients (32.1%). All patients with other types of pulmonary fibrosis were assessed within a year of the referral.

Stage 4: From First Hospital Appointment to Diagnosis Pulmonary Fibrosis

The 273 respondents underwent a total of 1,232 diagnostic tests in the hospital (**Table 1**). The majority of patients reported having performed spirometry ($n = 246$), blood tests ($n = 222$) and

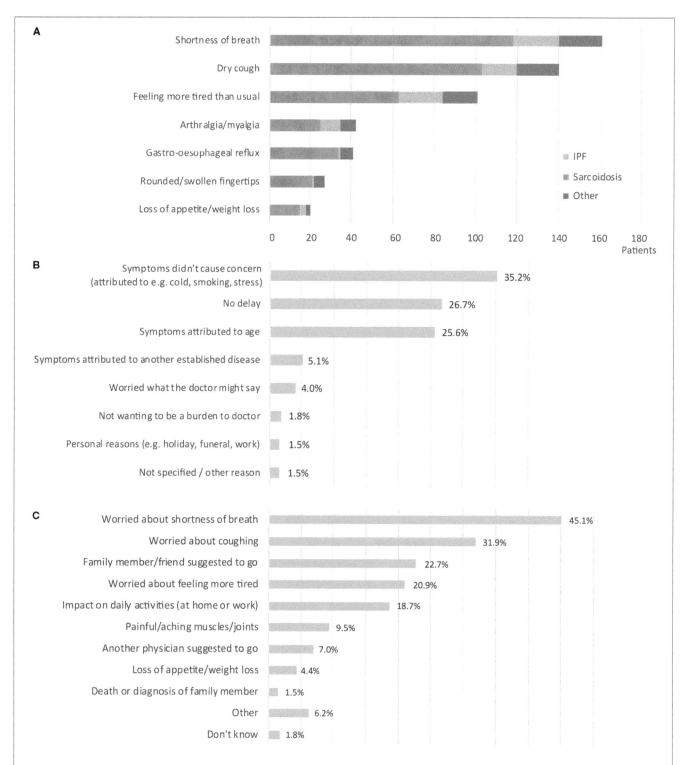

FIGURE 2 | Patient symptoms and motives in stage 1. **(A)** Number of patients (*n* =) reporting a specific symptom at onset. Bars are divided into diagnosis groups (total responses *n* = 532). **(B)** Reason to delay the initial primary care appointment (*n* = 277). **(C)** Reason to schedule the initial primary care appointment (*n* = 463). Percentages do not add up to 100% as more than one response was allowed. IPF, idiopathic pulmonary fibrosis.

chest imaging (X-ray *n* = 209; CT scan *n* = 201) without large differences in proportions between the diagnosis subgroups. Other tests reported included assessment of 6-min walk test (*n* = 149), lung biopsy (*n* = 125), and bronchoaveolar lavage (*n* = 74). Lung biopsy was more frequently reported by sarcoidosis patients compared to the other subgroups.

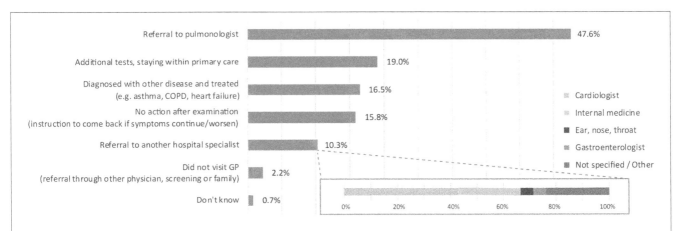

FIGURE 3 | Action of physician at first visit primary care. Percentages do not add up to 100% as more than one response was allowed. Total responses *n* = 306. COPD, chronic obstructive pulmonary disease; GP, general practitioner.

TABLE 1 | Performed tests in hospital before diagnosis.

Tests	IPF (*n* = 214)		Sarcoidosis (*n* = 28)		Other type (*n* = 31)	
	n =	% of patients in subgroup	*n* =	% of patients in subgroup	*n* =	% of patients in subgroup
Spirometry	194	90.7%	24	85.7%	28	90.3%
Blood tests	168	78.5%	26	92.9%	28	90.3%
Chest X-ray	161	75.2%	22	78.6%	26	83.9%
CT scan	156	72.9%	19	67.9%	26	83.9%
6-min walk test	120	56.1%	10	35.7%	19	61.3%
Lung biopsy	93	43.5%	19	67.9%	13	41.9%
Bronchoaveolar lavage	49	22.9%	11	39.3%	14	45.2%
Other/Don't know	5	2.3%	1	3.6%	-	-
Tests per patient (mean)	*4.4*		*4.7*		*5.0*	

Number of patients (n =) reporting a specific diagnostic test. Percentages do not add up to 100% as more than one response was allowed. CT, Computed tomography; IPF, idiopathic pulmonary fibrosis.

Although the final diagnosis was made within 3 months of the first hospital appointment for 62.6% of the 273 patients (**Figure 1B**, stage 4), 21.6% took between 3 months and 1 year, and 13.2% took over 1 year; 2.6% did not know how long this took. Small differences were found between the proportion of patients in each diagnosis group who were diagnosed within 3 months (IPF 64.5%, sarcoidosis 50.0%, and other pulmonary fibrosis types 61.3%) and more than 1 year after the first hospital appointment (IPF 11.2%, sarcoidosis 21.4%, and other pulmonary fibrosis types 19.4%).

Experiences and Recommendations
Information Provision
We assessed the patient perceptions on the information provided at the different stages in the diagnostic pathway. During assessment at the hospital (stage 4), 13.6% of patients reported not knowing why certain diagnostic tests were being performed. Almost a quarter (23.6%) of all patients felt they received insufficient information. At diagnosis, most patients (75.6%) received an explanation about their diagnosis from a physician and/or specialist nurse during a consultation. However, only 6.0% percent of patients received educational materials and 6.0%

received information related to support groups. A small number (3.0%) reported not having received any information at the time of diagnosis. In response to an open-ended question, patients reported that the discussion with their doctor or nurse was particularly valuable, as well as ongoing follow up appointments at the hospital and contact details to enable them to ask questions or reach out if they were feeling unwell.

The patients stated that they would have benefitted from more information during the diagnostic process, not only after the diagnosis was established. They would have welcomed more information before, at and after diagnosis on the following topics: differential diagnosis, diagnostic tests, available pharmacological, and non-pharmacological therapies, disease course, and prognosis. Respondents would have also liked more information on living with pulmonary fibrosis day-to-day, future perspectives, access to a psychologist, and information on peer support groups for patients and carers.

Emotional Experiences
Patients' perceptions and experiences were retrospectively assessed at different time points during their diagnostic journey. When describing their feelings after the onset of symptoms

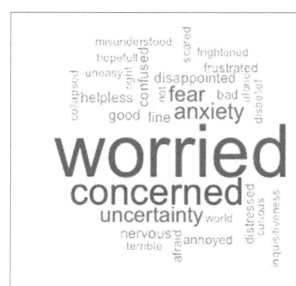

FIGURE 4 | Reported feelings during stage 3. Words grouped after coding, ones with minimum frequency of 2 are included in figure (*n* = 28). Full list (*n* = 62) can be found in **Supplementary Material 3**.

before their first doctor's visit (*n* = 179 responses), 65.4% of the respondents experienced negative emotions, 5.6% positive emotions, and the remainder (29.1%) were neutral. When asked to describe feelings after referral to the hospital (*n* = 240 responses), 74.6% of the responding patients experienced negative emotions at that time (16.7% neutral, 8.8% positive) (**Figure 4**).

Recommendations to Patients

Overall, the advice and tips offered by patients to those undiagnosed or living with pulmonary fibrosis were: seeking help early when you experience symptoms, pushing for a speedier diagnosis, seeking as much information as possible from healthcare professionals at all stages, taking regular exercise, joining pulmonary rehabilitation classes to assist with breathlessness, joining patient support groups, remaining positive, pacing themselves, and making the most of their time. General tips for fellow patients regarding mental well-being contained phrases such as: stay calm, stay positive, no stress, don't despair, don't give up, focus on the present, and don't get agitated, frustrated or anxious.

Recommendations to Healthcare

Advices to healthcare workers included performing tests earlier, providing more information and lifestyle advice, gaining more knowledge about pulmonary fibrosis, improving communication between healthcare workers, structuring the diagnostic process better, and earlier start of pharmacological and palliative treatment. More recommendations are listed as quotes in **Supplementary Material 4**.

DISCUSSION

The purpose of this survey was to document the time taken to diagnosis and to identify potential causes of delays at different

stages of the diagnostic pathway for pulmonary fibrosis patients in Europe. The second aim was to describe patients' experiences during this journey.

We found that the time to diagnosis varies widely. Only 30% of patients were diagnosed with pulmonary fibrosis within 3 months of symptom onset, while for over 40% of patients it took more than 1 year to be diagnosed. Other studies observed a median time from onset of first symptoms to diagnosis of 7 months (range 0–252) based on a patient survey (9) and 2.1 years (IQR 0.9–5.0) from a retrospective cohort study (5). In 2020, a group of ILD specialists reported a mean time from symptom onset to pulmonary fibrosis diagnosis of 2.3 years (Q1–Q3: 2–3) (19). The proportion of patients in our cohort who took more than a year to be diagnosed is smaller than that reported by other studies of pulmonary fibrosis patients (9, 11). Moreover, in a study of IPF patients, the median time to diagnosis was 13.6 months (range 5.9–39.5; max. 274.3) but 49% of the cohort received a diagnosis after more than 1 year (17). In another study, the median time for establishing a diagnosis was 1.5 years (range <1 week to 12 years) but this was calculated from the time of the first doctors' appointment rather than onset of symptoms (12). Compared to these historical studies, our results suggest fewer patients had such long delays from symptom onset to diagnosis.

Delays in diagnosis can occur at each stage of the patient journey and may be due to both patient- and healthcare-related causes. The longest delay we observed occurred in stage 1 (**Figure 1B**). More delay in this stage translated into a prolonged time to the final diagnosis. Our results show that only a quarter (26.7%) of all patients did not delay their initial appointment with their primary care physician. These findings are similar to results from a patient survey conducted in 2015 (9). A more recent survey amongst IPF patients reported a median delay of 0.1 years for this stage (5). From our survey, those who delayed their appointment reported they had not been concerned about their symptoms. This highlights the need to raise awareness of pulmonary fibrosis amongst the general public, so that individuals seek medical assistance earlier.

The time taken by people being treated in primary care (stage 2) varies. In our survey, almost 40% of patients were referred to a hospital specialist after their first primary care appointment, which is greater than that observed in a study conducted in the USA in 2015 (27.8%) (9). However, Hoyer et al. found that 80% of patients in Denmark (between 2016 and 2019) were referred after 1 or 2 visits to their general practitioner (5). These observations may reflect differences in healthcare systems or in awareness of pulmonary fibrosis between countries.

Of all respondents, 15.3% were referred after 4 or more appointments. Several factors may contribute to delays in primary care. Firstly, initial symptoms in the early stage of the disease can be non-specific and not yet known to be life threatening. In support of this, 42% of IPF patients had a normal lung function when initially assessed in primary care (18). Secondly, primary care physicians may suspect the symptoms to be due to more common respiratory diseases (such as asthma, pneumonia, bronchitis, allergies, and COPD [9]) and decide on a period of observation (20). Such misdiagnosis occurs in up to 41% of patients (5) and can prolong time to establish an ILD diagnosis (9, 10). Thirdly, primary care physicians may lack knowledge about pulmonary fibrosis. A study in Finland found almost half of referral letters lack key information related to possible ILD diagnosis (18). An e-learning for General Practitioners has recently been launched by the Royal College of General Practitioners in the United Kingdom and patient organisation APF to increase knowledge about symptoms and treatment of pulmonary fibrosis (21). In other countries, similar initiatives are evolving.

Stage 3 is the time between being referred and the patient's actual hospital appointment. Based on our data, 76.9% were assessed by a pulmonologist within 3 months, compared to 91% reported from a Finnish cohort (18). In this Finnish study only referral letters to tertiary care centres were evaluated, which may explain the higher percentage. However, in the United Kingdom and Ireland the time to secondary care respiratory clinic visit [47 days (25–84)] was significantly less than the time to an ILD specialist clinic visit [290 days (133–773)] (16). Given differences in the structure and complexities of healthcare systems, it is difficult to compare data from different countries. To our knowledge, there are no published data as to why delays in stage 3 occur. It may reflect waiting times or patients postponing a hospital clinic appointment.

Delays occurring from the first hospital appointment to final diagnosis (stage 4) can be partly explained by the number of diagnostic tests, access to them (22) and challenges in confirming a specific diagnosis accurately. Patients in our survey underwent on average 4.5 tests per person. The most common were spirometry, blood tests, and radiological chest imaging, similar to those reported by others (9, 14). The proportion of reported lung biopsies was surprisingly high in our cohort (41.9–67.9%), which may reflect variation in healthcare practises, as biopsy rates differ between countries [16.1–1.2% (2013–2019) in England (23), 34.1% in Germany (2012–2014) (24), 20.1% in Italy (2015–2017) (25)].

Several parameters may predict potential delays, as they are associated with an increased time to diagnosis. In our cohort patients with a final diagnosis of IPF experience shorter delays and undergo less invasive diagnostic testing than patients with other diagnoses. These differences may be due to IPF patients presenting with more severe symptoms initially, availability of the IPF international diagnostic guidelines, or availability of tests (22, 26). We can only speculate on this as we did not collect data on disease severity nor have powered for separate subgroup analyses. Another parameter that may influence time to diagnosis are the specific presenting symptoms. When patients present with dyspnoea, the median time to confirm an ILD diagnosis was 307 days, which increased for symptoms as cough and fatigue, to 563 and 639 days, respectively (15). Similarly, Pritchard et al. found an association between dyspnoea and a shorter time to hospital referral, which was not observed for lung crackles or chronic cough (8). Other factors that may contribute to a delayed diagnosis include presence of specific comorbidities, male sex, increased body mass index, older age, previous inhalation therapy use, preserved diffusing capacity and better St. George's Respiratory Questionnaire scores (5, 7, 16, 17). Lastly, abnormal chest imaging is one of the main reasons to

initiate a hospital referral from primary care (8, 18) and naming ILD on the thoracic CT radiologic report doubled the likelihood of a referral to a pulmonologist within 6 months (8). Interestingly, performing lung function tests in primary care, which indicated the possibility of ILD did not significantly influence time to CT scan or hospital referral (8).

Patients' Experiences

The pulmonary fibrosis journey to diagnosis generally involves extensive, repetitive, and sometimes invasive testing. Most patients in the survey reported that this causes a considerable burden, which can impact on emotional health, finances, and personal and professional life (9). Shortening the diagnostic journey and assessment at an ILD expert centre results in higher patient satisfaction (12). In addition, our survey highlighted the need to better inform patients during their diagnostic journey, to provide information on how to live with pulmonary fibrosis and advice on lifestyle changes at diagnosis. After diagnosis, providing information on perspectives, and options and discussions concerning symptom management should also be a priority as identified by our respondents. These observations are similar to those reported from surveys and in-depth patient interviews (27, 28). In one paper, authors highlighted that patients need time to come to terms with their diagnosis and that repeated provision of information was essential to fully understand the consequences and implications of their disease (11). However, a survey of ILD professionals in Europe showed that although two-thirds of specialist centres offered patient education only a few patients attended these existing programmes (10). Furthermore, only 6% of patients from our survey were informed about support groups, despite the value of peer support to patients and carers reported not only by our respondents but also from a previous patient survey (12). However, scientific evidence for the benefits of peer support is scarce (29). Regarding caregivers' needs, several patients in our survey highlighted the need to provide them with more information on the patient's experience and practical help on how best to support them (30). Finally, providing details of websites which offer reliable and accurate information is important as many websites contain incorrect or out-dated information (31).

Limitations

In this study, we used a variety of survey methods, which resulted in a good understanding of patients' perceptions and experiences. Nevertheless, using patient reported data is also a weakness of this study. A general limitation of open-ended questions is the variety of responses, which could not be included in the quantitative analysis. Limitations also include patient recall, non-response, and misinformation bias. These factors could have influenced the lung biopsies reported in our cohort, as patients may not differentiate between procedures such as endobronchial biopsies, surgical biopsies, or only bronchoscopy. As the responses were anonymous, we could not confirm information from medical records.

TABLE 2 | Strategies for improving the diagnostic pathway of pulmonary fibrosis patients.

	Stage 1	Stage 2	Stage 3	Stage 4	After diagnosis
Education and information	Increase awareness of PF amongst the general public.	Increase awareness of PF symptoms amongst primary care physicians and nurses.	Inform patients and policy makers on the need for urgency in hospital referral.	Inform patients about the reasons for diagnostic investigation and the differential diagnosis.	Inform patients about drug treatment, non-pharmaceutical treatment (rehabilitation, oxygen therapy, palliative care, lung transplant), prognosis and lifestyle
Improving standard care		Develop criteria for referral for chest CT scan or to a specialist when abnormalities on examination suggest PF.	Regular (virtual) MDDs between general hospital specialist and ILD experts.	Day case assessment with diagnostic investigations and clinical assessment.	Introduce psychological support, helplines and peer groups for patients as part of standard care.
		Better communication between primary care physician and ILD specialist.	Increase the number of ILD specialists in general hospitals.	Availability of DLCO measurement in all hospitals.	Discuss duration and frequency of follow-up visit.
Research areas	Identify the optimum way to provide information about PF to the general population.	Cost-effectiveness of performing chest CT scan in primary care or at community facilities.	Comparing waiting times and diagnostic pathway of PF to other uncommon diseases or disorders with poor prognosis [e.g., cancer (39)]		Assess caregivers' needs on counselling and support.

Content is based on survey outcomes, available literature, and authors' opinions. CT, computed tomography; DLCO, diffusing capacity for carbon monoxide; ILD, interstitial lung disease; IPF, idiopathic pulmonary fibrosis; MDD, multidisciplinary discussion; PF, pulmonary fibrosis.

Several factors prevent generalisation of these results to the overall population of patients with pulmonary fibrosis. We used a non-random sample of self-selecting pulmonary fibrosis patients invited via patient associations without a pre-defined number of invited patients, target, or countries. Most organisations have, until recently, focused on supporting and representing IPF patients, which likely accounts for the high number of IPF participants in this survey. Furthermore, patient characteristics, such as gender, age, comorbidities, and stage and/or severity of disease were not collected.

Although there are European guidelines for the diagnostic pathway of IPF and other ILDs, differences exist between countries (10). This may be related to the organisation of healthcare and options for primary care physicians to refer for CT scans or to ILD expertise centres. In our survey, we did not take these differences into account nor collect information on whether a CT chest scan was performed in primary care.

Recommendations Clinical Practice

There is an urgent need to improve the diagnostic journey and recommendations on how to achieve this have been raised in several papers (10, 12, 13). Our findings on patient satisfaction and diagnostic delay endorse this and encourage further improvement. Rapid diagnosis is becoming increasingly important because several treatments are currently available to slow disease progression, improve quality of life, and may extend life expectancy (32–34). Although there are guidelines and other guidance documents on

features, diagnosis, and management of ILD (26, 35–37) many patients have a diagnosis that is not confirmed by a multidisciplinary discussion and do not receive treatment (38). Additionally, geographical differences that may influence time to diagnosis and access to treatment still exists between countries (10).

In **Table 2**, we provide concrete strategies for each stage of the diagnostic journey to improve the standard clinical practise and patient satisfaction in order to promote a more rapid pathway for patients with pulmonary fibrosis throughout Europe. These strategies are based upon our survey outcomes, available literature, and expert authors' opinions. Awareness and education in general public, patients, and healthcare workers is a major topic in this field, as well as for other rare lung diseases (40).

CONCLUSION

From the onset of symptoms to diagnosis of pulmonary fibrosis, the patient journey involves delays at each stage of the diagnostic pathway. Most of these delays are avoidable. Based upon our findings, there is a particular need to raise awareness of pulmonary fibrosis in the general population. Additionally, patients' experiences highlight the need for understandable information concerning the diagnostic tests performed, differential diagnosis, final diagnosis, and treatments as well as peer support groups. Improving several aspects of the diagnostic pathway for pulmonary fibrosis is therefore warranted to minimise delays and improve patient satisfaction throughout Europe.

ETHICS STATEMENT

Ethical review and approval was not required for the study on human participants in accordance with the local legislation and institutional requirements. The patients/participants provided their written informed consent to participate in this study.

AUTHOR CONTRIBUTIONS

IvS organised the database and performed the statistical analysis. IvS and SJ wrote the first draught of the manuscript. IvS, SJ, DC

and HP wrote sections of the manuscript. All authors contributed to conception and design of the study and contributed to manuscript revision, read, and approved the submitted version.

ACKNOWLEDGEMENTS

The authors wish to thank W. M. Bramer from the Erasmus Medical Center Medical Library for developing the search strategies. The authors also wish to thank all patients and their carers for participating in the survey.

REFERENCES

1. Wijsenbeek M, Cottin V. Spectrum of fibrotic lung diseases. *N Engl J Med.* (2020) 383:958–68. doi: 10.1056/NEJMra2005230
2. Khor YH, Ng Y, Barnes H, Goh NSL, McDonald CF, Holland AE. Prognosis of idiopathic pulmonary fibrosis without anti-fibrotic therapy: a systematic review. *Eur Respir Rev.* (2020) 29:190158. doi: 10.1183/16000617.0158-2019
3. Olson AL, Gifford AH, Inase N, Fernandez Perez ER, Suda T. The epidemiology of idiopathic pulmonary fibrosis and interstitial lung diseases at risk of a progressive-fibrosing phenotype. *Eur Respir Rev.* (2018) 27:180077. doi: 10.1183/16000617.0077-2018
4. Gulati M. Diagnostic assessment of patients with interstitial lung disease. *Prim Care Respir J.* (2011) 20:120–7. doi: 10.4104/pcrj.2010.00079
5. Hoyer N, Prior TS, Bendstrup E, Wilcke T, Shaker SB. Risk factors for diagnostic delay in idiopathic pulmonary fibrosis. *Respir Res.* (2019) 20:103. doi: 10.1186/s12931-019-1076-0
6. Vasakova M, Mogulkoc N, Sterclova M, Zolnowska B, Bartos V, Plackova M, et al. Does timeliness of diagnosis influence survival and treatment response in idiopathic pulmonary fibrosis? Real-world results from the EMPIRE registry. *Eur Respir J.* (2017) 50. doi: 10.1183/1393003.congress-2017.PA4880
7. Lamas DJ, Kawut SM, Bagiella E, Philip N, Arcasoy SM, Lederer DJ. Delayed access and survival in idiopathic pulmonary fibrosis: a cohort study. *Am J Respir Crit Care Med.* (2011) 184:842–7. doi: 10.1164/rccm.201104-0668OC
8. Pritchard D, Adegunsoye A, Lafond E, Pugashetti JV, Digeronimo R, Boctor N, et al. Diagnostic test interpretation and referral delay in patients with interstitial lung disease. *Respir Res.* (2019) 20:253. doi: 10.1186/s12931-019-1228-2
9. Cosgrove GP, Bianchi P, Danese S, Lederer DJ. Barriers to timely diagnosis of interstitial lung disease in the real world: the INTENSITY survey. *BMC Pulm Med.* (2018) 18:9. doi: 10.1186/s12890-017-0560-x
10. Moor CC, Wijsenbeek MS, Balestro E, Biondini D, Bondue B, Cottin V, et al. Gaps in care of patients living with pulmonary fibrosis: a joint patient and expert statement on the results of a europe-wide survey. *ERJ Open Res.* (2019) 5:00124–2019. doi: 10.1183/23120541.00124-2019
11. Collard HR, Tino G, Noble PW, Shreve MA, Michaels M, Carlson B, et al. Patient experiences with pulmonary fibrosis. *Respir Med.* (2007) 101:1350–4. doi: 10.1016/j.rmed.2006.10.002
12. Schoenheit G, Becattelli I, Cohen AH. Living with idiopathic pulmonary fibrosis: an in-depth qualitative survey of European patients. *Chron Respir Dis.* (2011) 8:225–31. doi: 10.1177/1479972311416382
13. Bonella F, Wijsenbeek M, Molina-Molina M, Duck A, Mele R, Geissler K, et al. European IPF Patient Charter: unmet needs and a call to action for healthcare policymakers. *Eur Respir J.* (2016) 47:597–606. doi: 10.1183/13993003.01204-2015
14. Mooney J, Chang E, Lalla D, Papoyan E, Raimundo K, Reddy SR, et al. Potential delays in diagnosis of idiopathic pulmonary fibrosis in Medicare beneficiaries. *Ann Am Thorac Soc.* (2019) 16:393–6. doi: 10.1513/AnnalsATS.201806-376RL
15. Sköld CM, Arnheim-Dahlström L, Bartley K, Janson C, Kirchgaessler KU, Levine A, et al. Patient journey and treatment patterns in adults with IPF based on health care data in Sweden from 2001 to 2015. *Respir Med.* (2019) 155:72–8. doi: 10.1016/j.rmed.2019.06.001

16. Brereton CJ, Wallis T, Casey M, Fox L. Time taken from primary care referral to a specialist centre diagnosis of idiopathic pulmonary fibrosis: an opportunity to improve patient outcomes? *ERJ Open.* (2020) 6:00120–2020.doi: 10.1183/23120541.00120-2020
17. Snyder LD, Mosher C, Holtze CH, Lancaster LH, Flaherty KR, Noth I, et al. Time to diagnosis of idiopathic pulmonary fibrosis in the IPF-pro registry. *BMJ Open Respir Res.* (2020) 7(1):e000567. doi: 10.1136/bmjresp-2020-000567
18. Purokivi M, Hodgson U, Myllärniemi M, Salomaa ER, Kaarteenaho R. Are physicians in primary health care able to recognize pulmonary fibrosis? *Eur Clin Respir J.* (2017) 4:1290339. doi: 10.1080/20018525.2017.1290339
19. Wuyts WA, Papiris S, Manali E, Kilpeläinen M, Davidsen JR, Miedema J, et al. The burden of progressive fibrosing interstitial lung disease: a DELPHI approach. *Adv Ther.* (2020) 37:3246–64. doi: 10.1007/s12325-020-01384-0
20. Heins MJ, Schermer TRJ, de Saegher MEA, van Boven K, van Weel C, Grutters JC. Diagnostic pathways for interstitial lung diseases in primary care. *Prim Care Respir J.* (2012) 21:253–4. doi: 10.4104/pcrj.2012.00074
21. *Royal College of General Practitioners.* Available online at: https://elearning.rcgp.org.uk/course/view.php?id=409
22. Cottin V. Current approaches to the diagnosis and treatment of idiopathic pulmonary fibrosis in Europe: the AIR survey. *Eur Respir Rev.* (2014) 23:225–30. doi: 10.1183/09059180.00001914
23. Spencer LG, Loughenbury M, Chaudhuri C, Spiteri M, Parfrey H. Idiopathic pulmonary fibrosis in the United Kingdom: analysis of the british thoracic society electronic registry between 2013 and 2019. *ERJ Open Res.* (2020) 7:187–2020. doi: 10.1183/23120541.00187-2020
24. Behr J, Kreuter M, Hoeper MM, Wirtz H, Klotsche J, Koschel D, et al. Management of patients with idiopathic pulmonary fibrosis in clinical practice: the INSIGHTS-IPF registry. *Eur Respir J.* (2015) 46:186–96. doi: 10.1183/09031936.00217614
25. Poletti V, Vancheri C, Albera C, Harari S, Pesci A, Metella RR, et al. Clinical course of IPF in Italian patients during 12 months of observation: results from the FIBRONET observational study. *Respir Res.* (2021) 22:66. doi: 10.1186/s12931-021-01643-w
26. Raghu G, Remy-Jardin M, Myers JL, Richeldi L, Ryerson CJ, Lederer DJ, et al. Diagnosis of idiopathic pulmonary fibrosis. an official ATS/ERS/JRS/ALAT clinical practice guideline. *Am J Respir Crit Care Med.* (2018) 198:e44–68. doi: 10.1164/rccm.201807-1255ST
27. Senanayake S, Harrison K, Lewis M, McNarry M, Hudson J. Patients' experiences of coping with Idiopathic Pulmonary Fibrosis and their recommendations for its clinical management. *PLOS ONE.* (2018) 13:e0197660. doi: 10.1371/journal.pone.0197660
28. Overgaard D, Kaldan G, Marsaa K, Nielsen TL, Shaker SB, Egerod I. The lived experience with idiopathic pulmonary fibrosis: a qualitative study. *Eur Respir J.* (2016) 47:1472–80. doi: 10.1183/13993003.01566-2015
29. Magnani D, Lenoci G, Balduzzi S, Artioli G, Ferri P. Effectiveness of support groups to improve the quality of life of people with idiopathic pulmonary fibrosis a pre-post test pilot study. *Acta Biomed.* (2017) 88:5–12. doi: 10.23750/abm.v88i5-S.6870
30. Ramadurai D, Corder S, Churney T, Graney B, Harshman A, Meadows

S, et al. Understanding the informational needs of patients with IPF and their caregivers: 'You get diagnosed, and you ask this question right away, what does this mean?'. *BMJ Open Qual.* (2018) 7:e000207. doi: 10.1136/bmjoq-2017-000207

31. Fisher JH, O'Connor D, Flexman AM, Shapera S, Ryerson CJ. Accuracy and reliability of internet resources for information on idiopathic pulmonary fibrosis. *Am J Respir Crit Care Med.* (2016) 194:218–25. doi: 10.1164/rccm.201512-2393OC

32. Bolton CE, Bevan-Smith EF, Blakey JD, Crowe P, Elkin SL, Garrod R, et al. British Thoracic Society guideline on pulmonary rehabilitation in adults: accredited by NICE. *Thorax.* (2013) 68:ii1–ii30. doi: 10.1136/thoraxjnl-2013-203808

33. Susan SJ, Jerry AK, David JL, Marya G, Tanzib H, Ai-Yui MT, et al. Home oxygen therapy for adults with chronic lung disease. an official american thoracic society clinical practice guideline. *Am J Respir Crit Care Med.* (2020) 202:e121–41. doi: 10.1164/rccm.202009-3608ST

34. Flaherty KR, Wells AU, Cottin V, Devaraj A, Walsh SLF, Inoue Y, et al. Nintedanib in progressive fibrosing interstitial lung diseases. *N Engl J Med.* (2019) 381:1718–27. doi: 10.1056/NEJMoa1908681

35. Raghu G, Remy-Jardin M, Ryerson CJ, Myers JL, Kreuter M, Vasakova M, et al. Diagnosis of hypersensitivity pneumonitis in adults. an official ATS/JRS/ALAT clinical practice guideline. *Am J Respir Crit Care Med.* (2020) 202:e36–69. doi: 10.1164/rccm.202005-2032ST

36. Hoffmann-Vold AM, Maher TM, Philpot EE, Ashrafzadeh A, Distler O. Assessment of recent evidence for the management of patients with systemic sclerosis-associated interstitial lung disease: a systematic review. *ERJ Open Res.* (2021) 7: 00235–2020. doi: 10.1183/23120541.00235-2020

37. Travis WD, Costabel U, Hansell DM, King TE Jr, Lynch DA, Nicholson AG, et al. An official American Thoracic Society/European Respiratory Society statement: update of the international multidisciplinary classification of the idiopathic interstitial pneumonias. *Am J Respir Crit Care Med.* (2013) 188:733–48. doi: 10.1164/rccm.201308-1483ST

38. Maher TM, Molina-Molina M, Russell A-M, Bonella F, Jouneau S, Ripamonti E, et al. Unmet needs in the treatment of idiopathic pulmonary fibrosis—insights from patient chart review in five European countries. *BMC Pulm Med.* (2017) 17:124. doi: 10.1186/s12890-017-0468-5

39. van Harten WH, Goedbloed N, Boekhout AH, Heintzbergen S. Implementing large scale fast track diagnostics in a comprehensive cancer center, pre- and post-measurement data. *BMC Health Serv Res.* (2018) 18:85. doi: 10.1186/s12913-018-2868-5

40. Alfaro TM, Wijsenbeek MS, Powell P, Stolz D, Hurst JR, Kreuter M, et al. Educational aspects of rare and orphan lung diseases. *Respir Res.* (2021) 22:92. doi: 10.1186/s12931-021-01676-1

10

Efficiency of Therapeutic Plasma-Exchange in Acute Interstitial Lung Disease, Associated With Polymyositis/Dermatomyositis Resistant to Glucocorticoids and Immunosuppressive Drugs

Yaogui Ning[1,2], Guomei Yang[2], Yuechi Sun[3], Shiju Chen[3], Yuan Liu[3*] and Guixiu Shi[3*]*

Department of Intensive Care Unit, The First Affiliated Hospital of Xiamen University, Xiamen, China, [2] Medical College, Xiamen University, Xiamen, China, [3] Department of Rheumatology and Clinical Immunology, The First Affiliated Hospital of Xiamen University, Xiamen, China

*Correspondence:
Shiju Chen
shiju@xmu.edu.cn
Yuan Liu
liuyuan@xmu.edu.cn
Guixiu Shi
gshi@xmu.edu.cn

Interstitial lung disease (ILD) is a life-threating complication, commonly associated with polymyositis (PM), and dermatomyositis (DM). A subset of acute ILD associated with PM/DM patients are refractory to conventional treatment, and leads to a high rate of mortality. The efficacy of therapeutic plasma-exchange (TPE) as a PM/DM treatment to improve muscle involvement is controversial due to a lack of evidence. However, in recent reports, TPE has been effective in improving lung involvement. To evaluate the efficacy of this therapy, we retrospectively studied TPE treatment outcomes for in 18 acute PM/DM-ILD patients who were resistant to conventional therapies. Five patients were diagnosed with DM (27.8%), 11 with CADM (61.1%), and two with PM (11.1%). Among 18 patients, 11 (61.1%) achieved satisfactory improvement after four or more rounds of TPE, whereas seven died due to respiratory failure. We also analyzed risk factors to predict unresponsiveness to TPE in these patients. Notably, the prevalence of subcutaneous/mediastinal emphysema was significantly higher in the non-responsive group (6/7, 85.7%) than in the responsive group (2/11, 18.2%; $P = 0.013$); moreover, patients with this complication were mainly in the CADM subgroup (6/8, 75%). Subcutaneous/mediastinal emphysema and increased serum ferritin levels were shown to be poor prognostic factors, predictive of unresponsiveness to TPE, in PM/DM patients. No autoantibodies were found to be associated with TPE outcome, although we only investigated anti-Jo-1 and anti-Ro antibodies; the clinical significance of other myositis-specific autoantibodies, especially anti-melanoma differentiation-associated gene 5 (MDA5) antibody, is not known. Our results indicate that TPE might be an alternative treatment for acute PM/DM-ILD patients resistant to conventional therapies, except for those with subcutaneous/mediastinal emphysema and high serum ferritin levels.

Keywords: therapeutic plasma exchange, interstitial lung disease, dermatomyositis, polymyositis, efficiency

INTRODUCTION

Idiopathic inflammatory myopathy (IIM) is a group of heterogeneous inflammatory muscle disorders, which includes subacute, chronic, and acute IIM. IIM is characterized by low muscle strength and endurance, as well as inflammatory cell infiltration into the skeletal muscles (1). Based on distinct clinical features, IIM can be subdivided into dermatomyositis (DM), polymyositis (PM), and inclusion body myositis (IBM). Clinically amyopathic dermatomyositis (CADM) is also defined in recent years and classified as a subgroup of DM. DM and PM are the most common forms of IIM and are also life-threating in rheumatic diseases. Besides the muscle and skin, other vital organs such as the lung and heart can also be involved in PM/DM, and complications in these organs contribute to the high rate of mortality associated with these conditions. Interstitial lung disease (ILD) is one of the most common and life-threating complications of PM/DM, with a prevalence up to 86% (2–6). The survival rate of patients with PM/DM-ILD is 56.7% during the first year, and even lower in those with acute ILD (7). Further, patients with rapidly progressive ILD are often resistant to high-dose glucocorticoids and immunosuppressive agents (8), thereby resulting in acute fatal respiratory failure with a 6-months survival rate of 40.8–45.0% (9, 10). The lack of effective treatment strategies for PM/DM-ILD patients who are resistant to glucocorticoids and immunosuppressive agents is the main contributor to high mortality rates.

Therapeutic plasma exchange (TPE) is a blood purification method that removes circulating cytokines, immune complexes, immunoglobulins, and complement components. Since the 1980s, it has been used to manage autoimmune diseases (11). However, the efficiency of TPE as a treatment for IIM remains controversial, due to a lack of evidence regarding its significant effects on improving muscle involvement (12–15). TPE is still not considered a standard treatment procedure for IIM. However, in recent years, it has shown promise. A patient with acute ILD associated with PM/DM was successfully treated and several case studies reported significant improvements in lung involvement after TPE treatment (16–20). Although evidence for TPE efficacy in PM/DM-ILD is limited, its potential as an effective treatment strategy for this disease is worth exploring, especially for patients who are resistant to glucocorticoids, and immunosuppressive agents. For a better understanding of the benefits of this treatment, we retrospectively studied the efficacy of this therapy based on 18 patients with acute PM/DM-ILD who were resistant to conventional therapies and specifically focused on the clinical characteristics of those who benefited from TPE.

METHODS

Subjects

In this study, patients who were diagnosed with PM/DM-ILD resistant to conventional therapies and treated with TPE from January 2011 to May 2018 at the First Affiliated Hospital of Xiamen University were included. The conventional therapies included glucocorticoids and immunosuppressive agents. A total of 18 patients met the following inclusion criteria: (1) patients admitted into the intensive care unit (ICU) for ILD aggravation after failure of intensive treatment; (2) patients treated with TPE for more than four rounds. Patients with malignancy-associated disease, inclusion body myositis, and overlapping cases were excluded. The diagnosis of PM/DM was based on the Bohan and Peter diagnostic criteria, and diagnosis of clinically amyopathic dermatomyositis (CADM) was based on the diagnostic criteria of the European Neuromuscular Center international workshop (21), and the diagnosis of CADM, as a subtype of DM characterized by typical skin manifestations with little or no myositis, was based on the diagnostic criteria of the European Neuromuscular Center international workshop (22). CADM included both amyopathic dermatomyositis and hypomyopathic dermatomyositis. Amyopathic dermatomyositis is characterized by heliotrope rash, Gottron's papules, or Gottron's sign, and with normal creatine kinase (CK) and muscle biopsy results and no muscle weakness. Hypomyopathic dermatomyositis bears similar characteristic skin findings mentioned with no clinical evidence of muscle disease but mild changes in CK, magnetic resonance imaging (MRI), EMG, or muscle biopsy. Patients classified as having premyopathic dermatomyositis for whom fatal ILD developed within the first 6 months of their disease course were also included as CADM. All patients underwent muscle biopsies in the quadriceps. A chest high-resolution computed tomography (HRCT) was performed on each patient. ILD was diagnosed using HRCT imaging with the following qualitative criteria: signs of ground glass opacities, reticular abnormalities, traction bronchiectasis, irregular linear opacities, subpleural curvilinear shadows, and honeycombing. This retrospective study was approved by the Ethics Committee of the First Affiliated Hospital of Xiamen University, in accordance with the World Medical Association Declaration of Helsinki. Informed consent was obtained from either the patient or their authorized relative.

Data Collection

The electronic medical record of each patient was retrospectively reviewed. The following data were collected: information of patients' characteristics, such as age, sex, and disease course of PM/DM; clinical symptoms including IIM-related and pulmonary symptoms; occurrence of subcutaneous/mediastinal emphysema; Acute Physiology and Chronic Health Evaluation (APACHE) II score (23) during the first 24 h after admission to the ICU; type of immunosuppressive therapy administered; use of ventilator assistance; laboratory findings.

TPE Procedures

TPE procedures were performed every day for 3 days, and every other day after that, using the AQUARIUS multifiltrate machine (Edwards Lifesciences AG, Irvine, CA, USA). Intravenous methylprednisolone (40–80 mg/days) and oral immunosuppressive agents were administered as a combined maintenance therapy. For vascular access, a double coaxial lumen 14-Fr catheter was inserted percutaneously, either through the right or left femoral vein, using the Seldinger technique. The blood flow rate was 80 mL/min for TPE. Plasma (40–60 mL plasma/kg) was exchanged for the same volume of normal fresh frozen plasma each time. The duration of TPE was 3–4 h. The procedures were performed by trained nurses and supervised by senior physicians at the ICU. Treatment was suspended when a significant improvement in CT or death occurred.

Statistical Analysis

All statistical calculations were conducted using SPSS 23.0 software. Data are presented as the mean ± standard error of mean (SEM), or median (range) for continuous variables, and numbers (percentages) for qualitative variables. For comparisons between two groups, the chi-squared, or Fisher's exact tests were used for binary data and the Student's t- or Mann-Whitney U-tests were used for continuous data. Results of the logistic regression models are shown as the odds ratio (OR) and 95% confidence interval (CI). A $p < 0.05$ indicated statistical significance.

RESULTS

Efficacy of TPE for Acute PM/DM-ILD Patients Resistant to Conventional Therapies

This retrospective study included 18 patients who received TPE for the aggravation of ILD after treatment with a combination of high-dose glucocorticoids, cyclophosphamide, a calcineurin inhibitor, or intravenous immunoglobulin G. Five patients were diagnosed with DM (27.8%), 11 with CADM (61.1%), and two with PM (11.1%). The main respiratory symptom was dyspnea on exertion. Fine crackles were also observed in these patients. Although seven patients (38.9%) died from respiratory failure after TPE, the other 11 patients (61.1%) showed great improvement in lung involvement, reduced HRCT scores (24, 25), and their conditions were not life-threatening after treatment (**Figure 1**). These data suggested that TPE might be an alternative treatment strategy for acute PM/DM-ILD patients resistant to conventional therapies.

Clinical Characteristics of PM/DM-ILD Patients Responsive to TPE

We analyzed the characteristics and clinical profiles of the PM/DM-ILD patients whose conditions were improved by TPE. We divided PM/DM-ILD patients into responsive ($n = 11$) and non-responsive ($n = 7$) groups. Responsiveness was defined as improved or controlled lung involvement and rescue from life-threating complications, whereas non-responsiveness was defined as aggressive lung involvement and death. The clinical characteristics of the patients are summarized in **Table 1**.

No significant differences were observed between the responsive and non-responsive groups in terms of other clinical parameters such as age, types of IIM, and disease duration (**Table 1**). In the two groups, the most common IIM type was CADM (54.5 and 71.4%, respectively). Skin lesions were observed in nine cases in the responsive group (81.8%) and six in the non-responsive group (85.7%), including skin ulceration (three and three, respectively), palmar papules (four and three), oral erosions (one and zero), heliotrope rash (four and two), and Gottron papules (six and five). Skin ulceration, palmar papules,

and oral erosions are unique cutaneous phenotypes associated with the anti-melanoma differentiation associated protein 5 (MDA5) antibody (26); regarding these rashes, there were no significant differences between the two groups.

Notably, six patients (five CADM and one DM) of seven patients in the non-responsive group suffered from mediastinal emphysema; only two (one CADM and one DM) of 11 patients in the responsive-group had this complication. Patients with SP were mainly in the CADM subgroup (6/8, 75%). Three cases in the non-responsive group had SP concomitant subcutaneous emphysema. The prevalence of subcutaneous/mediastinal emphysema was significantly higher in the non-responsive group (85.7%) than in the responsive group (18.2%), suggesting that subcutaneous/mediastinal emphysema might be a treatment response predictor for TPE.

Laboratory Characteristics of PM/DM-ILD Patients Responsive to TPE

Laboratory findings of PM/DM-ILD patients receiving TPE are shown in **Table 2**. Antinuclear antibodies ($\geq$1: 100) were detected in three patients (16.7%). The myositis-specific autoantibody, anti-Jo-1, was present in only one patient (5.6%). Regarding myositis-associated autoantibodies, anti-SSA/Ro antibodies were identified in 12 patients (66.7%). In four patients (22.2%), no antibodies were detected. The CD4+/CD8+ T ratio was significantly higher in the responsive group than in the non-responsive group ($p = 0.049$), implying that TPE might have exerted little effects on PM/DM-ILD patients whose pathogeneses were mainly attributed to CD8+ T cells. Levels of C-reactive protein and serum ferritin were significantly lower in the responsive group than in the non-responsive group ($p = 0.031$ and $p = 0.002$, respectively). Besides the three mentioned parameters, no other significant differences between the groups were identified.

HRCT Findings in PM/DM-ILD Patients Responsive to TPE

HRCT imaging characteristics of all patients are shown in **Table 3**. Ground glass opacities, irregular linear opacities, and consolidation were the main image findings in these patients. No significant differences in HRCT features of PM/DM-ILD were observed between the responsive and non-responsive groups. The condition of most patients was too serious for them to undergo pulmonary function tests. **Figure 1** shows improvements in the CT scores of survivors before and after TPE treatment (2.414 ± 0.1379 and 1.073 ± 0.1236, respectively, $p < 0.0001$).

Risk Factors to Predict TPE Efficiency

We next evaluated the risk factors that could predict the unresponsiveness of PM/DM-ILD patients to TPE treatment. The results of univariate analysis revealed that four parameters, namely subcutaneous/mediastinal emphysema, CD4+/8+ ratio, and CRP and serum ferritin levels, were significantly different between the responsive and non-responsive groups. A multivariable logistic model was then established to predict the risk factors related to patient unresponsiveness to TPE

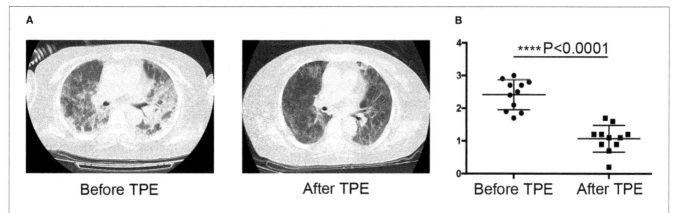

FIGURE 1 | Effect of therapeutic plasma exchange (TPE) on polymyositis (PM) and dermatomyositis interstitial lung disease (PM/DM-ILD) improvement. **(A)** Representative CT images of the lung before and after TPE. Lung CT scans of one patient before and after TPE. Interstitial opacities with multifocal ground glass opacities and consolidations (left panel). Follow-up CT scan indicating the frank regression of interstitial pneumonia (right panel). **(B)** CT score before and after TPE treatment in the responsive group ($n = 11$), ****$p < 0.0001$.

(**Table 4**). The results of logistic regression analyses showed that subcutaneous/mediastinal emphysema and serum ferritin levels were significantly associated with this in acute PM/DM-ILD patients who were resistant to conventional therapies. CRP levels and the CD4+/8+ ratio were found to be risk factors for death.

DISCUSSION

ILD is very common in PM/DM patients and can cause life-threatening complications even after standard treatments. A large proportion of patients with acute PM/DM-ILD show no response to conventional therapies including glucocorticoids and immunosuppressive agents, leading to uncontrolled and aggressive lung involvement and finally death due to respiratory failure. This is the first and largest retrospective study to analyze the efficacy of TPE therapy for acute PM/DM-ILD patients who were resistant to conventional therapies and to evaluate the risk factors that can predict unresponsiveness to this treatment. Our study showed that TPE might be an alternative treatment for acute PM/DM-ILD patients who are resistant to conventional therapies.

TPE was initially developed to treat liver failure and immune diseases. The use of TPE against PM/DM has been controversial for years. The American Society for Apheresis' indication category for TPE use in PM/DM was IV in the latest 2016 Therapeutic Apheresis guideline (27). To date, this recommendation is based on the results of a unique randomized controlled trial comprising 39 PM/DM patients by Miller et al. (12). In that study, there was no significant difference in final muscle strength or functional capacity following plasma exchange, leukapheresis, or sham apheresis. No concomitant immunosuppressants except glucocorticoids were administered to all patients. In 1981, Dau, in an uncontrolled trial, treated 35 inflammatory myopathy patients with TPE combined with immunosuppressants (cyclophosphamide or chlorambucil), and found improvement in muscle strength without significant side effects in 32 of them (13). Other retrospective multicenter studies have also demonstrated the efficiency of TPE in PM/DM.

Herson examined 38 PM/DM patients who were treated with TPE as a rescue therapy when conventional treatment failed, and observed improvements in muscle strength in 24 (63%) patients (14). Cherin investigated 27 patients who suffered from severe pharyngeal muscle weakness and were resistant to conventional therapy; eight (30%) reported the disappearance of symptoms, whereas the other 19 (70%) reported the stabilization of dysphagia after receiving TPE (15). Some case reports have also showed that TPE in association with immunosuppressant agents could play a relevant role in severe pharyngo-esophageal muscle weakness (28).

The effects of TPE on acute respiratory failure during ILD have not been fully established. In 2015, Omotoso published a report in which TPE was found to be beneficial for the treatment of a patient with ILD-associated antisynthetase syndrome who was refractory to glucocorticoids and other immunosuppressive therapeutics (17). Bozkirli also reported a case of antisynthetase syndrome with ILD who benefited from double-filtration plasmapheresis (16). The therapeutic effects of TPE also include the removal of pathological substances from the blood, such as autoantibodies, cytokines, complement components, and paraproteins. Further, other possible mechanisms include alterations to lymphocyte proliferation, the immune system, and cell sensitivity to immunosuppressants or chemotherapeutic agents (29–31). Although more data are necessary, TPE might be an immediate treatment option for acute PM/DM-ILD patients who are resistant to conventional therapies. Moreover, because TPE substitutes fresh frozen plasma components such as anti-idiotypic antibodies and immunoglobulins, which target host antigens, this therapy might provide additional therapeutic benefits (29). Clearly, TPE is only a short-term solution, because immune cells that secrete antibodies, complement components, and cytokines will continue to function in response to repeated antigenic stimulation after TPE. Moreover, the transient effects of TPE require additional long-term immunosuppression treatment. Another disadvantage of this therapy is risks associated with the use of blood products, including sexually transmitted diseases. Despite these drawbacks,

TABLE 1 | Comparison of clinical characteristics between PM/DM-ILD patients who were responsive and non-responsive to TPE.

Variables	Responsive group (n = 11)	Non-responsive group (n = 7)	P-value
Sex, male/female, n (%)	3/8 (27.3/72.7)	3/4 (42.9/57.1)	0.627
Age, years, mean ± SEM	55.70 ± 11.08	52.71 ± 11.46	0.540
DISEASE DURATION, WEEKS, MEDIAN (RANGE)			
at ILD diagnosis	3.0 (1–4)	3.2 (1.57–5.71)	0.328
at PM/DM/CADM diagnosis	13 (2.43–96)	6.86 (4–528)	0.536
IIM TYPE, n (%)			
PM/DM	2/3 (18.2/27.3)	0/2 (0/28.6)	0.952
CADM	6 (54.5)	5 (71.4)	0.637
CLINICAL SYMPTOM, n (%)			
Arthritis/arthralgia	4 (36.4)	1 (14.3)	0.596
Skin rash	9 (81.8)	6 (85.7)	1.000
Fever	3 (27.3)	2 (28.6)	1.000
Cough	4 (36.4)	3 (42.9)	1.000
Dyspnea on exertion	9 (81.8)	6 (85.7)	1.000
Dysphagia	3 (27.3)	1 (14.3)	1.000
Muscle weakness/myalgia	5 (45.5)	1 (14.3)	0.316
Subcutaneous/mediastinal emphysema n (%)	2 (18.2)*	6 (85.7)	0.013
APACHE II Score, median (range)	17 (11–24)	18.5 (15–31)	0.126
P/F ratio	218.8 ± 13.38	173.3 ± 21.38	0.074
THERAPY, n (%)			
High-dose steroids	11 (100)	7 (100)	NA
Cyclosporine A	8 (72.7)	5 (71.4)	1.000
Cyclophosphamide	6 (54.5)	2 (28.6)	0.367
Intravenous immunoglobulin G	6 (54.5)	5 (71.4)	0.637
Hydroxychloroquine	1 (9.1)	1 (14.3)	1.000
Methotrexate	1 (9.1)	0	0.611
Thalidomide	2 (18.2)	0	0.137
Total dosage of MP before TPE, mg (mean ± SEM)	460.9 ± 49.88	341.4 ± 61.81	0.153
Duration of MP use before TPE, days (mean ± SEM)	6.6 ± 0.3	6.4 ± 0.4	0.676
PLASMA EXCHANGE			
Times, median (range)	5 (4–24)	6 (4–10)	0.724
Plasma amount, mL, median (range)	3,000 (2,500–3,000)	3,000 (2,500–3,000)	0.724
Use of ventilator, n (%)	4 (36.4)	6 (85.7)	0.066

ILD, Interstitial lung disease; PM, polymyositis; DM, dermatomyositis; CADM, clinically amyopathic dermatomyositis; IIM, idiopathic inflammatory myopathy; SEM, standard error of mean; TPE, therapeutic plasma-exchange; APACHE II, Acute Physiology and Chronic Health Evaluation; MP, methylprednisolone; P/F, arterial partial pressure of oxygen /fraction of inspired oxygen. *p < 0.05.

no plasma-related adverse events were observed in patients after short-term treatment in the current study.

In the present study, a multivariable logistic model showed that subcutaneous/mediastinal emphysema and serum ferritin levels were significantly associated with unresponsiveness to TPE. A previous study showed that serum ferritin level is the most significant prognostic factor for PM/DM (32). Moreover, serum ferritin was found to predict the disease severity and prognosis for anti-MDA5 antibody-associated ILD with DM; a serum ferritin concentration cut-off value of 1,600 μg/L was suggested to be the best indicator of survival in this subgroup (33). In the present study, the average ferritin level in the unresponsiveness group was 1518.6 μg/L, almost equal to that value. However, the lack of an anti-MDA5 antibody test did not allow us to conclude whether patients in the unresponsiveness group had anti-MDA5

antibody-associated ILD. In addition, PM/DM-ILD patients with hyperferritinemia might be unresponsive to TPE when resistant to conventional therapies.

Subcutaneous/mediastinal emphysema was found to be another potential prognostic factor associated with TPE outcome in our study. DM/PM patients are mostly predisposed to develop spontaneous pneumomediastinum with a prevalence ranging from 2.2 to 8.6% (10, 34–36). Spontaneous pneumomediastinum can be fatal if unrecognized and can lead to death within 2 months in approximately 25% of patients (34, 35); further, it is more prevalent in patients with CADM (34). In this retrospective study, six patients with spontaneous pneumomediastinum (6/8, 75%) were diagnosed with CADM. CADM patients should be carefully screened for spontaneous pneumomediastinum since the latter is a prognostic factor. A previous study also

TABLE 2 | Comparison of laboratory characteristics between responsive and non-responsive groups of PM/DM-ILD patients.

Clinical parameters	Responsive group (*n* = 11)	Non-responsive group (*n* = 7)	P-value
Lymphocytes, ×10⁹/L, median (range)	0.69 (0.38–9.50)	0.60 (0.12–1.16)	0.285
CD4+/8+ T ratio, mean ± SEM	2.01 + 0.58*	1.29 ± 0.87	0.049
Platelet count, ×10⁹/L, mean ± SEM	224.819 ± 85.427	203.571 ± 91.874	0.894
Erythrocyte sedimentation rate, mm/h, median (range)	29 (2–105)	30 (1–64)	0.660
C-reactive protein, mg/L, mean ± SEM	6.506 ± 5.056*	15.281 ± 8.170	0.031
Serum ferritin, μg/L, median (range)	414.6 (78.1–3659.4)*	1518.6 (984.2–3819.2)	0.002
IL-6, pg/mL, median (range)	3.58 (0.07–35.50)	19.77 (5.99–832)	0.247
Procalcitonin (PCT), ng/mL, median (range)	0.710 (0.037–0.655)	0.125 (0.036–7.520)	0.151
Serum albumin (ALB), mg/L, mean ± SEM	31.960 ± 3.289	32.486 ± 3.023	0.204
Alanine aminotransferase (ALT), IU/L, median (range)	99 (20–142)	60 (26–439)	0.659
Aspartate aminotransferase (AST), IU/L, median (range)	64 (20–100.5)	60 (24–467)	0.860
Creatine kinase, IU/L, median (range)	80 (10–3,794)	83 (46–770)	0.930
Lactate dehydrogenase (LDH), IU/L, median (range)	412 (58–1,337)	491 (312–2,032)	0.375
Creatine, IU/L, mean ± SEM	54.82 ± 21.10	107.14 ± 128.4	0.325
Positive antinuclear antibody, *n* (%)	3(27.3)	0	0.245
Positive anti-Jo-1 antibody, *n* (%)	1(9.1)	0	0.611
Anti-SSA antibody, positivity, *n* (%)	7 (63.5)	5 (71.4)	1.000
Anti Ro-52 antibody, *n* (%)	7 (63.5)	4 (57.1)	1.000
Immunoglobulin A, mg/dL, median (range)	1.78 (1.39–3.55)	1.91 (0.72–3.65)	1.000
Immunoglobulin M, mg/dL, median (range)	1.45 (0.765–2.05)	1.100 (0.245–8.900)	0.425
Immunoglobulin G, mg/dL, mean ± SEM	14.84 ± 5.97	8.75 ± 6.15	0.894

*$p < 0.05$. SEM, standard error of mean; ILD, interstitial lung disease; PM, polymyositis; DM, dermatomyositis.

TABLE 3 | Comparison of HRCT findings between responsive and non-responsive groups of PM/DM-ILD patients.

CT findings	Responsive group (*n* = 11)	Non-responsive group (*n* = 7)	P-value
Consolidation, *n* (%)	9 (81.8)	6 (85.7)	1.000
Ground glass opacities, *n* (%)	5 (45.5)	5 (71.4)	0.367
Irregular linear opacities, *n* (%)	8 (72.7)	5 (71.4)	1.000
Traction bronchiectasis, *n* (%)	0	2 (28.6)	0.137
Honeycombing, *n* (%)	1 (9.1)	1 (14.3)	1.000
Subpleural curvilinear shadows, *n* (%)	0	1 (14.3)	0.389

ILD, interstitial lung disease; PM, polymyositis; DM, dermatomyositis; HRCT, high-resolution computed tomography.

TABLE 4 | Adjusted odds ratios (ORs) with associated 95% confidence interval (95%CI) for death.

Variables	Death		
	OR	95%CI	P-value
CD4+/8+ T cell ratio	0.188	0.030–1.164	0.072
C-reactive protein (mg/L)	1.351	0.972–1.878	0.073
Subcutaneous/mediastinal emphysema	15.185	1.233–186.983	0.034*
Serum ferritin (μg/L)†	5.683	1.110–29.101	0.037*

*$p < 0.05$. Model was adjusted for sex and age.
†OR and 95% CI are expressed by standard deviation increases in serum ferritin.

demonstrated that anti-MDA5 antibodies are associated with spontaneous pneumomediastinum (35). Spontaneous pneumomediastinum increases the risk of death in DM patients with anti-MDA5 antibody-associated ILD (37). These findings again indicate that anti-MDA5 antibodies might be associated with TPE outcome. However, anti-MDA5 and other myositis-specific autoantibodies were not investigated in the present study. In the responsive group, two patients suffered from spontaneous pneumomediastinum and one patient died due to respiratory failure several months after discharge from the hospital. Taken together, these results suggest that spontaneous pneumomediastinum is a poor prognostic factor for TPE and

that patients who suffer from this could comprise a population that should be excluded from TPE treatment.

There are some limitations to the present retrospective study. The high cost of TPE imposed restrictions on its application, thus limiting the size of our patient sample size. Further, the lack of data on most myositis-specific antibodies, and especially anti-MDA5 antibody testing, in these patients did not allow us to conclude whether the anti-MDA5 antibody was a predictive factor of TPE outcome. It was reported that forced vital capacity is a poor predictive factor for survival with ILD (38). In this retrospective study, pulmonary function tests including carbon monoxide-diffusing capacity were unavailable due to the patients' severe disease states. Moreover, measurements of Krebs von den Lungen-6 levels were not performed; therefore, the severity of

ILD could not be assessed. Those limitations resulted in these important parameters being excluded from predictive evaluation.

In conclusion, this retrospective study shows promise regarding the use of TPE in addition to glucocorticoids and immunosuppressants for early-stage PM/DM-ILD. Further, subcutaneous/mediastinal emphysema and serum ferritin levels might serve as poor prognostic factors of responsiveness to TPE. More controlled trials and long-term observations are required in the future.

ETHICS STATEMENT

This study was carried out in accordance with the recommendations of the Ethics Committee of the First Affiliated Hospital of Xiamen University with written informed consent

from all subjects. All subjects gave written informed consent in accordance with the Declaration of Helsinki.

AUTHOR CONTRIBUTIONS

YN, SC, and GS conceived and designed this study. YN and YL were responsible for the integrity of the study, interpretation of data, and drafting of the manuscript. YN, GY, and YS participated in medical record collection. All authors reviewed and approved the manuscript for submission.

ACKNOWLEDGMENTS

We are extremely grateful to all the patients and their authorized relatives who participated in this study, as well as the complete rheumatology and ICU teams and medical record system personnel.

REFERENCES

1. Plotz PH, Dalakas M, Leff RL, Love LA, Miller FW, Cronin ME. Current concepts in the idiopathic inflammatory myopathies: polymyositis, dermatomyositis, and related disorders. Ann Intern Med. (1989) 111:143–57.
2. Fathi M, Lundberg IE. Interstitial lung disease in polymyositis and dermatomyositis. Curr Opin Rheumatol. (2005) 17:701–6. doi: 10.1097/01.bor.0000179949.65895.53
3. Fathi M, Lundberg IE, Tornling G. Pulmonary complications of polymyositis and dermatomyositis. Semin Respir Crit Care Med. (2007) 28:451–8. doi: 10.1055/s-2007-985666
4. Morisset J, Johnson C, Rich E, Collard HR, Lee JS. Management of myositis-related interstitial lung disease. Chest. (2016) 150:1118–28. doi: 10.1016/j.chest.2016.04.007
5. Marie I, Lahaxe L, Benveniste O, Delavigne K, Adoue D, Mouthon L, et al. Long-term outcome of patients with polymyositis/ dermatomyositis and anti-PM-Scl antibody. Br J Dermatol. (2010) 162:337–44. doi: 10.1111/j.1365-2133.2009.09484.x
6. Douglas WW, Tazelaar HD, Hartman TE, Hartman RP, Decker PA, Schroeder DR, et al. Polymyositis-dermatomyositis-associated interstitial lung disease. Am J Respir Crit Care Med. (2001) 164:1182–5. doi: 10.1164/ajrccm.164.7.2103110
7. Chen IJ, Jan Wu YJ, Lin CW, Fan KW, Luo SF, Ho HH, et al. Interstitial lung disease in polymyositis and dermatomyositis. Clin Rheumatol. (2009) 28:639–46. doi: 10.1007/s10067-009-1110-6
8. Schnabel A, Reuter M, Biederer J, Richter C, Gross WL. Interstitial lung disease in polymyositis and dermatomyositis: clinical course and response to treatment. Semin Arthritis Rheum. (2003) 32:273–84. doi: 10.1053/sarh.2002.50012
9. Mukae H, Ishimoto H, Sakamoto N, Hara S, Kakugawa T, Nakayama S, et al. Clinical differences between interstitial lung disease associated with clinically amyopathic dermatomyositis and classic dermatomyositis. Chest. (2009) 136:1341–7. doi: 10.1378/chest.08-2740
10. Ye S, Chen XX, Lu XY, Wu MF, Deng Y, Huang WQ, et al. Adult clinically amyopathic dermatomyositis with rapid progressive interstitial lung disease: a retrospective cohort study. Clin Rheumatol. (2007) 26:1647–54. doi: 10.1007/s10067-007-0562-9
11. Dequeker J, Geusens P, Wielands L. Short and longterm experience with plasmapheresis in connective tissue diseases. Biomedicine. (1980) 32:189–94.
12. Miller FW, Leitman SF, Cronin ME, Hicks JE, Leff RL, Wesley R, et al. Controlled trial of plasma exchange and leukapheresis in polymyositis and dermatomyositis. N Engl J Med. (1992) 326:1380–4. doi: 10.1056/NEJM199205213262102
13. Dau PC. Plasmapheresis in idiopathic inflammatory myopathy: experience with 35 patients. JAMA Neurol. (1981) 38:544–52. doi: 10.1001/archneur.1981.00510090038003
14. Herson S, Lok C, Roujeau JC, Coutellier A, Etienne SD, Revuz J, et al. Plasma exchange in dermatomyositis and polymyositis. Retrospective study of 38 cases of plasma exchange. Ann Med Interne. (1989) 140:453–5.
15. Cherin P, Auperin I, Bussel A, Pourrat J, Herson S. Plasma exchange in polymyositis and dermatomyositis: a multicenter study of 57 cases. Clin Exp Rheumatol. (1995) 13:270–1.
16. Bozkirli DEE, Kozanoglu I, Bozkirli E, Yucel E. Antisynthetase syndrome with refractory lung involvement and myositis successfully treated with double filtration plasmapheresis. J Clin Apher. (2013) 28:422–5. doi: 10.1002/jca.21285
17. Omotoso BA, Ogden MI, Balogun RA. Therapeutic plasma exchange in antisynthetase syndrome with severe interstitial lung disease. J Clin Apher. (2015) 30:375–9.
18. Fujita Y, Fukui S, Suzuki T, Ishida M, Endo Y, Tsuji S, et al. Anti-MDA5 antibody-positive dermatomyositis complicated by autoimmune-associated hemophagocytic syndrome that was successfully treated with immunosuppressive therapy and plasmapheresis. Intern Med. (2018) 57:3473–78. doi: 10.2169/internalmedicine.1121-18
19. Endo Y, Koga T, Suzuki T, Hara K, Ishida M, Fujita Y, et al. Successful treatment of plasma exchange for rapidly progressive interstitial lung disease with anti-MDA5 antibody-positive dermatomyositis: a case report. Medicine. (2018) 97:e0436. doi: 10.1097/MD.0000000000010436
20. Yagishita M, Kondo Y, Terasaki T, Terasaki M, Shimizu M, Honda F, et al. Clinically amyopathic dermatomyositis with interstitial pneumonia that was successfully treated with plasma exchange. Intern Med. (2018) 57:1935–8. doi: 10.2169/internalmedicine.0297-17
21. Bohan A, Peter JB, Bohan A, Peter JB. Polymyositis and dermatomyositis. Parts 1 and 2. N Engl J Med. (1975) 292:344–7. doi: 10.1056/NEJM197502132920706
22. Bailey EE, Fiorentino DF. Amyopathic dermatomyositis: definitions, diagnosis, and management. Curr Rheumatol Rep. (2014) 16:1–7. doi: 10.1007/s11926-014-0465-0
23. Knaus WA, Draper EA, Wagner DP, Zimmerman JE. APACHE II: a severity of disease classification system. Crit Care Med. (1985) 13:818–29. doi: 10.1097/00003246-198510000-00009
24. Ichikado K, Suga M, Muranaka H, Gushima Y, Miyakawa H, Tsubamoto M, et al. Prediction of prognosis for acute respiratory distress syndrome with thin-section CT: validation in 44 cases. Radiology. (2006) 238:321–9. doi: 10.1148/radiol.2373041515
25. Ichikado K, Suga M, Muller NL, Taniguchi H, Kondoh Y, Akira M, et al. Acute interstitial pneumonia: comparison of high-resolution computed tomography findings between survivors and non-survivors. Am J Respir Crit Care Med. (2002) 165:1551–6. doi: 10.1164/rccm.2106157
26. Muro Y, Sugiura K, Akiyama M. Cutaneous manifestations in dermatomyositis: Key clinical and serological features-a comprehensive review. Clin Rev Allergy Immunol. (2016) 51:293–302. doi: 10.1007/s12016-015-8496-5

27. Schwartz J, Padmanabhan A, Aqui N, Balogun RA, Connelly-Smith L, Delaney M, et al. Guidelines on the use of therapeutic apheresis in clinical practice—evidence-based approach from the Writing Committee of the American society for apheresis: the seventh special issue. *J Clin Apher.* (2016) 31:149–62. doi: 10.1002/jca.21470

28. Cozzi F, Marson P, Pigatto E, Tison T, Polito P, Galozzi P, et al. Plasma-exchange as a "rescue therapy" for dermato/polymyositis in acute phase. Experience in three young patients. *Transfus Apher Sci.* (2015) 53:368–72. doi: 10.1016/j.transci.2015.07.005

29. Reeves HM, Winters JL. The mechanisms of action of plasma exchange. *Br J Haematol.* (2014) 164:342–51. doi: 10.1111/bjh.12629

30. Nakamura T, Ushiyama C, Suzuki S, Shimada N, Ebihara I, Suzaki M, et al. Effect of plasma exchange on serum tissue inhibitor of metalloproteinase 1 and cytokine concentrations in patients with fulminant hepatitis. *Blood Purif.* (2000) 18:50–4. doi: 10.1159/000014407

31. Toft P, Schmidt R, Broechner AC, Nielsen BU, Bollen P, Olsen KE. Effect of plasmapheresis on the immune system in endotoxin-induced sepsis. *Blood Purif.* (2008) 26:145–50. doi: 10.1159/000113507

32. Ishizuka M, Watanabe R, Ishii T, Machiyama T, Akita K, Fujita Y, et al. Long-term follow-up of 124 patients with polymyositis and dermatomyositis: statistical analysis of prognostic factors. *Mod Rheumatol.* (2016) 26:115–20. doi: 10.3109/14397595.2015.1054081

33. Gono T, Kawaguchi Y, Satoh T, Kuwana M, Katsumata Y, Takagi K,
et al. Clinical manifestation and prognostic factor in anti-melanoma differentiation-associated gene 5 antibody-associated interstitial lung disease as a complication of dermatomyositis. *Rheumatology.* (2010) 49:1713–9. doi: 10.1093/rheumatology/keq149

34. Le Goff B, Cherin P, Cantagrel A, Gayraud M, Hachulla E, Laborde F, et al. Pneumomediastinum in interstitial lung disease associated with dermatomyositis and polymyositis. *Arthritis Rheum.* (2009) 61:108–18. doi: 10.1002/art.24372

35. Ma X, Chen Z, Hu W, Guo Z, Wang Y, Kuwana M, et al. Clinical and serological features of patients with dermatomyositis complicated by spontaneous pneumomediastinum. *Clin Rheumatol.* (2016) 35:489–93. doi: 10.1007/s10067-015-3001-3

36. Kono H, Inokuma S, Nakayama H, Suzuki M. Pneumomediastinum in dermatomyositis: association with cutaneous vasculopathy. *Ann Rheum Dis.* (2000) 59:372–6. doi: 10.1136/ard.59.5.372

37. Yamaguchi K, Yamaguchi A, Itai M, Kashiwagi C, Takehara K, Aoki S, et al. Clinical features of patients with anti-melanoma differentiation-associated gene-5 antibody-positive dermatomyositis complicated by spontaneous pneumomediastinum. *Clin Rheumatol.* (2019). doi: 10.1007/s10067-019-04729-5. [Epub ahead of print].

38. Kang EH, Lee EB, Shin KC, Im CH, Chung DH, Han SK, et al. Interstitial lung disease in patients with polymyositis, dermatomyositis and amyopathic dermatomyositis. *Rheumatology.* (2005) 44:1282–6. doi: 10.1093/rheumatology/keh723

11

Hypersensitivity Pneumonitis: Diagnostic and Therapeutic Challenges

Maria Laura Alberti [1], Emily Rincon-Alvarez [2], Ivette Buendia-Roldan [3] and Moises Selman [3]*

[1] *Hospital María Ferrer, Buenos Aires, Argentina,* [2] *Fundación Neumológica Colombiana, Bogotá, Colombia,* [3] *Instituto Nacional de Enfermedades Respiratorias "Ismael Cosío Villegas", Mexico City, Mexico*

*Correspondence:
Moises Selman
mselmanl@yahoo.com.mx

Hypersensitivity pneumonitis (HP) is one of the most common interstitial lung diseases (ILD), that presents unique challenges for a confident diagnosis and limited therapeutic options. The disease is triggered by exposure to a wide variety of inciting antigens in susceptible individuals which results in T-cell hyperactivation and bronchioloalveolar inflammation. However, the genetic risk and the pathogenic mechanisms remain incompletely elucidated. Revised diagnostic criteria have recently been proposed, recommending to classify the disease in fibrotic and non-fibrotic HP which has strong therapeutic and outcome consequences. Confident diagnosis depends on the presence of clinical features of ILD, identification of the antigen(s), typical images on high-resolution computed tomography (HRCT), characteristic histopathological features, and lymphocytosis in the bronchoalveolar lavage. However, identifying the source of antigen is usually challenging, and HRCT and histopathology are often heterogeneous and not typical, supporting the notion that diagnosis should include a multidisciplinary assessment. Antigen removal and treating the inflammatory process is crucial in the progression of the disease since chronic persistent inflammation seems to be one of the mechanisms leading to lung fibrotic remodeling. Fibrotic HP has a few therapeutic options but evidence of efficacy is still scanty. Deciphering the molecular pathobiology of HP will contribute to open new therapeutic avenues and will provide vital insights in the search for novel diagnostic and prognostic biomarkers.

Keywords: lung fibrosis, risk factors, hypersensitivity pneumonitis, prognostic factors, diagnosis

INTRODUCTION

Hypersensitivity Pneumonitis (HP) is an immune-mediated disease that manifests as interstitial lung disease (ILD) in susceptible individuals after exposure to identified or unidentified inciting agent(s) (1). The disease has a heterogeneous clinical presentation, as well as varied radiological and morphological patterns likely associated with the individual genetic susceptibility, type of antigen, the extent of exposure, and the interaction with other injuring factors (2, 3).

The genetic susceptibility that increases the risk to develop the disease is unclear, and most studies have focuses on polymorphisms in the Major Histocompatibility Complex class II (HLA-DR and HLA-DQ) molecules which are involved in the presentation of antigens by antigen-presenting cells (APCs) and recognized by the respective T-cell receptor on the CD4+ T-cell surface (2–5). More recently, it was found that several interactions involving polymorphisms of either the *SFTPA1* and/or *SFTPA2*, increase HP risk whereas their interactions with the hydrophobic surfactant proteins (*SFTPB* and *SFTPC*) were associated with a decreased risk to develop the disease (6).

On the other hand, exposure to damaging agents, such as cigarette smoke, air pollution, viral infections, and pesticides also influences the development of the disease as well as the heterogeneous behavior (2, 3, 7–9).

EPIDEMIOLOGY

The definite incidence and prevalence of HP are uncertain because it varies according to the countries and customs, and importantly due to the lack of consensus over a definition of the disease, and the inability to detect the source of antigen exposure leading to a misdiagnosis attributing the patient's findings to another ILD. The incidence of HP has been reported in some countries such as the UK population, where is recorded as ~1 per 100,000 (10). In the US, a yearly incidence in the range of 1.7–2.7 per 100,000 population, has been recently reported (11), while Japan and France estimate an incidence between 0.3 and 0.9 per 100,000 individuals (12, 13). However, the incidence could be much higher according to one study that reported bird breeder's disease in 4.9 per 100,000 individuals over 10 years or 54.6 per 100,000 bird breeders (1, 14). The proportion of HP among all ILD cases could be higher and may represents around half of the newly diagnosed patients in high prevalent regions. The high variability in incidence and prevalence likely depends of many factors including differences in geographical conditions, local customs and occupational factors of each region and also because only until recently, there is a consensus over a definition of the disease.

ANTIGENS AND SOURCES OF EXPOSURE

Numerous antigens able to induce the disease have been identified and the list is constantly being expanded. The most studied antigens are avian antigens, fungi and thermophilic bacteria in the home or the working environment (15, 16); but there are also numerous reports revealing the association with other type of bacteria, protozoal, other animal proteins, and low-molecular-weight chemical compounds. For this reason, it is very important to investigate the presence of visible mold indoors; occupational environments such as where greenhouses, mushroom farming, compost, other food production methods, and metalworking fluids that could be contaminated by bacterial, mycobacterial, and fungal organisms (17). Even hobby activities may be a source of HP antigens, for example, non-tuberculous mycobacteria have been identified in patients exposed to indoor hot tubs and outdoor pools (18). Finally, specific chemicals used in industry, such as isocyanates and anhydrides, should also be considered as causal antigens. A list with most of the antigens and sources of exposure identified so far can be found in ATS/JRS/ALAT Guidelines (1).

PATHOGENIC MECHANISMS
The Inflammatory Response
The first step is the sensitization to the inhaled antigens which is associated with repeated exposure in individuals with genetic susceptibility to HP. The immunopathological response to the antigens involves T- and B-cells. Progression from sensitization to HP requires the accumulation of CD4+ TH1 cells in the lung, creating a pro-inflammatory microenvironment. Importantly, the suppressive activity of regulatory T cells is impaired, resulting in the amplification of the inflammatory response. IFNγ and TNF promote the accumulation, activation, and aggregation of macrophages, resulting in the development of granulomatous inflammation (4, 19). Also, immune complex-mediated lung injury with specific IgG antibodies may contribute to the inflammatory response.

The Fibrotic Response
Several factors may hamper the resolution of the inflammation, including further exposure to the antigen, which occurs mainly when it has not been identified (20), cigarette smoking, a genetic predisposition that may enhance the development of autoantibodies (21), and other unknown factors.

Several changes in T cell subsets are found in fibrotic HP, which may contribute to the non-resolution of inflammation triggering a fibrotic response, including a decrease of the immunoregulatory and antifibrotic γδ T cells, an increase of CD4+ cells, and a switch from a predominant TH1-like phenotype to a TH2-like phenotype (4, 19). TH2 cells secrete, among others, IL-4 and mainly IL-13 that contribute to a fibrotic response stimulating the TGFβ1 signaling pathway and activating the expansion of fibroblasts population (19, 22, 23). Fibroblasts arrive at the injured areas and differentiate into myofibroblasts, which are responsible for the accumulation of extracellular matrix. At the initial stages of fibrosis, the disease may stabilize or even improve in the pulmonary functional status, however, a subset of patients develops an aggressive phenotype called progressive pulmonary fibrosis that results in the destruction of the lung architecture (24). The mechanisms triggering this devastating phenotype are unclear but may include the type of fibrosis (UIP vs. non-UIP pattern), the aberrant composition and stiffness of the extracellular matrix, and the emergence of some unique profibrotic cell subsets (25).

CLINICAL FEATURES

It has been recently proposed that HP can be classified in fibrotic and non-fibrotic phenotypes (1). This proposal was considered to be more consistently associated with the clinical course, outcomes, and treatment efficiency.

Dyspnea is the main symptom of both non-fibrotic and fibrotic HP. Occasionally, patients with the non-fibrotic disease may present an acute influenza-like syndrome occurring a few hours after a (usually) substantial exposure. In these cases, symptoms gradually decrease over hours/days but may recur with re-exposure. More often, patients with non-fibrotic HP present progressive dyspnea during weeks or a few months together with constitutional symptoms, including fever, chills, chest tightness, wheezing, and weight loss (3). Patients with fibrotic HP show progressive (usually insidious) exertional dyspnea and chronic cough that develops over months to years. Clubbing may be present and on auscultation may yield inspiratory "velcro" crackles. Some patients display a high-pitched wheeze at the end of inspiration ("chirping" rales) while others describe the presence of inspiratory squeaks, caused by airways involvement (26). Pulmonary function test (PFT) reveal in both fibrotic and non-fibrotic HP a predominantly restrictive defect with DL_{CO} impairment, although some small airway obstruction may be detected in non-fibrotic patients. Finally, in the advanced stage of the disease patients may develop pulmonary arterial hypertension which is more prevalent in hypoxemic patients with greater impairment in lung function and lower exercise capacity (27).

DIAGNOSTIC APPROACH

HP represents a diagnostic challenge and requires a high index of suspicion by the clinician evaluating by the first time a patient with ILD (28, 29). Targeted diagnostic steps should include a thorough evaluation of the ILD patient's history of occupational and environmental antigenic exposures, chest high resolution computed tomography (HRCT), serum specific IgGs for confirmation of exposure or as a screening tool, bronchioalveolar lavage (BAL), and histopathological study in some cases (1, 30, 31).

Evidence of Exposure

Identification of the source of exposure and putative antigen(s) can be difficult. Validated and regionally relevant questionnaires that include occupational, residential, and avocational environments are mandatory (30, 32). Questions should also consider indirect exposures through contact with individuals who may carry antigens on their clothing or other materials. If an exposure is identified, details of duration, extent, and frequency should be obtained and importantly putative cause-effect relationship with symptoms. Evidence-based guidance has been published by WHO suggesting questions that may help clinicians to find out indoor dampness and molds (33). The on-site visual inspection is also useful for identifying obvious exposure sources (30).

Diagnostic Detection of Cellular and Humoral Immune Responses to HP Antigens

Identification of serum-specific Immunoglobulins (ssIGg) may help to recognize the inciting antigen (1, 30). According to the ATS Workshop Report, serum IgG testing against potential antigens associated with HP distinguish this disease from other ILDs with a sensitivity and specificity of 83 and 68%, respectively (30). However, it is important to emphasize that the presence of positive circulating antibodies, is only evidence of exposure to a potential HP antigen but does not prove causality and it may be worthy of further consideration to explore the source (30, 34).

On the other hand, since antigen T-cell mediated immune response plays a pivotal role in the pathogenesis of HP it has been proposed that lymphocyte proliferation testing may be a diagnostic tool (30, 35, 36).

However, studies using this method are scant, usually performed in small cohorts, and primarily in patients suspected to have bird-related HP. In addition, there is no standardized methodology to recommend in clinical practice. Nevertheless, this technique may be a promissory diagnostic tool in the future, mainly in patients with fibrotic HP that do not have detectable antibodies to causative antigens (37).

Chest HRCT Scanning

HRCT plays a pivotal role in the diagnosis of HP. In both fibrotic and non-fibrotic HP, images should be acquired at deep inspiration and after prolonged expiration.

The presence of centrilobular nodules, ground-glass opacities, mosaic attenuation, air trapping, mosaic perfusion are recognized as the principal findings in both fibrotic a non-fibrotic HP (**Figure 1**). The "three-density pattern" which describes a form of mosaic attenuation that combines areas of ground-glass opacification, lobular areas of low attenuation, and normal lung has a specificity of 93% for a diagnosis of fibrotic HP (38). For the fibrotic HP pattern, coexisting lung fibrosis and inflammation with signs of bronchiolar obstruction are highly suggestive. Honeycombing and traction bronchiectasis can be present and may be extensive in severe forms of fibrotic HP. Lung fibrosis can be more severe in the mid or mid and lower lung zones or equally distributed in the three lung zones with relative basal sparing (**Figure 2**) (39).

In general terms, the ATS/JRS/ALAT Guidelines and CHEST Guideline and Expert Panel Report 2021, show similar recommendations to classify HRCT images in the context of fibrotic or non-fibrotic HP (1, 31).

Cell Profile in the Bronchoalveolar Lavage Fluid (BAL)

BAL is a safe and well-tolerated diagnostic tool to evaluate alveolar inflammation. Increased cellularity with lymphocytosis is an important piece to improve the diagnostic likelihood of HP, where a higher percentage of lymphocytes could reflect the degree of alveolitis (**Figure 3**). However, the threshold proportion of BAL fluid lymphocytes that distinguishes HP from non-HP ILD is unclear and is strongly associated with the presence and extent of fibrotic changes (1, 31). Important for interpretation, BAL lymphocytosis may also be influenced by several variables, including, timing relative to antigen exposure, smoking status, and others (40). In general, and according to the ATS/JRS/ALA and CHEST guidelines, and to our own experience, we consider that a 30% threshold is reasonable for use in the differential diagnosis of HP vs. non-HP ILD.

Lung Biopsy

When the diagnosis is uncertain even after multidisciplinary discussion, lung biopsy is indicated. The histological specimen can be obtained by transbronchial cryobiopsy (if the Institution

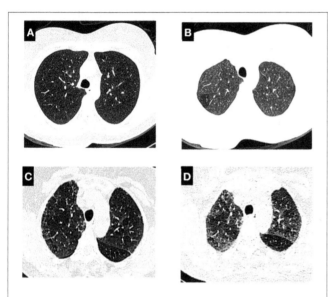

FIGURE 1 | High-resolution computed tomography scan in patients with non-fibrotic HP: **(A)** show inspiratory phase with diffuse centrilobular nodules, **(B)** expiratory phase in the same patient with centrilobular nodules and air trapping in right side; **(C)** in inspiratory phase present subpleural reticular pattern, with mosaic attenuation which is highlighted in the expiratory phase **(D)**.

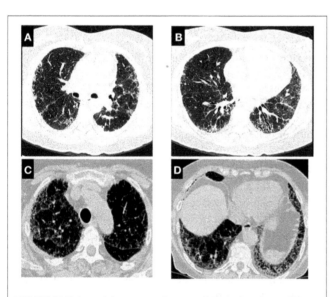

FIGURE 2 | High-resolution computed tomography scan in patients with fibrotic HP. In **(A)**, it is observed bilateral subpleural reticulation and in **(B)** traction bronchiectasis, honey combing and discrete ground-glass opacification and volume loss in left lung; **(C)** show lung fibrosis and areas of low attenuation and the same patient in **(D)** bronchiectasis and persistence of mosaic attenuation.

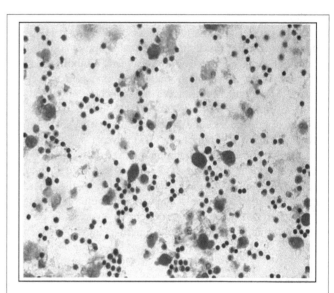

FIGURE 3 | Differential cell count in bronchoalveolar lavage fluid from a patient with hypersensitivity pneumonitis showing strong lymphocytosis. Hematoxylin and eosin staining, magnification: 40×.

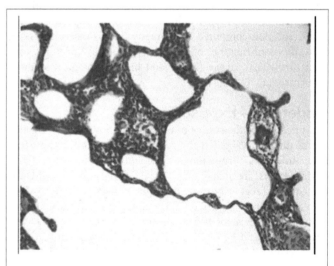

FIGURE 4 | Lung biopsy sample from a patient with non-fibrotic hypersensitivity pneumonitis showing cellular chronic interstitial pneumonia and a poorly formed non-necrotizing granuloma. Hematoxylin and eosin staining, magnification: 40×.

has experience with this technique), or surgical lung biopsy where samples of two different lobes are indicated (41–43).

The histopathological features vary according to the phenotypes. In the case of the non-fibrotic HP, characteristic findings include bronchiolocentric cellular interstitial pneumonia and cellular bronchiolitis of lymphocyte-predominant inflammatory infiltrate, as well as loosely formed granulomas and randomly scattered multinucleated giant cells within the interstitial inflammation (**Figure 4**) (1, 31).

Fibrotic HP differs from non-fibrotic HP in that the underlying chronic interstitial pneumonia and/or bronchiolitis is complicated by fibrosis, which occasionally may overlap with a UIP pattern hindering the differential diagnosis with IPF. In other cases, interstitial pneumonia shows a more uniform and diffuse distribution mimicking fibrotic non-specific interstitial pneumonia or may display features compatible with interstitial airway-centered fibrosis (1, 31, 44). Findings of non-fibrotic HP may help to distinguish fibrotic HP from other fibrotic lung disorders. Moreover, UIP-like pattern is related with worst survival (1, 45, 46).

Multidisciplinary Discussion

As recommended in all newly diagnosed ILD, multidisciplinary evaluation of patients with suspected HP is advised. Diagnosis is guided by the integration of clinical history and questionnaire, environmental assessment and sampling, HRCT, and BAL, and in select cases, immunologic testing, and histopathological evaluation, which likely will provide the most precise approach to diagnosis. Two recently published guidelines, from ATS/JRS/ALAT (1), and from CHEST (31) recommended diagnostic algorithms based in three domains: exposure identification, HRCT findings, and BAL lymphocytosis, which in the case of the ATS/JRS/ALAT diagnostic criteria is strengthened by histopathologic findings. A recent study showed that the agreement between them in a real-life setting was low for definitive/high-confidence diagnosis (47). Accordingly, we proposed an algorithm for the diagnostic evaluation of HP, based in the same domains used by both guidelines (**Figure 5**).

PROGNOSTIC FACTORS

HRCT and Morphological Phenotypes

The type of fibrotic structural remodeling may indicate an increased risk of early mortality. Particularly, the usual interstitial pneumonia (UIP) pattern either by HRCT or biopsy carry-out the worst prognosis. For example, a study that involved a large cohort of patients, showed that CT honeycombing is highly prevalent in diverse forms of ILD, including HP, and that is associated with marked increased in long-term mortality rate compared with those without honeycombing (48). Likewise, in another study where three radiologically defined phenotypes were identified, it was found that patients with typical UIP-like pattern (that included honeycombing) displayed a median survival similar to IPF (the most aggressive ILD), and significantly lower than in patients with non-honeycomb fibrosis (2.8 vs. 7.95 years) (49). Therefore, CT honeycombing is prevalent in fibrotic HP and identifies a progressive fibrotic phenotype that is associated with increased mortality rates.

UIP findings in the lung biopsy also predict prognosis (1, 45). Interestingly, a biomarker that distinguishes UIP from a non-UIP pattern has been proposed for the diagnosis of IPF. The Envisia Genomic Classifier, through the detection of a 190-gene machine-learning classifier in lung samples obtained from transbronchial biopsies, could assist in the confident diagnosis of UIP (50). However, if this molecular biomarker will be useful (and accessible) in UIP of other fibrotic lung disorders, such as HP, is largely unknown.

Interestingly, some HP patients may present features of pleuroparenchymal fibroelastosis (PPFE) an unusual biopathological process characterized by upper-lobe-dominant progressive pulmonary fibrosis consisting of visceral pleural thickening with collagenous matrix and subpleural elastosis (51), and this association is linked to worsened HP survival (52).

Importantly, using automated computer-based quantitative imaging it was shown that patients with a pulmonary vessel volume above $6 \cdot 5\%$ of the total lung volume, had a rate of disease progression, nearly identical to that of IPF (53).

Genomic and Molecular Risk Factors

There are significant inter-individual differences in the severity and progression of the pulmonary disease in patients with HP that otherwise seem to share similar antigen exposure and other demographic characteristics indicating that some genetic or molecular modifiers may contribute.

For example, it was found that an exaggerated shortening of telomeres was associated with fibrosis and was a strong predictor of poor survival in HP patients. Moreover, short telomere length was also linked to radiographic and histopathologic changes similar to IPF (54).

More recently, it was demonstrated that around 10% of patients with HP carry rare protein-altering variants in telomere-related genes, such as *TERT*, *RTEL1*, and *PARN* (55). Importantly, this finding was associated with shorter peripheral blood telomere length and significantly reduced transplant-free survival.

Likewise, The MUC5B promoter polymorphism rs35705950 minor allele was associated with HRCT evidence of fibrosis and traction bronchiectasis, and in contrast to IPF, showed a statistical tendency toward poorer survival among patients with HP (54).

There is some evidence that some biomarkers may be an independent predictor of disease progression and mortality in HP. The relative change in the serum levels of KL-6/MUC1, a human mucin protein expressed by type 2 alveolar epithelial cells, is associated with rapid progression in patients with fibrotic HP (56). Interestingly, raised KL-6 is associated with early-stage HP suggesting a mechanistic link with the behavior of the lung epithelium (57).

YKL-40 is a chitinase-like protein mainly secreted by inflammatory and epithelial cells, which is involved in the inflammatory response to tissue damage. HP patients who experienced disease progression had higher baseline serum YKL-40 levels than those who remained stable during follow-up. Likewise, HP patients who died had higher baseline serum YKL-40 levels than those who survived (58).

A serum chemokine profile showed that a lower CXCL9, in combination with higher CCL17, was an important predictor of worsening lung function (59). However, is important to emphasize that studies of prognostic biomarkers in HP are scanty, performed in small cohorts, and usually without verification cohorts.

Two recent studies have demonstrated that a subset of patients with HP presents circulating present autoantibodies, without features of autoimmune disease (21, 60). In both studies, the presence of autoantibodies was an independent predictor of increased mortality. Patients carrying the

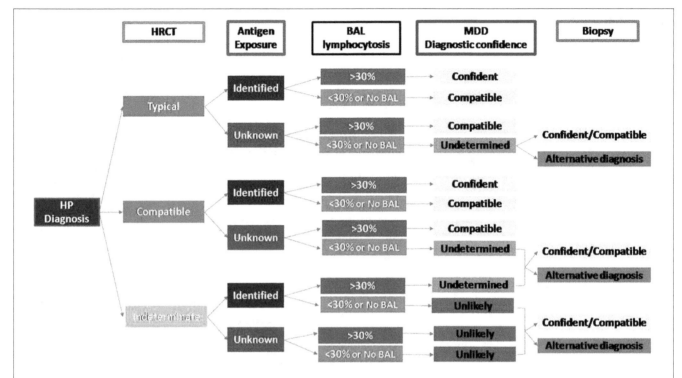

FIGURE 5 | Hypersensitivity pneumonitis diagnostic algorithm. The diagnosis of HP diagnosis relies primarily on three domains: HRCT pattern (according to ATS guideline classification), antigen exposure, and BAL lymphocytosis. This approach is followed by multidisciplinary team discussion where the diagnostic confidence is made. Undetermined or Unlikely HP may require the lung biopsy to orientate to an alternative diagnosis, or occasionally, reveal a hidden HP. Diagnostic confidence: Confident (>90%), Compatible (70%-89%), Undetermined (50%-69%), Unlikely (<50%). NO BAL (Not performed, e.g., patients with comorbidities and/or very low pulmonary function tests, patient's refusal to do the procedure; BAL not available, or other reasons). HP, hypersensitivity pneumonitis; HRCT, high resolution computed tomography; BAL, bronchoalveolar lavage; MDD, multidisciplinary discussion.

haplotype DRB1*03:01-DQB1*02:01, which is part of the 8.1 ancestral haplotype, and a major genetic determinant of autoimmune diseases showed a significant higher risk to develop autoantibodies (21).

Several studies have reported acute exacerbation (AE) in patients with fibrotic HP, following the same definition used in IPF, which results in poor prognosis (61). Recently it was reported as risk factors lower DLco, the presence of UIP-like pattern on HRCT at diagnosis, and cumulative incidence rates of AE showed high in-hospital mortality rate (62).

Finally, some demographic characteristics, such as aging and smoking may contribute to disease progression (3, 19).

THERAPEUTIC APPROACHES

There is no consensus or guidelines for HP management, and most of the evidence arises from retrospective cohort studies or case reports. The therapeutic approach consists mainly of antigen avoidance and pharmacological treatment with corticosteroids/immunosuppressive drugs and, more recently, antifibrotic therapy depending on HP phenotype. In advanced disease with severe clinical and functional deficiency, a lung transplant is indicated.

Antigen Avoidance

Identification and complete antigen avoidance are the mainstays of treatment and patients should be strongly advised to avoid further exposure (1, 19, 30). However, in 40–50% of HP patients the antigen(s) is not identified.

In non-fibrotic HP antigen-avoidance is associated with improved lung function but in fibrotic forms, the effectiveness remains controversial (63). In a cohort of patients with fibrotic HP, FVC remained stable and median survival was greater in patients who reported antigen avoidance while in another study no difference was found suggesting a self-perpetuating mechanism of the disease in fibrotic forms (63, 64). Despite these observations, it is important to make continuous efforts to identify the antigens' source and strongly recommend avoid exposure.

PHARMACOLOGICAL TREATMENT
Non-fibrotic HP

Corticosteroids are often used but the evidence supporting this approach is very limited and comes from studies in farmers lung disease, where pulmonary function improved during early follow-up protecting against progression but without beneficial effect on long term prognosis (65, 66). Recently De Sadeleer et al., showed that corticosteroid initiation in progressive patients resulted in a reversal with an improvement of lung function (63). An empiric treatment scheme may consist of prednisone (or equivalents) of 0.5 mg/kg/d for 1–2 weeks followed by a gradual tapering until maintenance of 10 mg/d (67). To ameliorate adverse events related to the prolonged corticosteroid use, sparing agents, mycophenolate (MMF) and azathioprine (AZA), might be a treatment option for patients showing progression and/or frequent relapses or in whom antigen avoidance is not possible.

Fibrotic HP

For many reasons, pharmacological treatment in fibrotic HP is challenging. Despite the lack of evidence, corticosteroids alone or associated with AZA or MMF are the most common immunosuppressants used for treating fibrotic HP, with fewer adverse events with combination therapy. In a retrospective study, a modest but significant improvement in DL_{CO} without changes in FVC was observed after 1-year treatment of MMF or AZA (68). The presence of BAL lymphocytosis seems to be associated with a favorable response to corticosteroids alone or in combination, especially with AZA, but only during the first 6 to 12 months of treatment, with FVC decline after this period (63, 69). HRCT honeycombing, low BAL lymphocytosis, and the presence of short telomeres could be factors associated with no response to immunosuppressive therapy (63, 70). Moreover, treatment with corticosteroids alone or in combination with AZA/MMF was associated with increased mortality risk after adjustment in two cohorts of patients with fibrotic HP. This finding is similar to those reported in IPF, probably reflecting a final common pathway in the pathophysiologic processes of advanced fibrosis that underlies these two diseases (25, 71, 72).

There is emerging evidence that Rituximab, an anti CD20 monoclonal antibody, seems to be well-tolerated and may lead to stabilization or improvement of lung function in some patients with fibrotic HP, particularly those without UIP or NSIP pattern (73, 74). Finally, leflunomide, a prototype member of dihydroorotate dehydrogenase (DHODH) enzyme inhibitors, could be an effective sparing immunomodulatory drug with a significant pulmonary function improvement in fibrotic HP, with a most pronounced effect in patients without >20% extent of fibrosis on HRCT (75).

Antifibrotics, pirfenidone and nintedanib, recently became a plausible option for patients who experience disease progression despite antigen avoidance and immunosuppressive treatment. The efficacy and safety of pirfenidone were evaluated in the RELIEF study that was prematurely terminated due to slow recruitment (76). Despite this, 45% of the patients included in the study had fibrotic HP and the addition of pirfenidone to ongoing medication showed slower disease progression as measured by loss of FVC. This data is similar to another real-life study where pirfenidone reduced the decline of vital capacity in a cohort of patients with fibrotic HP (77). By contrast, in a small cohort of patients with fibrotic, advanced HP, we found that adding pirfenidone to the immunosuppressive drugs, showed no effect on FVC compared with the patients using only immunosuppressive therapy, but displayed a tendency to DLCO

improvement and a significant improvement in the quality of life evaluated through the total score on the Saint George's Respiratory Questionnaire (78).

The INBUILD trial demonstrated that in patients with progressive fibrosing interstitial disease the annual rate decline in the FVC was significantly lower among patients who received nintedanib than those who received placebo (79). In the fibrotic HP subgroup (26% of the overall population) there was no statistical difference in the rate of FVC decline between nintedanib and placebo, likely because the study was not designed to provide evidence in specific subgroups (80). Finally, in patients with progressive and severe fibrotic HP, it should be considered for a lung transplant (81).

In summary, the management of HP patients should include, antigen avoidance in both HP phenotypes. For patients with non-fibrotic HP who don't have a full recovery after antigen removal, it is suggested corticosteroid treatment with a gradual tapering to achieve a low dose with or without AZA or MMF for patients with frequent relapses or when antigen avoidance it's not possible. In light of the evidence, in fibrotic HP and preferable after careful evaluation with multidisciplinary team discussion using HRCT, BAL, and histopathology findings to identify those with mixed inflammatory plus fibrotic or purely fibrotic disease, immunosuppressive therapy, and antifibrotic treatment should be considered and in advance disease, patients should be included for a lung transplant.

PALLIATIVE CARE

As in many interstitial lung disease that present progressive pulmonary fibrosis phenotype and end-stage disease, the decrease in quality of life of patients with HP represents an additional problem. Quality of life is not only affected by the disease but also by the presence of adverse events associated with the treatment, inability to continue with work or recreational activities and the economic impact for the family. Palliative care should be discussed and initiated early in the disease course, and should be focused not only according patient's needs and preferences but also include caregivers which should be supported throughout the disease trajectory (82).

CONCLUSIONS

The diagnosis and treatment of HP remain complex and challenging because the absence of a single diagnostic gold standard and lack of prospective clinical trials.

For a long time, HP was characterized by duration of symptoms at the time of diagnosis, as acute, subacute, or chronic which was not reliably associated with the prognosis. Consequently, a recently published guideline has proposed that patients should be classified as having fibrotic or non-fibrotic HP, according to the radiological or histopathological findings. These two phenotypes are clearly identifiable and likely show a better association with outcome. The pathogenic mechanisms have not been fully elucidated, and diagnostic and prognostic biomarkers are lacking. The prognosis of fibrotic HP is poor as in other fibrotic lung disorders, and questions remain unanswered about the optimal therapeutic strategy mainly for fibrotic HP for which large-scale clinical trials are necessary.

REFERENCES

1. Raghu G, Remy-Jardin M, Ryerson CJ, Myers JL, Kreuter M, Vasakova M, et al. Diagnosis of hypersensitivity pneumonitis in adults. An official ATS/JRS/ALAT clinical practice guideline. *Am J Respir Crit Care Med.* (2020) 202:e36–69. doi: 10.1164/rccm.202005-2 032ST

2. Vasakova M, Morell F, Walsh S, Leslie K, Raghu G. Hypersensitivity pneumonitis: perspectives in diagnosis and management. *Am J Respir Crit Care Med.* (2017) 196:680–9. doi: 10.1164/rccm.201611-2 201PP

3. Selman M, Pardo A, King TE Jr. Hypersensitivity pneumonitis: insights in diagnosis and pathobiology. *Am J Respir Crit Care Med.* (2012) 186:314–24. doi: 10.1164/rccm.201203-0513CI

4. Vasakova M, Selman M, Morell F, Sterclova M, Molina-Molina M, Raghu G. Hypersensitivity pneumonitis: current concepts of pathogenesis and potential targets for treatment. *Am J Respir Crit Care Med.* (2019) 200:301–8. doi: 10.1164/rccm.201903-0541PP

5. Zakharova MY, Belyanina TA, Sokolov AV, Kiselev IS, Mamedov AE. The contribution of major histocompatibility complex class II genes to an association with autoimmune diseases. *Acta Nat.* (2019) 11:4–12. doi: 10.32607/20758251-2019-11-4-4-12

6. Gandhi CK, Chen C, Amatya S, Yang L, Fu C, Zhou S, et al. SNP and haplotype interaction models reveal association of surfactant protein gene polymorphisms with hypersensitivity pneumonitis of mexican population. *Front Med.* (2021) 7:588404. doi: 10.3389/fmed.2020.588404

7. Singh S, Collins BF, Bairwa M, Joshi JM, Talwar D, Singh N, et al. Hypersensitivity pneumonitis and its correlation with ambient air pollution in urban India. *Eur Respir J.* (2019) 53:1801563. doi: 10.1183/13993003.01563-2018

8. Dakhama A, Hegele RG, Laflamme G, Israël-Assayag E, Cormier Y. Common respiratory viruses in lower airways of patients with acute hypersensitivity pneumonitis. *Am J Respir Crit Care Med.* (1999) 159:1316–22. doi: 10.1164/ajrccm.159.4.9807085

9. Hoppin JA, Umbach DM, Kullman GJ, Henneberger PK, London SJ, Alavanja MC, et al. Pesticides and other agricultural factors associated with self-reported farmer's lung among farm residents in the Agricultural Health Study. *Occup Environ Med.* (2007) 64:334–42. doi: 10.1136/oem.2006.028480

10. Solaymani-Dodaran M, West J, Smith C, Hubbard R. Extrinsic allergic alveolitis: incidence and mortality in the general population. *QJM.* (2007) 100:233–7. doi: 10.1093/qjmed/hcm008

11. Fernández Pérez ER, Kong AM, Raimundo K, Koelsch TL, Kulkarni R, Cole AL. Epidemiology of hypersensitivity pneumonitis among an insured population in the United States: a claims-based cohort analysis. *Ann Am Thorac Soc.* (2018) 15:460–9. doi: 10.1513/AnnalsATS.201704-288OC

12. Yoshida K, Suga M, Nishiura Y, Arima K, Yoneda R, Tamura M, et al. Occupational hypersensitivity pneumonitis in Japan: data on a nationwide epidemiological study. *Occup Environ Med.* (1995) 52:570–4. doi: 10.1136/oem.52.9.570

13. Dalphin JC. Extrinsic allergic alveolitis in agricultural environment. *Rev Prat.* (1992) 42:1790–6.

14. Morell F, Villar A, Ojanguren I, Muñoz X, Cruz MJ, Sansano I, et al. Hypersensitivity pneumonitis and (Idiopathic) pulmonary fibrosis due to feather duvets and pillows. *Arch Bronconeumol.* (2021) 57:87–93. doi: 10.1016/j.arbres.2019.12.003

15. Lacasse Y, Selman M. Clinical diagnosis of hypersensitivity pneumonitis. Am J Respir Crit Care Med (2003) 168:952–8. doi: 10.1164/rccm.200301-137OC

16. Kouranos V, Jacob J, Nicholson A, Renzoni E. Fibrotic hipersensitivity pneumonits: key issues in diagnosis and management. *J Clin Med.* (2017) 6:62. doi: 10.3390/jcm6060062

17. Cullinan P, D'Souza, E. Lesson of the month: extrinsic allergic (bronchiolo) alveolitis and metal working fluids. *Thorax.* (2014) 69:1059–60. doi: 10.1136/thoraxjnl-2014-205251

18. Glazer CS, Martyny JW. Nontuberculous mycobacteria in aerosol droplets and bulk water samples from therapy pools and hot tubs. *J Occup Environ Hyg.* (2007) 4:831–40. doi: 10.1080/15459620701634403

19. Costabel U, Miyazaki Y, Pardo A, Koschel D, Bonella F, Spagnolo P, et al. Hypersensitivity pneumonitis. *Nat Rev Dis Primers.* (2020) 6:65. doi: 10.1038/s41572-020-0191-z

20. Fernández Pérez ER, Swigris JJ, Forssén AV, Tourin O, Solomon JJ, Huie TJ, et al. Identifying an inciting antigen is associated with improved survival in patients with chronic hypersensitivity pneumonitis. *Chest.* (2013) 144:1644–51. doi: 10.1378/chest.12-2685

21. Buendía-Roldán I, Santiago-Ruiz L, Pérez-Rubio G, Mejía M, Rojas-Serrano J, Ambrocio-Ortiz E, et al. A major genetic determinant of autoimmune diseases is associated with the presence of autoantibodies in hypersensitivity pneumonitis. *Eur Respir J.* (2020) 56:1901380. doi: 10.1183/13993003.01380-2019

22. Barrera L, Mendoza F, Zuñiga J, Estrada A, Zamora AC, Melendro EI, et al. Functional diversity of T-cell subpopulations in subacute and chronic hypersensitivity pneumonitis. *Am J Respir Crit Care Med.* (2008) 177:44–55. doi: 10.1164/rccm.200701-093OC

23. Lee CG, Homer RJ, Zhu Z, Lanone S, Wang X, Koteliansky V, et al. Interleukin-13 induces tissue fibrosis by selectively stimulating and activating transforming growth factor beta(1). *J Exp Med.* (2001) 194:809–21. doi: 10.1084/jem.194.6.809

24. Kolb M, Vašáková M. The natural history of progressive fibrosing interstitial lung diseases. *Respir Res.* (2019) 20:57. doi: 10.1186/s12931-019-1022-1

25. Selman M, Pardo A. When things go wrong: exploring possible mechanisms driving the progressive fibrosis phenotype in interstitial lung diseases. *Eur Respir J.* (2021) 4:2004507. doi: 10.1183/13993003.04507-2020

26. Varone F, Iovene B, Sgalla G, Calvello M, Calabrese A, Larici AR, et al. Fibrotic hypersensitivity pneumonitis: diagnosis and management. *Lung.* (2020) 198:429–40. doi: 10.1007/s00408-020-00360-3

27. Oliveira RKF, Pereira CAC, Ramos RP, Ferreira EVM, Messina CMS, Kuranishi LT, et al. A haemodynamic study of pulmonary hypertension in chronic hypersensitivity pneumonitis. *Eur Respir J.* (2014) 44:415–24. doi: 10.1183/09031936.00010414

28. Salisbury ML, Myers JL, Belloli EA, Kazerooni EA, Martinez FJ, Flaherty KR. Diagnosis and treatment of fibrotic hypersensitivity pneumonia. where we stand and where we need to go. *Am J Respir Crit Care Med.* (2017) 196:690–9. doi: 10.1164/rccm.201608-1675PP

29. Morisset J, Johannson KA, Jones KD, Wolters PJ, Collard HR, Walsh SLF. Identification of diagnostic criteria for chronic hypersensitivity pneumonitis. an international modified Delphi survey. *Am J Respir Crit Care Med.* (2018) 197:1036–44. doi: 10.1164/rccm.201712-2403ED

30. Johannson KA, Barnes H, Bellanger A-P, Dalphin J-C, Fernández Pérez ER, Flaherty KR, et al. Exposure assessment tools for hypersensitivity pneumonitis. An official American thoracic society workshop report. *Ann Am Thorac Soc.* (2020) 17:1501–9. doi: 10.1513/AnnalsATS.202008-942ST

31. Fernández Pérez ER, Travis WD, Lynch DA, Brown KK, Johannson KA, Selman M, et al. Executive summary: diagnosis and evaluation of hypersensitivity pneumonitis: CHEST guideline and expert panel report. *Chest.* (2021) 160:595–615. doi: 10.1016/j.chest.2021.03.067

32. Chew GL, Horner WE, Kennedy K, Grimes C, Barnes CS, Phipatanakul W, et al. Procedures to assist healthcare providers to determine when home assessments for potential mold exposure are warranted. *J Allergy Clin Immunol Pract.* (2016) 4:417–22.e2. doi: 10.1016/j.jaip.2016.01.013

33. *World Health Organization Guidelines for Indoor Air Quality: Dampness and Mould.* (2021). Available online at: https://www.euro.who.int/en/health-

AUTHOR CONTRIBUTIONS

MS: conceptualization and writing the first draft. IB-R, MA, and ER-A: review and writing. All authors contributed to the article and approved the submitted version.

topics/environment-and-health/air-quality/publications/2009/damp-and-mould-health-risks-prevention-and-remedial-actions2/who-guidelines-for-indoor-air-quality-dampness-and-mould (accessed Apr 25,2021).

34. *FHPP2 - Clinical: Hypersensitivity Pneumonitis FEIA Panel II.* (2021). Available online at: https://www.mayocliniclabs.com/test-catalog/Clinical+and+Interpretive/57595 (accessed Apr 28, 2021).

35. Center DM, Berman JS, Kornfeld H, Theodore AC, Cruikshank WW. Mechanisms of lymphocyte accumulation in pulmonary disease. *Chest.* (1993) 103:88S–91. doi: 10.1378/chest.103.2_Supplement.88S

36. Yoshizawa Y, Miyake S, Sumi Y, Hisauchi K, Sato T, Kurup V. A follow-up study of pulmonary function tests, bronchoalveolar lavage cells, and humoral and cellular immunity in bird fancier's lung. *J Allergy Clin Immunol.* (1995) 96:122–9. doi: 10.1016/S0091-6749(95)70041-2

37. Ohtani Y, Saiki S, Sumi Y, Inase N, Miyake S, Costabel U, et al. Clinical features of recurrent and insidious chronic bird fancier's lung. *Ann Allergy Asthma Immunol.* (2003) 90:604–10. doi: 10.1016/S1081-1206(10)61863-7

38. Walsh S, Richeldi L. Demystifying fibrotic hypersensitivity pneumonitis diagnosis: it's all about shades of grey. *Eur Respir J.* (2019) 54:1900906. doi: 10.1183/13993003.00906-2019

39. Silva CIS, Müller NL, Lynch DA, Curran-Everett D, Brown KK, Lee KS, et al. chronic hypersensitivity pneumonitis: differentiation from idiopathic pulmonary fibrosis and nonspecific interstitial pneumonia by using thin-section CT. *Radiology.* (2008) 246:288–97. doi: 10.1148/radiol.2453061881

40. Meyer KC, Raghu G, Baughman RP, Brown KK, Costabel U, du Bois RM, et al. An official American Thoracic Society clinical practice guideline: the clinical utility of bronchoalveolar lavage cellular analysis in interstitial lung disease. *Am J Respir Crit Care Med.* (2012) 185:1004–14. doi: 10.1164/rccm.201202-0320ST

41. Ohshimo S, Bonella F, Guzman J, Costabel U. Hypersensitivity pneumonitis. *Immunol Allergy Clin North Am.* (2012) 32:537–56. doi: 10.1016/j.iac.2012.08.008

42. Johannson KA, Marcoux VS, Ronksley PE, Ryerson CJ. diagnostic yield and complications of transbronchial lung cryobiopsy for interstitial lung disease: a systematic review and meta-analysis. *Ann Am Thorac Soc.* (2016) 13:1828–38. doi: 10.1513/AnnalsATS.201606-461SR

43. Iftikhar IH, Alghothani L, Sardi A, Berkowitz D, Musani AI. transbronchial lung cryobiopsy and video-assisted thoracoscopic lung biopsy in the diagnosis of diffuse parenchymal lung disease: a meta-analysis of diagnostic test accuracy. *Ann Am Thorac Soc.* (2017) 14:1197–211. doi: 10.1513/AnnalsATS.201701-086SR

44. Churg A, Muller NL, Flint J, Wright JL. Chronic hypersensitivity pneumonitis. *Am J Surg Pathol.* (2006) 30:201–8. doi: 10.1097/01.pas.0000184806.38037.3c

45. Gaxiola M, Buendía-Roldán I, Mejía M, Carrillo G, Estrada A, Navarro MC, et al. Morphologic diversity of chronic pigeon breeder's disease: clinical features and survival. Respir Med (2011) 105:608–14. doi: 10.1016/j.rmed.2010.11.026

46. Churg A, Sin DD, Everett D, Brown K, Cool C. Pathologic patterns and survival in chronic hypersensitivity pneumonitis. *Am J Surg Pathol.* (2009) 33:1765–70. doi: 10.1097/PAS.0b013e3181bb2538

47. Buendia-Roldan I, Aguilar-Duran H, Johannson KA, Selman M. Comparing the performance of two recommended criteria for establishing a diagnosis for hypersensitivity pneumonitis. *Am J Respir Crit Care Med.* (2021). doi: 10.1164/rccm.202105-1091LE. [Epub ahead of print].

48. Adegunsoye A, Oldham JM, Bellam SK, Montner S, Churpek MM, Noth I, et al. Computed tomography honeycombing identifies a progressive fibrotic phenotype with increased mortality across diverse interstitial lung diseases. *Ann Am Thorac Soc.* (2019) 16:580–8. doi: 10.1513/AnnalsATS.201807-443OC

49. Salisbury ML, Gu T, Murray S, Gross BH, Chughtai A, Sayyouh M, et al. Hypersensitivity pneumonitis: radiologic phenotypes are associated with distinct survival time and pulmonary function trajectory. *Chest.* (2019) 155:699–711. doi: 10.1016/j.chest.2018.08.1076

50. Richeldi L, Scholand MB, Lynch DA, Colby TV, Myers JL, Groshong SD, et al. Utility of a molecular classifier as a complement to high-resolution computed tomography to identify usual interstitial pneumonia. *Am J Respir Crit Care Med.* (2021) 203:211–20. doi: 10.1164/rccm.202003-0877OC

51. Chua F, Desai SR, Nicholson AG, Devaraj A, Renzoni E, Rice A, et al. Pleuroparenchymal fibroelastosis. A review of clinical, radiological, and pathological characteristics. *Ann Am Thorac Soc.* (2019) 16:1351–9. doi: 10.1513/AnnalsATS.201902-181CME

52. Jacob J, Odink A, Brun AL, Macaluso C, de Lauretis A, Kokosi M, et al. Functional associations of pleuroparenchymal fibroelastosis and emphysema with hypersensitivity pneumonitis. *Respir Med.* (2018) 138:95–101. doi: 10.1016/j.rmed.2018.03.031

53. Jacob J, Bartholmai BJ, Egashira R, Brun AL, Rajagopalan S, Karwoski R, et al. Chronic hypersensitivity pneumonitis: identification of key prognostic determinants using automated CT analysis. *BMC Pulm Med.* (2017) 17:81. doi: 10.1186/s12890-017-0418-2

54. Ley B, Newton CA, Arnould I, Elicker BM, Henry TS, Vittinghoff E, et al. The MUC5B promoter polymorphism and telomere length in patients with chronic hypersensitivity pneumonitis: an observational cohort-control study. *Lancet Respir Med.* (2017) 5:639–47. doi: 10.1016/S2213-2600(17)30216-3

55. Ley B, Torgerson DG, Oldham JM, Adegunsoye A, Liu S, Li J, et al. rare protein-altering telomere-related gene variants in patients with chronic hypersensitivity pneumonitis. *Am J Respir Crit Care Med.* (2019) 200:1154–63. doi: 10.1164/rccm.201902-0360OC

56. Hanzawa S, Tateishi T, Ishizuka M, Inoue Y, Honda T, Kawahara T, et al. Changes in serum KL-6 levels during short-term strict antigen avoidance are associated with the prognosis of patients with fibrotic hypersensitivity pneumonitis caused by avian antigens. *Respir Investig.* (2020) 19:S2212-5345(20)30092-7. doi: 10.1016/j.resinv.2020.05.007

57. Ji Y, Bourke SJ, Spears M, Wain LV, Boyd G, Lynch PP, et al. Krebs von den Lungen-6 (KL-6) is a pathophysiological biomarker of early-stage acute hypersensitivity pneumonitis among pigeon fanciers. *Clin Exp Allergy.* (2020) 50:1391–9. doi: 10.1111/cea.13744

58. Long X, He X, Ohshimo S, Griese M, Sarria R, Guzman J, et al. Serum YKL-40 as predictor of outcome in hypersensitivity pneumonitis. *Eur Respir J.* (2017) 49:1501924. doi: 10.1183/13993003.01924-2015

59. Nukui Y, Yamana T, Masuo M, Tateishi T, Kishino M, Tateishi U, et al. Serum CXCL9 and CCL17 as biomarkers of declining pulmonary function in chronic bird-related hypersensitivity pneumonitis. *PLoS ONE.* (2019) 14:e0220462. doi: 10.1371/journal.pone.0220462

60. Adegunsoye A, Oldham JM, Demchuk C, Montner S, Vij R, Strek ME. Predictors of survival in coexistent hypersensitivity pneumonitis with autoimmune features. *Respir Med.* (2016) 114:53–60. doi: 10.1016/j.rmed.2016.03.012

61. Miyazaki Y, Tateishi T, Akashi T, Ohtani Y, Inase N, Yoshizawa Y. Clinical predictors and histologic appearance of acute exacerbations in chronic hypersensitivity pneumonitis. *Chest.* (2008) 134:1265–70. doi: 10.1378/chest.08-0866

62. Kang J, Kim YJ, Choe J, Chae EJ, Song JW. Acute exacerbation of fibrotic hypersensitivity pneumonitis: incidence and outcomes. *Respir Med.* (2021) 22:152. doi: 10.1186/s12931-021-01748-2

63. De Sadeleer L, Hermans F, De Dycker E, Yserbyt J, Verschakelen J, Verbeken E, et al. Effects of corticosteroid treatment and antigen avoidance in a large hypersensitivity pneumonitis cohort: a single-centre cohort study. *J Clin Med.* (2018) 8:14. doi: 10.3390/jcm8010014

64. Gimenez A, Storrer K, Kuranishi L, Soares MR, Ferreira RG, Pereira CAC. Change in FVC and survival in chronic fibrotic hypersensitivity pneumonitis. *Thorax.* (2018) 73:391–2. doi: 10.1136/thoraxjnl-2017-210035

65. Kokkarinen J, Tukiainen H TE. Recovery of pulmonary function in farmer's lung. *Am Rev Respir Dis.* (1993) 147:793–6. doi: 10.1164/ajrccm/147.4.793

66. Cano-Jiménez E, Rubal D, Pérez de Llano LA, Mengual N, Castro-Añón O, Méndez L, et al. Farmer's lung disease: analysis of 75 cases. *Med Clin.* (2017) 149:429–35. doi: 10.1016/j.medcle.2017.10.009

67. Spagnolo P, Rossi G, Cavazza A, Paladini I, Paladini I, Bonella F, et al. Hypersensitivity pneumonitis: a comprehensive review. *J Investig Allergol Clin Immunol.* (2015) 25:237–50.

68. Morisset J, Johannson KA, Vittinghoff E, Aravena C, Elicker BM, Jones KD, et al. Use of mycophenolate mofetil or azathioprine for the management of chronic hypersensitivity pneumonitis. *Chest.* (2017) 151:619–25. doi: 10.1016/j.chest.2016.10.029

69. Raimundo S, Pimenta AC, Cruz-Martins N, Rodrigues MC, Melo N, Mota PC, et al. Insights on chronic hypersensitivity pneumonitis' treatment: factors associated with a favourable response to azathioprine. *Life Sci.* (2021) 272:1–6. doi: 10.1016/j.lfs.2021.119274

70. Adegunsoye A, Morisset J, Newton CA, Oldham JM, Vittinghoff E, Linderholm AL, et al. Leukocyte telomere length and mycophenolate therapy in chronic hypersensitivity pneumonitis. *Eur Respir J.* (2021) 57:2002872. doi: 10.1183/13993003.02872-2020

71. Adegunsoye A, Oldham JM, Fernández Pérez ER, Hamblin M, Patel N, Tener M, et al. Outcomes of immunosuppressive therapy in chronic hypersensitivity pneumonitis. *ERJ Open Res.* (2017) 3:00016-2017. doi: 10.1183/23120541.00016-2017

72. Raghu G, Anstrom KJ, King TE Jr, Lasky JA, Martinez FJ. idiopathic pulmonary fibrosis clinical research network. prednisone, azathioprine, and N-acetylcysteine for pulmonary fibrosis. *N Engl J Med.* (2012) 366:1968–77. doi: 10.1056/NEJMoa1113354

73. Ferreira M, Borie R, Crestani B, Rigaud P, Wemeau L, Israel-Biet D, et al. Efficacy and safety of rituximab in patients with chronic hypersensitivity pneumonitis (cHP): a retrospective, multicentric, observational study. *Respir Med.* (2020) 172:6–11. doi: 10.1016/j.rmed.2020.106146

74. Keir GJ, Maher TM, Ming D, Abdullah R, De Lauretis A, Wickremasinghe M, et al. Rituximab in severe, treatment-refractory interstitial lung disease. *Respirology.* (2014) 19:353–9. doi: 10.1111/resp.12214

75. Noh S, Yadav R, Li M, Wang X, Sahoo D, Culver DA, et al. Use of leflunomide in patients with chronic hypersensitivity pneumonitis. *BMC Pulm Med.* (2020) 20:1–10. doi: 10.1186/s12890-020-01227-2

76. Behr J, Prasse A, Kreuter M, Johow J, Rabe KF, Bonella F, et al. Pirfenidone in patients with progressive fibrotic interstitial lung diseases other than idiopathic pulmonary fibrosis (RELIEF): a double-blind, randomised, placebo-controlled, phase 2b trial. *Lancet Respir Med.* (2021) 9:478–86. doi: 10.1016/S2213-2600(20)30554-3

77. Shibata S, Furusawa H, Inase N. Pirfenidone in chronic hypersensitivity pneumonitis: a real-life experience. *Sarcoidosis Vasc Diffus Lung Dis.* (2018) 35:139–42. doi: 10.36141/svdld.v35i2.6170

78. Mateos-Toledo H, Mejía-Ávila M, Rodríguez-Barreto Ó, Mejía-Hurtado JG, Rojas-Serrano J, Estrada A, et al. An open-label study with pirfenidone on chronic hypersensitivity pneumonitis. *Arch Bronconeumol.* (2020) 56:163–9. doi: 10.1016/j.arbr.2019.08.008

79. Flaherty KR, Wells AU, Cottin V, Devaraj A, Walsh SLF, Inoue Y, et al. Nintedanib in progressive fibrosing interstitial lung diseases. *N Engl J Med.* (2019) 381:1718–27. doi: 10.1056/NEJMoa1908681

80. Wells AU, Flaherty KR, Brown KK, Inoue Y, Devaraj A, Richeldi L, et al. Nintedanib in patients with progressive fibrosing interstitial lung diseases—subgroup analyses by interstitial lung disease diagnosis in the INBUILD trial: a randomised, double-blind, placebo-controlled, parallel-group trial. *Lancet Respir Med.* (2020) 8:453–60. doi: 10.1016/S2213-2600(20)30036-9

81. Kern RM, Singer JP, Koth L, Mooney J, Golden J, Hays S, et al. Lung transplantation for hypersensitivity pneumonitis. *Chest.* (2015)147:1558–65. doi: 10.1378/chest.14-1543

82. Kreuter M, Bendstrup E, Russell AM, Bajwah S, Lindell K, Adir Y, et al. Palliative care in interstitial lung disease: living well. *Lancet Respir Med.* (2017) 5:968–80. doi: 10.1016/S2213-2600(17)30383-1

Inflammatory Myopathy-Related Interstitial Lung Disease: From Pathophysiology to Treatment

Baptiste Hervier[1,2]* and Yurdagül Uzunhan[3,4]

[1] *Internal Medicine and Clinical Immunology Department, French Referral Centre for Rare Neuromuscular Disorders, Hôpital Pitié-Salpêtrière, APHP, Paris, France,* [2] *INSERM UMR-S 1135, CIMI-Paris, UPMC & Sorbonne Université, Paris, France,*
[3] *Pneumology Department, Reference Center for Rare Pulmonary Diseases, Hôpital Avicenne, APHP, Bobigny, France,*
[4] *INSERM UMR1272, Université Paris 13, Bobigny, France*

*Correspondence:
Baptiste Hervier
baptiste.hervier@aphp.fr

Inflammatory myopathies (IM) are auto-immune connective tissue diseases characterized by muscle involvement and by extramuscular manifestations. As such, pulmonary manifestations, which mainly include interstitial lung disease (ILD), often darken two out of four distinct IM, namely dermatomyositis and overlapping myositis. Being the initiation site of the disease and being the leading cause of morbidity and mortality, ILD is of major importance in this context. ILD has a heterogeneous expression among the patients, with various onset mode, various radiological pattern, various severity and finally with different prognoses, which are particularly difficult to predict at the time of IM diagnosis. Therefore, ILD is a challenging issue. Treatments are based on steroids and immunosuppressive or targeted therapies. Their respective place is yet poorly codified however and remains often based on clinician expertise. Dedicated clinical trials are lacking to date and are also difficult to build, due to difficulty of constituting large and homogeneous patient groups and to rigorously evaluate disease outcomes. Indeed, pulmonary function tests alone are being regularly defeated in IM, in which respiratory muscles are often involved. Composite scores, bringing together several lung parameters, should thus be developed and validated in the future, to better assess the disease response to treatment. This review aims to describe the current knowledge of IM immuno-pathogenesis, the clinical features associated with IM related-ILD, focusing of both severity and prognosis, and the actual therapeutic approaches.

Keywords: inflammatory myopathy, myositis, interstitial lung disease, auto-immunity, antisynthetase, anti-MDA-5 autoantibody

INTRODUCTION

Interstitial lung disease (ILD) and inflammatory myopathy (IM) are intimately (1). Diagnosing ILD in patients with IM is associated with worse morbidity and higher mortality than in patients without and therefore conditions the strength of the treatments (2).

In contrast, diagnosing autoimmune features in patients with ILD is of importance, as it confers a better prognosis than idiopathic forms: ILD with autoimmune features but without classification criteria for connective tissue diseases (CTD) as well as connective tissue disease (CTD)-related ILD have a better prognosis than idiopathic ILD (3–5).

The description of IMs has largely evolved over the past decades (6, 7). Based on clinical, immunological and histological features, five groups can be distinguished to date (**Figure 1**): (i) overlap myositis, which is the most common (ii) dermatomyositis, which often associates a specific skin involvement, (iii) immune mediated necrotizing myopathy (iv) sporadic inclusion body myositis and (v) polymyositis (8–11). These three latter are most of the time restricted to the muscles. The occurrence of ILD is more strongly associated with two out of five IM subtypes (**Figure 1**). As such, ILD commonly occurs in overlap myositis, among which the anti-synthetase syndrome (aSyS) is the most frequent and can be individualized in many ways (10–14). Other overlap disorders, with myositis-associated autoantibodies (anti-PM-Scl, anti-RNP, anti-Ku etc.) also belongs to this IM subgroup. It is considered that ¾ of the patients with aSyS present with an ILD, whereas this proportion is nearly 1/3 for the other overlap disorders (**Table 1**). Importantly, ILD may be associated with some phenotype of DM, especially the hypo- or amyopathic forms that are associated with anti-MDA-5 (melanoma differentiation-associated protein 5) auto-antibodies, in which its prevalence reaches up to 90% (15, 24, 25) especially in Asian populations. In association with anti-MDA-5, two distinct types of ILD may be distinguished: the rapidly progressive ILD vs. the chronic ILD. In all other cases, ILD occurs more seldom (<10% of the cases) and is most of the time non-severe (26–30).

However, classifying the patients as IM-related ILD is still difficult do date. Indeed, the EULAR-ACR classification criteria for adult and juvenile IM has just been validated, but has many limitations (8, 31, 32). Hence, these classification criteria do not take into account lung involvement and many myositis specific antibodies (MSA). Some patients could thus be misclassified, especially those that are hypo- or amyopathic. Hence, some could classify the patients with ILD, MSA and an hypo- or amyopathic disease as interstitial pneumonia with auto-immune features (IPAF) (33). Obviously, IPAF must not yet be considered as a diagnosis at all, and IPAF classification criteria remain controversial and need to be better defined (34). For instance, some series reported MSA in more than 30% of patients with ILD (35). It is however worth noting that considering IM-related-ILD diagnosis is in fact very important to drive pulmonary and extra-pulmonary management of the patients. Indeed, IM-related ILD has a heterogeneous spectrum, regarding the clinical and radiological features. In the absence of robust markers, prognosis is difficult to predict at diagnosis. Treatments are not standardized, as they have not yet been evaluated rigorously.

By focusing on the two main entities, aSyS and anti-MDA-5 dermatomyositis, the purpose of this review is to describe their immunopathogenesis, the means of assessing ILD activity and progression, as well as severity and prognosis, in order to provide insight into current and future treatments.

IMMUNOPATHOGENESIS

Autoimmune diseases are multifactorial diseases, tolerance breakdown being the results of various genetic susceptibilities, endocrinal and environmental factors that affect both the innate and adaptive immune system. As one of the largest areas of exchange of the individual with the elements of the environment,

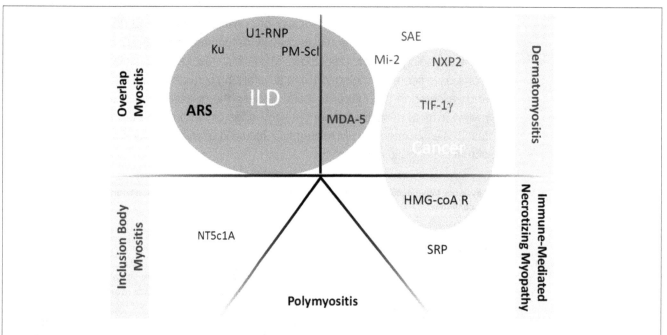

FIGURE 1 | Current classification of inflammatory myopathies and the respective autoantibodies. ILD, Interstitial Lung Disease; ARS, anti-tRNA-antisynthetase autoantidodies, including anti-Jo-1, PL7, PL12, OJ, EJ, Zo, KS, YRS. NXP2: example of myositis specific autoantibody or myositis associated autoantibody; when appearing inside gray circles, the autoantibodies have been shown to correlate with occurrence of either ILD or Cancer, respectively.

TABLE 1 | Prevalence of ILD in the context of Inflammatory-myopathy.

Diseases	Autoantibodies	Prevalence of the ILD	References
	Myositis-specific autoantibodies		
Dermatomyositis	MDA-5	90%	(15–17)
Antisynthetase syndrome	All ARS	80%	(18, 19)
	Jo-1	70%	
	Non-Jo-1	85%	
	Myositis-associated autoantibodies		
Overlap myositis	RNP	50%	(20)
	PM-Scl	25%	(21, 22)
	Ku	35%	(23)

ARS, anti-ARNt synthetase auto-antibodies; ILD, Interstitial Lung Disease.

some hypothesize that the lungs could be the initiation site of different IMs.

MDA-5 is a protein which functions as an intracellular pattern recognition receptor, recognizing double-strand RNA as danger signals. Upon activation, MDA-5 drives the production of large amounts of type I interferons (36). Anti-MDA-5 dermatomyositis is indeed associated with large amounts of type I interferons and mimics some monogenic interferonopathies (37, 38). However, the reasons leading to type I interferon pathway activation remains unknown to date and anti-MDA-5 autoantibodies have not been demonstrated as being pathogenic. Very little is known regarding the causes and consequences of such direct activation on lung parenchyma and on innate and adaptive immunity, but different data argue for the involvement of macrophages, as it has been reported in various autoimmune diseases (39). These cells may play important roles in immune-regulation and tissue-repair. As such, recent data have revealed that non-inflammatory macrophages (previously called M2 macrophages, which produce IL-10 and TGFβ) are involved in the progression of lung fibrosis (40, 41). Interestingly, soluble macrophage-mannose receptor, sCD206, a serum marker for M2 polarization, is increased in MDA-5 DM-associated ILD and its titer correlated with a poor outcome (42). Interleukin(IL)-18 (43), a potent macrophage activating molecule could be involved in the development of ILD. In addition, several macrophage activation markers, including ferritin (44), NOS2 or neopterin are increased in the patients with anti-MDA-5 dermatomyositis.

ASyS is a heterogeneous disease, immunologically characterized by MSA directed against different ARNt-synthetases, among which anti-hystidyl-tRNA-synthetase (also called anti-Jo-1) is the most common (18, 45). To date, seven auto-antibodies directed against other tRNAsynthetases, including anti-Alanyl (PL-12), anti Threonyl (PL-7), anti-Glycyl (EJ) -t-RNA-synthetases have been described. Although dark areas persist, the immunopathogenesis of Jo-1 positive aSyS is best described and could nowadays be drawn as follows:

following environmental exposure to tabacco smoke (46), airborne contaminants (47) including mineral particles (such as asbestiform amphiboles) or respiratory tract infections (48), the lung tissue is aggressed. This leads to cellular stress, danger signal pathway activation and cell death with microparticle release. Innate immune cells–such as NK cells- are unspecifically activated and release proteolytic enzymes, including Granzyme B (49). The antigen, Histidyl-tRNA-synthetase, which is expressed into a specific conformation within the lungs, is then released in the extracellular milieu and has many immune properties, including activity in inflammatory response with its cytokine like domains, chemoattractant properties with $CCR5^+$ cell recruitment and capacity to activate other immune cells (50, 51). All the immune cells are present within the lungs of patients with aSyS (52). Tolerance breakdown may occur when the different adaptive immune cells are successively activated. The cascade of events is efficiently favored by a certain genetic background, like HLA-B*08.01 (53), and includes antigen presentation, CD8-T cell priming and CD4-T cell-B-cell crosstalk. As a witness of these processes, type I/II interferons, B lymphocyte stimulator and other cytokines are increased in the sera of aSyS patients. Finally, anti-Histidyl-tRNA-synthetase autoantibodies are produced. The way the disease propagates to other organs remains largely unexplained: although histydyl-tRNA-synthetase could be abnormally expressed in various tissues, the pathogenicity of anti-Jo-1 is still matter of controversies and the presence of Jo-1 specific T cells within extra-pulmonary target tissues has to be further determined.

INITIAL EVALUATION

Clinical Evaluation of the ILD

Patients with IM-related ILD may present with clinical symptoms, including fever (1/4), cough (1/3) or dyspnea (>1/2), which could be either related to ILD or not, especially when gastro-esophageal reflux or respiratory muscle involvement also occurs as part of the aSyS (18, 19). Regarding the shortness of breath, it is immediately important to evaluate (i) the rapidity of onset, as the (sub)acute forms settling within 3 months –defining rapidly-progressive (RP)-ILD are of worse prognosis (54, 55) and (ii) the severity, as some patients require intensive care support (56). In contrast, the patients with mild ILD or in which ILD will develop later in the follow-up (1/5) can be asymptomatic, justifying careful explorations.

Explorations of the ILD

The severity of ILD can also be assessed by oximetry and blood gases to evaluate hypoxemia and/or hypercapnia.

CT-Scan is the major tool of the evaluation (**Figure 2**), revealing different types of lesions and helping in classifying ILD into different patterns, as defined by the ATS/ERS consensus for idiopathic interstitial pneumonias (**Table 2**) (61). As such, bi-basal ground glass opacities and linear reticulations are associated with non-specific interstitial pneumonia (NSIP) and are the most common, as found in other connective tissue disorders like systemic sclerosis. Alveolar condensations -willingly bilateral-also occur, especially in the RP-ILD subset and define organizing

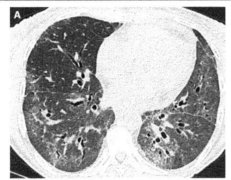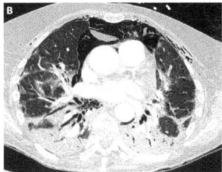

FIGURE 2 | Examples of lung CT findings in patients with IM-related ILD. **(A)** NSIP pattern in a patient with PL12+ antisynthetase syndrome: ground glass opacities with bilateral proximal bronchiectasis. **(B)** OP pattern in a patient with MDA5+ dermatomyositis: extensive parenchymal consolidation and pneumomediastinum.

pneumonia (OP). Both patterns may also mix together (NSIP-OP). Usual interstitial pneumonia (UIP), with sub-pleural honey combing lesions, is less frequent and dramatically more seldom in IM-related ILD than in rheumatoid arthritis-related ILD. In the worse cases with acute lung injury, often leading to acute respiratory distress syndrome (ARDS), CT-scan may show features of acute interstitial pneumonia with consolidations and extensive ground glass opacities.

CT-scan is also important to evaluate (i) the presence of fibrosing lesions, including traction bronchiectasis and reticulations, which are present at first evaluation in high proportion (57, 62), and (ii) the extension of the lesions (63) -usually bilateral and starting in posterior and basal regions-within all the lung parenchyma.

The distribution of these patterns partially depends on the IM subtype, NSIP predominating in aSyS and OP in MDA-5-dermatomyositis (**Table 2**) (58).

At diagnosis (as well as in any case of worsening during follow-up), endoscopy and broncho-alveolar lavage (BAL) could be discussed. It might help in distinguishing specific deterioration from intercurrent factors that may have caused respiratory decline, including aspiration pneumonia in newly diagnosed patients, or opportunistic infections, which occur mostly in patients under immunosuppressive therapy. In addition, rare cases of bronchiolo-alveolar cancer can be thus detected. BAL fluid discloses aspecific alveolitis with high counts of lymphocytes, neutrophils, eosinophils or with mixed cellularity.

Lung histology is no longer recommended due to the low benefit/risk ratio of the biopsy procedure, and ILD subtype could be almost easily determined on CT-scan rather than on histological features.

When possible, pulmonary function tests help in evaluating ILD severity, as well as detecting a possible respiratory muscle involvement. Restrictive syndrome, defined by a total lung capacity (TLC) <80% with a more or less severe decrease of forced vital capacity (FVC), is almost constantly observed. Severity of restriction may be appreciated by TLC impairment on plethysmography. However, the FVC impairment is more routinely followed as it is more easily measured on spirometry. Muscle impairment and especially diaphragmatic involvement

TABLE 2 | ILD-patterns on lung CT-scan: lesion types and prevalence in IM-related ILD.

ILD pattern		Predominant lesions on CT-scan	Prevalence in ASyS	Prevalence in MDA5*
Non-Specific Interstitial Pneumonia	NSIP	Basal ground glass opacities, linear reticulations	50%	20%
Organizing Pneumonia	OP	Alveolar consolidations	20%	50%**
	NSIP-OP	Associations of NSIP & OP lesions	25%	30%
Usual Interstitial Pneumonia	UIP	Basal subpleural reticulations with bronchectasis and honeycombing lesions	10%	<5%
Acute Interstitial Pneumonia	AIP	Consolidations and extensive ground-glass opacities	<5%	30%**
Other associated anomalies				
Signs of Fibrosis		Reticulations, Traction Bronchectasis	>75%	40%
Non-significant adenopathies			30%	30%

*To be confirmed in larger series, ** OP and AIP are often difficult to distinguish. Adapted from (56–60).

may worsen this parameter and is suggested when FVC is dramatically lower than expected as compared to CT-scan lesions or when decubitus FVC is significantly lower than conventional FVC. Diffusing capacity of the lung for carbon monoxide (DLCO) impairment often precede TLC and FVC decrease. DLCO is also useful to evaluate the ILD severity at any time of the disease course and/or to suspect pulmonary hypertension when excessively reduced in comparison to FVC deterioration. In this context, the screening for pulmonary hypertension by trans-thoracic echocardiography is recommended (64).

Exploring diaphragmatic involvement might be useful. Measurement of maximal static inspiratory pressure (PI max) and of maximal static expiratory pressure (PE max) are low invasive parameters that could be combined with radioscopic assessment of diaphragmatic course and electromyography of the diaphragm to explore significant diaphragmatic dysfunction (65, 66).

Six-minutes walk test (6MWT) may be useful to estimate ILD severity in the absence of significant muscle involvement. Dyspnea, nadir of oxygen saturation and walking distance are the main parameters evaluated during the test.

FVC, DLCO and in a lesser extend 6MWT are therefore main physiologic parameters for assessing respiratory severity at diagnosis and also to evaluate response to therapy during the disease course.

Extra-Pulmonary Evaluation

Besides pulmonary evaluation, muscle, skin, heart, joint, and vessel involvement must be carefully assessed. Above all, severe myositis with dysphagia and respiratory muscle involvement may complicate the management of ILD and biased the ILD evaluation.

A particular attention should be paid for skin manifestations, as ulcerations are found especially in MDA-5+ dermatomyositis (16).

In all patients with newly identified ILD, the last ATS/ERS/ALAT/JRS recommendations indicated an overwhelming agreement to perform serological testing to achieve a diagnosis rigorously. The majority of panelists acknowledged routine testing for C-reactive protein, antinuclear antibodies, myositis linear-dot panel or immunoprecipitation, as well as rheumatoid factor and anti–cyclic citrullinated peptide for Rheumatoid arthritis (67). Other detailed tests, such as creatine kinase, have to be performed on a case-by-case basis according to the associated clinical signs.

EVOLUTION

Short-Term Prognosis

Three factors, that are linked together, could be identified as short-term prognosis factors: (i) the severity of the ILD itself, (ii) the rapidity of onset (RP-ILD) (54, 55) and (iii) the presence of anti-MDA-5 auto-antibodies (15). Even in the absence of any comparative study, it is admitted that the most severe patients with either aSyS or anti-MDA-5 dermatomyositis, notably those requiring intensive care, are of worse prognosis. In these patients, the severity is evaluated clinically or with the CT-scan (showing extended OP or acute interstitial pneumonia lesions), but rarely with the pulmonary function tests, often impossible to perform. In intensive care unit, the mortality ratio reaches 50% (56). Most of the severe patients presented a RP-ILD, which is itself associated with a high mortality risk ratio, as compared to patients with chronic onset of ILD, both during aSyS and anti-MDA-5 dermatomyositis. When comparing patients according to the nature of the myositis specific autoantibodies, it has been clearly shown that the presence of MDA-5 autoantibodies is by itself a risk factor of early mortality, as compared to anti-ARNt-synthetases (15).

Long-Term Prognosis

General Outcome

Despite early mortality in the severe forms, the 5-year survival ratio is >85% in IM-ILD (18, 19, 59). Although some patients could worsen during the first year of treatment, the time to disease progression usually counts in years (57, 58). As examples, in long-term follow-up series, 20% of the patients with IM-related ILD (not including patients with anti-MDA-5) worsen despite immunosuppressive treatments, with the risk of developing respiratory failure. The remaining patients being stable (35–55%) or improved (25–45%) (59, 68, 69). It is thus important to find factors predictive of ILD progression over time, especially during the first months of treatment. However, the heterogeneity of IM-related ILD makes assessment of prognosis particularly difficult, not allowing us to clearly stratify the patient and adjust the treatment to the potential of aggravation. Such attitude is still a real challenge and should be the subject of future studies.

Evaluations

The severity of the ILD on pulmonary functions tests is probably not sufficient to predict long-term evolution. Some retrospective studies suggested a correlation between the PFTs at onset (such as low DLCO or FVC) and the long-term ILD prognosis (59, 70). However, in a prospective cohort, the first value of either FVC or DLCO did not correlate with improvement or worsening over time (71). This was at least partly due to the existence of respiratory muscle involvement, which is a confusing factor to interpret FVC as a marker of lung involvement only. It could be thus more relevant to evaluate the kinetic of FVC variations between two early time points, as a predictive factor of long-term response to treatment. However, such option has not been validated prospectively in large cohorts.

It has been demonstrated in studies dedicated to IPF, that serial decline in the FVC over 6–12 months is a powerful predictor of mortality (72). An absolute change in the FVC of 10% of the predicted normal value is a predictor of mortality but this large amplitude of change is less prevalent than relative change in a given time period, which has been shown to be also predictive of mortality in the majority of IPF studies. More recently, Goh et al. (73) have examined correlations between short-term pulmonary function trends and long-term outcome in ILD associated with systemic sclerosis, which is very close to chronical forms of IM-related ILD. Disease severity at baseline and subsequent pulmonary function trends were independent prognostic determinants. At 1 year, categorical FVC trends provide the most accurate prognostic information, especially when integrated with DLCO trends. Thus, the optimal definition of categorical decline in FVC for trial purposes may consist of either a ≥10% decline in the FVC or a 5–9% marginal decline in the FVC in association with a ≥15% decline in the DLCO for systemic sclerosis. However, such studies are lacking in IM-related ILD (74).

Thus, as suggested by these studies, it would be probably more accurate in IM-related ILD also to at least consider these parameters as qualitative variable, taking into account the proportion of patients improving/worsening FVC and/or DLCO for at least 10 and 15%, respectively.

Furthermore, defining time to ILD progression or event-free survival could be relevant and should be rigorously evaluated in the future as end-points. Composite scores including dyspnea score, muscle and physiologic parameters would probably be of great interest for evaluating disease progression and treatment response in IM-related ILD. Defining and validating such scores will be a challenge in the future.

Valuable information coming from CT-scan analyses is also insufficiently robust to date. Regarding the ILD radiologic pattern, some suggested UIP was worse than NSIP, especially in terms of disease progression (68). Although histology of UIP is more frequent than expected in the autopsy series, the corresponding radiologic pattern has however a better prognosis than IPF (75). A recent large study showed that the UIP pattern on lung-CT-scan is significantly associated with mortality. As opposed to acute interstitial pneumonia, the OP pattern was associated with the lowest mortality on long-term follow-up (76). No study has demonstrated yet a worse prognosis according to either fibrosing scores and/or extension scores assessed on CT-scan in IM-related ILD, as it has been for example reported in systemic sclerosis (63). At least, anti-rheumatic drug modifications (DMARDs) overtime correlated with the initial extension of the ILD within the lung parenchyma (60).

Different biomarkers could correlate with ILD prognosis. However, further studies are required to validate on a large scale the promising interest of KL-6 (77), Ferritin (44), C-RP or IL-18 serum dosage (43) alone or mixed together, to perform them routinely and stratify the patient with IM-related ILD early, according to their potential prognosis value. In ASyS patients, it has been shown that patients with non-Jo-1 had a worse prognosis in terms of mortality as compared to Jo-1 patients (18, 19). Although not rigorously demonstrated, these data could be at least due to higher proportions of hypo- or amyopathic patients in the non-Jo1 group, in which the ILD could therefore be more severe upon diagnosis. The concomitant positivity of anti-Ro 52 kilo-daltons, which is quite common in IM and especially in ASyS (78) might worsens the ILD prognosis (79). Using unsupervised analyses, three distinct subgroups with different prognoses can be observed on a large French multicentric cohort of MDA-5 dermatomyositis (Allenbach et al. unpublished data). The first cluster with severe lung involvement and a dramatically poor prognosis corresponded to the well-recognized "anti-MDA5+ RP-ILD." In addition, two other overlapping forms were isolated: the "anti-MDA5+ arthro-DM," with a good prognosis, and the "anti-MDA5+ vasculo-DM," with an intermediate prognosis. The decisional algorithm showed that only three variables (Raynaud phenomenon, arthralgia/arthritis and gender) are good predictors for cluster appurtenance and their related outcome.

ILD Complications

Besides progression of fibrosing ILD, aspiration or opportunistic pneumonia, IM-related ILD has two major complications.

Although rare (<8% of the cases) and often associated with pneumothorax, pneumomediastinum is non-fortuitously associated with IM-related ILD, as it occurs more commonly than in other connective tissue-related ILD (80). Association with MDA-5 auto-antibodies, long suspected from various reports

(81–83) has been rigorously demonstrated only recently (84). Pneumomediastinum is an aggravating factor, that usually occurs early (<24 months) in the course of the disease. Its underlying mechanism remains unknown to date.

Pulmonary hypertension is the second feared ILD complication. In contrast to pneumomediastinum, pulmonary hypertension occurs lately in the course of ILD and witnesses its severity. Indeed, during aSyS and conversely to other connective tissue diseases, pulmonary hypertension belongs to group III only and is diagnosed in almost 8% of the cases (64). However, in the severe forms, a contribution of a vascular component is not excluded. Even though there is no recommendation for pulmonary hypertension specific treatments in this context, its screening with repeated echocardiography is recommended. When necessary, right heart catheterization will confirm the diagnosis. In a French series, patients with pulmonary hypertension had a significantly lower survival rate.

Thus, finding efficient prognosis factors (or prognosis scores pooling the different parameters), correlating with long-term disease severity is of major importance, and should be the prospect of future studies. Indeed, the development of patient stratification according to the risk of progression, in order to manage therapeutic strategies for each patient. Such personalized medicine remains a challenge in the field of IM-related ILD.

TREATMENTS

Adjuvant Therapies

Besides different possibilities of medical treatment, patients with IM-related ILD must benefit from the update of the vaccines, like annual vaccination against flu, anti- pneumococcal vaccination. Such attitude is indeed justified by a recent study showing that antibody response rates in the connective tissue-related ILD patients (including those receiving immunosuppressants) were comparable with those of a control group without ILD (85). In addition, no acute exacerbation was observed after pneumococcal immunization, indicating pneumococcal vaccines in ILD patients are efficient and safe (85).

Occurrence of opportunistic infections in IM-related ILD is significant and could be at least associated with the disease itself and its treatments (86). Thus, preventive treatment of *pneumocystis jirovecii* with trimethoprime + sulfamethoxazole or in case of contraindication with atovaquone, should be prescribed as soon as patients received steroids >20 mg/d during >4 weeks and especially for the most severe patients (87).

Pulmonary rehabilitation as well as muscle physiotherapy may also be beneficial (88). Since nutrition-related factors have been noticed as a prognostic factor for patients with chronic respiratory diseases, including patients with ILD, particular attention should also be paid to this aspect of the patients' care (89). When clearly implicated and if possible, exposure to cigarette smoke and other airborne contaminants should be avoided.

All patients should benefit from this personalized treatment approach. Therapeutic education programs should address symptom management, oxygen therapy and medications. Patients emphasized the importance of understanding what the future might hold and were generally supportive of discussing advance care planning and end-of-life care.

Steroids and Classical Immunosuppressive Drugs

In the absence of randomized clinical trials, treatments of IM-related LD are based on small retrospective studies. Treatment efficacy is difficult to evaluate in this context and requires sufficiently long evaluation period. In most of the studies, the outcome measures are improvement of pulmonary function tests between two time points (FVC and/or DCLO being considered as quantitative variables). However, FVC also depends on respiratory muscle involvement and make respiratory evaluations difficult when the IM is severe.

Even though we noticed the absence of dedicated trial, treatment of IM-related ILD is based on steroids. Intravenous high doses are initially given in the most severe forms or RP-ILD.

Addition of an immunosuppressive drug as a first line treatment progressively became consensual, being now a cornerstone of the treatment, as ¾ of the patients could develop steroid resistance or relapse when tapering the doses (90), irrespectively of the initial severity. As such, cyclophosphamide and tacrolimus have been reported in retrospective studies to improve FVC and/or DLCO in almost all patients (91–93). Although less commonly reported, azathioprine and methotrexate could also be efficient (94, 95). Interestingly, tacrolimus and mycophenolate mophetil have shown interest in reducing steroid doses. Recently, one study has compared aztioprine vs. mycophenolate mophetil: both improved PFTs in similar proportions (96). Azathioprine allowed a greater decrease in the dose of steroids as compared to mycophenolate mophetil, while being associated with more side effects. Among these immunosupressants, intravenous cyclophosphamide, mycophenolate mofetil, and azathioprine have been reported to be efficient in similar proportions (97).

Some reports emphasize the interest of immunosuppressive treatment associations (98), especially when ILD is severe. However, such attitude exposes the patients to higher infectious risks.

IM-related ILD is a chronical disease and requires prolonged treatment duration, often exceeding several years. There is however no clear information to date regarding the most appropriate time and modalities to stop the treatments.

Single case reports indicated some benefit from plasma exchange for IM associated severe ILD, especially those with anti-MDA-5 autoantibodies, but no conclusion could be drawn to date. While some reported its use as an initial treatment in severe ASyS patients (99), no data support the long-term efficacy of intravenous immunoglobulin treatment for ILD in the context of IM.

Biologics

Over the past decades, the relative place of biologics to treat IM-related ILD has increased a lot. Among them, the anti-CD20 targeting B-cell therapy has become the most documented. In one of the few prospective studies, 50% of refractory AsyS patients receiving rituximab as a third line therapy improved

their FVC at 1 year (100). Several retrospective studies (101–103) and a meta-analysis (104) reported promising results of rituximab on pulmonary function tests. On the other hand, efficacy of rituximab based on the improvement of CT-score was less clear. However, the cost in terms of risk of infections, with sometimes fatal complications, is high (101). In these retrospective series, rituximab was most of the time used as at least a second line treatment and there was no comparison with other treatments. Thus, the place of anti-CD20 monoclonal antibodies in the therapeutic arsenal needs further clarifications, which will emerge from prospective trials currently in progress.

Other targeted therapies have been tried in severe RP-ILD associated with anti-MDA5 dermatomyositis. On the faith of a small case series of four patients, basiliximab, a monoclonal antibody targeting CD25+ activated T cells, could improve patients' survival (105). Similarly, JAK-inhibitors (in this case tofacitinib), which blocks interferon pathways and other pro-inflammatory cytokine pathways, has shown a promising survival rate improvement (17, 106).

Of note, anti-TNFα targeting therapies are usually not recommended in the context of IM (107), partly due to the occurrence of muscular aggravations under treatment.

Future Directions

Depending on a better understanding of the immune mechanisms leading to ASyS and MDA-5 dermatomyositis, new immune-based therapeutic strategies could emerge in the future. As such, different existing biologics could find a place to treat IM-related ILD, including anti-IL12/23, anti-IFNα and anti-IFNα receptors antibodies, anti-IL-6 or other anti-B cell therapy like ibrutinib etc. However, the rational to use these treatments lack translational data to date showing a clear involvement of these pathways in ILD pathogenesis. New directions could also be developed in the future according to these immunological researches and help in developing new treatments. As examples, blocking pattern recognition receptor-dependent immune cell activation or macrophage activation pathways, which seems specifically involved in ILD associated with MDA-5 positivity might become real and might open a new era in the future. Future immunotherapies have to integrate innovative approaches based on selective and oriented immunomodulations as well as on concomitant therapies promoting tissue repair. Anti-fibrotic agents could be a new treatment option: (i) fibrotic mechanisms are at work in the lung of patients with IM-related ILD, (ii) the recent results obtained in patients treated with nintedanib for systemic sclerosis-related ILD, another connective tissue disease associated with fibrosing ILD, are promising (108). Although such clinical trials required a large number of patients to be informative, efforts should be done to define eligible patients and to build international and randomized prospective trials, at least in ASyS-related ILD.

Lung Transplantation

Few cases of lung transplantation have been reported in patients with IM-related ILD (109). Of note, comorbidities as well as immune fragility of the patients, related to the previous immunosuppressive treatment they received, negatively impact the prognosis of the procedure. In addition, involvement of respiratory muscles, especially in ASyS, and/or skin vascular sequelae in MDA-5 positive patients are probably factors of transplantation failure. However, in patients carefully selected the reported risk of IM-related ILD recurrence is not higher than that of other connective tissue disorders, including systemic sclerosis, and a 5-year survival rate of 75% has been described in a small case series (110). Thus, lung transplantation is possible in IM-related ILD and its prognosis factors for success should be more largely studied worldwide. Extracorporeal membrane oxygenation (ECMO) may be interesting as a bridge to lung transplantation in selected patients already considered as candidates for lung transplantation. Thus, referring severe patients to transplantation centers early in the course of the disease is important.

CONCLUSION

Although the knowledge of IM-related ILD has tremendously progressed over the past decades, its management remains a challenge to date. Based on basic and clinical research, the future objectives will need to focus on the IM-related ILD definition of classification criteria, the development of reliable disease activity and progression scores that can be used as robust end-point for the future clinical trials and the finding of early prognosis biomarkers. The aims will be to adapt therapeutic strategies to individual risk factors (patients' stratification) and to find new efficient immune-based biologics as well as to prospectively study the relevance of innovative anti-fibrotic agents.

AUTHOR CONTRIBUTIONS

BH and YU wrote the manuscript and built the tables and figures, which are original.

REFERENCES

1. Mecoli CA, Christopher-Stine L. Management of interstitial lung disease in patients with myositis specific autoantibodies. *Curr Rheumatol Rep.* (2018) 20:27. doi: 10.1007/s11926-018-0731-7

2. Cottin V, Thivolet-Béjui F, Reynaud-Gaubert M, Cadranel J, Delaval P, Ternamian PJ, et al. Interstitial lung disease in amyopathic dermatomyositis, dermatomyositis and polymyositis. *Eur Respir J.* (2003) 22:245–50. doi: 10.1183/09031936.03.00026703

3. Park JH, Kim DS, Park I-N, Jang SJ, Kitaichi M, Nicholson AG, et al. Prognosis of fibrotic interstitial pneumonia: idiopathic versus collagen vascular disease-related subtypes. *Am J Respir Crit Care Med.* (2007) 175:705–11. doi: 10.1164/rccm.200607-912OC

4. Navaratnam V, Ali N, Smith CJP, McKeever T, Fogarty A, Hubbard RB. Does the presence of connective tissue disease modify survival in patients with pulmonary fibrosis? *Respir Med.* (2011) 105:1925–30. doi: 10.1016/j.rmed.2011.08.015

5. Yoshimura K, Kono M, Enomoto Y, Nishimoto K, Oyama Y, Yasui H, et al. Distinctive characteristics and prognostic significance of interstitial pneumonia with autoimmune features in patients with chronic fibrosing interstitial pneumonia. *Respir Med.* (2018) 137:167–75. doi: 10.1016/j.rmed.2018.02.024

6. Betteridge Z, Tansley S, Shaddick G, Chinoy H, Cooper RG, New RP, et al. Frequency, mutual exclusivity and clinical associations of myositis autoantibodies in a combined European cohort of idiopathic inflammatory myopathy patients. *J Autoimmun.* (2019) 101:48–55. doi: 10.1016/j.jaut.2019.04.001

7. Mariampillai K, Granger B, Amelin D, Guiguet M, Hachulla E, Maurier F, et al. Development of a new classification system for idiopathic inflammatory myopathies based on clinical manifestations and myositis-specific autoantibodies. *JAMA Neurol.* (2018) 75:1528–37. doi: 10.1001/jamaneurol.2018.2598

8. Lundberg IE, Tjärnlund A, Bottai M, Werth VP, Pilkington C, de Visser M, et al. 2017 European League Against Rheumatism/American College of Rheumatology classification criteria for adult and juvenile idiopathic inflammatory myopathies and their major subgroups. *Ann Rheum Dis.* (2017) 76:1955–64. doi: 10.1136/annrheumdis-2017-211468

9. Lilleker JB, Vencovsky J, Wang G, Wedderburn LR, Diederichsen LP, Schmidt J, et al. Response to: 'Antisynthetase syndrome or what else? Different perspectives indicate the need for new classification criteria' by Cavagna et al. *Ann Rheum Dis.* (2018) 77:e51.

10. Selva-O'Callaghan A, Pinal-Fernandez I, Trallero-Araguás E, Milisenda JC, Grau-Junyent JM, Mammen AL. Classification and management of adult inflammatory myopathies. *Lancet Neurol.* (2018) 17:816–28. doi: 10.1016/S1474-4422(18)30254-0

11. Noguchi E, Uruha A, Suzuki S, Hamanaka K, Ohnuki Y, Tsugawa J, et al. Skeletal Muscle Involvement in Antisynthetase Syndrome. *JAMA Neurol.* (2017) 74:992–9. doi: 10.1001/jamaneurol.2017.0934

12. Stenzel W, Preuße C, Allenbach Y, Pehl D, Junckerstorff R, Heppner FL, et al. Nuclear actin aggregation is a hallmark of anti-synthetase syndrome-induced dysimmune myopathy. *Neurol.* (2015) 84:1346–54. doi: 10.1212/WNL.0000000000001422

13. Aouizerate J, De Antonio M, Bassez G, Gherardi RK, Berenbaum F, Guillevin L, et al. Myofiber HLA-DR expression is a distinctive biomarker for antisynthetase-associated myopathy. *Acta Neuropathol Commun.* (2014) 2:154. doi: 10.1186/s40478-014-0154-2

14. Mescam-Mancini L, Allenbach Y, Hervier B, Devilliers H, Mariampillay K, Dubourg O, et al. Anti-Jo-1 antibody-positive patients show a characteristic necrotizing perifascicular myositis. *Brain J Neurol.* (2015) 138:2485–92. doi: 10.1093/brain/awv192

15. Labrador-Horrillo M, Martinez MA, Selva-O'Callaghan A, Trallero-Araguas E, Balada E, Vilardell-Tarres M, et al. Anti-MDA5 antibodies in a large Mediterranean population of adults with dermatomyositis. *J Immunol Res.* (2014) 2014:290797. doi: 10.1155/2014/290797

16. Narang NS, Casciola-Rosen L, Li S, Chung L, Fiorentino DF. Cutaneous ulceration in dermatomyositis: association with anti-melanoma differentiation-associated gene 5 antibodies and interstitial lung disease. *Arthritis Care Res.* (2015) 67:667–72. doi: 10.1002/acr.22498

17. Kurasawa K, Arai S, Namiki Y, Tanaka A, Takamura Y, Owada T, et al. Tofacitinib for refractory interstitial lung diseases in anti-melanoma differentiation-associated 5 gene antibody-positive dermatomyositis. *Rheumatol.* (2018) 57:2114–9. doi: 10.1093/rheumatology/key188

18. Hervier B, Devilliers H, Stanciu R, Meyer A, Uzunhan Y, Masseau A, et al. Hierarchical cluster and survival analyses of antisynthetase syndrome: phenotype and outcome are correlated with anti-tRNA synthetase antibody specificity. *Autoimmun Rev.* (2012) 12:210–7. doi: 10.1016/j.autrev.2012.06.006

19. Aggarwal R, Cassidy E, Fertig N, Koontz DC, Lucas M, Ascherman DP, et al. Patients with non-Jo-1 anti-tRNA-synthetase autoantibodies have worse survival than Jo-1 positive patients. *Ann Rheum Dis.* (2013) doi: 10.1136/annrheumdis-2012-201800

20. Szodoray P, Hajas A, Kardos L, Dezso B, Soos G, Zold E, et al. Distinct phenotypes in mixed connective tissue disease: subgroups and survival. *Lupus.* (2012) 21:1412–22. doi: 10.1177/0961203312456751

21. D'Aoust J, Hudson M, Tatibouet S, Wick J, Mahler M, Baron M, et al. Clinical and serologic correlates of anti-PM/Scl antibodies in systemic sclerosis: a

multicenter study of 763 patients. *Arthritis Rheumatol.* (2014) 66:1608–15. doi: 10.1002/art.38428

22. De Lorenzo R, Pinal-Fernandez I, Huang W, Albayda J, Tiniakou E, Johnson C, et al. Muscular and extramuscular clinical features of patients with anti-PM/Scl autoantibodies. *Neurology.* (2018) 90:e2068–76. doi: 10.1212/WNL.0000000000005638

23. Rigolet A, Musset L, Dubourg O, Maisonobe T, Grenier P, Charuel J-L, et al. Inflammatory myopathies with anti-Ku antibodies: a prognosis dependent on associated lung disease. *Medicine.* (2012) 91:95–102. doi: 10.1097/MD.0b013e31824d9cec

24. Moghadam-Kia S, Oddis CV, Sato S, Kuwana M, Aggarwal R. Antimelanoma differentiation-associated Gene 5 antibody: expanding the clinical spectrum in North American patients with Dermatomyositis. *J Rheumatol.* (2017) 44:319–25. doi: 10.3899/jrheum.160682

25. Hall JC, Casciola-Rosen L, Samedy L-A, Werner J, Owoyemi K, Danoff SK, et al. Anti-melanoma differentiation-associated protein 5-associated dermatomyositis: expanding the clinical spectrum. *Arthritis Care Res.* (2013) 65:1307–15. doi: 10.1002/acr.21992

26. Miller T, Al-Lozi MT, Lopate G, Pestronk A. Myopathy with antibodies to the signal recognition particle: clinical and pathological features. *J Neurol Neurosurg Psychiatry.* (2002) 73:420–8. doi: 10.1136/jnnp.73.4.420

27. Hengstman GJD, Vree Egberts WTM, Seelig HP, Lundberg IE, Moutsopoulos HM, Doria A, et al. Clinical characteristics of patients with myositis and autoantibodies to different fragments of the Mi-2 beta antigen. *Ann Rheum Dis.* (2006) 65:242–5. doi: 10.1136/ard.2005.040717

28. Tarricone E, Ghirardello A, Rampudda M, Bassi N, Punzi L, Doria A. Anti-SAE antibodies in autoimmune myositis: identification by unlabelled protein immunoprecipitation in an Italian patient cohort. *J Immunol Methods.* (2012) 384:128–34. doi: 10.1016/j.jim.2012.07.019

29. Betteridge ZE, Gunawardena H, Chinoy H, North J, Ollier WER, Cooper RG, et al. Clinical and human leucocyte antigen class II haplotype associations of autoantibodies to small ubiquitin-like modifier enzyme, a dermatomyositis-specific autoantigen target, in UK Caucasian adult-onset myositis. *Ann Rheum Dis.* (2009) 68:1621–5. doi: 10.1136/ard.2008.097162

30. Allenbach Y, Drouot L, Rigolet A, Charuel JL, Jouen F, Romero NB, et al. Anti-HMGCR autoantibodies in European patients with autoimmune necrotizing myopathies: inconstant exposure to statin. *Medicine.* (2014) 93:150–7. doi: 10.1097/MD.0000000000000028

31. Lundberg IE, Tjärnlund A, Bottai M, Werth VP, Pilkington C, de Visser M, et al. 2017 European League Against Rheumatism/American College of Rheumatology classification criteria for adult and juvenile idiopathic inflammatory myopathies and their major subgroups. *Arthritis Rheumatol.* (2017) 69:2271–82. doi: 10.1002/art.40320

32. Lundberg IE, de Visser M, Werth VP. Classification of myositis. *Nat Rev Rheumatol.* (2018) 14:269–78. doi: 10.1038/nrrheum.2018.41

33. Fischer A, Antoniou KM, Brown KK, Cadranel J, Corte TJ, du Bois RM, et al. An official European Respiratory Society/American Thoracic Society research statement: interstitial pneumonia with autoimmune features. *Eur Respir J.* (2015) 46:976–87. doi: 10.1183/13993003.00150-2015

34. Sambataro G, Sambataro D, Torrisi SE, Vancheri A, Pavone M, Rosso R, et al. State of the art in interstitial pneumonia with autoimmune features: a systematic review on retrospective studies and suggestions for further advances. *Eur Respir Rev.* (2018) 27: doi: 10.1183/16000617.0139-2017

35. Chartrand S, Swigris JJ, Peykova L, Chung J, Fischer A. A Multidisciplinary evaluation helps identify the antisynthetase syndrome in patients presenting as idiopathic interstitial pneumonia. *J Rheumatol.* (2016) 43:887–92. doi: 10.3899/jrheum.150966

36. Rodero MP, Crow YJ. Type I interferon-mediated monogenic autoinflammation: the type I interferonopathies, a conceptual overview. *J Exp Med.* (2016) 213:2527–38. doi: 10.1084/jem.20161596

37. Horai Y, Koga T, Fujikawa K, Takatani A, Nishino A, Nakashima Y, et al. Serum interferon-α is a useful biomarker in patients with anti-melanoma differentiation-associated gene 5 (MDA5) antibody-positive dermatomyositis. *Mod Rheumatol.* (2014) doi: 10.3109/14397595.2014.900843

38. Allenbach Y, Leroux G, Suárez-Calvet X, Preusse C, Gallardo E, Hervier B, et al. Dermatomyositis with or without anti-melanoma differentiation-associated gene 5 antibodies: common interferon

signature but distinct NOS2 expression. *Am J Pathol.* (2016) 186:691–700. doi: 10.1016/j.ajpath.2015.11.010

39. Ma W-T, Gao F, Gu K, Chen D-K. The role of monocytes and macrophages in autoimmune diseases: a comprehensive review. *Front Immunol.* (2019) 10:1140. doi: 10.3389/fimmu.2019.01140

40. Prasse A, Pechkovsky DV, Toews GB, Jungraithmayr W, Kollert F, Goldmann T, et al. A vicious circle of alveolar macrophages and fibroblasts perpetuates pulmonary fibrosis via CCL18. *Am J Respir Crit Care Med.* (2006) 173:781–92. doi: 10.1164/rccm.200509-1518OC

41. Zhang L, Wang Y, Wu G, Xiong W, Gu W, Wang C-Y. Macrophages: friend or foe in idiopathic pulmonary fibrosis? *Respir Res.* (2018) 19:170. doi: 10.1186/s12931-018-0864-2

42. Horiike Y, Suzuki Y, Fujisawa T, Yasui H, Karayama M, Hozumi H, et al. Successful classification of macrophage-mannose receptor CD206 in severity of anti-MDA5 antibody positive dermatomyositis associated ILD. *Rheumatology.* (2019) 58:2143–52. doi: 10.1093/rheumatology/kez185

43. Gono T, Sato S, Kawaguchi Y, Kuwana M, Hanaoka M, Katsumata Y, et al. Anti-MDA5 antibody, ferritin and IL-18 are useful for the evaluation of response to treatment in interstitial lung disease with anti-MDA5 antibody-positive dermatomyositis. *Rheumatology.* (2012) 51:1563–70. doi: 10.1093/rheumatology/kes102

44. Yamada K, Asai K, Okamoto A, Watanabe T, Kanazawa H, Ohata M, et al. Correlation between disease activity and serum ferritin in clinically amyopathic dermatomyositis with rapidly-progressive interstitial lung disease: a case report. *BMC Res Notes.* (2018) 11:34. doi: 10.1186/s13104-018-3146-7

45. Gallay L, Gayed C, Hervier B. Antisynthetase syndrome pathogenesis: knowledge and uncertainties. *Curr Opin Rheumatol.* (2018) 30:664–73. doi: 10.1097/BOR.0000000000000555

46. Chinoy H, Adimulam S, Marriage F, New P, Vincze M, Zilahi E, et al. Interaction of HLA-DRB1*03 and smoking for the development of anti-Jo-1 antibodies in adult idiopathic inflammatory myopathies: a European-wide case study. *Ann Rheum Dis.* (2012) 71:961–5. doi: 10.1136/annrheumdis-2011-200182

47. Webber MP, Moir W, Zeig-Owens R, Glaser MS, Jaber N, Hall C, et al. Nested case-control study of selected systemic autoimmune diseases in World Trade Center rescue/recovery workers. *Arthritis Rheumatol.* (2015) 67:1369–76. doi: 10.1002/art.39059

48. Svensson J, Holmqvist M, Lundberg IE, Arkema EV. Infections and respiratory tract disease as risk factors for idiopathic inflammatory myopathies: a population-based case-control study. *Ann Rheum Dis.* (2017) 76:1803–8. doi: 10.1136/annrheumdis-2017-211174

49. Levine SM, Raben N, Xie D, Askin FB, Tuder R, Mullins M, et al. Novel conformation of histidyl-transfer RNA synthetase in the lung: the target tissue in Jo-1 autoantibody-associated myositis. *Arthritis Rheum.* (2007) 56:2729–39. doi: 10.1002/art.22790

50. Howard OMZ, Dong HF, Yang D, Raben N, Nagaraju K, Rosen A, et al. Histidyl-tRNA synthetase and asparaginyl-tRNA synthetase, autoantigens in myositis, activate chemokine receptors on T lymphocytes and immature dendritic cells. *J Exp Med.* (2002) 196:781–91. doi: 10.1084/jem.20020186

51. Lo W-S, Gardiner E, Xu Z, Lau C-F, Wang F, Zhou JJ, et al. Human tRNA synthetase catalytic nulls with diverse functions. *Science.* (2014) 345:328–32. doi: 10.1126/science.1252943

52. Gayed C, Uzunhan Y, Cremer I, Vieillard V, Hervier B. Immunopathogenesis of the Anti-Synthetase Syndrome. *Crit Rev Immunol.* (2018) 38:263–78. doi: 10.1615/CritRevImmunol.2018025744

53. Rothwell S, Cooper RG, Lundberg IE, Miller FW, Gregersen PK, Bowes J, et al. Dense genotyping of immune-related loci in idiopathic inflammatory myopathies confirms HLA alleles as the strongest genetic risk factor and suggests different genetic background for major clinical subgroups. *Ann Rheum Dis.* (2016) 75:1558–66. doi: 10.1136/annrheumdis-2015-208119

54. Fujisawa T, Hozumi H, Kono M, Enomoto N, Hashimoto D, Nakamura Y, et al. Prognostic factors for myositis-associated interstitial lung disease. *PLoS ONE.* (2014) 9:e98824. doi: 10.1371/journal.pone.0098824

55. Tillie-Leblond I, Wislez M, Valeyre D, Crestani B, Rabbat A, Israel-Biet D, et al. Interstitial lung disease and anti-Jo-1 antibodies: difference between acute and gradual onset. *Thorax.* (2008) 63:53–9. doi: 10.1136/thx.2006.069237

56. Vuillard C, Pineton de Chambrun M, de Prost N, Guérin C, Schmidt M, Dargent A, et al. Clinical features and outcome of patients with acute respiratory failure revealing anti-synthetase or anti-MDA-5 dermato-pulmonary syndrome: a French multicenter retrospective study. *Ann Intensive Care.* (2018) 8:87. doi: 10.1186/s13613-018-0433-3

57. Debray M-P, Borie R, Revel M-P, Naccache J-M, Khalil A, Toper C, et al. Interstitial lung disease in anti-synthetase syndrome: initial and follow-up CT findings. *Eur J Radiol.* (2015) 84:516–23. doi: 10.1016/j.ejrad.2014.11.026

58. Tanizawa K, Handa T, Nakashima R, Kubo T, Hosono Y, Watanabe K, et al. HRCT features of interstitial lung disease in dermatomyositis with anti-CADM-140 antibody. *Respir Med.* (2011) 105:1380–7. doi: 10.1016/j.rmed.2011.05.006

59. Obert J, Freynet O, Nunes H, Brillet P-Y, Miyara M, Dhote R, et al. Outcome and prognostic factors in a French cohort of patients with myositis-associated interstitial lung disease. *Rheumatol Int.* (2016) 36:1727–35. doi: 10.1007/s00296-016-3571-7

60. Stanciu R, Guiguet M, Musset L, Touitou D, Beigelman C, Rigolet A, et al. Antisynthetase syndrome with anti-Jo1 antibodies in 48 patients: pulmonary involvement predicts disease-modifying antirheumatic drug use. *J Rheumatol.* (2012) 39:1835–9. doi: 10.3899/jrheum.111604

61. Travis WD, Costabel U, Hansell DM, King TE, Lynch DA, Nicholson AG, et al. An official American Thoracic Society/European Respiratory Society statement: Update of the international multidisciplinary classification of the idiopathic interstitial pneumonias. *Am J Respir Crit Care Med.* (2013) 188:733–48. doi: 10.1164/rccm.201308-1483ST

62. MacDonald SL, Rubens MB, Hansell DM, Copley SJ, Desai SR, du Bois RM, et al. Nonspecific interstitial pneumonia and usual interstitial pneumonia: comparative appearances at and diagnostic accuracy of thin-section CT. *Radiology.* (2001) 221:600–5. doi: 10.1148/radiol.2213010158

63. Goh NSL, Desai SR, Veeraraghavan S, Hansell DM, Copley SJ, Maher TM, et al. Interstitial lung disease in systemic sclerosis: a simple staging system. *Am J Respir Crit Care Med.* (2008) 177:1248–54. doi: 10.1164/rccm.200706-877OC

64. Hervier B, Meyer A, Dieval C, Uzunhan Y, Devilliers H, Launay D, et al. Pulmonary hypertension in antisynthetase syndrome: prevalence, aetiology and survival. *Eur Respir J.* (2013) 42:1271–82. doi: 10.1183/09031936.00156312

65. Bachasson D, Dres M, Niérat M-C, Gennisson J-L, Hogrel J-Y, Doorduin J, et al. Diaphragm shear modulus reflects transdiaphragmatic pressure during isovolumetric inspiratory efforts and ventilation against inspiratory loading. *J Appl Physiol.* (2019) 126:699–707. doi: 10.1152/japplphysiol.01060.2018

66. Teixeira A, Cherin P, Demoule A, Levy-Soussan M, Straus C, Verin E, et al. Diaphragmatic dysfunction in patients with idiopathic inflammatory myopathies. *Neuromuscul Disord.* (2005) 15:32–9. doi: 10.1016/j.nmd.2004.09.006

67. Raghu G, Remy-Jardin M, Myers JL, Richeldi L, Ryerson CJ, Lederer DJ, et al. Diagnosis of Idiopathic Pulmonary Fibrosis. An Official ATS/ERS/JRS/ALAT Clinical Practice Guideline. *Am J Respir Crit Care Med.* (2018) 198:e44–68.

68. Marie I, Josse S, Hatron PY, Dominique S, Hachulla E, Janvresse A, et al. Interstitial lung disease in anti-Jo-1 patients with antisynthetase syndrome. *Arthritis Care Res.* (2013) 65:800–8. doi: 10.1002/acr.21895

69. Marie I, Hatron PY, Dominique S, Cherin P, Mouthon L, Menard J-F. Short-term and long-term outcomes of interstitial lung disease in polymyositis and dermatomyositis: a series of 107 patients. *Arthritis Rheum.* (2011) 63:3439–47. doi: 10.1002/art.30513

70. Rojas-Serrano J, Herrera-Bringas D, Mejía M, Rivero H, Mateos-Toledo H, Figueroa JE. Prognostic factors in a cohort of antisynthetase syndrome (ASS): serologic profile is associated with mortality in patients with interstitial lung disease (ILD). *Clin Rheumatol.* (2015) 34:1563–9. doi: 10.1007/s10067-015-3023-x

71. Fathi M, Vikgren J, Boijsen M, Tylen U, Jorfeldt L, Tornling G, et al. Interstitial lung disease in polymyositis and dermatomyositis: longitudinal evaluation by pulmonary function and radiology. *Arthritis Rheum.* (2008) 59:677–85. doi: 10.1002/art.23571

72. du Bois RM, Weycker D, Albera C, Bradford WZ, Costabel U, Kartashov A, et al. Six-minute-walk test in idiopathic pulmonary fibrosis: test validation and minimal clinically important difference. *Am J Respir Crit Care Med.* (2011) 183:1231–7. doi: 10.1164/rccm.201105-0840OC

73. Goh NS, Hoyles RK, Denton CP, Hansell DM, Renzoni EA, Maher TM, et al. Short-term pulmonary function trends are predictive of mortality in interstitial lung disease associated with systemic sclerosis. *Arthritis Rheumatol.* (2017) 69:1670–8. doi: 10.1002/art.40130

74. Trallero-Araguás E, Grau-Junyent JM, Labirua-Iturburu A, García-Hernández FJ, Monteagudo-Jiménez M, Fraile-Rodriguez G, et al. Clinical manifestations and long-term outcome of anti-Jo1 antisynthetase patients in a large cohort of Spanish patients from the GEAS-IIM group. *Semin Arthritis Rheum.* (2016) 46:225–31. doi: 10.1016/j.semarthrit.2016.03.011

75. Aggarwal R, McBurney C, Schneider F, Yousem SA, Gibson KF, Lindell K, et al. Myositis-associated usual interstitial pneumonia has a better survival than idiopathic pulmonary fibrosis. *Rheumatol.* (2017) 56:384–9. doi: 10.1093/rheumatology/kew426

76. Cobo-Ibáñez T, López-Longo F-J, Joven B, Carreira PE, Muñoz-Fernández S, Maldonado-Romero V, et al. Long-term pulmonary outcomes and mortality in idiopathic inflammatory myopathies associated with interstitial lung disease. *Clin Rheumatol.* (2019) 38:803–15. doi: 10.1007/s10067-018-4353-2

77. Fathi M, Barbasso Helmers S, Lundberg IE. KL-6: a serological biomarker for interstitial lung disease in patients with polymyositis and dermatomyositis. *J Intern Med.* (2012) 271:589–97. doi: 10.1111/j.1365-2796.2011.02459.x

78. Koenig M, Fritzler MJ, Targoff IN, Troyanov Y, Senécal J-L. Heterogeneity of autoantibodies in 100 patients with autoimmune myositis: insights into clinical features and outcomes. *Arthritis Res Ther.* (2007) 9:R78. doi: 10.1186/ar2276

79. La Corte R, Lo Mo Naco A, Locaputo A, Dolzani F, Trotta F. In patients with antisynthetase syndrome the occurrence of anti-Ro/SSA antibodies causes a more severe interstitial lung disease. *Autoimmunity.* (2006) 39:249–53. doi: 10.1080/08916930600623791

80. Le Goff B, Chérin P, Cantagrel A, Gayraud M, Hachulla E, Laborde F, et al. Pneumomediastinum in interstitial lung disease associated with dermatomyositis and polymyositis. *Arthritis Rheum.* (2009) 61:108–18. doi: 10.1002/art.24372

81. Selva-O'Callaghan A, Labrador-Horrillo M, Muñoz-Gall X, Martínez-Gomez X, Majó-Masferrer J, Solans-Laque R, et al. Polymyositis/dermatomyositis-associated lung disease: analysis of a series of 81 patients. *Lupus.* (2005) 14:534–42. doi: 10.1191/0961203305lu2158oa

82. Machuca JS, Cos J, Niazi M, Fuentes G-D. Spontaneous pneumomediastinum in a patient with facial rash. *J Bronchol Interv Pulmonol.* (2010) 17:59–63. doi: 10.1097/LBR.0b013e3181ca6b6c

83. Powell C, Kendall B, Wernick R, Heffner JE. A 34-year-old man with amyopathic dermatomyositis and rapidly progressive dyspnea with facial swelling. Diagnosis: pneumomediastinum and subcutaneous emphysema secondary to amyopathic dermatomyositis-associated interstitial lung disease. *Chest.* (2007) 132:1710–3. doi: 10.1378/chest.07-0286

84. Ma X, Chen Z, Hu W, Guo Z, Wang Y, Kuwana M, et al. Clinical and serological features of patients with dermatomyositis complicated by spontaneous pneumomediastinum. *Clin Rheumatol.* (2016) 35:489–93. doi: 10.1007/s10067-015-3001-3

85. Kuronuma K, Honda H, Mikami T, Saito A, Ikeda K, Otsuka M, et al. Response to pneumococcal vaccine in interstitial lung disease patients: influence of systemic immunosuppressive treatment. *Vaccine.* (2018) 36:4968–72. doi: 10.1016/j.vaccine.2018.06.062

86. Redondo-Benito A, Curran A, Villar-Gomez A, Trallero-Araguas E, Fernández-Codina A, Pinal-Fernandez I, et al. Opportunistic infections in patients with idiopathic inflammatory myopathies. *Int J Rheum Dis.* (2018) 21:487–96. doi: 10.1111/1756-185X.13255

87. Park JW, Curtis JR, Moon J, Song YW, Kim S, Lee EB. Prophylactic effect of trimethoprim-sulfamethoxazole for pneumocystis pneumonia in patients with rheumatic diseases exposed to prolonged high-dose glucocorticoids. *Ann Rheum Dis.* (2018) 77:644–9. doi: 10.1136/annrheumdis-2017-211796

88. Dowman LM, McDonald CF, Hill CJ, Lee AL, Barker K, Boote C, et al. The evidence of benefits of exercise training in interstitial lung disease: a randomised controlled trial. *Thorax.* (2017) 72:610–9. doi: 10.1136/thoraxjnl-2016-208638

89. Zisman DA, Kawut SM, Lederer DJ, Belperio JA, Lynch JP, Schwarz MI, et al. Serum albumin concentration and waiting list mortality in idiopathic interstitial pneumonia. *Chest.* (2009) 135:929–35. doi: 10.1378/chest.08-0754

90. Troyanov Y, Targoff IN, Tremblay J-L, Goulet J-R, Raymond Y, Senécal J-L. Novel classification of idiopathic inflammatory myopathies based on overlap syndrome features and autoantibodies: analysis of 100 French Canadian patients. *Medicine.* (2005) 84:231–49. doi: 10.1097/01.md.0000173991.74008.b0

91. Wilkes MR, Sereika SM, Fertig N, Lucas MR, Oddis CV. Treatment of antisynthetase-associated interstitial lung disease with tacrolimus. *Arthritis Rheum.* (2005) 52:2439–46. doi: 10.1002/art.21240

92. Yamasaki Y, Yamada H, Yamasaki M, Ohkubo M, Azuma K, Matsuoka S, et al. Intravenous cyclophosphamide therapy for progressive interstitial pneumonia in patients with polymyositis/dermatomyositis. *Rheumatology.* (2007) 46:124–30. doi: 10.1093/rheumatology/kel112

93. Sharma N, Putman MS, Vij R, Strek ME, Dua A. Myositis-associated interstitial lung disease: predictors of failure of conventional treatment and response to tacrolimus in a US cohort. *J Rheumatol.* (2017) 44:1612–8. doi: 10.3899/jrheum.161217

94. Marie I, Hatron P-Y, Cherin P, Hachulla E, Diot E, Vittecoq O, et al. Functional outcome and prognostic factors in anti-Jo1 patients with antisynthetase syndrome. *Arthritis Res Ther.* (2013) 15:R149. doi: 10.1186/ar4332

95. Douglas WW, Tazelaar HD, Hartman TE, Hartman RP, Decker PA, Schroeder DR, et al. Polymyositis-dermatomyositis-associated interstitial lung disease. *Am J Respir Crit Care Med.* (2001) 164:1182–5. doi: 10.1164/ajrccm.164.7.2103110

96. Huapaya JA, Silhan L, Pinal-Fernandez I, Casal-Dominguez M, Johnson C, Albayda J, et al. Long-term treatment with azathioprine and mycophenolate mofetil for myositis-related interstitial lung disease. *Chest.* (2019) doi: 10.1016/j.chest.2019.05.023

97. Mira-Avendano IC, Parambil JG, Yadav R, Arrossi V, Xu M, Chapman JT, et al. A retrospective review of clinical features and treatment outcomes in steroid-resistant interstitial lung disease from polymyositis/dermatomyositis. *Respir Med.* (2013) 107:890–6. doi: 10.1016/j.rmed.2013.02.015

98. Kurita T, Yasuda S, Oba K, Odani T, Kono M, Otomo K, et al. The efficacy of tacrolimus in patients with interstitial lung diseases complicated with polymyositis or dermatomyositis. *Rheumatol.* (2015) 54:39–44. doi: 10.1093/rheumatology/keu166

99. Huapaya JA, Hallowell R, Silhan L, Pinal-Fernandez I, Casal-Dominguez M, Johnson C, et al. Long-term treatment with human immunoglobulin for antisynthetase syndrome-associated interstitial lung disease. *Respir Med.* (2019) 154:6–11. doi: 10.1016/j.rmed.2019.05.012

100. Allenbach Y, Guiguet M, Rigolet A, Marie I, Hachulla E, Drouot L, et al. Efficacy of Rituximab in Refractory Inflammatory Myopathies Associated with Anti- Synthetase Auto-Antibodies: An Open-Label, Phase II Trial. *PLoS ONE.* (2015) 10:e0133702. doi: 10.1371/journal.pone.0133702

101. Andersson H, Sem M, Lund MB, Aaløkken TM, Günther A, Walle-Hansen R, et al. Long-term experience with rituximab in anti-synthetase syndrome-related interstitial lung disease. *Rheumatol.* (2015) 54:1420–8. doi: 10.1093/rheumatology/kev004

102. Sharp C, McCabe M, Dodds N, Edey A, Mayers L, Adamali H, et al. Rituximab in autoimmune connective tissue disease-associated interstitial lung disease. *Rheumatol.* (2016) 55:1318–24. doi: 10.1093/rheumatology/kew195

103. Doyle TJ, Dhillon N, Madan R, Cabral F, Fletcher EA, Koontz DC, et al. Rituximab in the treatment of interstitial lung disease associated with antisynthetase syndrome: a multicenter retrospective case review. *J Rheumatol.* (2018) 45:841–50. doi: 10.3899/jrheum.170541

104. Fasano S, Gordon P, Hajji R, Loyo E, Isenberg DA. Rituximab in the treatment of inflammatory myopathies: a review. *Rheumatol.* (2017) 56:26–36. doi: 10.1093/rheumatology/kew146

105. Zou J, Li T, Huang X, Chen S, Guo Q, Bao C. Basiliximab may improve the survival rate of rapidly progressive interstitial pneumonia in patients with clinically amyopathic dermatomyositis with anti-MDA5 antibody. *Ann Rheum Dis.* (2014) 73:1591–3. doi: 10.1136/annrheumdis-2014-205278

106. Chen Z, Wang X, Ye S. Tofacitinib in amyopathic dermatomyositis-associated interstitial lung disease. *N Engl J Med.* (2019) 381:291–3. doi: 10.1056/NEJMc1900045

107. Dastmalchi M, Grundtman C, Alexanderson H, Mavragani CP, Einarsdottir H, Helmers SB, et al. A high incidence of disease flares in an open pilot study of infliximab in patients with refractory inflammatory myopathies. *Ann Rheum Dis.* (2008) 67:1670–7. doi: 10.1136/ard.2007.077974

108. Distler O, Highland KB, Gahlemann M, Azuma A, Fischer A, Mayes MD, et al. Nintedanib for systemic sclerosis-associated interstitial lung disease. *N Engl J Med.* (2019) 380:2518–28. doi: 10.1056/NEJMoa1903076

109. Courtwright AM, El-Chemaly S, Dellaripa PF, Goldberg HJ. Survival and outcomes after lung transplantation for non-scleroderma connective tissue-related interstitial lung disease. *J Heart Lung Transplant.* (2017) 36:763–9. doi: 10.1016/j.healun.2016.12.013

110. Ameye H, Ruttens D, Benveniste O, Verleden GM, Wuyts WA. Is lung transplantation a valuable therapeutic option for patients with pulmonary polymyositis? Experiences from the Leuven transplant cohort. *Transplant Proc.* (2014) 46:3147–53. doi: 10.1016/j.transproceed.2014.09.163

13

Differences in Baseline Characteristics and Access to Treatment of Newly Diagnosed Patients With IPF in the EMPIRE Countries

Abigél Margit Kolonics-Farkas[1], Martina Šterclová[2], Nesrin Mogulkoc[3],
Katarzyna Lewandowska[4], Veronika Müller[1*], Marta Hájková[5], Mordechai Kramer[6],
Dragana Jovanovic[7], Jasna Tekavec-Trkanjec[8], Michael Studnicka[9], Natalia Stoeva[10],
Simona Littnerová[11] and Martina Vašáková[2]

[1] Department of Pulmonology, Semmelweis University, Budapest, Hungary, [2] Department of Respiratory Diseases of the First Faculty of Medicine Charles University, University Thomayer Hospital, Prague, Czechia, [3] Department of Pulmonary Medicine, Ege University Medical School, Izmir, Turkey, [4] First Department of Pulmonary Diseases, Institute of Tuberculosis and Lung Diseases, Warsaw, Poland, [5] Clinic of Pneumology and Phthisiology, University Hospital Bratislava, Bratislava, Slovakia, [6] Rabin Medical Center, Institute of Pulmonary Medicine, Petah Tikva, Israel, [7] Internal Medicine Clinic "Akta Medica", Belgrade, Serbia, [8] Pulmonary Department, University Hospital Dubrava, Zagreb, Croatia, [9] Clinical Research Centre Salzburg, Salzburg, Austria, [10] Tokuda Hospital Sofia, Sofia, Bulgaria, [11] Faculty of Medicine, Institute of Biostatistics and Analyses, Masaryk University, Brno, Czechia

*Correspondence:
Veronika Müller
muller.veronika@
med.semmelweis-univ.hu
orcid.org/0000-0002-1398-3187

Idiopathic pulmonary fibrosis (IPF) is a rare lung disease with poor prognosis. The diagnosis and treatment possibilities are dependent on the health systems of countries. Hence, comparison among countries is difficult due to data heterogeneity. Our aim was to analyse patients with IPF in Central and Eastern Europe using the uniform data from the European Multipartner IPF registry (EMPIRE), which at the time of analysis involved 10 countries. Newly diagnosed IPF patients ($N = 2{,}492$, between March 6, 2012 and May 12, 2020) from Czech Republic ($N = 971$, 39.0%), Turkey ($N = 505$, 20.3%), Poland ($N = 285$, 11.4%), Hungary ($N = 216$, 8.7%), Slovakia ($N = 149$, 6.0%), Israel ($N = 120$, 4.8%), Serbia ($N = 95$, 3.8%), Croatia ($N = 87$, 3.5%), Austria ($N = 55$, 2.2%), and Bulgaria ($N = 9$, 0.4%) were included, and Macedonia, while a member of the registry, was excluded from this analysis due to low number of cases ($N = 5$) at this timepoint. Baseline characteristics, smoking habit, comorbidities, lung function values, CO diffusion capacity, high-resolution CT (HRCT) pattern, and treatment data were analysed. Patients were significantly older in Austria than in the Czech Republic, Turkey, Hungary, Slovakia, Israel, and Serbia. Ever smokers were most common in Croatia (84.1%) and least frequent in Serbia (39.2%) and Slovakia (42.6%). The baseline forced vital capacity (FVC) was >80% in 44.6% of the patients, between 50 and 80% in 49.3%, and <50% in 6.1%. Most IPF patients with FVC >80% were registered in Poland (63%), while the least in Israel (25%). A typical usual interstitial pneumonia (UIP) pattern was present in 67.6% of all patients, ranging from 43.5% (Austria) to 77.2% (Poland). The majority of patients received antifibrotic therapy (64.5%); 37.4% used pirfenidone (range 7.4–39.8% between countries); and 34.9% nintedanib (range 12.6–56.0% between countries) treatment.

In 6.8% of the cases, a therapy switch was initiated between the 2 antifibrotic agents. Significant differences in IPF patient characteristics and access to antifibrotic therapies exist in EMPIRE countries, which needs further investigation and strategies to improve and harmonize patient care and therapy availability in this region.

Keywords: IPF, treatment, regional accessibility, registry analysis, Central−Eastern Europe

INTRODUCTION

Idiopathic pulmonary fibrosis (IPF) is a rare, chronic, progressive, fibrotic lung disease associated with poor prognosis and high mortality (1–3). The median survival is between 2 and 5 years (1). Despite the largely undefined etiology, several exogenous environmental, and microbial factors seem to play key roles in the disease (4–7). The natural course of the disease is variable, and the factors that influence disease progression are unknown at an individual level (8).

The incidence of IPF has risen over time, it is between 3 and 9 cases per 1,00,000 per year (9). Regarding the systematic review of J. Hutchinson et al., there is a high variety in incidence and mortality rates depending on the geographic region (9). The overall prevalence of IPF is estimated at 30.2 cases per 1,00,000 (10).

Diagnosis and treatment possibilities of IPF are dependent on the health systems of countries as confirmed by several previous studies (11–13). Healthcare systems deal differently with diagnostic possibilities and availability. Considering treatment, expensive therapies are often introduced later as in wealthier countries and might be limited to a selected population of IPF (14, 15). Many off-label treatments are applied in rare diseases with potentially serious side effects (16).

Uniformity in diagnosis and treatment is crucial to patients dealing with persistent symptoms and uncertainty about the prognosis of their disease with a great impact on their quality of life (17). IPF has a considerable impact on the lives of the patients and the healthcare system (18). Medical professionals play an important role in the care of patients with IPF through patient education, monitoring medication compliance and safety, ensuring optimized medications for comorbidities, and preventive strategies. Patient education and counseling play key role in the shared decision-making model and are necessary for the management of this chronic disease (19).

Patient registries are organized systems that use observational study methods to collect uniform data (clinical and other) to evaluate specified outcomes for a population defined by a particular disease, condition, or exposure, and serve predetermined scientific, clinical, or policy purpose(s). Studies derived from well-designed and well-performed patient registries can provide a real-world view of clinical practice, patient outcomes, safety, and clinical comparative and cost-effectiveness analyses, and can serve as important tools for decision-making purposes (20–22). Comparison among countries is difficult due to data collection heterogeneity.

The aim of our study is to assess the baseline characteristics and treatment possibilities of patients with IPF in the same geographical—Central and Eastern Europe—region, by analysing the data of the European Multipartner IPF Registry (EMPIRE) countries (23).

PATIENT SELECTION AND METHODS

Study Design and Participants

The EMPIRE is a non-interventional, international, multicenter database of patients with IPF in Central and Eastern Europe (23). The objective of the registry is to evaluate the incidence, prevalence, and mortality of IPF in this area in Europe, and to determine the basic characteristics of patients with IPF. Another valuable outcome is the possibility of the comparison of different diagnostic and therapeutic differences among countries and assessment of the baseline characteristics of patients with IPF that participate in the EMPIRE using a uniform database platform.

Patients with IPF included in EMPIRE were diagnosed according to the American Thoracic Society/European Respiratory Society (ATS/ERS) consensus classification (1).

All participants were included in the analysis from the EMPIRE registry between March 6, 2012 and May 12, 2020. Overall, 2,492 newly diagnosed patients were involved from 10 countries: Czech Republic (N = 971, 39.0%), Turkey (N = 505, 20.3%), Poland (N = 285, 11.4%), Hungary (N = 216, 8.7%), Slovakia (N = 149, 6.0%), Israel (N = 120, 4.8%), Serbia (N = 95, 3.8%,) Croatia (N = 87, 3.5%), Austria (N = 55, 2.2%), and Bulgaria (N = 9, 0.4%). The detailed patient selection process is shown in **Figure 1**.

Baseline characteristics, high-resolution CT (HRCT) pattern, and treatment data were analysed. Patient baseline demographics, including Gender-Age-Physiology (GAP) score, smoking history, symptoms, detailed lung function values [forced vital capacity (FVC), forced expiratory volume in 1 s (FEV1), total lung capacity (TLC), diffusing capacity of the lung for carbon monoxide (DLCO)], diffusing capacity for carbon monoxide (KLCO) and HRCT pattern were analyzed. In addition, information regarding comorbidities was obtained using chart reviews and was included in the analyses. Body mass index (BMI) and the 6-min walk test (6MWT) results were examined. Additionally, the number of patients in the respective groups was provided according to country (**Table 1**).

The study was performed in accordance with the Declaration of Helsinki and ethical approval was obtained in each country according to respective regulations.

Statistical Analysis

The study aimed to evaluate the differences and/or similarities in clinical data and treatment in patients with IPF in Central

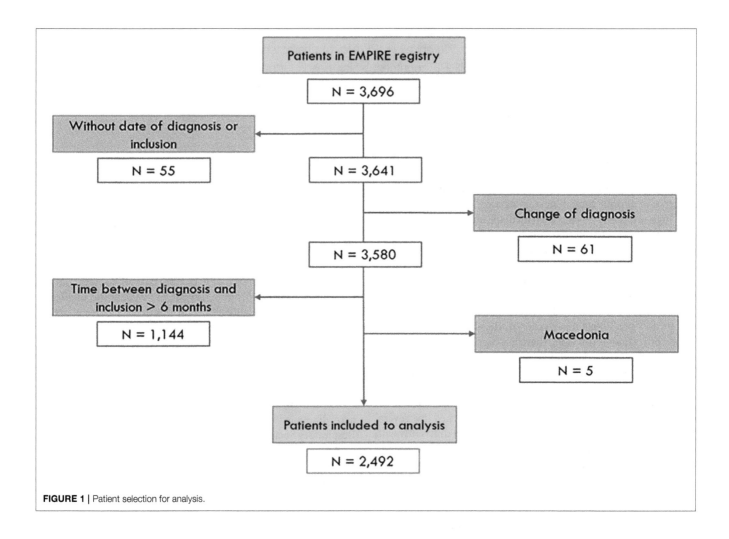

FIGURE 1 | Patient selection for analysis.

and Eastern Europe. A descriptive statistical analysis was performed and included absolute and relative frequencies for categorical variables and medians, with 5th−95th percentile ranges calculated for quantitative variables (in plots that were completed with interquartile range [IQR]). Significant differences among groups were analysed using the χ^2-test for categorical variables and Kruskal–Wallis tests for quantitative variables. If differences were statistically significant, *post-hoc* testing with a Bonferroni correction was used to identify homogeneous groups. The level of statistical significance was set at $p < 0.05$. Analyses were performed using SPSS v25 (IBM Corporation, Armonk, NY, USA) and Stata 14.2. (StataCorp., Lakeway Drive, TX, USA).

RESULTS

Patient Characteristics

Overall, 3,696 patients with IPF participated in the study. Information about the enrollment is shown in **Figure 1**. The final analysis included 2,492 patients. Exclusion of patients where the time of diagnosis and inclusion was over 6 months represented prevalent cases and not incident cases. To analyse the longitudinal outcome, newly diagnosed patients were included in the registry, defined by <6 months between inclusion and

diagnosis. Participants with no date of inclusion in the study ($N = 55$) or with an inclusion time that had been more than 6 months compared with the time of diagnosis ($N = 1,144$) or who had a change in diagnosis ($N = 61$) were excluded from the analysis.

Information on EMPIRE member distribution is summarized in **Table 1**. Patients with the highest average age came from Austria; Austrian IPF patients were typically older than patients from most of the other countries. Patients from Serbia were the youngest and appeared to be significantly younger than participants from the Czech Republic, Poland, and Austria. Patients with IPF were more frequently men, and a significantly higher ratio of women was noted in Hungary as in the Czech Republic, Turkey, and Poland. The highest percentile contribution of men was noted in Bulgaria and Austria. In almost every country, more than 50% of patients had a smoking history. Across all countries, patients in Croatia had the highest ratio of patients with a history of smoking, whereas this number was the lowest in Serbia. BMI had the highest average value in Bulgaria, followed by the Czech Republic, and the lowest in Serbia. New York Heart Association (NYHA) class IV dyspnea was very rare among the patients; most frequently, NYHA class II dyspnea occurred, and it was most common among the Slovakian patients. Cough was present in more than two-thirds of the

TABLE 1 | Patient characteristics in individual countries.

	Total N = 2,492	Czech Republic N = 971	Turkey N = 505	Poland N = 285	Hungary N = 216	Slovakia N = 149	Israel N = 120	Serbia N = 95	Croatia N = 87	Austria N = 55	Bulgaria N = 9
Median age, years (range)											
All	2492/69 (54;82)	971/70 (54;82) T, S, R, A	505/68 (52;81) C, A	285/69 (57;84) S, R, A	216/70 (53;82) A	149/67 (48;79) C, P, A	120/67 (55;82) A	95/65 (48;79) C, P, A	87/70 (53;82) A	55/74 (63;87) C, T, P, HU, S, I, R, HR	9/69 (57;83)
Men	1786/69 (54;82)	719/70 (54;82)	383/68 (51;79)	206/69 (57;84)	125/69 (53;82)	97/68 (50;78)	83/69 (57;82)	57/67 (50;79)	64/71 (54;83)	45/74 (64;87)	7/71 (57;83)
Women	706/68 (54;82)	252/71 (54;82)	122/68 (54;83)	79/70 (57;84)	91/70 (54;82)	52/67 (40;81)	37/64 (50;78)	38/63 (44;81)	23/69 (51;76)	10/69 (62;81)	2/69 (68;69)
Sex, N (%)											
Men	1786 (71.7%)	719 (74.0%)	383 (75.8%)	206 (72.3%)	125 (57.9%)	97 (65.1%)	83 (69.2%)	57 (60.0%)	64 (73.6%)	45 (81.8%)	7 (77.8%)
Women	706 (28.3%)	252 (26.0%) HU	122 (24.2%) HU	79 (27.7%) HU	91 (42.1%) C, T, P	52 (34.9%)	37 (30.8%)	38 (40.0%)	23 (26.4%)	10 (18.2%)	2 (22.2%)
Smoking, N (%)											
Never-smoker	919 (37.1%)	395 (40.7%) T, P, R, HR	155 (30.7%) C, S, R	70 (24.6%) C, HU, S, R	90 (44.3%) P, HR	81 (55.1%) T, P, HR, A	50 (41.7%) HR	53 (56.4%) C, T, P, HR, A	12 (13.8%) C, HU, S, I, R	11 (20.0%) S, R	2 (22.2%)
Ever-smoker	1496 (60.4%)	562 (57.9%)	336 (66.5%)	206 (72.5%)	106 (52.2%)	62 (42.2%)	66 (55.0%)	36 (38.3%)	73 (83.9%)	42 (76.4%)	7 (77.8%)
Current smoker	60 (2.4%)	14 (1.4%)	14 (2.8%)	8 (2.8%)	7 (3.4%)	4 (2.7%)	4 (3.3%)	5 (5.3%)	2 (2.3%)	2 (3.6%)	0 (0.0%)
BMI, kg/m^2 (range)	2443/28.0 (21.7;36.0)	967/28.6 (22.2;36.1) T, R, A	496/27.7 (21.3;34.9) C, R	281/28.0 (22.8;35.9) R	187/27.6 (20.8;37.7)	146/28.1 (22.2;37.1) R	120/27.7 (20.7;36.8)	95/26.1 (21.0;32.0) C, T, P, S	87/27.4 (21.5;34.0)	55/26.4 (21.5;34.2) C	9/29.2 (23.5;35.8) C
Dyspnea—NYHA											
I	113 (4.9%)	13 (1.4%) T, P, HU, I, R, HR, A	23 (4.7%) C, P, HU, S, I, R, HR, A	20 (8.3%) C, T, S	31 (16.1%) C, T, S	0 (0.0%) T, P, HU, R, HR, A, M	9 (7.6%) C, T	4 (4.8%) C, T, S	8 (9.9%) C, T, S	5 (11.1%) C, T, S	0 (0.0%)
II	1325 (57.1%)	582 (62.7%)	172 (35.5%)	159 (66.3%)	106 (54.9%)	96 (68.6%)	73 (61.9%)	49 (59.0%)	56 (69.1%)	28 (62.2%)	4 (44.4%)
III	848 (36.5%)	325 (35.0%)	285 (58.8%)	55 (22.9%)	53 (27.5%)	44 (31.4%)	33 (28.0%)	22 (26.5%)	15 (18.5%)	11 (24.4%)	5 (55.6%)
IV	36 (1.6%)	8 (0.9%)	5 (1.0%)	6 (2.5%)	3 (1.6%)	0 (0.0%)	3 (2.5%)	8 (9.6%)	2 (2.5%)	1 (2.2%)	0 (0.0%)
Cough, N (%)											
Yes	1,594 (68.0%)	664 (73.0%) S	335 (66.7%) S	180 (64.7%)	118 (65.6%)	69 (51.1%) C, T, R	77 (68.8%)	60 (75.9%) S	53 (60.9%)	31 (57.4%)	7 (87.5%)
Dry	966 (60.6%)	459 (69.1%) T, I, A, B	175 (52.2%) C, A, B	106 (58.9%) A, B	64 (54.2%) A, B	50 (72.5%) A, B	33 (42.9%) C, A, B	42 (70.0%) A, B	25 (47.2%) A, B	8 (25.8%) C, T, P, HU, S, I, R, HR	4 (57.1%) C, T, P, HU, S, I, R, HR
Productive	599 (37.6%)	195 (29.4%)	159 (47.5%)	73 (40.6%)	53 (44.9%)	19 (27.5%)	43 (55.8%)	18 (30.0%)	28 (52.8%)	11 (35.5%)	0 (0.0%)
Unknown	29 (1.8%)	10 (1.5%)	1 (0.3%)	1 (0.6%)	1 (0.8%)	0 (0.0%)	1 (1.3%)	0 (0.0%)	0 (0.0%)	12 (38.7%)	3 (42.9%)
Crackles, N (%)	2254 (90.7%)	947 (97.5%) T, P, HU, S, R, A	392 (77.6%) C, P, HU, I, HR	264 (93.0%) C, T	192 (91.0%) C, T	127 (85.2%) C	112 (93.3%) T	83 (87.4%) C	84 (96.6%) T	44 (80.0%) C	9 (100.0%)
Finger clubbing, N (%)	874 (35.2%)	423 (43.6%) T, P, S, A	135 (26.7%) C, I, HR	70 (24.6%) C, HU, I, HR	81 (38.6%) P, S, A	26 (17.4%) C, HU, I, HR, B	55 (45.8%) T, P, S, A	27 (28.4%) HR	47 (54.0%) T, P, S, R, A	4 (7.3%) C, HU, I, HR, B, M	6 (66.7%) S, A

(Continued)

TABLE 1 | Continued

	Total N = 2,492	Czech Republic N = 971	Turkey N = 505	Poland N = 285	Hungary N = 216	Slovakia N = 149	Israel N = 120	Serbia N = 95	Croatia N = 87	Austria N = 55	Bulgaria N = 9
GAP Score, N (%)											
I	897(45.0%)	331 (42.1%)	163 (43.8%)	130 (53.5%)	83 (55.3%)	76 (58.5%)	38 (35.8%)	25 (38.5%)	31 (39.7%)	17 (31.5%)	3 (37.5%)
II	904 (45.4%)	380 (48.3%)	164 (44.1%)	97 (39.9%)	57 (38.0%)	46 (35.4%)	56 (52.8%)	33 (50.8%)	42 (53.8%)	27 (50.0%)	2 (25.0%)
III	192 (9.6%)	76 (9.7%)	45 (12.1%)	16 (6.6%)	10 (6.7%)	8 (6.2%)	12 (11.3%)	7 (10.8%)	5 (6.4%)	10 (18.5%)	3 (37.5%)
HRCT pattern, N (%)											
UIP	1523 (67.5%)	647 (73.8%) T, HU, S, R, A	284 (62.1%) C, P, A	207 (77.2%) T, HU, S, R, A	119 (58.3%) C, P	76 (56.3%) C, P	75 (76.5%) R, A	42 (49.4%) C, P, I	48 (61.5%)	19 (43.2%) C, T, P, I	6 (66.7%)
Possible UIP	653 (29.0%)	218 (24.9%)	138 (30.2%)	60 (22.4%)	78 (38.2%)	53 (39.3%)	19 (19.4%)	32 (37.6%)	27 (34.6%)	25 (56.8%)	3 (33.3%)
Inconsistent with UIP	79 (3.5%)	12 (1.4%)	35 (7.7%)	1 (0.4%)	7 (3.4%)	6 (4.4%)	4 (4.1%)	11 (12.9%)	3 (3.8%)	0 (0.0%)	0 (0.0%)
Comorbidities											
0	211 (8.5%)	77 (7.9%) P, HU, S, I, R, M	29 (5.7%) P, HU, S, I, R, M	27 (9.5%) C, T, I, R, HR, M	32 (14.8%) C, T, I, HR, M	24 (16.1%) C, T, I, HR, M	0 (0.0%) C, T, P, HU, S, R, A, B, M	16 (16.8%) C, T, P, I, HR, M	2 (2.3%) P, HU, S, R, A, M	3 (5.5%) I, HR, M	1 (11.1%) I
1	449 (18.0%)	144 (14.8%)	73 (14.5%)	65 (22.8%)	55 (25.5%)	45 (30.2%)	5 (4.2%)	35 (36.8%)	8 (9.2%)	15 (27.3%)	4 (44.4%)
2	463 (18.6%)	179 (18.4%)	94 (18.6%)	63 (22.1%)	43 (19.9%)	27 (18.1%)	10 (8.3%)	25 (26.3%)	8 (9.2%)	13 (23.6%)	1 (11.1%)
>2	1369 (54.9%)	571 (58.8%)	309 (61.2%)	130 (45.6%)	86 (39.8%)	53 (35.6%)	105 (87.5%)	19 (20.0%)	69 (79.3%)	24 (43.6%)	3 (33.3%)

Data are N (%) or median (range); GAP, Gender-Age-Physiology.

cases; patients in Serbia and Bulgaria complained about it in most of the cases. Dry cough was more typical than productive cough in every country. Crackles were present in more than 90% of the cases with the highest ratio in the Czech Republic and Bulgaria.

GAP scores I and II had almost the same frequency among all countries and together they accounted for more than 90% of the cases. Slovakian patients had GAP score I most frequently, GAP score II was mostly observable in Croatia, while GAP score III was most common in Bulgaria and Austria.

HRCT lung imaging was described according to the ATS/ERS consensus classification in all patients (1). Usual interstitial pneumonia (UIP) pattern was present in approximately two-thirds of the patients with the highest prevalence in Poland. A possible UIP pattern was the most frequent in Austria, whereas a pattern inconsistent with UIP was most common in Serbia.

Analysis of Lung Function

Baseline lung function values are summarized in **Table 2**. FVC was between 50 and 80% in 49.3% and >80% in 49.3% of the patients. Most IPF-patients with FVC > 80% were registered in Poland, while the lowest number frequency was in Israel. Baseline FEV1% predicted was between 70% and 90% in 40.1% of the cases and >90% in 32.8% of the patients. Most cases with

FEV1% > 90% were registered in Slovakia and Poland, while the lowest was in Israel. FEV1/FVC was between 70% and 80% in 22.3%, >80% in 70.6%, and <70% in 7.1% of the patients at the time of enrollment. Most patients with FEV1/FVC > 80% were registered in Slovakia and the highest number of patients with FEV1/FVC < 70% values came from Austria (20%). TLC% predicted had the highest average value in Poland and Slovakia, while the lowest average value in Israel. DLCO% and KLCO% predicted values were the highest in Hungary and the lowest in Serbia. Patients from Slovakia had the biggest average distance of 6MWT, whereas this value was the lowest in the Czech Republic.

In our study, the FVC% predicted values were tested in 91.8% of the total population. The highest ratio appeared in Croatia and Austria as patients in both countries underwent testing for FVC in 100% and the lowest ratio could be seen in Serbia (76.8%). FEV1% predicted was measured in all cases in Croatia (100%), whereas the lowest ratio of patients was in Hungary (76.4%). FEV1/FVC was calculated in most cases in Croatia and the least in Serbia. TLC% predicted evaluation had the highest percentage in Austria (100%), whereas, in Bulgaria, there was no evaluation of TLC% predicted. DLCO% predicted was entered into the registry with the highest patient participation in Austria (98.2%) and the lowest in Hungary (69.0%). KLCO% predicted testing ratios were the following: highest test proportion in Austria and no tested patient for KLCO% predicted in Bulgaria. 6MWT was performed

TABLE 2 | Lung function values and 6-min walk test in individual countries.

Valid N/median (5th;95th percentile)	Total N = 2,497	Czech Republic N = 971	Turkey N = 505	Poland N = 285	Hungary N = 216	Slovakia N = 149	Israel N = 120	Serbia N = 95	Croatia N = 87	Austria N = 55	Bulgaria N = 9
FVC (L)	2293/2.59 (1.36;4.10)	911/2.56 (1.45;3.91) T, P, I	454/2.37 (1.19;3.87) C, P, S, I, HR, A	271/2.92 (1.61;4.54) C, T, HU, I	189/2.35 (1.29;4.05) P, S, HR	131/2.83 (1.55;4.35) T, HU, I	114/1.96 (0.91;3.53) C, T, P, S, R, HR, A	73/2.70 (1.37;4.15) I	87/2.79 (1.53;4.33) T, HU, I	55/2.68 (1.68;4.43) T, I,	8/2.57 (1.43;3.66)
FVC (% predicted)	2267/77 (48;114)	910/76 (50;106) P, S, I, HR	450/74 (45;110) P, S, I, HR	271/87 (59;127) C, T, HU, I	168/76 (43;115) P, S, I	131/85 (52;121) C, T, HU, I	114/63 (34;104) C, T, P, HU, S, R, HR, A	73/81 (47;115) I	87/86 (52;123) C, T, I	55/84 (49;120) I	8/76 (42;115)
FEV1 (L)	2286/2.14 (1.16;3.31)	910/2.20 (1.27;3.27) T, HU, I	451/1.96 (1.03;3.08) C, P, S, I, R	270/2.32 (1.33;3.62) T, HU, I	186/1.97 (1.15;3.32) C, P, S, I	132/2.41 (1.38;3.68) T, HU, I	114/1.71 (0.82;2.90) C, T, P, HU, S, R, HR, A	73/2.34 (1.22;3.54) T, I	87/2.18 (1.28;3.23) I	55/2.26 (1.28;3.35) I	8/2.19 (1.04;2.92)
FEV1 (% predicted)	2258/81 (51;114)	909/81 (55;110) T, P, S, I	448/77 (48;110) C, P, S, I	268/89 (59;122) C, T, HU, I	165/79 (45;115) P, S, I	132/89 (57;124) C, T, HU, I	114/70 (39;103) C, T, P, HU, S, R, HR, A	73/84 (50;115) I	87/81 (55;113) I	54/85 (43;107) I	8/78 (46;110)
FEV1/FVC	2274/84 (68; 97)	900/86 (71; 98) T, P, HR, A	457/83 (70; 96) C, P, HR, AT	270/81 (65; 91) C, T, HU, S, I, R	184/84 (70; 95) P, HR, A	130/85 (68; 96) P, HR, A	114/86 (68; 97) P, HR, A	70/85 (69; 99) P, HR, A	87/78 (56; 94) C, T, HU, S, I, R	54/79 (52; 91) C, T, HU, S, I, R	8/81 (73; 91)
TLC (L)	1984/4.23 (2.21;6.60)	853/4.28 (2.62;6.51) T, S, I, A	280/3.85 (2.08;5.89) C, P, S, A	233/4.67 (0.00;6.98) T, HU, I	181/3.96 (2.11;6.32) P, S, A	124/4.68 (3.06;7.76) C, T, HU, I, R	105/3.77 (2.13;6.16) C, P, S, A	71/4.23 (0.00;6.50) S, A	82/4.19 (2.42;6.92)	55/4.77 (3.20;6.72) C, T, HU, I, R	0/0
TLC (% predicted)	1963/70 (41;100)	854/69 (46;97) T, P, S	279/64 (43;95) C, P, S, A	231/78 (0;109) C, T, HU, I	162/67 (38;100) P, S	124/78 (54;151) C, T, HU, I, R, HR	105/62 (44;92) P, S, A	71/67 (0;100) S	82/69 (45;98) S	55/76 (52;108) T, I	0/0
DLCO%	2126/46.8 (0.0;80.5)	895/46.4 (23.7;73.0) HU, R	384/46.1 (0.0;80.7) HU, R	250/47.9 (0.0;86.6) HU, R	149/59 (24;104) C, T, P, S, I, R, HR, A	130/51 (0;78) HU, R	107/45.4 (20.6;87.0) HU, R	70/30.2 (0.0;59.2) C, T, P, HU, S, I, HR, A	79/42.2 (9.2;72.3) HU, R	54/45.9 (0.0;72.9) HU, R	8/35.6 (19.4;69.7)
KLCO%	2041/75 (0;119)	850/76 (13;115) P, HU, I, R, HR	388/77 (0;123) P, R	220/65 (0;105) C, T, HU, S	153/86 (14;140) C, P, I, R, HR, A	131/76 (0;176) P, R	88/67 (0;104) C, HU	73/53 (0;188) C, T, HU, S	81/65 (15;103) C, HU	54/73 (0;111) HU	0/0
6MWT Distance (m)	1231/390 (168;560)	274/360 (160;530) P, S	373/375 (135;511) P, S	189/420 (235;600) C, T, S	129/400 (170;578) S	72/495 (355;590) C, T, P, HU, I, R, HR	72/403 (90;540) S	39/400 (140;545) S	66/401 (190;540) S	17/460 (196;635)	0/0

in most cases in Croatia, while no 6MWT was done in the case of Bulgarian patients.

Patient Comorbidities

Significant alterations were noted in comorbidities in the different countries. The leading comorbidities were cardiovascular diseases followed by gastrointestinal and pulmonary disorders. Overall, more than half of the patients had more than 2 comorbidities. In general, patients in Serbia had the lowest rate of comorbidities, whereas patients from Israel had a medical history with at least 2 co-occurring disorders. A detailed analysis of comorbidities is shown in **Figure 2**.

Antifibrotic Treatment

More than 50% of the patients received antifibrotic therapy. Pirfenidone and nintedanib use showed significant differences between countries. The use of pirfenidone was the most frequent in Turkey; a significantly higher proportion of Turkish patients received pirfenidone at the time of investigation as compared with the other countries participating in the study. The application of nintedanib was most frequent in Hungary:

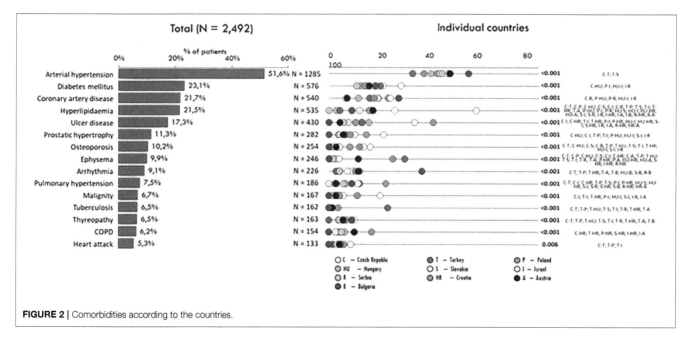

FIGURE 2 | Comorbidities according to the countries.

TABLE 3 | Antifibrotic treatment in individual countries.

	Total N = 2492	Czech Republic N = 971	Turkey N = 505	Poland N = 285	Hungary N = 216	Slovakia N = 149	Israel N = 120	Serbia N = 95	Croatia N = 87	Austria N = 55	Bulgaria N = 9
Pirfenidone	750 (30.1%)	364 (37.5%) T, P, HU, S, I, R, HR, A	201 (39.8%) C, P, HU, S, I, A	73 (25.6%) C, T, HU, S, I, A	22 (10.2%) C, T, P, S, R, HR	11 (7.4%) C, T, P, HU, I, R, HR	20 (16.7%) C, T, P, S, R, HR	27 (28.4%) C, HU, S, I, A	25 (28.7%) C, HU, S, I, A	6 (10.9%) C, T, P, R, HR	1 (11.1%)
Nintedanib	689 (27.6%)	246 (25.3%)	72 (14.3%)	58 (20.4%)	121 (56.0%)	74 (49.7%)	52 (43.3%)	19 (20.0%)	11 (12.6%)	34 (61.8%)	2 (22.2%)
Switch	169 (6.8%)	94 (9.7%)	22 (4.4%)	8 (2.8%)	15 (6.9%)	0 (0.0%)	18 (15.0%)	3 (3.2%)	6 (6.9%)	3 (5.5%)	0 (0.0%)
None	884 (35.5%)	267 (27.5%)	210 (41.6%)	146 (51.2%)	58 (26.9%)	64 (43.0%)	30 (25.0%)	46 (48.4%)	45 (51.7%)	12 (21.8%)	6 (66.7%)

Data are N (%) or median (range). Data are only expressed as absolute number of patients and corresponding proportion percentage.

more than half of the patients received it as antifibrotic treatment. The summary of antifibrotic treatment can be found in **Table 3**.

As the availability of different antifibrotics might be dependent on the healthcare provider regulation of the individual country, reimbursement, and country-specific regulations are described in **Table 4**.

DISCUSSION

Our data are the first to compare intercountry differences in patients with IPF using the common platform of EMPIRE enabling uniform data input and analysis. While real-world registries have limitations, our results confirm profound differences in baseline characteristics, lung function, HRCT pattern, and comorbidities in the patients with IPF from 10 Central and Eastern European countries.

Maximizing the potential of precision medicine for patients and healthcare services is a major social challenge. Disease registries have great potential to provide insight into real-world data and, consequently, provide information for planning healthcare services (24, 25). With their help, it is easier to collect data about complaints, symptoms, and quality of life of the patients, to investigate the effects and adverse effects of different treatments and to evaluate the disease development. However, registry data may suffer from bias and vary between countries as a result of incomplete registration, precluding measurement of true incidence and prevalence (26). Previously, the European Respiratory Journal emphasized the importance of registry data in IPF: prospective cohorts mean a solution to support patient care and research in complex chronic diseases (26).

Data collected from clinical trials are often misleading due to selection bias. Globally, there are significant differences in the incidence, prevalence, diagnostic approach, therapies, and survival for patients with IPF according to continents and countries. For example, the prevalence of IPF varies widely depending on location, identifying criteria, and year of study, ranging from 3 to 6 per 1,00,000 in the United Kingdom

TABLE 4 | Antifibrotic treatment availability in individual countries.

Country	Year of joining EMPIRE	Number of patients receiving antifibrotic treatment, N (% all patients in the given country)	Reimbursement specifics
Czech Republic	2015 (2012–2015 as National Czech Registry of IPF)	• nintedanib: 246 (25.3) ○ pirfenidone: 364 (37.5)	• 2015–2018 covered on individual request Reimbursed since 2018 in patients fulfilling predefined criteria covered by health insurance ○ 2014–2017 covered on individual request Reimbursed since 2017 in patients fulfilling predefined criteria covered by health insurance
Turkey	2016	• nintedanib: 72 (14.3) ○ pirfenidone: 201 (39.8)	• September 23, 2017 Nintedanib received a refund. Free for those with FVC more than 50%, DLCO more than 30%, <10% FVC loss in 6 months ○ October 11, 2016–267 mg capsules and 200 mg tablets received a refund 01 April 2020–600 mg tablets received a refund September 9, 2020–267 mg tablets and 801 mg tablets received a refund. Free for those with FVC more than 50%, DLCO more than 30%, <10% FVC loss in 6 months
Poland	2015	• nintedanib: 58 (20.4) ○ pirfenidone: 73 (25.6)	• 2018 Therapeutic program (fully reimbursed in patients with: FVC ≥ 50% DLCO ≥ 30%). Stopping rule: decrease of 10% in FVC in first year of treatment and then in 6 months assessed every 6 months ○ 2017 Therapeutic program (fully reimbursed in patients with: FVC ≥ 50% DLCO ≥ 30%) Stopping rule: decrease of 10% in FVC in first year of treatment and then in 6 months assessed every 6 months
Hungary	2015	• nintedanib: 121 (56.0) ○ pirfenidone: 22 (10.2)	• 2015–2017: individual request coverage by national insurance Since 2017 according label fully covered by national insurance ○ 2017: According label fully covered by national insurance
Slovakia	2015	• nintedanib: 74 (49.7) ○ pirfenidone: 11 (7.4)	• Available since 2015 based on individual reimbursement ○ Available since 2015 based on individual reimbursement
Israel	2018	• nintedanib: 52 (43.3) ○ pirfenidone: 20 (16.7)	• 2014–2016: Compassionate use program 2016: Fully covered ○ 2016: Fully covered
Serbia	2015	• nintedanib: 19 (20.0) ○ pirfenidone: 27 (28.4)	• 2017: According label, not covered by national insurance, but at the cost of referral institutions (4 University hospitals of Pulmonology) based on decisions of their Consilia for Fibrosis ○ 2016: For all cases of IPF, not covered by national insurance, but at the cost of referral institutions (4 University hospitals of Pulmonology) based on decisions of their Consilia for Fibrosis
Croatia	2016	• nintedanib: 11 (12.6) ○ pirfenidone: 25 (28.7)	• 2017: Fully covered by National Health insurance fund for patients with FVC between 50% and 80% Stopping rule: decrease of FVC >10% at any time during 12 months Reassessment: every 12 months ○ 2017: Fully covered by National Health insurance fund for patients with FVC between 50 and 80% Stopping rule: decrease of FVC >10% at any time during 12 months Reassessment: every 12 months
Austria	2018	• nintedanib: 34 (61.8) ○ pirfenidone: 6 (10.9)	• Available since 2015, the access for patients is based on individual reimbursement. Full reimbursement for IPF no restrictions—systemic sclerosis/progressive fibrosing ILD individual reimbursement ○ Available since 2011, only individual reimbursement for IPF with FVC ≥ 50 and ≤ 80 and stopping rule (10% in 6 months)—new indications still under discussion
Bulgaria	2018	• nintedanib: 2 (22.2) ○ pirfenidone: 1 (11.1)	• Since April 2018 Reimbursed by National Health insurance fund for patients over 50 year old and with FVC between 50 and 80% and DLCO between 79 and 30%. Stopping rule for patients reached DLCO or FVC bellow lower limit Reassessment every 6 month ○ Since April 2018 Reimbursed by National Health insurance fund for patients over 50 year old and with FVC between 50–80% and DLCO between 79 and 30%. Stopping rule for patients reached DLCO or FVC bellow lower limit Reassessment every 6 month

up to 16–18 per 1,00,000 in Finland (27, 28). Individual registries, generally, differ from each other, thus there might be differences regarding inclusion criteria, frequency, and outcome of IPF exacerbations, comorbidities, genetic factors and variance, efficacy and safety of pharmaceutical therapy, predictors of outcome, etc. With international registries, it is possible to create large datasets that enable clinicians and researchers to compare regions, countries, and time periods. According to McCormick et al., who made a comparative analysis of Cystic Fibrosis Registry data from the United Kingdom with other countries, the development of national cystic fibrosis databases has enabled a comparison between countries in key clinical outcomes. However, the authors highlighted the limitation of the study and urged a standardization of data collection between national cystic fibrosis registries to obtain a greater understanding from international and intercontinental comparisons (29).

In this study, we present clinical data from EMPIRE, the registry of patients with IPF from Central and Eastern Europe (23). We evaluated patient baseline characteristics, clinical symptoms, radiological features, spirometric values, and therapeutic solutions to emphasize similarities and differences between 10 countries. Despite living in the same geographical area, there were statistically significant differences regarding all the examined features and parameters. However, through this study, similarities and main differences could be highlighted and the shortcomings in terms of uniformity can be improved in the future. Currently, there are 2 IPF-registries in which Central and Eastern Europe is a partaker, namely EMPIRE and eurIPFreg. There are 12 other IPF-registries in Europe, however, they only include patients from one country (24).

The quality of healthcare system of a country can be estimated, for example, by the proportion of the structured clinical examinations performed (30). While not comparable, clinical data from well-structured IPF national registries might give some hints about diversities in different countries. The national IPF-registry of Spain, the SEPAR National Registry analysed the data from 608 patients between 2012 and 2017 (31). The electronic registry of IPF in the United Kingdom, the UK IPF Registry has counted 2,474 registered patients in the time period of 2013–2019 (32). To the INSIGHTS-IPF registry of Germany, 588 patients were entered between 2012 and 2018 (33). Between 2012 and 2016, 647 patients were registered to the Australian Idiopathic Pulmonary Fibrosis Registry (AIPFR) (8). For example, dyspnea was less frequent in the UK IPF registry, in comparison with the other 4 registries. In AIPFR, better baseline lung function was noted than in the other cohorts. GAP stage I was the rarest in EMPIRE compared with the other 4 registries, while UIP HRCT pattern appeared more often in our analysis. Our data show comparable lung function values for the most published registry data.

The organization of detailed evidence is considered to be a very strict measure as its purpose is also to create clinical practice guidelines (34, 35). Clinical practice guidelines are by their nature general recommendations aimed for broad applicability in the clinical setting. The applicability, however, is limited by numerous factors. The challenge of using guidelines on daily basis is that these guidelines are likely to be disease-oriented and not patient-oriented. Guideline recommendations are mainly based on the disease severity without taking coexistent conditions and other factors (e.g., factors that are used by physicians to individualize diagnosis and treatment), into consideration (36). High-quality meta-analyses and systematic reviews of randomized control trials (RCTs) or RCTs with a very low risk of bias stand in first place on the hierarchy of levels of evidence from published papers (34, 37). RCTs are created to maximize internal validity by studying a strictly defined population in a controlled setting, hence, establishing the efficacy of treatment (36, 38). Their results may have limited applicability to patients in clinical settings (39). These trials generally register a thoroughly selected patient population that meets strict inclusion criteria and exclusion criteria, including regular laboratory and clinical monitoring and measure objective parameters of efficacy. In "real world" clinical practice, however, the patients are unselected, monitoring is likely to be less frequent, and effectiveness is the most relevant outcome (36, 40). Pragmatic trials and observational studies can play an important role in addition to RCTs as they are created to recreate conditions in the daily clinical practice (40). Observational studies examine large groups of patients to evaluate long-term outcomes, examine very important consequences, such as mortality, and examine outcomes that may not be easily assessed by RCTs (e.g., pharmacoeconomic data). Recent analyses of data gained by RCTs and observational studies concluded that the effects of treatment revealed in observational studies were not greater or qualitatively different from those of RCT comparing the same treatments (41, 42). The reliance on RTCs as the highest level of evidence is thus challenged (43). Although observational studies should not replace RCTs, they can be useful in complementing the results of such trials. Well-designed observational studies can identify clinically important differences among therapeutic options and provide information on long-term drug effectiveness and safety (39). As a result of a review that compared the two methods used in good clinical practice concluded that the development of country-specific guidelines or local guidelines for each region would provide more suitable practical solutions. Besides, factors, such as social factors and expenses—that influence choice of the patients—and therapy adherence would be better considered (36).

Randomized control trials play the leading role and are inevitable when developing and testing new pharmaceutical substances. Over the last years—despite being a rare disease—numerous large, multicenter RCTs have been conducted culminating in the approval of 2 drugs for the treatment of IPF (44).

Our data confirmed, that in IPF, significant differences exist in drug availability according to countries, possibly resulting from high costs when introducing new treatments. As we summarized data for nintedanib and pirfenidone, there were no two countries with the same policy for providing these drugs to patients. As a result, regional differences in survival might be observed due to treatment differences arising from national regulations. Comparisons of the effectivity of antifibrotics might be further challenged, as availability changes over time and over regions. For example, in Australia, antifibrotic treatment was available through clinical trials, special access programs, and private purchase by the time of inclusion in the published AIPFR document (8). Further studies are needed to evaluate the long-term outcome in patients treated with antifibrotics by stratifying cases according to already developed prognostic factors (45).

Healthcare specialists, patient organizations, and EU regulatory bodies should work to cease inequalities in patient care also highlighted in our data.

The limitation of our study is the disproportion in the number of patients from different countries, as it varied from 971 (Czech Republic) to 9 patients (Bulgaria) and 55 (Austria) mainly representing the time of being in the Registry. Differences in center size, the number of centers, time to enrollment and operator practice, and ethnic/cultural heterogeneity might all affect the outcome of the analysis.

CONCLUSIONS

Well-organized and unified registries for patients with IPF are indispensable to achieve better outcomes. In this study, we proved significant differences in the characteristics of patients with IPF and described differences in availability to antifibrotic therapies in EMPIRE countries that needs

further investigation and strategies to improve patient care in this region. Equal participation rates and complete data registration in EMPIRE are fundamental to maximize precision. Unified methods and maximal accuracy are key elements to better understanding and more effective treatment of IPF. Inequalities resulting from differences in the availability of antifibrotics should be managed with international cooperation.

ETHICS STATEMENT

The studies involving human participants were reviewed and approved by the EMPIRE registry protocol was approved in each country by the respective Ethical Committee. Written informed consent was obtained from all individual patients, who were enrolled in accordance with the Helsinki Declaration. The patients/participants provided their written informed consent to participate in this study.

AUTHOR CONTRIBUTIONS

AK-F wrote the first draft of the manuscript. MŠte, NM, KL, VM, MH, MK, DJ, JT-T, MStu, NS, and MV contributed to conception and the design of the study. SL worked out the concept of statistical evaluation and performed statistical analysis. All authors contributed to the data collection, manuscript revision, read, and approved the submitted version.

REFERENCES

1. Raghu G, Collard HR, Egan JJ, Martinez FJ, Behr J, Brown KK, et al. An official ATS/ERS/JRS/ALAT statement: idiopathic pulmonary fibrosis: evidence-based guidelines for diagnosis and management. *Am J Respir Crit Care Med.* (2011) 183:788–824. doi: 10.1164/rccm.2009-040GL
2. Molina-Molina M, Aburto M, Acosta O, Ancochea J, Rodríguez-Portal JA, Sauleda J, et al. Importance of early diagnosis and treatment in idiopathic pulmonary fibrosis. *Expert Rev Respir Med.* (2018) 12:537–9. doi: 10.1080/17476348.2018.1472580
3. Raghu G, Remy-Jardin M, Myers JL, Richeldi L, Ryerson CJ, Lederer DJ, et al. Diagnosis of idiopathic pulmonary fibrosis. an official ATS/ERS/JRS/ALAT clinical practice guideline. *Am J Respir Crit Care Med.* (2018) 198:e44–68. doi: 10.1164/rccm.201807-1255ST
4. Taskar VS, Coultas DB. Is idiopathic pulmonary fibrosis an environmental disease? *Proc Am Thorac Soc.* (2006) 3:293–8. doi: 10.1513/pats.200512-131TK
5. Taskar V, Coultas D. Exposures and idiopathic lung disease. *Semin Respir Crit Care Med.* (2008) 29:670–9. doi: 10.1055/s-0028-1101277
6. Spira A, Beane J, Shah V, Liu G, Schembri F, Yang X, et al. Effects of cigarette smoke on the human airway epithelial cell transcriptome. *Proc Natl Acad Sci USA.* (2004) 101:10143–8. doi: 10.1073/pnas.0401422101
7. Chioma OS, Drake WP. Role of microbial agents in pulmonary fibrosis. *Yale J Biol Med.* (2017) 90:219–27.
8. Jo HE, Glaspole I, Grainge C, Goh N, Hopkins PM, Moodley Y, et al. Baseline characteristics of idiopathic pulmonary fibrosis: analysis from the Australian Idiopathic Pulmonary Fibrosis Registry. *Eur Respir J.* (2017) 49:1601592. doi: 10.1183/13993003.01592-2016
9. Hutchinson J, Fogarty A, Hubbard R, McKeever T. Global incidence and mortality of idiopathic pulmonary fibrosis: a systematic review. *Eur Respir J.* (2015) 46:795–806. doi: 10.1183/09031936.00185114
10. Duchemann B, Annesi-Maesano I, Jacobe de Naurois C, Sanyal S, Brillet PY, Brauner M, et al. Prevalence and incidence of interstitial lung

diseases in a multi-ethnic county of Greater Paris. *Eur Respir J.* (2017) 50:1602419. doi: 10.1183/13993003.02419-2016
11. Bendstrup E, Hyldgaard C, Altraja A, Sjåheim T, Myllärniemi M, Gudmundsson G, et al. Organisation of diagnosis and treatment of idiopathic pulmonary fibrosis and other interstitial lung diseases in the Nordic countries. *Eur Clin Respir J.* (2015) 2:1. doi: 10.3402/ecrj.v2.28348
12. Behr J, Günther A, Bonella F, Dinkel J, Fink L, Geiser T, et al. S2K-Leitlinie zur Diagnostik der idiopathischen Lungenfibrose [German Guideline for Idiopathic Pulmonary Fibrosis]. *Pneumologie.* (2020) 74:e1–2. doi: 10.1055/a-1179-2905
13. Richeldi L, Rubin AS, Avdeev S, Udwadia ZF, Xu ZJ. Idiopathic pulmonary fibrosis in BRIC countries: the cases of Brazil, Russia, India, and China. *BMC Med.* (2015) 13:237. doi: 10.1186/s12916-015-0495-0
14. Farrand E, Iribarren C, Vittinghoff E, Levine-Hall T, Ley B, Minowada G, et al. Impact of idiopathic pulmonary fibrosis on longitudinal health-care utilization in a community-based cohort of patients. *Chest.* (2021) 159:219–27. doi: 10.1016/j.chest.2020.07.035
15. Quinn C, Wisse A, Manns ST. Clinical course and management of idiopathic pulmonary fibrosis. *Multidiscip Respir Med.* (2019) 14:35. doi: 10.4081/mrm.2019.484
16. Wijsenbeek M, Cottin V. Spectrum of fibrotic lung diseases. *N Engl J Med.* (2020) 383:958–68. doi: 10.1056/NEJMra2005230
17. Wijsenbeek MS, Holland AE, Swigris JJ, Renzoni EA. Comprehensive supportive care for patients with fibrosing interstitial lung disease. *Am J Respir Crit Care Med.* (2019) 200:152–9. doi: 10.1164/rccm.201903-0614PP
18. Diamantopoulos A, Wright E, Vlahopoulou K, Cornic L, Schoof N, Maher TM. The burden of illness of idiopathic pulmonary fibrosis: a comprehensive evidence review. *Pharmacoeconomics.* (2018) 36:779–807. doi: 10.1007/s40273-018-0631-8
19. Pleasants R, Tighe RM. Management of idiopathic pulmonary fibrosis. *Ann Pharmacother.* (2019) 53:1238–48. doi: 10.1177/1060028019862497
20. Patient Registries. *Registries for Evaluating Patient Outcomes - NCBI Bookshelf.* Available online at: https://www.ncbi.nlm.nih.gov/books/NBK208643/ (accessed February 8, 2021).

21. Kolonics-Farkas AM, Šterclová M, Mogulkoc N, Kus J, Hájková M, Müller V, Jovanovic D, et al. Anticoagulant use and bleeding risk in central European patients with Idiopathic Pulmonary Fibrosis (IPF) treated with antifibrotic therapy: real-world data from EMPIRE. *Drug Saf.* (2020) 43:971–80. doi: 10.1007/s40264-020-00978-5

22. Barczi E, Starobinski L, Kolonics-Farkas A, Eszes N, Bohacs A, Vasakova M, et al. Long-term effects and adverse events of nintedanib therapy in idiopathic pulmonary fibrosis patients with functionally advanced disease. *Adv Ther.* (2019) 36:1221–32. doi: 10.1007/s12325-019-00906-9

23. *EMPIRE Registry: Homepage.* Available online at: http://empire.registry.cz/index-en.php (accessed November 23, 2018).

24. Culver DA, Behr J, Belperio JA, Corte TJ, de Andrade JA, Flaherty KR, et al. Patient registries in idiopathic pulmonary fibrosis. *Am J Respir Crit Care Med.* (2019) 200:160–7. doi: 10.1164/rccm.201902-0431CI

25. Chorostowska-Wynimko J, Wencker M, Horváth I. The importance of effective registries in pulmonary diseases and how to optimize their output. *Chron Respir Dis.* (2019) 16:1479973119881777. doi: 10.1177/1479973119881777

26. Cottin V, Wuyts W. Insights into idiopathic pulmonary fibrosis in the real world. *Eur Respir J.* (2015) 46:16–8. doi: 10.1183/09031936.00036815

27. Wilson JW, du Bois RM, King TE Jr. Challenges in pulmonary fibrosis: 8–the need for an international registry for idiopathic pulmonary fibrosis. *Thorax.* (2008) 63:285–7. doi: 10.1136/thx.2004.031062

28. Ferrara G, Arnheim-Dahlström L, Bartley K, Janson C, Kirchgässler KU, Levine A, et al. Epidemiology of pulmonary fibrosis: a cohort study using healthcare data in Sweden. *Pulm Ther.* (2019) 5:55–68. doi: 10.1007/s41030-019-0087-9

29. McCormick J, Sims EJ, Green MW, Mehta G, Culross F, Mehta A. Comparative analysis of cystic fibrosis registry data from the UK with USA, France and Australasia. *J Cyst Fibros.* (2005) 4:115–22. doi: 10.1016/j.jcf.2005.01.001

30. Donev D, Kovacic L, Laaser U. The role and organization of health care systems. *Heal Syst. Lifestyles Policies.* Lage: Jacobs Verlag (2013) 1:3–14.

31. Fernández-Fabrellas E, Molina-Molina M, Soriano JB, Portal JAR, Ancochea J, Valenzuela C, et al. Demographic and clinical profile of idiopathic pulmonary fibrosis patients in Spain: the SEPAR National Registry. *Respir Res.* (2019) 20:127. doi: 10.1186/s12931-019-1084-0

32. Spencer LG, Loughenbury M, Chaudhuri N, Spiteri M, Parfrey H. Idiopathic pulmonary fibrosis in the UK: analysis of the British Thoracic Society electronic registry between 2013 and 2019. *ERJ Open Res.* (2021) 7:00187–2020. doi: 10.1183/23120541.00187-2020

33. Behr J, Prasse A, Wirtz H, Koschel D, Pittrow D, Held M, et al. Survival and course of lung function in the presence or absence of antifibrotic treatment in patients with idiopathic pulmonary fibrosis: long-term results of the INSIGHTS-IPF registry. *Eur Respir J.* (2020) 56:1902279. doi: 10.1183/13993003.02279-2019

34. SIGN 50: *A Guideline Developer's Handbook. Scottish Intercollegiate Guidelines 2011 Network.* Available online at: https://www.sign.ac.uk/assets/sign50_2011.pdf (accessed November 11, 2020).

35. Atkins D, Best D, Briss PA, Eccles M, Falck-Ytter Y, Flottorp S, et al. Grading quality of evidence and strength of recommendations. *BMJ.* (2004) 328:1490. doi: 10.1136/bmj.328.7454.1490

36. Price D, Thomas M. Breaking new ground: challenging existing asthma guidelines. *BMC Pulm Med.* (2006) 6 (Suppl. 1):S6. doi: 10.1186/1471-2466-6-S1-S6

37. Bousquet J, Van Cauwenberge P. A critical appraisal of 'evidence-based medicine' in allergy and asthma. *Allergy.* (2004) 59(Suppl 78):12–20. doi: 10.1111/j.1398-9995.2004.00654.x

38. Miravitlles M, Roche N, Cardoso J, Halpin D, Aisanov Z, Kankaanranta H, et al. Chronic obstructive pulmonary disease guidelines in Europe: a look into the future. *Respir Res.* (2018) 19:11. doi: 10.1186/s12931-018-0715-1

39. Silverman SL. From randomized controlled trials to observational studies. *Am J Med.* (2009) 122:114–20. doi: 10.1016/j.amjmed.2008.09.030

40. Roland M, Torgerson DJ. What are pragmatic trials? *BMJ.* (1998) 316:285. doi: 10.1136/bmj.316.7127.285

41. Benson K, Hartz AJ. A comparison of observational studies and randomized, controlled trials. *N Engl J Med.* (2000) 342:1878–86. doi: 10.1056/NEJM200006223422506

42. Concato J, Shah N, Horwitz RI. Randomized, controlled trials, observational studies, and the hierarchy of research designs. *N Engl J Med.* (2000) 342:1887–92. doi: 10.1056/NEJM200006223422507

43. Concato J. Observational versus experimental studies: what's the evidence for a hierarchy? *NeuroRx.* (2004) 1:341–7. doi: 10.1602/neurorx.1.3.341

44. Raghu G. Idiopathic pulmonary fibrosis: lessons from clinical trials over the past 25 years. *Eur Respir J.* (2017) 50:1701209. doi: 10.1183/13993003.01209-2017

45. Tran T, Šterclová M, Mogulkoc N, Lewandowska K, Müller V, Hájková M, et al. The European MultiPartner IPF registry (EMPIRE): validating long-term prognostic factors in idiopathic pulmonary fibrosis. *Respir Res.* (2020) 21:11. doi: 10.1186/s12931-019-1271-z

14

Acute Exacerbation of Interstitial Lung Disease in Adult Patients With Idiopathic Inflammatory Myopathies: A Retrospective Case-Control Study

Junyu Liang[†], Heng Cao[†], Yini Ke, Chuanyin Sun, Weiqian Chen and Jin Lin*

Department of Rheumatology, The First Affiliated Hospital, College of Medicine, Zhejiang University, Hangzhou, China

*Correspondence:
Jin Lin
linjinzju@zju.edu.cn

[†]These authors have contributed equally to this work

Objective: This study aimed at clarifying the prevalence, risk factors, outcome, and outcome-related factors of acute exacerbation of interstitial lung disease (AE-ILD) in patients with idiopathic inflammatory myopathy (IIM).

Methods: Data of IIM patients who were admitted to the First Affiliated Hospital of Zhejiang University (FAHZJU) from September 2007 to September 2019 were retrospectively collected. And the IIM patients with AE-ILD formed the case group. In addition, age and sex matched IIM patients without AE-ILD were randomly selected to constitute the control group. A 1:2 case-control study and intragroup analysis were performed to identify risk factors for development of AE-ILD in IIM patients and unfavorable short-term outcome in AE-ILD patients through comparison, univariate and multivariate logistic regression analysis.

Results: AE-ILD occurred in 64 out of 665 IIM patients (9.6%) with a short-term mortality rate of 39.1%. And the 64 IIM patients with AE-ILD formed the case group. Besides, 128 age and sex matched IIM patients without AE-ILD were randomly selected to constitute the control group. The retrospective case-control study revealed that elevated on-admission disease activity ($P < 0.001$), lower percent-predicted diffusing capacity of the lung for carbon monoxide (DLCO%, $P = 0.013$) and diagnosis of clinically amyopathic dermatomyositis (CADM, $P = 0.007$) were risk factors for development of AE-ILD in IIM patients. The following intragroup analysis indicated that elevated on-admission disease activity ($P = 0.008$) and bacterial infection ($P = 0.003$) were significantly correlated with the unfavorable short-term outcome of patients complicated with AE-ILD. In addition, combined use of steroid and disease modifying antirheumatic drugs (DMARDs, $P = 0.006$) was found to significantly reduce the short-term mortality in IIM patients with AE-ILD.

Conclusion: AE-ILD is a less frequent but fatal complication in IIM patients with elevated on-admission disease activity, lower DLCO% and diagnosis of CADM working as risk factors, indicating the potential roles of autoimmune abnormality and hypoxia in development of AE-ILD. Elevated on-admission disease activity and bacterial infection could predict unfavorable short-term outcome of IIM patients with AE-ILD. A therapeutic regimen of steroid and DMARDs was found to reduce short-term death in these patients.

Keywords: interstitial lung disease, dermatomyositis, polymyositis, complication, outcome

INTRODUCTION

Idiopathic inflammatory myopathies (IIM) are a group of autoimmune diseases that primarily target the skeleton muscles (1, 2). Dermatomyositis (DM) and polymyositis (PM) are two conventional subtypes of IIM, while clinically amyopathic dermatomyositis (CADM) is a newly recognized subset of DM with typical skin rash of DM and slight muscular damage. Although the incidence of DM, PM, and CADM was considerably low in common people, the high mortality rate, the various clinical manifestations, and multiple complications have drawn much attention from clinicians and researchers. In published studies, the 10-year survival rate for patients with DM, PM, or CADM ranged from 51 to 91% (3). An ~4.5% in-hospital mortality rate was seen in two retrospective studies (3, 4).

Multiple organs apart from muscle are often affected as well, leading to critical worsening of the life quality and outcome of these patients (5). Among the multiple extramuscular complications of IIM, interstitial lung disease (ILD) was identified as both the most frequent and severe involvement, leading to a significant elevation in mortality rate (6). Moreover, acute exacerbation of ILD (AE-ILD), which used to be mainly studied in patients with idiopathic pulmonary fibrosis, has also been noticed in patients with connective tissue disease (CTD). In CTD patients, AE-ILD was reported to occur at a 1-year frequency of 1.25–3.3%, at a lifetime incidence of 7.2% in CTD patients, and contributed to a high mortality rate within these patients (7, 8). In the past few years, there existed a few reports and small-sample studies of AE-ILD, or rapid progression of ILD, in IIM patients. However, systemic understandings including the incidence of AE-ILD, its risk factors and outcome in IIM patients remained unclear. It is thus necessary to uncover the enigma by figuring out factors correlated with AE-ILD in patients with DM, PM, or CADM, and factors associated with outcome of patients with AE-ILD.

In this study, we retrospectively reviewed the medical records of 424 patients with DM, PM, and CADM who were admitted to our center from February 2011 to February 2019, and performed a case-control analysis to identify potential related risk factors for AE-ILD among these patients. Besides, factors affecting the short-term outcome of patients with AE-ILD were as well-probed into via subgroup analysis.

MATERIALS AND METHODS
Patients

Medical records of adult patients who were admitted to the inpatient department of the Qingchun division of the First Affiliated Hospital of Zhejiang University (FAHZJU) with the diagnosis of DM, PM, or CADM from September 2007 to September 2019 was reviewed and collected. The approval (Reference Number: 2019-646) of the Institutional Review Board (IRB) of the FAHZJU was acquired before the initiation of the study, and written informed consent from each patient involved was acquired as well. The inclusion criteria of this study were: (1) age over 18 years old; (2) the diagnosis of DM or PM fulfilled the diagnostic criteria of Bohan and Peter (9), and the diagnosis of CADM met the criteria developed by Sontheimer (10). Exclusion criteria were: (1) overlap syndromes with other connective tissue diseases; (2) hospitalization for causes unrelated to myositis and its complications, such as fracture, pregnancy, cataract, and appendicitis etc.; (3) myopathies that might be related to thyroid dysfunction, excessive exercises, inherited, or metabolic disorders, recent use of muscle-impairment drugs including statins, chloroquine, colchicine, entecavir, traditional Chinese medicine, etc.; (4) loss to follow-up within 2 weeks after discharge.

Methods

Medical records of all patients enrolled were retrospectively collected by reviewing the electronic medical record (EMR) system. Data including demographic information, course of disease, duration of diagnosis delay, clinical manifestations, or complications, on-admission disease activity, results of pulmonary function test, preceding comorbidities, harmful hobbies, imaging reports, laboratory findings, medications, as well as short-term outcome were acquired and analyzed. ILD, subtype of ILD and AE-ILD were evaluated by radiologists using high-resolution computed tomography (HRCT). In absence of diagnostic criteria dedicated to AE-ILD in patients with CTD, an updated criteria of acute exacerbation of idiopathic pulmonary fibrosis (AE-IPF) was adopted based on the experience of published studies on AE-ILD in CTD patients. The updated criteria included previous or concurrent diagnosis of ILD, acute worsening or development of dyspnea typically <1 month duration, computed tomography with new bilateral ground-glass opacity and/or consolidation superimposed on a background pattern consistent with usual interstitial pneumonia (UIP) pattern, and deterioration not fully explained by cardiac failure or fluid overload (11). Compared with the previous diagnostic criteria for AE-ILD proposed in 2007 (12), the new criteria does not demand thorough exclusion of infection. And infection has been found to participate in the pathogenesis and progression of idiopathic pulmonary fibrosis (IPF) (13). As previously suggested, the occurrence of this clinical and radiological manifestation in a background of possible or inconsistent with UIP pattern was also considered diagnostic for AE in CTD patients (14, 15). Cases manifested as UIP pattern were identified based on their radiologic appearance on HRCT: the presence of basal-dominant reticular opacities and predominantly basal and subpleural distribution of honeycomb lesions, with multiple equal-sized cystic lesions of 2–10 mm diameter with a thick wall (16). Diagnosis of bacterial, fungal, or tuberculosis infection was a comprehensive decision based on the essential positive result of etiological detection, HRCT manifestation, clinical symptoms, infection-related laboratory abnormalities, treatment of intravenous antibiotics, and antifungal drugs, positive response after treatment, etc. The etiological detection was defined as the culture of bronchoalveolar lavage fluid (BALF) and sputum. Sputum culture result counted only if >25 squamous epithelial cells per low-power field were observed (17). In bacterial infections, the thresholds for positivity of quantitative cultures were applied: 10^5 cfu/ml for sputum culture (17), 10^4 cfu/mL for bronchoalveolar lavage (18). For patients with infection of *Candida albican* or *Candida glabrata*, the BALF or sputum culture should show a visually medium to large amount of *C. albicans* or *C. glabrata* in the sample. The repeated cultures of BALF or sputum were routinely initiated before intravenous use of antibiotics or anti-fungal medications. Meanwhile diagnosis of virus infection, to be specific, Epstein-Barr virus (EBV) or Cytomegalo virus (CMV) infection, relied on the screening of serum antibody and DNA of these two viruses. Identification of gastrointestinal hemorrhage was based on repeated positive results of fecal occult blood test. To minimize omission of lymphadenectasis, hepatomegaly, and splenomegaly, the identification was based on records of physical examination together with reports of ultrasound examination, computed tomography and positron emission tomography. On-admission disease activity was routinely assessed by the Myositis Disease Activity Assessment Visual Analog Scales (MYOACT) within the first week of admission (19). Immunosuppressive regimens used during hospitalization were categorized into four groups: (1) steroid monotherapy; (2) steroid + disease-modifying antirheumatic drugs (DMARDs); (3) steroid + intravenous immunoglobulin (IVIG); (4) steroid + DMARDs +IVIG. In this study, usage of DMARDs included usage of mycophenolate mofetil (MMF), thalidomide, hydroxychloroquine, cyclosporine, azathioprine, methotrexate, cyclophosphamide, etc. Short-term mortality, or unfavorable short-term outcome, referred to in-hospital mortality or death within 2 weeks of hospital discharge.

To probe into factors exerting significant influence on development of AE-ILD within patients with DM, PM, or CADM, a case-control study was performed. Patients diagnosed with AE-ILD constituted the case group. And ILD patients without AE-ILD were selected using a systematic sampling method by matching age and sex with cases with AE-ILD at a proportion of 1:2. Comparisons, univariate and multivariate logistic regression analysis were performed between the case group and the control group. To clarify the time axis of risk factors and results, only clinical manifestations or complications that happened before the diagnosis of AE-ILD would be taken into account for patients with AE-ILD. In order to identity potential factors affecting the short-term outcome of the AE-ILD patients involved, the AE-ILD patients were further divided into two groups: patients who died in hospital or within 2 weeks of hospital discharge were defined as the mortality group, and those who survived after 2 weeks of hospital discharge were categorized as the survival group. Comparisons and logistic regression analysis were made between the two groups of patients regarding age, sex, clinical features, disease activity, laboratory findings, etc.

Statistical Analysis

Statistical analysis was performed using SPSS 22.0 (Chicago, IL, USA) and R 3.6.1. The normality of continuous variables was tested by the Kolmogorov-Smirnov goodness-of-fit model. Continuous variables were expressed as mean ± SD if normally distributed and median (quartiles) if skewed. Ordinal categorical variables were as well shown as median (quartiles). Unordered categorical variables were presented as numbers and percentages. Independent sample t-test was used to compare normally distributed continuous variables. And Mann-Whitney U-test was applied to compare skewed continuous variables or ordinal categorical variables. Chi-square test and Fisher's exact test were used to compare unordered categorical variables. All tests were two-sided and a $P < 0.05$ was considered statistically significant. Univariate and multivariate logistic regression analyses were subsequently adopted to identify risk factors for AE-ILD in patients with PM, DM or CADM as well as risk factors for unfavorable short-term outcome in AE-ILD. In the study of risk factors for AE-ILD, explanatory factors with $P < 0.1$ in the univariate logistic regression analysis were entered into the multivariate logistic regression analysis. In the process of figuring out risk factors for unfavorable short-term outcome, however, factors with $P < 0.05$ in univariate analysis were enrolled into the multivariate logistic regression analysis owing to the limited number of AE-ILD patients. For normally distributed continuous variables with missing values, inputation using expectation maximization (EM) algorithm was performed for those that passed univariate screening. Multivariate logistic regression analysis with a stepwise forward likelihood ratio (LR) method was used to determine the statistically significant factors. Results from the multivariate logistic regression were presented as an odds ratio (OR) with 95% confidence interval (CI). A two-sided $P < 0.05$ was considered to be statistically significant. If there existed any positive result in serum biomarkers or disease activity in multivariate logistic regression analysis, a receiver operating characteristic (ROC) curve analysis would be performed to evaluate its predictive value for development and outcome of AE-ILD.

RESULTS

A total of 665 patients treated at FAHZJU with a diagnosis of DM, PM, or CADM between September 2007 and September 2019 were enrolled into this study, including 334 with DM, 264 with PM, and 67 with CADM. Four hundred and eighty-three patients (72.6%) were identified to be complicated with ILD. Sixty-four out of 665 patients were diagnosed with AE-ILD during their stay in hospital (**Figure 1**). The incidence of AE-ILD was 9.6% in patients with DM, PM, or CADM, and 13.3% in patients who were complicated with ILD at the same time. To be specific, the incidence of AE-ILD in patient with DM, PM, and CADM were 10.8, 5.7, and 19.4%, respectively. In the 665 patients, the average age for AE-ILD patients was 57.7 ± 11.9 years, which was significantly higher than that of the patients without AE-ILD (53.1 ± 13.7 years, $P = 0.011$). Among the 64 AE-ILD patients, 25 were males and 39 were females. The proportion of males in AE-ILD patients was not significantly different from that in non-AE-ILD patients (39.1 vs. 32.3%, $P = 0.272$). Short-term mortality rate for AE-ILD and non-AE-ILD patients were 39.1 vs. 5.7% ($P < 0.001$).

In total, 64 AE-ILD patients and 128 ILD patients without occurrence of AE-ILD were included in the case-control analysis to identify risk factors for AE-ILD in patients with DM, PM, or CADM. Due to the retrospective nature of this study, only 137 patients (54 of AE-ILD patients and 83 of patients without

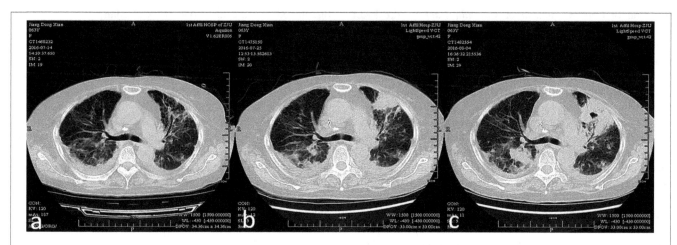

FIGURE 1 | Acute exacerbation of interstitial lung disease of a patient within 3 weeks (from **a–c** chronologically).

AE-ILD) received pulmonary function test within the first week of hospitalization. The case group presented more frequently with treatment of steroid + IVIG ($P = 0.034$), diagnosis of CADM ($P = 0.034$) and less frequently with allergic history ($P = 0.049$). Higher levels of serum ferritin ($P = 0.027$) and C reactive protein (CRP, $P = 0.004$) were seen in patients with AE-ILD. On-admission disease activity, which was evaluated by MYOACT score, was as well-significantly higher for patients in the case group ($P < 0.001$). In addition, AE-ILD patients were found to present with lower level of percent-predicted diffusing capacity of the lung for carbon monoxide (DLCO%, $P = 0.009$; **Table 1, Supplementary Data 1**).

Univariate analysis showed that there were eight factors associated with AE-ILD at the level of $P < 0.1$. These factors included elevated on-admission disease activity ($P < 0.001$), lower DLCO% ($P = 0.010$), serum ferritin ($P = 0.058$), CRP ($P = 0.037$), hypertension ($P = 0.065$), allergic history ($P = 0.058$), treatment of steroid + IVIG ($P = 0.038$), and diagnosis of CADM ($P = 0.038$) (**Supplementary Table 1**). Inputation was performed for DLCO% before multivariate logistic regression analysis. Using Kolmogorov-Smirnov test, DLCO% was found a continuous variable that was subject to normal distribution. EM inputation was hereby performed to handle the impact of missing values more appropriately. Afterwards, all variables with $P < 0.1$ were entered into the multivariate logistic regression analysis, and elevated on-admission disease activity ($P < 0.001$), lower DLCO% ($P = 0.013$), and diagnosis of CADM ($P = 0.007$) were found to be significantly different between the case group and the control group. The results were found similar to those without EM imputation (**Table 2**). As presented in **Figure 2**, the optimal cut-off value of the on-admission disease activity for AE-ILD was >7.5, with a sensitivity of 76.6% and a specificity of 57.0%. The area under the curve (AUC) was 0.705.

Of the 64 AE-ILD patients identified in the study, 25 (39.1%) died in hospital or within 2 weeks of hospital discharge. In addition to 36 AE-ILD patients with DM, we also found 15 PM patients and 13 CADM patients who as well-suffered from AE-ILD. And 15 of them (23.4%) manifested as UIP pattern

in HRCT. Infection happened to 30 out of 64 adult AE-ILD patients. Ten had bacterial infection, 12 had fungal infection, three were diagnosed with tuberculosis, one was found to have EBV infection. Three suffered from both bacterial and fungal infection, and one had both bacterial and EBV infection. Bacterial (21.9%) and fungal (23.4%) infections were hereby recognized as the two most common infections in AE-ILD patients. Only eight patients with infections (five in bacterial infection, two in fungal infection, and one in tuberculosis infection) were identified based on positive result of BALF smear or culture. To be specific, bacterial infection included four cases of *Acinetobacter baumannii*, four cases with *Stenotrophomonas maltophilia*, three case with *Klebsiella pneumonia*, onc case with *Pseudomonas* aeruginosa, one case with *Staphylococcus haemolyticus*, and one case with *Staphylococcus aureus*. And fungal infection included 10 cases with medium to large amount of *C. albicans*, three cases with *Aspergillus fumigatus*, one case with *Pneumocystis carinii* and one case with *C. glabrata*. Therefore, infections in patients with AE-ILD were mostly opportunistic infections. Details on infections in the matched control group was provided in **Supplementary Data 2**. In addition, the most commonly used therapy was a combined application of steroid and DMARDs (45.3%). And MMF (48.3%) was the most frequently used DMARD in this regimen. Patients with unfavorable short-term outcome presented more frequently with dysphagia ($P = 0.030$), bacterial infection ($P = 0.001$), hypertension ($P = 0.017$), treatment of steroid + IVIG ($P = 0.013$), and less frequently with treatment of steroid + DMARDs ($P = 0.001$). Higher on-admission disease activity ($P = 0.014$) was as well-seen in patients with unfavorable outcome (**Table 3**).

Univariate analysis showed that there were six factors associated with unfavorable short-term outcome in AE-ILD patients at the level of $P < 0.05$. These factors included dysphagia ($P = 0.019$) bacterial infection ($P = 0.002$), on-admission disease activity ($P = 0.012$), hypertension ($P = 0.020$), treatment of steroid + DMARDs ($P = 0.002$) and steroid + IVIG ($P = 0.018$) (**Supplementary Table 2**). The following multivariate logistic regression analysis revealed that higher on-admission

Acute Exacerbation of Interstitial Lung Disease in Adult Patients With Idiopathic Inflammatory...

139

TABLE 1 | Comparison of clinical characteristics between case group and control group.

Factors	AE-ILD (64)	Non-AE-ILD (128)	P-value
Age (y)	60.5 (48.0, 66.0)	60.0 (48.3, 65.0)	0.726
Sex (male/female)	25/39	50/78	1.000
Course of disease (m)	3.0 (1.0, 6.8)	4.0 (2.0, 8.8)	0.122
Duration of diagnosis delay (m)	2.0 (1.0, 4.5)	3.0 (1.0, 6.0)	0.113
Clinical manifestations or complications			
Fever	27 (42.2%)	40 (31.3%)	0.134
Lymphadenectasis	26 (40.6%)	47 (36.7%)	0.599
Hepatomegaly	1 (1.6%)	1 (0.8%)	1.000
Splenomegaly	14 (21.9%)	21 (16.4%)	0.355
Heliotrope rash	33 (51.6%)	63 (49.2%)	0.759
Gottron's sign	36 (56.3%)	65 (50.8%)	0.474
Periungual erythema	13 (20.3%)	21 (16.4%)	0.504
Mechanic's hands	9 (14.1%)	17 (13.3%)	0.881
Raynaud's phenomenon	4 (9.5%)	8 (9.5%)	1.000
Muscle pain	22 (34.4%)	53 (41.4%)	0.347
Muscle weakness	50 (78.1%)	111 (86.7%)	0.127
Joint pain	17 (26.6%)	24 (18.8%)	0.213
Joint swelling	8 (12.5%)	21 (16.4%)	0.476
Dysphagia	11 (17.2%)	27 (21.1%)	0.522
Dysarthria	5 (7.8%)	8 (6.3%)	0.919
Respiratory muscle involvement	2 (3.1%)	7 (5.5%)	0.717
Cardiac involvement	4 (6.3%)	10 (7.8%)	0.922
Gastrointestinal hemorrhage	9 (14.1%)	15 (11.7%)	0.643
Bacterial infection	14 (21.9%)	21 (16.4%)	0.355
Fungal infection	15 (23.4%)	22 (17.2%)	0.301
Tuberculosis infection	3 (4.7%)	3 (2.3%)	0.402
EBV or CMV infection	2 (3.1%)	6 (4.7%)	0.890
Carcinoma	6 (9.4%)	11 (8.6%)	0.857
UIP pattern	15 (23.4%)	23 (18.0%)	0.370
Pneumomediastinum	4 (6.3%)	6 (4.7%)	0.909
On-admission disease activity			
MYOACT score	10.0 (8.0,12.0)	7.0 (5.0,9.0)	<0.001
Pulmonary function test			
FVC% (%)	66.1 ± 17.9	67.4 ± 19.2	0.684
TLC (L)	3.1 (2.6,4.3)	3.6 (2.9,4.2)	0.107
FEV1% (%)	66.8 ± 15.8	70.4 ± 21.3	0.288
FEV1/FVC	0.8 (0.7,0.9)	0.8 (0.8,0.9)	0.335
DLCO% (%)	53.6 ± 15.4	62.3 ± 20.5	0.009
On-admission laboratory findings			
ALT (U/L)	49.0 (22.8,122.3)	50.0 (27.0,134.0)	0.710
AST (U/L)	48.0 (29.5,105.8)	61.5 (31.5,163.3)	0.283
Cr (μmol/L)	52.0 (43.0,69.0)	49.5 (43.0,59.0)	0.129
LDH (U/L)	421.0 (330.8,619.3)	401.0 (300.5,820.8)	0.844
CK (U/L)	179.0 (54.3,958.5)	484.5 (58.0,2465.5)	0.113
CK-MB (U/L)	31.5 (18.3,55.5)	32.0 (19.0,110.0)	0.210
CRP (mg/L)	10.1 (4.5,43.7)	6.1 (2.3,18.8)	0.004
Ferritin (ng/ml)	821.7 (342.9,2034.5)	532.7 (247.4,1205.9)	0.027

(Continued)

TABLE 1 | Continued

Factors	AE-ILD (64)	Non-AE-ILD (128)	P-value
ANA	40 (62.5%)	75 (58.6%)	0.603
Comorbidities/Harmful hobbies			
Smoking	14 (21.9%)	26 (20.3%)	0.802
Alcohol abuse	10 (15.6%)	24 (18.8%)	0.593
Hypertension	22 (34.4%)	28 (21.9%)	0.063
Diabetes	8 (12.5%)	12 (9.4%)	0.504
Hepatitis	4 (6.3%)	15 (11.7%)	0.232
Allergic History	4 (6.3%)	21 (16.4%)	0.049
Immunosuppressive therapy			
Steroid monotherapy	19 (29.7%)	37 (28.9%)	0.911
Steroid + DMARDs	29 (45.3%)	71 (55.5%)	0.184
Steroid + IVIG	13 (20.3%)	12 (9.4%)	0.034
Steroid + DMARDs + IVIG	3 (4.7%)	8 (6.3%)	0.913
IIM subtypes			
DM	36 (56.3%)	72 (56.3%)	1.000
PM	15 (23.4%)	44 (34.4%)	0.122
CADM	13 (20.3%)	12 (9.4%)	0.034

AE-ILD, Acute exacerbation of interstitial lung disease; y, years; m, months; EBV, Epstein-Barr virus; CMV, Cytomegalo virus; UIP pattern, Usual interstitial pneumonia pattern; MYOACT, Myositis Disease Activity Assessment Visual Analog Scales; FVC%, Percent-predicted forced vital capacity; TLC, Total lung capacity; FEV1%, Percent-predicted forced expiratory volume in 1 s; FEV1/FVC, Ratio of FEV1 over FVC; DLCO%, Percent-predicted diffusing capacity of the lung for carbon monoxide; ALT, Glutamic pyruvic transaminase; AST, Glutamic oxaloacetic transaminase; Cr, Serum creatinine; LDH, Lactate dehydrogenase; CK, Creatine kinase; CK-MB, Creatine kinase isoenzymes; ANA, Antinuclear antibody; DMARDs, Disease-modifying anti-rheumatic drugs; IVIG, Intravenous immunoglobulin; IIM, Idiopathic inflammatory myopathies; DM, dermatomyositis; PM, Polymyositis; CADM, Clinically amyopathic dermatomyositis.

TABLE 2 | Multivariate logistic regression analysis of risk factors for AE-ILD in patients with DM, PM, or CADM.

Factors	P-value	OR value	95% CI
On-admission disease activity (MYOACT score)	<0.001	1.243	1.127–1.371
DLCO%	0.013	0.972	0.950–0.994
CADM	0.007	3.781	1.444–9.903

DM, dermatomyositis; PM, Polymyositis; CADM, Clinically amyopathic dermatomyositis; OR value, Odds ratio value; 95%CI, 95% Confidence interval; MYOACT, Myositis Disease Activity Assessment Visual Analog Scales, DLCO%, Percent-predicted diffusing capacity of the lung for carbon monoxide.

disease activity ($P = 0.008$), bacterial infection ($P = 0.003$), and treatment of steroid+DMARDs ($P = 0.006$) were significantly correlated with unfavorable short-term outcome in AE-ILD patients (**Table 4**). As presented in **Figure 3**, the best cut-off value of the on-admission disease activity for unfavorable short-term outcome in patients with AE-ILD was >8.5, with a sensitivity of 84.0% and a specificity of 43.6%. The AUC was 0.682.

DISCUSSION

To date, this is the first study to systematically probe into the risk factors for development of AE-ILD in patients with

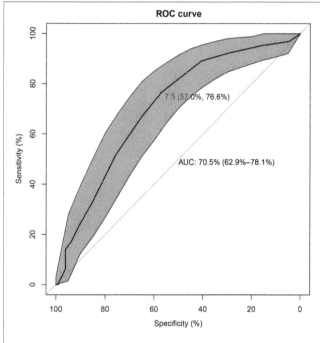

FIGURE 2 | The receiver operating characteristic curve of on-admission disease activity for development of AE-ILD in IIM patients. AE-ILD, Acute exacerbation of interstitial lung disease; IIM, Idiopathic inflammatory myopathies.

DM, PM, or CADM, and potential factors affecting the short-term outcome of the AE-ILD patients. Preceding studies on acute exacerbation mainly focused on AE-IPF. And the annual incidence of AE-IPF ranged from 7 to 19.1% in different clinical trials and retrospective studies (20–25). Knowledge on AE-ILD in non-IPF patients, namely connective-tissue-disease-related ILD (CTD-ILD), was limited. The reported incidence of AE-ILD in rheumatoid arthritis (RA) patients with ILD was 7.7–22% (26, 27). Tomiyama et al. revealed an AE-ILD incidence of 9.4% in systemic sclerosis (28). In this study, the incidence of AE-ILD was 9.6% in patients with DM, PM, or CADM, and 13.3% in patients complicated with ILD. And the mortality rate of AE-ILD was significantly higher than that in non-AE-ILD patients (39.1 vs. 5.7% $P < 0.001$). Besides, the average age for AE-ILD patients was as well-higher than that of the patients without AE-ILD (57.7 $\pm$ 11.9 vs. 53.1 $\pm$ 13.7 years, $P = 0.011$). Elevated on-admission disease activity, lower DLCO% and diagnosis of CADM were found to be risk factors for development of AE-ILD in patients with DM, PM, or CADM. Moreover, bacterial infection, elevated on-admission disease activity and treatment of steroid + DMARDs were significantly correlated with short-term outcome in AE-ILD patients.

Previous studies revealed that declined forced vital capacity (FVC), low diffusing capacity of the lung for carbon monoxide (DLCO), pulmonary hypertension, comorbid coronary artery disease, surgical resection of lung cancers and various infections etc. were found to be risk factors for AE-ILD (29–31). However, the results were not homogeneous in different studies. In

TABLE 3 | Comparison of clinical characteristics between mortality group and survival group.

Factors	Mortality group (25)	Survival group (39)	P-value
Age (y)	62.0 (47.0,67.0)	60.0 (51.0,65.0)	0.967
Sex (male/female)	12/13	13/26	0.241
Course of disease (m)	2.0 (1.0,4.5)	3.0 (1.0,9.0)	0.235
Duration of diagnosis delay (m)	2.0 (1.0,3.0)	3.0 (1.0,6.0)	0.332
Clinical manifestations or complications			
Fever	14 (56.0%)	13 (33.3%)	0.073
Lymphadenectasis	8 (32.0%)	18 (46.2%)	0.261
Hepatomegaly	1 (4.0%)	0 (0.0%)	0.391
Splenomegaly	6 (24.0%)	8 (20.5%)	0.742
Heliotrope rash	12 (48.0%)	21 (53.8%)	0.648
Gottron's sign	12 (48.0%)	24 (61.5%)	0.287
Periungual erythema	4 (16.0%)	9 (23.1%)	0.492
Mechanic's hands	4 (16.0%)	5 (12.8%)	1.000
Raynaud's phenomenon	0 (0.0%)	4 (10.3%)	0.149
Muscle pain	11 (44.0%)	11 (28.2%)	0.194
Muscle weakness	20 (80.0%)	30 (76.9%)	0.771
Joint pain	7 (28.0%)	10 (25.6%)	0.835
Joint swelling	3 (12.0%)	5 (12.8%)	1.000
Dysphagia	8 (32.0%)	3 (7.7%)	0.030
Dysarthria	4 (16.0%)	1 (2.6%)	0.072
Respiratory muscle involvement	1 (4.0%)	1 (2.6%)	1.000
Cardiac involvement	3 (12.0%)	1 (2.6%)	0.291
Gastrointestinal hemorrhage	5 (20.0%)	4 (10.3%)	0.468
Bacterial infection	11 (44.0%)	3 (7.7%)	0.001
Fungal infection	9 (36.0%)	6 (15.4%)	0.057
Tuberculosis infection	0 (0.0%)	3 (7.7%)	0.275
EBV or CMV infection	0 (0.0%)	2 (5.1%)	0.516
Carcinoma	0 (0.0%)	6 (15.4%)	0.074
UIP pattern	5 (20.0%)	10 (25.6%)	0.603
Pneumomediastinum	3 (12.0%)	1 (2.6%)	0.291
On-admission disease activity			
MYOACT score	10.0 (9.0, 14.5)	9.0 (7.0, 12.0)	0.014
Pulmonary function test			
FVC% (%)	61.7 (36.7, 85.1)	69.0 (58.8, 79.3)	0.248
TLC (L)	3.2 (2.6, 4.3)	3.1 (2.4, 4.4)	0.787
FEV1% (%)	64.0 (42.7, 77.2)	69.4 (60.9, 78.6)	0.205
FEV1/FVC	0.8 (0.7,0.9)	0.8 (0.7,0.9)	0.615
DLCO% (%)	51.1 (44.9, 61.8)	58.2 (42.8, 63.2)	0.533
On-admission laboratory findings			
ALT (U/L)	63.0 (29.5, 120.5)	39.0 (21.0, 139.0)	0.559
AST (U/L)	60.0 (34.5, 97.0)	44.0 (24.0, 215.0)	0.461
Cr (μmol/L)	67.0 (41.0, 98.0)	52.0 (43.0, 63.0)	0.198
LDH (U/L)	439.0 (369.0, 609.5)	403.0 (317.0, 625.0)	0.518
CK (U/L)	151.0 (38.0, 312.0)	193.0 (93.0, 1667.0)	0.128
CK-MB (U/L)	25.0 (17.0, 58.5)	37.0 (20.0, 54.0)	0.405
CRP (mg/L)	18.7 (5.4, 53.2)	9.5 (4.4, 27.2)	0.259
Ferritin (ng/ml)	834.9 (611.0, 2757.4)	811.6 (186.4, 1690.2)	0.139

(Continued)

TABLE 3 | Continued

Factors	Mortality group (25)	Survival group (39)	P-value
ANA	12 (48.0%)	28 (71.8%)	0.055
Comorbidities/Harmful hobbies			
Smoking	6 (24.0%)	8 (20.5%)	0.742
Alcohol abuse	4 (16.0%)	6 (15.4%)	1.000
Hypertension	13 (52.0%)	9 (23.1%)	0.017
Diabetes	4 (16.0%)	4 (10.3%)	0.701
Hepatitis	2 (8.0%)	2 (5.1%)	0.640
Allergic History	2 (8.0%)	2 (5.1%)	0.640
Immunosuppressive therapy			
Steroid monotherapy	8 (32.0%)	11 (28.2%)	0.746
Steroid + DMARDs	5 (20.0%)	24 (61.5%)	0.001
Steroid + IVIG	9 (36.0%)	4 (10.3%)	0.013
Steroid + DMARDs + IVIG	3 (12.0%)	0 (0.0%)	0.055
IIM subtypes			
DM	14 (56.0%)	22 (56.4%)	0.974
PM	7 (28.0%)	8 (20.5%)	0.490
CADM	4 (16.0%)	9 (23.1%)	0.960

y, years; m, months; EBV, Epstein-Barr virus; CMV, Cytomegalo virus; UIP pattern, Usual interstitial pneumonia pattern; MYOACT, Myositis Disease Activity Assessment Visual Analog Scales; FVC%, Percent-predicted forced vital capacity; TLC, Total lung capacity; FEV1%, Percent-predicted forced expiratory volume in 1 s; FEV1/FVC, Ratio of FEV1 over FVC; DLCO%, Percent-predicted diffusing capacity of the lung for carbon monoxide; ALT, Glutamic pyruvic transaminase; AST, Glutamic oxaloacetic transaminase; Cr, Serum creatinine; LDH, Lactate dehydrogenase; CK, Creatine kinase; CK-MB, Creatine kinase isoenzymes; ANA, Antinuclear antibody; DMARDs, Disease-modifying anti-rheumatic drugs; IVIG, Intravenous immunoglobulin; IIM, Idiopathic inflammatory myopathies; DM, dermatomyositis; PM, Polymyositis; CADM, Clinically amyopathic dermatomyositis.

TABLE 4 | Multivariate logistic regression analysis of risk factors for unfavorable short-term outcome in patients complicated with AE-ILD.

Factors	P-value	OR value	95% CI
On-admission disease activity (MYOACT score)	0.008	1.346	1.082–1.674
Bacterial infection	0.003	13.494	2.398–75.945
Steroid+DMARDs	0.006	0.137	0.033–0.565

AE-ILD, Acute exacerbation of interstitial lung disease; MYOACT, Myositis Disease Activity Assessment Visual Analog Scales; DMARDs, Disease-modifying anti-rheumatic drugs.

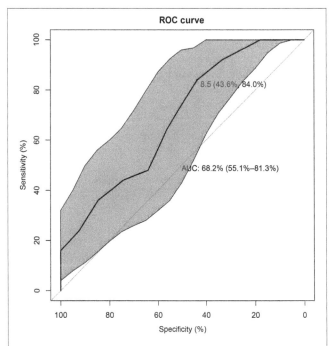

FIGURE 3 | The receiver operating characteristic curve of on-admission disease activity for unfavorable short-term outcome in IIM patients with AE-ILD. IIM, Idiopathic inflammatory myopathies; AE-ILD, Acute exacerbation of interstitial lung disease.

this study, decreased DLCO%, which reflected lower diffusing capacity, was found to be a risk factor for AE-ILD in patients with DM, PM, or CADM. The role of lower DLCO% in AE-ILD was not clear. On the one hand, lower DLCO% reflected decreased gas-exchanging function of lung. With no significant alteration in pulmonary ventilation function etc., decreased gas-exchanging function would lead to hypoxia, which could subsequently contribute to progress of ILD. Hypoxia have been recognized to induce progress of interstitial lung disease through augmenting oxidative and inflammatory pathways, increasing the total lung collagen content and heterogeneous structural alterations (32–34). On the other hand, decreased DLCO% could be an early-stage manifestation of AE-ILD since ILD and its progression could result in impaired diffuse capacity via alveolar structural alteration, thickening of alveolar capillary wall, etc. Lower DLCO% seemed to be both initiating factor and consequence of AE-ILD.

MYOACT score works as a systemic evaluation of disease activity of IIM (19, 35). After adjusting for other factors, elevated on-admission MYOACT score was found to be related to development of AE-ILD in IIM patients. The role of CTD disease activity in AE-ILD was disputable in published studies. In a retrospective study concerning RA patients receiving tocilizumab treatment, AE-ILD was found to be positively related to disease activity of RA (36). However, no similar association was seen in RA patients treated by corticosteroids and immunosuppressants. The predictive role of MYOACT score in this study might lie in the partially overlapped pathological mechanism between AE-ILD and IIM. Elevated levels of several cytokines and chemokines, namely IL-6, IL-8, IL-17, IL-23, etc., were seen in peripheral blood, muscle or skin of IIM patients, and were consistent with disease activity (37). Meanwhile several studies also observed significant elevation of cytokines and chemokines including IL-6, IL-8 in patients with ILD exacerbation, and the elevation was found to be related to worse outcome (38, 39). The partially overlapped pathological mechanism made baseline disease activity a valuable predictor of AE-ILD. Besides, after adjusting for factors including infections, medication, pulmonary function, etc., the significance of on-admission disease activity could, to some extent, demonstrated the role of autoimmune abnormality in development of AE-ILD. In 2011, Shu etc. found that initial disease activity, which was evaluated by MYOACT score, was not significantly correlated with long-term outcome of IIM patients (40). And no linkage between initial disease activity and short-term outcome of hospitalized IIM patients was reported previously. By narrowing down to DM, PM, or CADM patients complicated with AE-ILD, on-admission disease activity, which was evaluated by MYOACT score, was found to herald unfavorable short-term outcome in this study.

However, the evaluation of disease activity demands ability for communication, which would be difficult in patients with mental retardation or disturbed behavior. It would thus be of great significance to identify serum biomarkers for development and outcome of AE-ILD in IIM patients. Researchers in Hamamatsu University found that higher levels of ferritin predicted development of AE-IPF and unfavorable outcome (41). However, in this study, serum ferritin was not found to be significantly related to development of AE-ILD after adjusting for other clinical features. Nor was it identified to predict short-term outcome of IIM patients with AE-ILD. Preceding study also revealed that CRP could be used to predict development of AE-ILD in patients receiving non-pulmonary surgery (42). Nevertheless, no statistical significance for CRP was seen in IIM patients with regard to development and outcome of AE-ILD. Further studies would be demanded to identify serum biomarkers for development and outcome of AE-ILD in CTD patients.

In addition to the high prevalence of ILD in CADM patients, preceding studies proposed that rapidly progressive pattern of ILD was more frequently seen in CADM patients compared with patients with DM or PM (43, 44). After multivariate logistic regression analysis, diagnosis of CADM was found to be a risk factor for AE-ILD in patients with DM, PM or CADM, which was consistent with the past clinical findings. Although CD8+ T cells were found to play a key role in development of IIM-related ILD, high proportion of CD4+ T cells seemed to play a greater role in acute exacerbation of ILD. Suda and his colleagues focused on CADM patients and found that the CD4/CD8 ratio in bronchoalveolar lavage fluid (BALF) was higher in patients with rapidly progressive ILD in comparison to that in chronic ILD patients (45). Ito et al. demonstrated similar results in BALF and peripheral blood of patients with DM (46). Moreover, Mukae et al. uncovered a higher CD4/CD8 ratio in BALF of CADM-related ILD patients compared with that in ILD patients with classic DM (43). Taken together, the higher proportion of CD4+ T cells in BALF seem to link diagnosis of CADM with higher incidence of AE-ILD. Confirmation of the role of higher proportion of CD4+ T cells and exploration of its detailed mechanism in immune abnormality of AE-ILD in IIM patients demands further exploration.

In-hospital IIM patients regularly received immunosuppressive therapy, which greatly increased their vulnerability to bacterial, fungal, or viral infection. More infections, opportunistic bacterial and fungal infections in particular, were hereby identified in this study. Although infectious triggers were found in 10–30% of patients with AE in preceding study (47), no significant association was found between infections and development of AE-ILD after adjusting for disease activity, pulmonary function, medication, etc. In the following intragroup analysis, bacterial infection was found to be associated with unfavorable short-term outcome in DM, PM, or CADM patients complicated with AE-ILD. Similar linkage between infection and short-term outcome was seen in IIM patients (3, 4). And opportunistic infection was as well-recognized as a major cause of mortality in patients with IIM-related ILD (48). However, this is the first study identifying infection as risk factor for unfavorable short-term outcome in patients complicated with AE-ILD.

The mortality rate of patients with AE-ILD was relatively high. For patients with IPF, 46% of deaths are secondary to AE and median survival period after AE is 3-4 months (49). And a high mortality rate (55.6%) was as well-seen in CTD patients with AE-ILD (14). In this study, the short-term mortality rate of AE-ILD group was 39.1%. The relatively high mortality rate of AE-ILD patients indicated much room for improvement in therapeutic regimens. In IIM patients with AE-ILD, a combined use of steroid and DMARDs was found to reduce the short-term mortality rate of these patients. Meanwhile no significant effect was identified in the application of intravenous immunoglobulin. Preceding study revealed a favorable response of exacerbation of ILD in RA patients after receiving a combined therapy of steroid and DMARDs (50). And cyclosporine, tacrolimus, and cyclophosphamide were the major DMARDs used in this study. However, the mostly commonly used DMARD in our study was MMF, the use of which has been proved effective in myositis-related ILD (51). The combined use of steroid and MMF in CTD patients with AE-ILD deserved further exploration in the future. Intravenous immunoglobulin, which was as well-frequently used in patients with ILD or AE-ILD, still played a disputable role in treatment of AE-ILD, especially CTD-related AE-ILD (29, 52). Biologics could be viewed as a two-edge sword in AE-ILD. On the one hand, rituximab, etc. have shown optimistic result in therapy of several AE-ILD cases (52, 53). On the other hand, biologics have also been reported to induce AE-ILD (54, 55). Apart from immunosuppressant treatment, empirical antibiotic therapy is also considered for all patients (56). Application of azithromycin and prophylactic use of co-trimoxazole were found effective in several clinical trials (57–59). Besides, antifibrotic medication, anti-acid therapy, plasma exchange, Polymyxin-B-immobilized fiber column (PMX) and fluid management were as well-found to have potential, yet disputable effect on outcome of AE-ILD patients (29–31).

The most significant limitations of this study are the retrospective and observational nature of the study and the small sample size. Furthermore, absence of records of pulmonary hypertension and several myositis-associated antibodies in over half of the patients also restrained us from figuring out their roles in development of AE-ILD among IIM patients. A large prospective cohort study is essential to confirm our findings and fill in the gaps. In spite of all the limitations, we intended to shed some light on the future study of AE-ILD in patients with DM, PM, or CADM.

CONCLUSIONS

AE-ILD is a fatal complication in IIM patients. Elevated on-admission disease activity, lower DLCO% and diagnosis of CADM were found to be risk factor for development of AE-ILD in patients with DM, PM, or CADM. Speculations on the roles of autoimmune abnormality and hypoxia in development of AE-ILD were hereby brought up. In addition, elevated on-admission disease activity, bacterial infection could be used to predict unfavorable short-term outcome in AE-ILD patients. A therapeutic regimen of steroid and DMARDs was found to reduce short-term death in IIM patients with AE-ILD.

ETHICS STATEMENT

The studies involving human participants were reviewed and approved by the Institutional Review Board (IRB) of the First Affiliated Hospital of Zhejiang University. The patients/participants provided their written informed consent to participate in this study. Written informed consent was obtained from the individual(s) for the publication of any potentially identifiable images or data included in this article.

AUTHOR CONTRIBUTIONS

All authors met the criteria for authorship established by the International Committee of Medical Journal Editors. Specifically, JLia and HC were responsible for substantial contributions to the conception, design, analysis, drafting the work, revising the work, and reviewing of the manuscript. YK, CS, WC, and JLin assisted with the data gathering, revising the work, and reviewing of the manuscript. All the authors listed have approved for publication of the content and have agreed to be accountable for all aspects of the work in ensuring that questions related to the accuracy or integrity of any part of the work.

ACKNOWLEDGMENTS

The authors appreciate the assistance of Bei Xu and Yuli Wang in verification of ILD and AE-ILD.

REFERENCES

1. Dalakas MC. Pathogenesis and therapies of immune-mediated myopathies. *Autoimmun Rev.* (2012) 11:203–6. doi: 10.1016/j.autrev.2011.05.013
2. Marasco E, Cioffi E, Cometi L, Valentini V, Zanframundo G, Neri R, et al. One year in review 2018: idiopathic inflammatory myopathies. *Clin Exp Rheumatol.* (2018) 36:937–47.
3. Murray SG, Schmajuk G, Trupin L, Lawson E, Cascino M, Barton J, et al. A population-based study of infection-related hospital mortality in patients with dermatomyositis/polymyositis. *Arthritis Care Res.* (2015) 67:673–80. doi: 10.1002/acr.22501
4. Wu C, Wang Q, He L, Yang E, Zeng X. Hospitalization mortality and associated risk factors in patients with polymyositis and dermatomyositis: a retrospective case-control study. *PLoS ONE.* (2018) 13:e0192491. doi: 10.1371/journal.pone.0192491
5. Schmidt J. Current classification and management of inflammatory myopathies. *J Neuromuscul Dis.* (2018) 5:109–29. doi: 10.3233/JND-180308
6. Barba T, Fort R, Cottin V, Provencher S, Durieu I, Jardel S, et al. Treatment of idiopathic inflammatory myositis associated interstitial lung disease: a systematic review and meta-analysis. *Autoimmun Rev.* (2019) 18:113–22. doi: 10.1016/j.autrev.2018.07.013
7. Park IN, Kim DS, Shim TS, Lim CM, Lee SD, Koh Y, et al. Acute exacerbation of interstitial pneumonia other than idiopathic pulmonary fibrosis. *Chest.* (2007) 132:214–20. doi: 10.1378/chest.07-0323
8. Suda T, Kaida Y, Nakamura Y, Enomoto N, Fujisawa T, Imokawa S, et al. Acute exacerbation of interstitial pneumonia associated with collagen vascular diseases. *Respir Med.* (2009) 103:846–53. doi: 10.1016/j.rmed.2008.12.019
9. Bohan A, Peter JB. Polymyositis and dermatomyositis (first of two parts). *N Engl J Med.* (1975) 292:344–7. doi: 10.1056/NEJM197502132920706
10. Sontheimer RD. Would a new name hasten the acceptance of amyopathic dermatomyositis (dermatomyositis sine myositis) as a distinctive subset within the idiopathic inflammatory dermatomyopathies spectrum of clinical illness? *J Am Acad Dermatol.* (2002) 46:626–36. doi: 10.1067/mjd.2002.120621
11. Collard HR, Ryerson CJ, Corte TJ, Jenkins G, Kondoh Y, Lederer DJ, et al. Acute exacerbation of idiopathic pulmonary fibrosis. an international working group report. *Am J Respir Crit Care Med.* (2016) 194:265–75. doi: 10.1164/rccm.201604-0801CI
12. Collard HR, Moore BB, Flaherty KR, Brown KK, Kaner RJ, King TE Jr, et al. Acute exacerbations of idiopathic pulmonary fibrosis. *Am J Respir Crit Care Med.* (2007) 176:636–43. doi: 10.1164/rccm.200703-463PP
13. Invernizzi R, Molyneaux PL. The contribution of infection and the respiratory microbiome in acute exacerbations of idiopathic pulmonary fibrosis. *Eur Respir Rev.* (2019) 28:190045. doi: 10.1183/16000617.0045-2019
14. Manfredi A, Sebastiani M, Cerri S, Vacchi C, Tonelli R, Della Casa G, et al. Acute exacerbation of interstitial lung diseases secondary to systemic rheumatic diseases: a prospective study and review of the literature. *J Thorac Dis.* (2019) 11:1621–8. doi: 10.21037/jtd.2019.03.28
15. Papanikolaou IC, Drakopanagiotakis F, Polychronopoulos vs. Acute exacerbations of interstitial lung diseases. *Curr Opin Pulm Med.* (2010) 16:480–6. doi: 10.1097/MCP.0b013e32833ae49d
16. Sato T, Teramukai S, Kondo H, Watanabe A, Ebina M, Kishi K, et al. Impact and predictors of acute exacerbation of interstitial lung diseases after pulmonary resection for lung cancer. *J Thorac Cardiovasc Surg.* (2014) 147:1604–11.e3. doi: 10.1016/j.jtcvs.2013.09.050
17. Joyce SM. Sputum analysis and culture. *Ann Emerg Med.* (1986) 15:325–8. doi: 10.1016/S0196-0644(86)80576-5
18. Chastre J, Fagon JY, Bornet-Lecso M, Calvat S, Dombret MC, al Khani R, et al. Evaluation of bronchoscopic techniques for the diagnosis of nosocomial pneumonia. *Am J Respir Crit Care Med.* (1995) 152:231–40. doi: 10.1164/ajrccm.152.1.7599829
19. Isenberg DA, Allen E, Farewell V, Ehrenstein MR, Hanna MG, Lundberg IE, et al. International consensus outcome measures for patients with idiopathic inflammatory myopathies. Development and initial validation of myositis activity and damage indices in patients with adult onset disease. *Rheumatology.* (2004) 43:49–54. doi: 10.1093/rheumatology/keg427
20. Richeldi L, du Bois RM, Raghu G, Azuma A, Brown KK, Costabel U, et al. Efficacy and safety of nintedanib in idiopathic pulmonary fibrosis. *N Engl J Med.* (2014) 370:2071–82. doi: 10.1056/NEJMoa1402584
21. Ohshimo S, Ishikawa N, Horimasu Y, Hattori N, Hirohashi N, Tanigawa K, et al. Baseline KL-6 predicts increased risk for acute exacerbation of idiopathic pulmonary fibrosis. *Respir Med.* (2014) 108:1031–9. doi: 10.1016/j.rmed.2014.04.009
22. Judge EP, Fabre A, Adamali HI, Egan JJ. Acute exacerbations and pulmonary hypertension in advanced idiopathic pulmonary fibrosis. *Eur Respir J.* (2012) 40:93–100. doi: 10.1183/09031936.00115511
23. Kakugawa T, Sakamoto N, Sato S, Yura H, Harada T, Nakashima S, et al. Risk factors for an acute exacerbation of idiopathic pulmonary fibrosis. *Respir Res.* (2016) 17:79. doi: 10.1186/s12931-016-0400-1
24. Song JW, Hong SB, Lim CM, Koh Y, Kim DS. Acute exacerbation of idiopathic pulmonary fibrosis: incidence, risk factors and outcome. *Eur Respir J.* (2011) 37:356–63. doi: 10.1183/09031936.00159709
25. Kim DS, Park JH, Park BK, Lee JS, Nicholson AG, Colby T. Acute exacerbation

of idiopathic pulmonary fibrosis: frequency and clinical features. *Eur Respir J.* (2006) 27:143–50. doi: 10.1183/09031936.06.00114004

26. Toyoda Y, Hanibuchi M, Kishi J, Kawano H, Morizumi S, Sato S, et al. Clinical features and outcome of acute exacerbation of interstitial pneumonia associated with connective tissue disease. *J Med Invest.* (2016) 63:294–9. doi: 10.2152/jmi.63.294

27. Hozumi H, Nakamura Y, Johkoh T, Sumikawa H, Colby TV, Kono M, et al. Acute exacerbation in rheumatoid arthritis-associated interstitial lung disease: a retrospective case control study. *BMJ Open.* (2013) 3:e003132. doi: 10.1136/bmjopen-2013-003132

28. Tomiyama F, Watanabe R, Ishii T, Kamogawa Y, Fujita Y, Shirota Y, et al. High prevalence of acute exacerbation of interstitial lung disease in japanese patients with systemic sclerosis. *Tohoku J Exp Med.* (2016) 239:297–305. doi: 10.1620/tjem.239.297

29. Leuschner G, Behr J. Acute exacerbation in interstitial lung disease. *Front Med.* (2017) 4:176. doi: 10.3389/fmed.2017.00176

30. Azadeh N, Moua T, Baqir M, Ryu JH. Treatment of acute exacerbations of interstitial lung disease. *Expert Rev Respir Med.* (2018) 12:309–13. doi: 10.1080/17476348.2018.1446831

31. Azadeh N, Limper AH, Carmona EM, Ryu JH. The role of infection in interstitial lung diseases: a review. *Chest.* (2017) 152:842–52. doi: 10.1016/j.chest.2017.03.033

32. Barratt SL, Blythe T, Ourradi K, Jarrett C, Welsh GI, Bates DO, et al. Effects of hypoxia and hyperoxia on the differential expression of VEGF-A isoforms and receptors in Idiopathic Pulmonary Fibrosis (IPF). *Respir Res.* (2018) 19:9. doi: 10.1186/s12931-017-0711-x

33. Kim JS, Podolanczuk AJ, Borker P, Kawut SM, Raghu G, Kaufman JD, et al. Obstructive sleep apnea and subclinical interstitial lung disease in the multi-ethnic study of atherosclerosis (MESA). *Ann Am Thorac Soc.* (2017) 14:1786–95. doi: 10.1513/AnnalsATS.201701-091OC

34. Braun RK, Broytman O, Braun FM, Brinkman JA, Clithero A, Modi D, et al. Chronic intermittent hypoxia worsens bleomycin-induced lung fibrosis in rats. *Respir Physiol Neurobiol.* (2018) 256:97–108. doi: 10.1016/j.resp.2017.04.010

35. Alexanderson H, Lundberg IE. Disease-specific quality indicators, outcome measures and guidelines in polymyositis and dermatomyositis. *Clin Exp Rheumatol.* (2007) 25(6 Suppl 47):153–8.

36. Akiyama M, Kaneko Y, Yamaoka K, Kondo H, Takeuchi T. Association of disease activity with acute exacerbation of interstitial lung disease during tocilizumab treatment in patients with rheumatoid arthritis: a retrospective, case-control study. *Rheumatol Int.* (2016) 36:881–9. doi: 10.1007/s00296-016-3478-3

37. Rider LG, Aggarwal R, Machado PM, Hogrel JY, Reed AM, Christopher-Stine L, et al. Update on outcome assessment in myositis. *Nat Rev Rheumatol.* (2018) 14:303–18. doi: 10.1038/nrrheum.2018.33

38. Marchioni A, Tonelli R, Ball L, Fantini R, Castaniere I, Cerri S, et al. Acute exacerbation of idiopathic pulmonary fibrosis: lessons learned from acute respiratory distress syndrome? *Crit Care.* (2018) 22:80. doi: 10.1186/s13054-018-2002-4

39. Papiris SA, Tomos IP, Karakatsani A, Spathis A, Korbila I, Analitis A, et al. High levels of IL-6 and IL-8 characterize early-on idiopathic pulmonary fibrosis acute exacerbations. *Cytokine.* (2018) 102:168–72. doi: 10.1016/j.cyto.2017.08.019

40. Shu XM, Lu X, Xie Y, Wang GC. Clinical characteristics and favorable long-term outcomes for patients with idiopathic inflammatory myopathies: a retrospective single center study in China. *BMC Neurol.* (2011) 11:143. doi: 10.1186/1471-2377-11-143

41. Enomoto N, Oyama Y, Enomoto Y, Mikamo M, Karayama M, Hozumi H, et al. Prognostic evaluation of serum ferritin in acute exacerbation of idiopathic pulmonary fibrosis. *Clin Respir J.* (2018) 12:2378–89. doi: 10.1111/crj.12918

42. Takao S, Masuda T, Yamaguchi K, Sakamoto S, Horimasu Y, Nakashima T, et al. High preoperative C-reactive protein level is a risk factor for acute exacerbation of interstitial lung disease after non-pulmonary surgery. *Medicine.* (2019) 98:14296. doi: 10.1097/MD.0000000000014296

43. Mukae H, Ishimoto H, Sakamoto N, Hara S, Kakugawa T, Nakayama S, et al. Clinical differences between interstitial lung disease associated with clinically amyopathic dermatomyositis and classic dermatomyositis. *Chest.* (2009) 136:1341–7. doi: 10.1378/chest.08-2740

44. Saketkoo LA, Ascherman DP, Cottin V, Christopher-Stine L, Danoff SK, Oddis CV. Interstitial lung disease in idiopathic inflammatory myopathy. *Curr Rheumatol Rev.* (2010) 6:108–19. doi: 10.2174/157339710791330740

45. Suda T, Fujisawa T, Enomoto N, Nakamura Y, Inui N, Naito T, et al. Interstitial lung diseases associated with amyopathic dermatomyositis. *Eur Respir J.* (2006) 28:1005–12. doi: 10.1183/09031936.06.00038806

46. Ito M, Kaise S, Suzuki S, Kazuta Y, Sato Y, Miyata M, et al. Clinico-laboratory characteristics of patients with dermatomyositis accompanied by rapidly progressive interstitial lung disease. *Clin Rheumatol.* (1999) 18:462–7. doi: 10.1007/s100670050139

47. Atochina EN, Beck JM, Preston AM, Haczku A, Tomer Y, Scanlon ST, et al. Enhanced lung injury and delayed clearance of *Pneumocystis carinii* in surfactant protein A-deficient mice: attenuation of cytokine responses and reactive oxygen-nitrogen species. *Infect Immun.* (2004) 72:6002–11. doi: 10.1128/IAI.72.10.6002-6011.2004

48. Marie I, Hachulla E, Cherin P, Hellot MF, Herson S, Levesque H, et al. Opportunistic infections in polymyositis and dermatomyositis. *Arthritis Rheum.* (2005) 53:155–65. doi: 10.1002/art.21083

49. Suzuki A, Kimura T, Kataoka K, Matsuda T, Yokoyama T, Mori Y, et al. Acute exacerbation of idiopathic pulmonary fibrosis triggered by Aspergillus empyema. *Respir Med Case Rep.* (2018) 23:103–6. doi: 10.1016/j.rmcr.2018.01.004

50. Ota M, Iwasaki Y, Harada H, Sasaki O, Nagafuchi Y, Nakachi S, et al. Efficacy of intensive immunosuppression in exacerbated rheumatoid arthritis-associated interstitial lung disease. *Mod Rheumatol.* (2017) 27:22–8. doi: 10.3109/14397595.2016.1173816

51. Huapaya JA, Silhan L, Pinal-Fernandez I, Casal-Dominguez M, Johnson C, Albayda J, et al. Long-term treatment with azathioprine and mycophenolate mofetil for myositis-related interstitial lung disease. *Chest.* (2019) 156:896–906. doi: 10.1016/j.chest.2019.05.023

52. So H, Wong VTL, Lao VWN, Pang HT, Yip RML. Rituximab for refractory rapidly progressive interstitial lung disease related to anti-MDA5 antibody-positive amyopathic dermatomyositis. *Clin Rheumatol.* (2018) 37:1983–9. doi: 10.1007/s10067-018-4122-2

53. Tokunaga K, Hagino N. Dermatomyositis with rapidly progressive interstitial lung disease treated with rituximab: a report of 3 cases in Japan. *Internal Med.* (2017) 56:1399–403. doi: 10.2169/internalmedicine.56.7956

54. Kawashiri SY, Kawakami A, Sakamoto N, Ishimatsu Y, Eguchi K. A fatal case of acute exacerbation of interstitial lung disease in a patient with rheumatoid arthritis during treatment with tocilizumab. *Rheumatol Int.* (2012) 32:4023–6. doi: 10.1007/s00296-010-1525-z

55. Matsumoto T, Iwano S, Takahashi N, Asai S, Watanabe T, Asai N, et al. Association between chest computed tomography findings and respiratory adverse events in rheumatoid arthritis patients undergoing long-term biological therapy. *Int J Rheum Dis.* (2019) 22:626–35. doi: 10.1111/1756-185X.13434

56. Maher TM, Whyte MK, Hoyles RK, Parfrey H, Ochiai Y, Mathieson N, et al. Development of a consensus statement for the definition, diagnosis, and treatment of acute exacerbations of idiopathic pulmonary fibrosis using the delphi technique. *Adv Ther.* (2015) 32:929–43. doi: 10.1007/s12325-015-0249-6

57. Kawamura K, Ichikado K, Suga M, Yoshioka M. Efficacy of azithromycin for treatment of acute exacerbation of chronic fibrosing interstitial pneumonia: a prospective, open-label study with historical controls. *Respiration.* (2014) 87:478–84. doi: 10.1159/000358443

58. Shulgina L, Cahn AP, Chilvers ER, Parfrey H, Clark AB, Wilson EC, et al. Treating idiopathic pulmonary fibrosis with the addition of co-trimoxazole: a randomised controlled trial. *Thorax.* (2013) 68:155–62. doi: 10.1136/thoraxjnl-2012-202403

59. Wilson EC, Shulgina L, Cahn AP, Chilvers ER, Parfrey H, Clark AB, et al. Treating idiopathic pulmonary fibrosis with the addition of co-trimoxazole: an economic evaluation alongside a randomised controlled trial. *Pharmacoeconomics.* (2014) 32:87–99. doi: 10.1007/s40273-013-0112-z

15

Interstitial Lung Disease Associated With Autoimmune Rheumatic Diseases: Checklists for Clinical Practice

Silvia Laura Bosello[1], Lorenzo Beretta[2], Nicoletta Del Papa[3], Sergio Harari[4,5], Stefano Palmucci[6], Alberto Pesci[7], Gilda Rechichi[8], Francesco Varone[9] and Marco Sebastiani[10]*

[1] Rheumatology Unit, A. Gemelli University Hospital Foundation - Istituto di Ricerca e Cura a Carattere Scientifico (IRCCS), Catholic University of the Sacred Heart, Rome, Italy, [2] Scleroderma Unit, Istituto di Ricerca e Cura a Carattere Scientifico (IRCCS) Ca' Granda Foundation Ospedale Maggiore Policlinico di Milan, Milan, Italy, [3] Rheumatology Department, Scleroderma Clinic, ASST Pini-CTO, Milan, Italy, [4] Department of Medical Sciences, San Giuseppe Hospital MultiMedica Istituto di Ricerca e Cura a Carattere Scientifico (IRCCS), Milan, Italy, [5] Department of Clinical Sciences and Community Health, Università Degli Studi di Milano, Milan, Italy, [6] Radiology Unit I, Department of Medical Surgical Sciences and Advanced Technologies GF Ingrassia, University Hospital Policlinico "G. Rodolico-San Marco", University of Catania, Catania, Italy, [7] Pneumological Clinic of the University of Milan-Bicocca, ASST-Monza, Monza, Italy, [8] Radiology Unit, University Hospital San Gerardo, ASST-Monza, Monza, Italy, [9] Pneumology Unit, A. Gemelli University Hospital Foundation Istituto di Ricerca e Cura a Carattere Scientifico (IRCCS), Rome, Italy, [10] Rheumatology Unit, University of Modena and Reggio Emilia, Italy

*Correspondence:
Marco Sebastiani
marco.sebastiani@unimore.it

Background: Interstitial lung diseases (ILDs) are often associated with rheumatic diseases. Their early diagnosis and management are not only difficult, but also crucial, because they are associated with major morbidity and mortality and can be the first cause of death in autoimmune rheumatic diseases (ARDs).

Objectives: By using methodologies, such as Nominal Group Technique (NGT) and Delphi Survey, the aims of this study were (1) to measure consensus between pulmonologists, radiologists, and rheumatologists experienced in the management of ARD-ILD; (2) to highlight the importance of a multidisciplinary approach; and (3) to provide clinicians with a practical tool aimed at improving the prompt recognition and follow-up of ILD associated with ARDs and of any possible rheumatic conditions underlying ILD.

Results: During the NGT round, the Steering Committee defined 57 statements to be used in the Delphi survey. A total of 78 experts participated in the Delphi survey, namely 28 pulmonologists, 33 rheumatologists, and 17 radiologists. During this round, consensus on agreement was reached in 47 statements, while disagreement was not reached in any statements. A secondary questionnaire was drafted by the Steering Committee to obtain clearer indications on ILD-ARD "red-flags" and follow-up. Delphi Panelists took part also in the second-questionnaire survey. Answers from both surveys were used to draft two checklists of "red flags" sign or symptom suggestive of ILD and ARD, respectively, and two checklists on identification and monitoring of rheumatoid arthritis (RA) and systemic sclerosis (SSc) ILD.

Limitations: This study is a consensus work, which cannot produce empiric data, and is limited to the Italian scenario.

Conclusions: This work showed a high level of agreement, but also shows some divergent opinions between different experts. This underlines the importance of a multidisciplinary approach. Eventually, we believe the drafted checklists can help clinicians in the diagnosis and follow-up of ILD-ARD.

Keywords: interstitial lung disease, autoimmune rheumatic diseases, multidisciplinary team, nominal group technique, Delphi panel survey, red flags and referral indications, consensus, ARD-ILD

INTRODUCTION

Interstitial lung diseases (ILDs) encompass a heterogeneous group of clinical conditions characterized by fibrosis of and/or inflammation the lungs (1). A common cause of ILD is represented by rheumatic diseases; in these conditions, lung involvement is not only common, but can be the main organ involvement (2, 3). Systemic sclerosis (SSc), rheumatoid arthritis (RA), antisynthetase syndrome, Sjogren's syndrome, mixed connective tissue disease (CTD), idiopathic inflammatory myopathies, and systemic lupus erythematosus are often associated with ILD (4). Moreover, a recent international consensus statement proposed "interstitial pneumonia with autoimmune features" as a new definition for ILD underlined by systemic autoimmune condition and not classifiable as any definite CTD, emphasizing the relationship between ILD and autoimmune response (5, 6). In patients with rheumatic diseases, ILD is difficult to diagnose at an early stage, and can be associated with major morbidity and mortality, or even be the leading cause of death (7–13).

Interstitial lung diseases should be managed, from its diagnosis, by a multidisciplinary team (MDT) composed of at least one pulmonologist, one radiologist, and one pathologist (2–4, 14). However, since phenotypic features of both ILDs and systemic autoimmune disorders often overlap, the patient's assessment should not be limited to clinical, radiological, and pathological evaluation, but should also include a clinical–immunological evaluation. The inclusion of an expert rheumatologist to the MDT can significantly reduce invasive procedures and increase diagnostic accuracy (1, 3, 4, 15). Nonetheless, in daily practice, it could be of use having specific and easy-to-use recommendations to improve the diagnosis and follow-up even for clinicians without specific experience in ARD-ILD or when an MDT is not available. This would help reduce diagnostic timing, which is of outmost importance, since a prompt recognition of the pathology would result in better outcomes.

Aims of this work were (1) to measure consensus between pulmonologists, radiologists, and rheumatologists experienced in the management of ARD-ILD; (2) to highlight the importance and raise sensibility on the necessity of a multidisciplinary approach; and (3) to provide clinicians with a practical tool aimed at improving the prompt recognition and follow-up of ILD associated with autoimmune rheumatic diseases (ARDs) and of any possible rheumatic conditions underlying ILD.

METHODS

The project structure is shown in the flowchart (**Figure 1**).

Briefly, a Steering Committee reviewed the available literature and identified six key questions, which were used to generate some statements through the Nominal Group Technique (NGT) (16). The statements were used for a round of an adapted Delphi survey for an expert panel. Answers were used to draft a first checklist and as inputs to design a second, more specific questionnaire. Eventually, results from the second questionnaire were integrated with the result of the Delphi survey by the Steering Committee to define the check lists of red flags and the timing of ILD screening and monitoring.

Steering Committee and Delphi Expert Panel

The members of both the Steering Committee and Delphi Panel are experts on ARD-associated ILDs.

The Steering Committee included different healthcare professionals, namely three pneumologists (SH, AP, FV), three rheumatologists (SB, NDP, MS), one immunologist (LB), and two radiologists (SP, GR). The Steering Committee sought the assistance of a non-clinical chair from an independent scientific consultancy agency (Polistudium srl, Milan, Italy) in order to provide meeting facilitation, material preparation and scientific accuracy. The Steering Committee designed and developed the project, identified the expert panel, generated the statements, reviewed and discussed survey results, and drafted the checklists.

The expert panel comprised members of different therapeutic areas in order to achieve a multidisciplinary overview. Inclusion criteria were clinical experience in ARD associated-ILDs and proven activity in MDTs. Candidate experts were proposed, shared, and approved within the Steering Committee.

Literature Review and Key Questions

The Steering Committee with the help of the non-clinical chair reviewed the most recent literature on the topic and drafted six key questions to be used to generate statements through a NGT round. Domains of the questions comprised (1) risk factors; (2) pulmonary signs and symptoms; (3) rheumatological signs and symptoms; (4) monitoring timing and frequency of pulmonary symptoms in ARD and ARD-ILD patients; (5) rheumatologists' and pulmonologists' sensitivity and attention to the suspicion of ILD; and (6) how to implement multidisciplinary management.

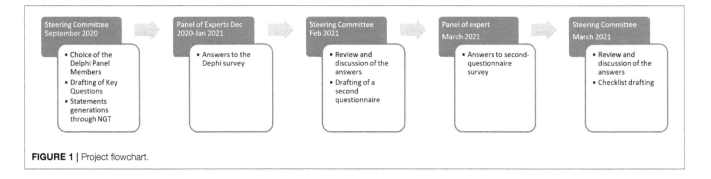

FIGURE 1 | Project flowchart.

Statement Definition

The NGT is a direct and structured technique, based on experts' opinion, aimed at managing meetings organized to make decisions on a specific topic on which there is no strong evidence (16). The NGT was used to generate the statements for the Delphi Panel. At first, the six key questions were asked to the members of the steering committee, who then had the opportunity to independently develop their own thoughts and opinions during the "silent generation" process. Their opinions were presented during an online meeting in September 2020, chaired by a Professional Facilitator. All the opinions (items) were collected and shared with the participants; with the help of the facilitator, items were re-elaborated and similar ones were merged according to a statistical clustering and participants' opinion to draft preliminary statements. Before reaching a final formulation, participants had the opportunity to review and/or comment all items. The so-drafted 57 statements were ranked through an online survey (due to COVID-19 pandemic) in terms of priority and relevance using a 1–5 scale during a second, remotely performed meeting. All 57 statements were considered relevant and kept, eventually drafting the complete list of items.

Adapted Delphi Process

The Delphi Method is a standard method of consensus, used to evaluate in an interactive and anonymous way, through online surveys, the level of agreement (consensus quantification) using a Likert scale (1–5; 1 = total disagreement; 5 = total agreement) and to resolve differences of opinion (consensus development). It takes place through several phases or rounds of expression and evaluation of opinions of a group of appropriately selected experts (17). Consensus on agreement is reached when at least 75% of voters express a vote equal to 4 or 5, according to the indications of the Ministry of Health (18).

Between December 2020 and January 2021, panelists participated to the Delphi online survey and indicated their level of agreement with the statements generated through the NGT.

Second Questionnaire

A qualitative second online survey aimed at outlining, more precisely, what the red flags are and the timing of ILD screening and monitoring was drafted by the Steering Committee after the first Delphi round. The members of the Delphi Panel participated in the online survey.

Statistical Analysis

All data were analyzed with descriptive statistics.

RESULTS

NGT and Delphi Survey

During the NGT round, the Steering Committee answered six key questions and defined 57 statements to be used in the Delphi survey. The key questions statements are reported in **Tables 1, 2**.

In total, 85 experts from different therapeutic areas were invited to join the Delphi Panel (**Supplementary Appendix A**); all the members were based in Italy.

A total of 78 total experts participated in the Delphi survey, composed of 28 pulmonologists, 33 rheumatologists, and 17 radiologists. During this round, consensus on agreement was reached in 47 statements, as shown in **Table 1**. Consensus on disagreement was not reached in any statements. Statements in which consensus was not reached ($n = 10$) are shown in **Table 2**. Due to the practical aim of this paper (i.e., the creation of a checklist regarding useful red flags to suspect ILD in ARD patients and vice versa and regarding screening and monitoring of ILD in ARD patients) this process was adapted by doing a single round; the first-round responses were analyzed by the Steering Committee, who reviewed statements in which consensus had not been reached, discussed the reasons, and provided inputs for the creation of the second, more-in-depth questionnaire.

Second Questionnaire

This first round led to some reflections and conclusions from the committee: (1) there were clear difficulties for reaching consensus in some cases (cf. statement 1.5); differences in views holds despite all members being expert on the topic and part of MDTs—but this is where, in our opinion, value of multidisciplinary resides; (2) some answers from the Delphi survey were conflicting and weren't suitable with our need to give clear indications on patient management; (3) some statements were less relevant for the aim of the paper and were decided not to be investigated with a second round, while others were vague and interpretable. A further reason resides on the practical aim of this paper, which lead us in asking more specific questions to give clearer indications based on opinions of the large number of experts of the Delphi Panel. A detailed questionnaire, with a different structure than the

TABLE 1 | Statements that reached overall consensus.

Statements that reached consensus	Level of agreement (%)			
	Total	**Pn**	**Rh**	**Ra**
Q1: What are the main risk factors for the development of ILD in ARDs?				
1.1—ARDs, in particular, systemic sclerosis, rheumatoid arthritis, and anti-synthetase syndrome, have to be considered important risk factors for the development of ILD.	98	100	94	100
1.2—In the presence of ARDs, the presence of some autoantibodies (anti-JO1, anti-PL 7, anti-PL12, anti-SSA Ro, anti-MDA 5, anti-Scl70, anti-PM/Scl, anti-Th/To) increase the risk of developing ILD.	94	90	97	94
1.3—Some gene variants are associated with a greater risk of developing ILD, particularly for some forms, such as usual interstitial pneumonia.	78	87	**67**	84
1.4—In the case of a patient suffering from systemic sclerosis, there are specific risk factors for the development of ILD, such as male gender, a diffuse form of the disease, and the presence of anti-Scl70 antibodies.	87	81	97	78
1.6—In patients with rheumatoid arthritis, the risk of developing ILD increases in males, smoking patients, with an older age of onset, in proportion to the duration of disease, and the titer of anti-citrulline antibodies.	83	84	88	**72**
Q2: What are the pulmonary signs, symptoms, and investigations that rheumatologists need to evaluate in generating a suspicion of ILD in patients with ARD?				
2.1—A careful anamnesis about the presence of respiratory symptoms is essential in the ARD work-up to evaluate any symptoms of ILD.	91	97	85	94
2.2—A careful thoracic physical examination is essential in the work up of systemic autoimmune diseases to assess the presence of ILD.	87	97	76	94
2.3—The presence of dry cough and exertional dyspnea, not justified by an infectious respiratory or cardiological pathology in progress, can generate the suspicion of ILD in a patient with ARD.	97	100	94	100
2.4—The presence of a feeling of fatigue or chest tightness or digital hippocratism or chest pain can raise the suspicion of ILD in a patient with ARD.	84	86	82	83
2.5—Presence of basal velcro crackles on chest auscultation may raise the suspicion of ILD in a patient with ARD.	92	100	88	89
2.6—Chest x-ray is a poorly specific and insensitive tool to check for the presence of ILD in a patient with ARD.	86	76	97	83
2.7—Spirometry coupled with the CO diffusion test is an investigation to be performed to monitor the course of ILD in a patient with ARD.	97	97	97	100
2.8—The high-resolution CT scan of the chest is the most sensitive and specific radiological method to validate the presence of ILD in a patient with ARD.	100	100	100	100
2.9—If ILD is suspected, a volumetric rather than axial CT scan should be performed, with multiplanar reconstructions and eventual scans in prone decubitus.	89	90	82	100
2.10—Blood–gas analysis allows to evaluate the degree of impairment of gas exchange at rest during ILD in a patient with ARD.	80	79	79	83
2.11—6MWT (Six-Minute Walking Test) allows to evaluate the functional consequences of cardio-pulmonary damage during ILD in a patient with ARD.	80	90	**67**	89
2.12—In case of systemic sclerosis and anti-synthetase syndrome, high-resolution CT of the chest is already recommended at diagnosis.	85	83	88	83
2.13—Within the framing work-up of a diffuse type of systemic sclerosis in early phase or in the presence of predisposing antibodies, high-resolution chest CT scan must always be considered.	92	93	100	78
Q3: What are the rheumatological signs and symptoms that pulmonologists need to evaluate in generating a suspicion of ARD in patients with ILD?				
3.1—Presence of Raynaud's phenomenon, digital edema, skin sclerosis, digital ulcers, telangiectasias, alone or in combination, can generate the suspicion of ARD in a patient with ILD.	91	90	94	88
3.2—Presence of skin manifestations (lower limbs purpura, Gottron's papules, vasculitis, photosensitivity, palmar erythema) can lead to suspicion of ARD in a patient with ILD.	87	83	91	88
3.3—Presence of skin cracks on fingers ("mechanic's hands") can lead to suspicion of ARD in a patient with ILD.	91	86	94	94
3.4—Presence of Sicca syndrome can raise suspicion of ARD in an ILD patient.	76	86	**73**	94
3.5—The presence of arthralgia and morning stiffness can generate suspicion of ARD in a patient with ILD.	77	80	76	77
3.7—Positivity to antinuclear antibodies of a significant titer or ≥1/320 may raise suspicion of ARD in a patient with ILD.	85	79	85	94
3.12—In patients with ILD, capillaroscopy should be required at least for patients with Raynaud's phenomenon and for those with specific autoantibodies for systemic sclerosis, mixed connective tissue disease and myositis (anticentromere, anti-Scl70, anti-RNP, specific anti-myositis, anti-synthetase)	100	100	100	100
Q4: What should be the monitoring timing and frequency of pulmonary symptoms in the patient with ARD?				
4.1—Pulmonary symptoms in the ARD patient should be assessed at each visit.	92	93	93	100
4.3—Timing and frequency of pulmonary symptoms monitoring in the ARD patient depend on the specific rheumatic disease.	78	76	82	77

TABLE 1 | Continued

Statements that reached consensus	Level of agreement (%)			
	Total	Pn	Rh	Ra
4.4—In the event of worsening respiratory symptoms in a patient with ARD, a high-resolution chest CT scan should be performed.	87	100	76	88
4.5—Respiratory function tests and carbon monoxide alveolar–capillary diffusion test (DLCO) should be performed every 12 months in patients with ARD, in case of systemic sclerosis every 6–12 months.	86	90	82	88
4.6—Pulmonary symptoms of patients with systemic sclerosis should be monitored every 6 months in case of progressive rheumatic disease.	81	90	**72**	88
4.7—Respiratory function tests and carbon monoxide alveolar–capillary diffusion test (DICO) should be performed every 12 months in the presence of clinical (systemic sclerosis) or laboratory (predisposing autoantibodies) risk factors in the absence of proven ILD.	90	93	88	88
Q4.1: What should be the monitoring timing and frequency of pulmonary symptoms in the patient with ARD–ILD?				
4.1.1—In case of patients with ARD and ILD, it is necessary, depending on the severity, to evaluate pulmonary symptoms every 3–6 months, carry out spirometry tests every 3–6 months, carry out carbon monoxide alveolar–capillary diffusion tests (DLCO), perform Six-Minute Walking Test (6MWT), and perform echocardiogram every 6–12 months.	85	90	90	**71**
4.1.2—Possible appearance or progression of ILD must be evaluated, in relation to the disease, by high-resolution CT scan of the chest as symptoms vary, in the presence of velcro crackles or worsening of functional tests.	98	97	97	100
Q5: What could be the approaches to increase rheumatologists' and pulmonologists' sensitivity and attention to the suspicion of ILD, in the Italian setting?				
5.1—The creation of a network between different centers of reference, which also favors the organization of national collaborative studies between pulmonologists, radiologists, and rheumatologists, can help to increase rheumatologists' and pulmonologists' sensitivity and attention to suspicion of ILD, in the Italian setting.	96	93	97	100
5.2—Webinar organization, seminars with MDT, and monothematic courses at regional and national level can be useful in increasing rheumatologists' and pulmonologists' sensitivity and attention to the suspicion of ILD, in the Italian setting.	87	90	79	100
5.3—Opportunity increase for meeting and updating with experts, through regional periodic scientific tables with simulation of MDT on paradigmatic cases or participation in multidisciplinary clinics, can be useful to increase rheumatologists' and pulmonologists' sensitivity and attention to the suspicion of ILD, in the Italian setting.	96	93	97	100
5.4—Sharing literature (e.g., creation of a six-monthly scientific bulletin to be distributed to level 1 centers) can be useful in increasing rheumatologists' and pulmonologists' sensitivity and attention to the suspicion of ILD, in the Italian setting.	77	79	**70**	88
5.5—The creation of an informatic platform, where level 1 centers can ask more specialized centers' opinion, can serve to increase rheumatologists' and pulmonologists' sensitivity and attention to the suspicion of ILD, in the Italian setting.	82	90	**73**	88
Q6: What can be ways to implement multidisciplinary management of ARD patients with suspicion of ILD?				
6.1—Creation of shared clinics between rheumatologists and pulmonologists can facilitate multidisciplinary management of rheumatology patients with suspicion of ILD.	95	93	100	82
6.2—Organization of joint training courses between rheumatologists, pulmonologists, radiologists can be useful for implementing multidisciplinary management of rheumatological patients with suspicion of ILD.	97	96	97	100
6.3—Creation of a preferential path of access to rheumatologists and pulmonologists for patients with suspected ILD, secondary to ARD, can favor multidisciplinary management of rheumatological patients with suspicion of ILD.	94	89	94	100
6.4—Sharing of diagnostic classification criteria of both ARD and ILD among the rheumatological and pneumological community, e.g., with the formulation of statements by scientific societies or the organization of regular meetings for the discussion of cases, would favor a multidisciplinary management of rheumatologic patients with suspicion of ILD.	95	100	88	100
6.5—In the case of patients with lung disease not classified with certainty by the pulmonologist, a rheumatological evaluation should also be performed.	82	75	82	94

Pn, pneumologists; Rh, rheumatologists; Ra, radiologists. Values in bold highlight an unmet consensus within a specialty.

Delphi, was thus drafted. This included four sections. In section A, which was addressed only to rheumatologists, the signs and symptoms they would report as red flags to pulmonologists to help suspect ILD in patients with ARD were ranked. Section B had the same structure but was only addressed to pulmonologists and which red flags they would report to the rheumatologist. Section C included questions regarding the tests—and their timing—to be performed on ARD patients without a diagnosis of ILD both in the presence and absence of risk factors for developing ILD. Section D questions were the same as section C but focused on ARD patients with a diagnosis of ILD and on risk factors for ILD progression rather than ILD developing. Questions in section C and D also asked to make the considered risk factors explicit, and to express any adjunctive comments; moreover, they did not only refer to a generic ARD patient, but specifically addressed the following rheumatic diseases: SSc, antisynthetase syndrome, Sjögren's syndrome, RA, and undifferentiated CTD.

TABLE 2 | Statements without overall consensus.

Statements that reached consensus	Level of agreement (%)			
	Total	Pn	Rh	Ra
Q1: What are the main risk factors for the development of ILD in ARDs?				
1.5—The severity of skin involvement in case of systemic sclerosis correlates with an increased risk of ILD.	51	26	**79**	44
1.7—The risk of developing ILD tends to increase with the age of onset of ARD, such as in the case of rheumatoid arthritis.	73	65	**79**	**78**
Q3: What are the rheumatological signs and symptoms that pulmonologists need to evaluate in generating a suspicion of ARD in patients with ILD?				
3.6—Presence of joint deformations can raise the suspicion of ARD in a patient with ILD.	71	**76**	61	**82**
3.8—Presence of alteration in phlogosis indexes can generate suspicion of ARD in a patient with ILD.	35	31	30	53
3.9—Morning functional impotence can raise suspicion of ARD in a patient with ILD.	53	55	49	59
3.10—Presence of subcutaneous nodules may raise suspicion of ARD in a patient with ILD.	66	62	58	**88**
3.11—Presence of a feeling of hyposthenia can generate suspicion of ARD in an ILD patient.	44	41	46	47
Q4: What should be the monitoring timing and frequency of pulmonary symptoms in the patient with ARD?				
4.2—Pulmonary symptoms in ARD patients should be monitored every 12 months for stable rheumatic disease or low-risk patients.	70	66	67	**82**
4.8—In the case of high-risk patients (i.e., diffuse systemic sclerosis with the presence of anti-scl70 antibodies) pulmonary symptoms should be evaluated every 3 months while high-resolution chest CT should be performed every 12 months.	72	**76**	67	**77**
Q6: What can be ways to implement multidisciplinary management of ARD patients with suspicion of ILD?				
6.6—Creation of "smart" digital platforms for each MDT group can facilitate multidisciplinary management of rheumatology patients with suspicion of ILD.	72	68	64	**94**

Pn, pneumologists; Rh, rheumatologists; Ra, radiologists; Values in bold highlight a reached consensus within a specialty.

TABLE 3 | Check list of red flags sign or symptom suggestive of ILD.

Presence of basal velcro crackles on chest auscultation.

Dry cough and exertional dyspnea, not justified by an infectious respiratory or cardiological pathology in progress.

TABLE 4 | Check list of red flags sign or symptom suggestive of ARD.

Skin manifestations (cutaneous sclerosis, purpura of the lower limbs, Gottron's papules, cutaneous vasculitis, photosensitivity, palmar erythema, "mechanic's hands").

Raynaud's phenomenon.

Digital ulcers and telangiectasias, alone or in combination.

Positivity to anti-nuclear antibodies with significant titer ($\geq 1/160$).

Presence of muscle weakness associated with an increase in CPK.

Arthralgia, joint swelling or swelling of the hands, morning stiffness.

Dry eyes and dry mouth.

A total of 76 clinicians (31 pulmonologists, 30 rheumatologists, and 15 radiologists) took part in the second survey. All the questions are available as **Supplementary Material (Supplementary Tables)**.

Red Flags of ILD in Patients With ARD

Rheumatologists should pose particular attention to signs and symptoms shown in **Table 3** since they are useful red flags to suspect an underlying ILD in patients with ARD. If any of these is present, a high-resolution computed tomography (HRCT) should be prescribed.

Red Flags of ARD in Patients With ILD

Pulmonologists should pose particular attention to signs and symptoms shown in **Table 4** since they are useful red flags to suspect an underlying ARD in patients with ILD. If any of these is present, patients should be referred to a rheumatologist.

Screening and Monitoring of ILD in Patients With ARD

Following indications given from the expert panel through the Delphi survey and the second questionnaire, pulmonary symptoms in the ARD patient should be assessed at each visit (item 4.1, **Table 1**). Considering that the ARD-intrinsic risk of onset and developing of ILDs changes according to specific ARDs (items 1, **Table 1**) (19), the timing and type of screening and monitoring must be evaluated according to the specific pathology, and the overall clinical condition of the patient.

ILD in Patients With RA

Clinically evident ILD is usually reported in 7–10% of patients with RA (20, 21), and lifetime risk of RA-ILD of 7.7% has been reported in a population-based cohort study conducted in the USA (22). However, prevalence largely varied according to the different studies and it is significantly higher when consecutive patients are evaluated by HRCT, recording abnormalities compatible with ILD in up to one-third of cases (23–25).

Although the few available data, generally based on retrospective studies, male sex, older age at RA onset, and ever-smokers are associated with RA-ILD in majority of studies (26, 27), mainly for patients with a usual interstitial pneumonia pattern.

TABLE 5 | Identification and monitoring of RA-ILD.

	Respiratory signs and symptoms*	Spirometry and DLCO	HRCT
Baseline/diagnosis time	Check	In presence of respiratory signs or symptoms*	In presence of respiratory signs or symptoms*
Follow-up in patients without a known ILD	Check at every examination*	In presence of respiratory signs or symptoms* or when a pulmonary arterial hypertension is suspected[a,b]	In presence of respiratory signs or symptoms* and/or in presence of significant deficit of functional tests[§]
Follow-up in patients with a known ILD	Check at every examination NB: Worsening of symptoms are suggestive of ILD progression or complications[o]	Every 3–6 months according to clinical status	Every 12 months according to clinical status[c]

[a] Do not delay spirometry if DLCO is not available in a short time.
[b] Discrepancy between FVC and DLCO deficiency may suggest the presence of pulmonary hypertension.
[c] HRCT should be performed (1) in case of a worsening of clinical symptoms or lung function tests or (2) in stable patients to exclude lung cancer and to monitor lung disease.
*Presence of basal Velcro crackles, dry cough, and exertional dyspnea, not justified by a respiratory infection or cardiological pathology in progress.
[§] FVC and/or TLC and/or DLCO deficit ≥20%.
[o] Infection, cancer, heart failure, drug toxicity.

TABLE 6 | Identification and monitoring of SSc-ILD.

	Signs and symptoms*	Spirometry and DLCO	HRCT
Baseline/diagnosis time	Check	Yes	Yes
Follow-up in patients without a known ILD	Check at every examination	Every 6–12 months or in case of onset of respiratory signs or symptoms^	Every 24 months Every 12 months in presence of risk factors[a]
Follow-up in patients with a known ILD	Check at every examination NB: Worsening of symptoms are suggestive of ILD progression or complications[o]	Every 6–12 months, or every 3–6 months, if risk factors[a] are present	To be performed every 12 months according to clinical status In case of rapid deterioration, re-evaluate the timing

[a] Risk factors should be assessed at every examination. Risk factors include male gender, diffuse skin disease, and presence of anti-Scl70 antibodies.
*Presence of basal velcro crackles, dry cough and exertional dyspnea, not justified by a respiratory infection or cardiological pathology in progress.
[o] Infection, cancer, heart failure, drug toxicity.
^Do not delay spirometry if DLCO is not available in a short time.

Despite contrasting results, anti-citrullinated peptide antibodies (ACPA) have been also associated to ILD. In particular, Correia reported a correlation between ACPA titer and the risk to develop ILD (28). Finally, Doyle reported that a combination of older age, male sex, ever-smoking, RF, and ACPA was strongly associated with RA-ILD (29).

The Steering committee analyzed the answers from both the Delphi and the second survey, discussed such answers, compared them with available literature, integrated them with its opinion, and drafted a practical checklist for screening and monitoring of ILD in patients with RA, as shown in **Table 5**.

ILD in Patients With SSc

Interstitial lung disease is a common manifestation of SSc, with approximately one-third of patients developing progressive ILD (30). Fibrotic non-specific interstitial pneumonia is the most common feature of parenchymal lung disease in patients with SSc-associated ILD, followed by usual interstitial pneumonia. Both the forms appear to have a similar survival in patients with SSc (31, 32). Despite significant improvement in the overall 10-year survival in SSc patients in the last few years, ILD represents a significant cause of morbidity and mortality. Risk factors for the development or progression of ILD among patients with SSc include diffuse cutaneous SSc, male sex, African–American race, older age at disease onset, shorter disease duration, and the presence of anti-Scl-70/anti-topoisomerase I antibody (33–36). However, none of these risk factors is absolute. Clinicians

should remember that ILD may develop even in patients with limited cutaneous SSc. In addition, SSc-ILD has a variable and not predictable clinical course. Most patients experience a slow decline in lung function, but others have a rapid progression just after disease onset (37). Different studies showed that the most important predictors of mortality in patients with SSc-ILD are the short-term changes in pulmonary functional parameters (38, 39) and extent of lung fibrosis on HRTC. Despite physicians knowing the established relationship between SSc-ILD and mortality and morbidity well, the lack of a consensus on ILD screening, and monitoring of disease progression raise important implications for a better therapeutic management of SSc-ILD patients, mainly for new available treatment options.

The Steering committee analyzed the answers from both the Delphi and the second survey, discussed such answers, compared them with available literature, integrated them with its opinion, and drafted a practical checklist for screening and monitoring of ILD in patients with RA, as shown in **Table 6**.

ILD in Patients With Other ARD

The other ARD considered in our questions are systemic lupus erythematosus, Sjögren's syndrome, mixed CTD, polymyositis/dermatomyositis, undifferentiated CTD. The risk to develop an ILD varies between different diseases, but in some the mortality related to interstitial lung involvement is very high (i.e., in the antisynthetase syndrome, 28% developed progressive respiratory failure and died) (40). The high heterogeneity spectrum of these diseases either in the risk to develop an ILD either in clinical manifestations and in progression of lung involvement reduced the consensus of the statement that varies from 5 to 75% in the timing of performing CT scan and from 4.5 to 70% in timing to a perform function test.

Regarding identification and monitoring of ILD associated with these ARDs, the respiratory signs and symptoms to be valued are the same as the ones presented for RA and SSc. Diffusing capacity of the lungs for carbon monoxide (DLCO) should be performed annually, or every 3–6 months in case of an already diagnosed ILD. In patients without an ILD diagnosis, HRCT should be performed when clinically indicated from symptoms, or, in patients at high risk for the clinical characteristics of the disease, every 12–24 months. If ILD has been already diagnosed, HRCT should be carried out at least annually.

The Multidisciplinary Approach

All statements addressing how to increase sensitivity and attention to the suspicion of ILD in the Italian setting (Q5 and Q6, **Table 1**) reached consensus. Their approaches include the creation of a network between different centers of reference, webinar/seminar with MDT, monothematic courses, regional periodic scientific tables with simulation of MDT on paradigmatic cases or participation in multidisciplinary clinics, sharing literature, and the creation of an informatic platform, where level 1 centers can ask more specialized centers' opinion.

Statements referring to key question number 6 addressed how to implement multidisciplinary management of ARD patients with suspicion of ILD. Statements that reached consensus suggest the creation of shared clinics between rheumatologists and pulmonologists, the organization of joint training courses between rheumatologists, pulmonologists, and radiologists, the creation of a preferential path of access to rheumatologists and pulmonologists for patients with suspected ILD secondary to ARD, and sharing of diagnostic classification criteria of both ARD and ILD among the rheumatological and pneumological community. The only statement (6.6, **Table 2**) that did not reach consensus suggested the creation of "smart" digital platforms for each MDT group. However, consensus for this statement was reached among the radiologists, likely because of them being more prone in working in a digital setting given their every-day work always involves computers.

DISCUSSION

Interstitial lung disease is often associated with rheumatic diseases. Its early diagnosis and management are not only difficult, but also crucial, because it is associated with major morbidity and mortality and can be the first cause of death in ARDs (7–13). We, therefore, aimed to measure consensus between specialists who can be involved in its management: this is one of the very first studies to address consensus between pulmonologists, rheumatologists, and radiologists. Consensus was high, with 42 out of 50 statements that reached the 75% threshold agreement. No statements reached the disagreement threshold. With this work we also aimed at highlighting the importance of a multidisciplinary approach that includes rheumatologists, and at providing the drafted checklists (see **Tables 3–6**) as a practical tool useful in the prompt recognition and in follow-up of ARD-ILD.

The main strength of this study is the combinations of techniques, such as NGT and Delphi Survey, which allow clinicians firstly to share their own opinion rising from their personal experience, and secondly to work toward an integration of such opinions. This methodology highlights the multidisciplinary approach of this work. The importance of multidisciplinary approaches has been consolidated in the clinical practice, and it is of utmost important to keep such an approach for diagnosis, therapy and follow-up. The evaluation of ILD by an MDT has been proposed as the gold standard for its management (41) but, while up to 20% of ILD cases can be referred to rheumatic conditions, only ~37% of MDT cases worldwide include a rheumatologist (42); this may create a vicious circle, where rheumatologist referral is up to pulmonologist, who may underestimate clinical manifestation of an ARD. Therefore, if we also consider that ILD can be the leading cause of death for some ARD, and the exclusion of any systemic ARD in any freshly diagnosed ILD is mandatory according to current guidelines, we believe that rheumatologists' non-inclusion in MDTs is not justifiable; their view could potentially complete the evaluation of a pulmonologist, who may overlook important details (15). With regards to this study, when comparing factors taken into account by pneumologists and rheumatologists to decide on the monitoring of the exams, it shows such factors are more lung-related for pneumologists, and more disease-specific for rheumatologists. Clinicians should be aware of this "bias" since it could lead them in taking a wider perspective on the pathology in exam.

Despite the high reached consensus, when we take a more in-depth look to data from the surveys, and consider discussions of the meetings of the steering committee, some discrepancies arose in terms of attitude and management methods of the disease among Delphi panelists, the steering committee, and among clinicians of different expertise. For example, statement 1.5 "The severity of skin involvement in the case of SSc correlates with an increased risk of ILD" reached a level of agreement of 77.8% within rheumatologists, 44.4% between radiologists and 25.8% within pneumologists. While it may be that disagreement occurred because of actual lack of general knowledge or evidence, it could also be argued that agreement occurred for the same reasons. However, we believe this is not the case, since members of the expert panel were chosen for their clinical experience in ARD associated-ILDs and proven activity in MDTs. We think result heterogenicity from the Delphi survey can be explained in several different ways: the presence of specialists with different backgrounds and sensitivities, and with specific experience on different rheumatic diseases; the heterogeneity of rheumatic diseases themselves, which require approaches that cannot be generalized tout-court; a lack of international guidelines (except, partially, on idiopathic pulmonary fibrosis), which may have led panelists in sharing what they can do to the best of the means at their disposal in the everyday clinical setting; the need to reconcile the evaluation of pulmonary involvement with that of the other systemic manifestations of the disease; the difficulties of working in an MDT. Despite discrepancies arising from the variability of different points of view, we managed to integrate such diverse opinions through several meetings in which statements were discussed, compared to available literature, and our clinical view, and we went so far as to give our opinion based on our experience in MDTs. Notwithstanding differences between specialists, some statements reach a really strong consensus, with one of those being number 2.8 stating that "the high-resolution CT scan of the chest is the most sensitive and specific radiological method to validate the presence of ILD in a patient with ARD," and reaching a level of agreement of 100%. This is coherent with HRCT driving therapeutic choices, given the fact that is useful to identify subclinical outlines, and differentiate ILA from subclinical forms of ARD-ILD (19).

Training clinicians and improving their sensitivity and attention to the suspicion of ARD-ILD can be a valuable solution when working with an MDT is not possible; this happens quite often in the Italian scenario, where the triplet pulmonologist, rheumatologist, and radiologist is not always available, or present within the same structure. Q5 of the Delphi survey addressed how to implement such training; results therefore show which ways clinicians would feel effective if they had to be instructed. The two most-agreed ways are the creation of a network between different centers of reference, which also favors the organization of national collaborative studies between pulmonologists, radiologists, and rheumatologists, and an opportunity increase for meeting and updating with experts, through regional periodic scientific tables with simulation of MDT on paradigmatic cases or participation in multidisciplinary clinics. Other solutions include webinars/seminars with MDT and monothematic courses at regional and national level, the creation of an informatic platform, where level 1 centers can ask more specialized centers' opinion, and sharing literature through scientific bulletin to be distributed to level 1 centers. Improving untrained physicians' sensitivity is the first step toward implementation of ARD-ILD multidisciplinary management. Q6 of the Delphi survey addressed ways for such implementations; statement consensus was reached for four out of five statements. According to the Delphi panelists, the most effective way to implement multidisciplinary management is the organization of joint training courses between rheumatologists, pulmonologists, and radiologists, followed by the creation of shared clinics between rheumatologists and pulmonologists, the sharing of diagnostic classification criteria of both ARD and ILD among the rheumatological and pneumological community (e.g., the formulation of statements by scientific societies or the organization of regular meetings for the discussion of cases), and eventually the creation of a preferential path of access to rheumatologists and pulmonologists for patients with suspected ILD secondary to ARD. On top of this, it must be remembered that being part of an MDT is an ongoing process. Even once multidisciplinary management has been implemented, clinicians need time to adapt to it: levels of agreement between different specialists rise over time, improving diagnostic, and managing performance (15, 43).

The solutions proposed in the statements from Q5 and Q6 could be effective, but they require a lot of time to be carried on and applied. Moreover, not all clinical settings are suitable for having an MDT. Because of this, and to provide all specialties with tools that are shared and recommended by other specialists. We propose some checklists to help recognition and follow up of ARD-ILD; these checklists arise from the integration of results from the Delphi survey, the second questionnaire, and our experience of MDT. Given the irreversibility and high morbidity and mortality rates of ILD (1, 44) a prompt diagnosis is extremely important; the red-flag checklist of respiratory signs and symptoms suggestive of ILD in ARD patients (**Table 3**) can be a useful tool for rheumatologists for the recognition of ILD. On the other hand, the red-flag checklist of systemic signs and symptoms suggestive of ARD in ILD patients (**Table 4**) is addressed to pulmonologist to help them recognize a rheumatic condition underlying ILD. A fast recognition of the presence of an ARD underlying ILD, and vice versa, can help guide therapy and give better outcomes. **Tables 5, 6** go more in-depth tackling identification and monitoring of ILD in RA and SSc, respectively. They explicit symptoms to be addressed and examinations to be performed and give indication on the timing depending on whether the rheumatic disease has just been diagnosed, or patients are in the follow-up phase with a diagnosed or undiagnosed ILD already. We believe these short, easy-to-consult checklists can help untrained physicians better address these pathologies in the wait of more robust, international guidelines.

This study has four main limitations. Firstly, drafting items and statement can often lead to them being redundant or already addressed in literature Secondly, Delphi panelists could not comment on the relevance or importance of the drafted statements, as well as they could not give a position of "non-opinion." Thirdly, it is limited to the Italian scenario; this may have yielded results that are not in line with other countries' reality, especially when considering every-day clinical practice, which can differ because of different regulations and resources. Finally, albeit based on the experience of a high number of clinicians, it is a consensus work and could not produce empiric data.

CONCLUSIONS

This consensus work showed a high level of agreement, but also shows some divergent opinions between different experts. This underlines the importance of a multidisciplinary approach and of a constant update in overcoming these differences and in enhancing the diagnosis timing and management of patients with ILD-ARD. Given the high morbidity and mortality rates of ILD-ARD, its early recognition is crucial. The expert-shared red-flag checklist of respiratory signs and symptoms suggestive of ILD in ARD patients (**Table 3**) can be a useful tool for rheumatologists for the recognition of ILD, while the expert-shared red-flag checklist of systemic signs and symptoms suggestive of ARD in ILD patients can help the pulmonologist to recognize a rheumatic condition underlying ILD (**Table 4**). Since RA and SSc are two of the most common ARDs that can be associated with ILD, we drafted related checklists on identification and monitoring (**Tables 5, 6**), which can help tackle these conditions.

AUTHOR CONTRIBUTIONS

All authors contributed equally to the planning, implementation, and drafting of the study.

REFERENCES

1. Ferri C, Manfredi A, Sebastiani M, Colaci M, Giuggioli D, Vacchi C, et al. Interstitial pneumonia with autoimmune features and undifferentiated connective tissue disease: our interdisciplinary rheumatology-pneumology experience, and review of the literature. *Autoimmun Rev.* (2016) 15:61–70. doi: 10.1016/j.autrev.2015.09.003
2. Sambataro D, Sambataro G, Pignataro F, Zanframundo G, Codullo V, Fagone E, et al. Patients with interstitial lung disease secondary to autoimmune diseases: how to recognize them? *Diagnostics.* (2020) 10:208. doi: 10.3390/diagnostics10040208
3. Levi Y, Israeli-Shani L, Kuchuk M, Epstein Shochet G, Koslow M, Shitrit D. Rheumatological assessment is important for interstitial lung disease diagnosis. *J Rheumatol.* (2018) 45:1509–14. doi: 10.3899/jrheum.171314
4. Furini F, Carnevale A, Casoni GL, Guerrini G, Cavagna L, Govoni M, et al. The role of the multidisciplinary evaluation of interstitial lung diseases: systematic literature review of the current evidence and future perspectives. *Front Med.* (2019) 6:246. doi: 10.3389/fmed.2019.00246
5. Fischer A, Antoniou KM, Brown KK, Cadranel J, Corte TJ, du Bois RM, et al. An official European Respiratory Society/American Thoracic Society research statement: interstitial pneumonia with autoimmune features. *Eur Respir J.* (2015) 46:976–87. doi: 10.1183/13993003.00150-2015
6. Varone F, Sgalla G, Iovene B, Richeldi L. Progressive fibrosing interstitial lung disease. a proposed integrated algorithm for management. *Ann Am Thorac Soc.* (2020) 17:1199–203. doi: 10.1513/AnnalsATS.202003-214PS
7. Giacomelli R, Liakouli V, Berardicurti O, Ruscitti P, Di Benedetto P, Carubbi F, et al. Interstitial lung disease in systemic sclerosis: current and future treatment. *Rheumatol Int.* (2017) 37:853–63. doi: 10.1007/s00296-016-3636-7
8. Silver KC, Silver RM. Management of systemic-sclerosis-associated interstitial lung disease. *Rheum Dis Clin North Am.* (2015) 41:439–57. doi: 10.1016/j.rdc.2015.04.006
9. Strickland G, Pauling J, Cavill C, Shaddick G, McHugh N. Mortality in systemic sclerosis-a single centre study from the UK. *Clin Rheumatol.* (2013) 32:1533–9. doi: 10.1007/s10067-013-2289-0
10. Olson AL, Swigris JJ, Sprunger DB, Fischer A, Fernandez-Perez ER, Solomon J, et al. Rheumatoid arthritis-interstitial lung disease-associated mortality. *Am J Respir Crit Care Med.* (2011) 183:372–8. doi: 10.1164/rccm.201004-0622OC
11. Ascherman DP. Interstitial lung disease in rheumatoid arthritis. *Curr Rheumatol Rep.* (2010) 12:363–9. doi: 10.1183/16000617.0011-2021
12. Kim EJ, Elicker BM, Maldonado F, Webb WR Ryu JH, Uden JHV, et al. Usual interstitial pneumonia in rheumatoid arthritis-associated interstitial lung disease. *Eur Respir J.* (2010) 35:1322–8. doi: 10.1183/09031936.00092309
13. Hoffmann-Vold AM, Maher TM, Philpot EE, Ashrafzadeh A, Barake R, Barsotti S., et al. The identification and management of interstitial lung disease in systemic sclerosis: evidence-based European consensus statements. *Lancet Rheumatol.* (2020) 2:e71–83. doi: 10.1016/S2665-9913(19)30144-4
14. Sebastiani M, Faverio P, Manfredi A, Cassone G, Vacchi C, Stainer A, et al. Interstitial pneumonia with autoimmune features: why rheumatologist-pulmonologist collaboration is essential. *Biomedicines.* (2020) 9:17. doi: 10.3390/biomedicines9010017
15. De Lorenzis E, Bosello SL, Varone F, Sgalla G, Calandriello L, Natalello G, et al. Multidisciplinary evaluation of interstitial lung diseases: new opportunities linked to rheumatologist involvement. *Diagnostics (Basel).* (2020) 10:664. doi: 10.3390/diagnostics10090664
16. Jones J, Hunter D. Consensus methods for medical and health services research. *BMJ.* (1995) 311:376. doi: 10.1136/bmj.311.7001.376

ACKNOWLEDGMENTS

Fabio Perversi, Aashni Shah, Sara di Nunzio, and Valentina Mirisola (Polistudium srl, Milan, Italy) provided writing, scientific and statistical assistance, under the authors' conceptual direction and based on feedback from the authors; Polistudium srl was contracted and compensated by Boehringer Ingelheim Italia SpA. Delphi Panelists took part in the Delphi survey and second-questionnaire survey.

17. Milholland AV, Wheeler SG, Heieck JJ. Medical assessment by a delphi group opinion technic. *N Engl J Med.* (1973) 288:1272–5. doi: 10.1056/nejm197306142882405
18. Candiani G, Colombo C, Daghini, R, Magrini, N, Mosconi P, Nonino F,et al. *Come Organizzare Una Conferenza di Consenso. Manuale Metodologico Sistema Nazionale per le Linee Guida* (2019).
19. Fischer A, Distler J. Progressive fibrosing interstitial lung disease associated with systemic autoimmune diseases. *Clin Rheumatol.* (2019) 38:2673–81. doi: 10.1007/s10067-019-04720-0
20. Hyldgaard C, Hilberg O, Pedersen AB, Ulrichsen SP, Løkke A, Bendstrup E, et al. population-based cohort study of rheumatoid arthritis-associated interstitial lung disease: comorbidity and mortality. *Ann Rheum Dis.* (2017) 76:1700–6. doi: 10.1136/annrheumdis-2017-211138
21. Raimundo K, Solomon JJ, Olson AL, Kong AM, Cole AL, Fischer A, et al. Rheumatoid arthritis-interstitial lung disease in the united states: prevalence, incidence, and healthcare costs and mortality. *J Rheumatol.* (2019) 46:360–9. doi: 10.3899/jrheum.171315
22. Bongartz T, Nannini C, Medina-Velasquez YF, Achenbach SJ, Crowson CS Ryu JH, et al. Incidence and mortality of interstitial lung disease in rheumatoid arthritis: a population-based study. *Arthritis Rheum.* (2010) 62:1583–91. doi: 10.1002/art.27405
23. Gabbay E, Tarala R, Will R, Carroll G, Adler B, Cameron D, et al. Interstitial lung disease in recent onset rheumatoid arthritis. *Am J Respir Crit Care Med.* (1997) 156:528–35. doi: 10.1164/ajrccm.156.2.9609016
24. Dawson JK, Fewins HE, Desmond J, Lynch MP, Graham DR. Fibrosing alveolitis in patients with rheumatoid arthritis as assessed by high resolution computed tomography, chest radiography, and pulmonary function tests. *Thorax.* (2001) 56:622–7. doi: 10.1136/thorax.56.8.622
25. Gochuico BR, Avila NA, Chow CK, Novero LJ, Wu HP, Ren P, et al. Progressive preclinical interstitial lung disease in rheumatoid arthritis. *Arch Intern Med.* (2008) 168:159–66. doi: 10.1001/archinternmed.2007.59
26. Kelly CA, Saravanan V, Nisar M, Arthanari S, Woodhead FA, Price-Forbes AN, et al. Rheumatoid arthritis-related interstitial lung disease: associations, prognostic factors and physiological and radiological characteristics–a large multicentre UK study. *Rheumatology (Oxford).* (2014) 53:1676–82. doi: 10.1093/rheumatology/keu165
27. Zhang Y, Li H, Wu N, Dong X, Zheng Y. Retrospective study of the clinical characteristics and risk factors of rheumatoid arthritis-associated interstitial lung disease. *Clin Rheumatol.* (2017) 36:817–23. doi: 10.1007/s10067-017-3561-5
28. Correia CS, Briones MR, Guo R, Ostrowski RA. Elevated anti-cyclic citrullinated peptide antibody titer is associated with increased risk for interstitial lung disease. *Clin Rheumatol.* (2019) 38:1201–6. doi: 10.1007/s10067-018-04421-0
29. Doyle TJ, Patel AS, Hatabu H, Nishino M, Wu G, Osorio JC, et al. Detection of rheumatoid arthritis-interstitial lung disease is enhanced by serum biomarkers. *Am J Respir Crit Care Med.* (2015) 191:1403–12. doi: 10.1164/rccm.201411-1950OC
30. Denton CP, Khanna D. Systemic sclerosis. *Lancet.* (2017) 390:1685–99. doi: 10.1016/S0140-6736(17)30933-9
31. Bouros D, Wells AU, Nicholson AG, Colby TV, Polychronopoulos V, Pantelidis P, et al. Histopathologic subsets of fibrosing alveolitis in patients with systemic sclerosis and their relationship to outcome. *Am J Respir Crit Care Med.* (2002) 165:1581–6. doi: 10.1164/rccm.2106012
32. Park JH, Kim DS, Park IN, Jang SJ, Kitaichi M, Nicholson AG, et al.

Prognosis of fibrotic interstitial pneumonia: idiopathic versus collagen vascular disease-related subtypes. *Am J Respir Crit Care Med.* (2007) 175:705–11. doi: 10.1164/rccm.200607-912OC

33. Ashmore P, Tikly M, Wong M, Ickinger C. Interstitial lung disease in South Africans with systemic sclerosis. *Rheumatol Int.* (2018) 38:657–62. doi: 10.1007/s00296-017-3893-0

34. Steen V. Predictors of end stage lung disease in systemic sclerosis. *Ann Rheum Dis.* (2003) 62:97–9. doi: 10.1136/ard.62.2.97

35. Wangkaew S, Euathrongchit J, Wattanawittawas P, Kasitanon N, Louthrenoo W. Incidence and predictors of interstitial lung disease (ILD) in Thai patients with early systemic sclerosis: inception cohort study. *Mod Rheumatol.* (2016) 26:588–93. doi: 10.3109/14397595.2015.1115455

36. Distler O, Assassi S, Cottin V, Cutolo M, Danoff SK, Denton CP, et al. Predictors of progression in systemic sclerosis patients with interstitial lung disease. *Eur Respir J.* (2020) 55:1902026. doi: 10.1183/13993003.02026-2019

37. Cottin V, Brown KK. Interstitial lung disease associated with systemic sclerosis (SSc-ILD). *Respir Res.* (2019) 20:13. doi: 10.1186/s12931-019-0980-7

38. Volkmann ER, Tashkin DP, Sim M, Li N, Goldmuntz E, Keyes-Elstein L, et al. Short-term progression of interstitial lung disease in systemic sclerosis predicts long-term survival in two independent clinical trial cohorts. *Ann Rheum Dis.* (2019) 78:122–30. doi: 10.1136/annrheumdis-2018-213708

39. Goh NS, Hoyles RK, Denton CP, Hansell DM, Renzoni EA, Maher TM, et al. Short-term pulmonary function trends are predictive of mortality in interstitial lung disease associated with systemic sclerosis. *Arthritis Rheumatol.* (2017) 69:1670–8. doi: 10.1002/art.40130

40. Solomon J, Swigris JJ, Brown KK. Myositis-related interstitial lung disease and antisynthetase syndrome. *J Bras Pneumol.* (2011) 37:100–9. doi: 10.1590/s1806-37132011000100015

41. Raghu G, Remy-Jardin M, Myers JL, Richeldi L, Ryerson CJ, Lederer DJ, et al. Diagnosis of idiopathic pulmonary fibrosis. An official ATS/ERS/JRS/ALAT clinical practice guideline. *Am J Respir Crit Care Med.* (2018) 198:e44–68. doi: 10.1164/rccm.201807-1255ST

42. Richeldi L, Launders N, Martinez F, Walsh SLF, Myers J, Wang B, et al. The characterisation of interstitial lung disease multidisciplinary team meetings: a global study. *ERJ Open Res.* (2019) 5:00209-2018. doi: 10.1183/23120541.00209-2018

43. Han Q, Wang HY, Zhang XX, Wu LL, Wang LL, Jiang Y, et al. The role of follow-up evaluation in the diagnostic algorithm of idiopathic interstitial pneumonia: a retrospective study. *Sci Rep.* (2019) 9:6452. doi: 10.1038/s41598-019-42813-7

44. Raghu G, Collard HR, Egan JJ, Martinez FJ, Behr J, Brown KK, et al. An official ATS/ERS/JRS/ALAT statement: idiopathic pulmonary fibrosis: evidence-based guidelines for diagnosis and management. *Am J Respir Crit Care Med.* (2011) 183:788–824. doi: 10.1164/rccm.2009-040GL

16

Multidisciplinary Approach in the Early Detection of Undiagnosed Connective Tissue Diseases in Patients With Interstitial Lung Disease

Claudio Tirelli[1†], Valentina Morandi[2†], Adele Valentini[3], Claudia La Carrubba[1], Roberto Dore[4], Giovanni Zanframundo[2], Patrizia Morbini[5], Silvia Grignaschi[2], Andrea Franconeri[3], Tiberio Oggionni[1], Emiliano Marasco[2], Ludovico De Stefano[2], Zamir Kadija[1], Francesca Mariani[1], Veronica Codullo[6], Claudia Alpini[7], Carlo Scirè[8], Carlomaurizio Montecucco[2], Federica Meloni[1] and Lorenzo Cavagna[2*]

[1] Division of Pneumology, University and IRCCS Policlinico S. Matteo Foundation, Pavia, Italy, [2] Division of Rheumatology, University and IRCCS Policlinico S. Matteo Foundation, Pavia, Italy, [3] Institute of Radiology, University and IRCCS Policlinico S. Matteo Foundation, Pavia, Italy, [4] Radiology Unit, Isituti Clinici Città di Pavia, Pavia, Italy, [5] Pathology Unit, University and IRCCS Policlinico S. Matteo Foundation, Pavia, Italy, [6] Rheumatology Department, Hopital Cochin, Paris, France, [7] Laboratory of Biochemical-Clinical Analyses, IRCCS Policlinico San Matteo Foundation, Pavia, Italy, [8] Division of Rheumatology, Arcispedale Sant'Anna, Ferrara, Italy

*Correspondence:
Lorenzo Cavagna
lorenzo.cavagna@unipv.it

These authors have contributed equally to this work

Interstitial lung disease (ILD) encompasses a wide range of parenchymal lung pathologies with different clinical, histological, radiological, and serological features. Follow-up, treatment, and prognosis are strongly influenced by the underlying pathogenesis. Considering that an ILD may complicate the course of any connective tissue disease (CTD) and that CTD's signs are not always easily identifiable, it could be useful to screen every ILD patient for a possible CTD. The recent definition of interstitial pneumonia with autoimmune features is a further confirmation of the close relationship between CTD and ILD. In this context, the multidisciplinary approach is assuming a growing and accepted role in the correct diagnosis and follow-up, to as early as possible define the best therapeutic strategy. However, despite clinical advantages, until now, the pathways of the multidisciplinary approach in ILD patients are largely heterogeneous across different centers and the best strategy to apply is still to be established and validated. Aims of this article are to describe the organization of our multidisciplinary group for ILD, which is mainly focused on the early identification and management of CTD in patients with ILD and to show our results in a 1 year period of observation. We found that 15% of patients referred for ILD had an underlying CTD, 33% had interstitial pneumonia with autoimmune feature, and 52% had ILD without detectable CTD. Furthermore, we demonstrated that the adoption of a standardized strategy consisting of a screening questionnaire, specific laboratory tests, and nailfold videocapillaroscopy in all incident ILD proved useful in making the right diagnosis.

Keywords: interstitial lung disease, connective tissue diseases, multidisciplinary team, early diagnosis, rheumatology, pulmonology, radiology

INTRODUCTION

Interstitial lung disease (ILD) includes a heterogeneous group of parenchymal lung pathologies with different clinical, histological, radiological, and serological features (1). To correctly classify ILD is crucial, since follow-up, treatment, and prognosis are strongly dependent on ILD subtype (2, 3). Considering that ILD may complicate the course of any connective tissue disease (CTD) and that signs of CTD are frequently not easy to identify (4–7), an underlying CTD should be ruled out in every ILD, even when the suspect is low or even absent. The recent definition of interstitial pneumonia with autoimmune features (IPAF) is a further confirmation of the close relationship between CTDs and ILD and of how the borders between the rheumatology and pulmonology practices are day by day less defined (8). In a similar context, the multidisciplinary approach is assuming a growing and accepted role, as the discussion of such cases may help to identify the sometime subtle signs or symptoms of CTD in ILD (9–14). However, despite the clinical advantages, the pathways of the multidisciplinary approach in ILD are largely heterogeneous across different centers and countries, and the best strategy to apply is still to be established and validated, as well as the composition of the multidisciplinary team (i.e., the rheumatologist is not included in many of the described multidisciplinary teams) (15). Furthermore, until now, no screening tools for the early identification of CTD signs and symptoms have been applied in ILD, although previous reports in other settings showed their potential usefulness (16). The inclusion of the rheumatology assessment is an added value for patients (9, 17, 18), and the possibility to start the multidisciplinary pathway from a screening tool seems to be effective in terms of health-care resources optimization. Despite these observations, the best strategy to apply in the multidisciplinary evaluation still has to be defined and validated (19). In this article, we want to describe the organization, and share the first results, of our Multidisciplinary Group for Interstitial Lung Disease (GI-ILD), focusing on the early identification of CTDs in ILD patients referring to our clinics.

MATERIALS AND METHODS

The Pavia Multidisciplinary Group for Interstitial Lung Disease

The GI-ILD is a multidisciplinary group first established in 2015 as a shared initiative between the Rheumatology, Pulmonology, and Radiology Divisions of the University and IRCCS Policlinico San Matteo Foundation of Pavia, a tertiary center of referral in the diagnosis and treatment of CTDs, ILD, and rare pulmonary diseases (4, 5, 20–32). The GI-ILD has been first created for the collegial discussion and revision of the most complex or intriguing cases of ILD through a multidisciplinary discussion (MDD). From 2015 to 2018 the selection of cases to be discussed was on individual basis, as every clinician identified independently the patients. To improve the GI-ILD diagnostic performance at the meantime reducing the risk of missed CTDs diagnosis, from 2018, we established a multistep assessment pathway for newly referred (incident)

ILD patients in our hospital. Actually, the process of selection is preliminary to MDD, and it is addressed to focus on patients at increased risk of CTDs, to facilitate the admission to our Multidisciplinary Rheumatology–Pulmonology outpatient clinic for the final assessment.

GI-ILD General Organization

The organization of the GI-ILD is represented in **Figure 1**. Our multidisciplinary group includes a team of six Pulmonology, three Rheumatology, two Radiology, and one Pathology specialists supported by their respective fellows. The group's meetings are regularly scheduled every 2 weeks. The GI-ILD is mainly focused on ILD patients first referred to the Pulmonology Unit and without a previous diagnosis of any CTD, to rule out the occurrence of an underlying autoimmune disorder. Patients with a previous diagnosis of CTD have a direct access to the Rheumatology CTD outpatient clinic for diagnosis confirmation. During the first pulmonology assessment, patients are asked to perform or repeat pulmonary function tests (PFT) with diffusion capacity test (DLCO) and to fill in a 12-item questionnaire addressed to identify CTDs features. A previous version of this questionnaire has been applied in another setting with good results (16). When available, all the high-resolution computed tomographies (HRCT) of the chest are evaluated and, if not performed in our center, a copy of the DICOM images are stored for future MDD. Further steps include nailfold videocapillaroscopy (NVC), which is performed independently of Raynaud's Phenomenon (RP) occurrence (25), and a locally established autoimmune and laboratory panel of tests (**Figure 2**). To avoid possible selection bias, NVC and laboratory tests are, respectively, performed in the Rheumatology and in the Laboratory Division of the IRCCS Policlinico S. Matteo Foundation, a tertiary structure with high skills in the analysis of autoimmune and laboratory tests (33–36). Patients with either a positive questionnaire, NVC, or autoimmune and laboratory panel enter the MDD. During the MDD, the baseline screening results are presented, and the clinical case is discussed, together with the evaluation of chest HRCT images, PFT, and DLCO results. At the end of the discussion, patients without the suspect of an underlying CTD are planned for the regular pulmonology follow-up and treatment according to the suspected or established diagnosis. In case of CTD/IPAF, the patients are referred to the Multidisciplinary Rheumatology–Pulmonology outpatient clinic (RP-OC) for the final diagnostic steps, treatment, and follow-up definition. According to guidelines or expert recommendations, every patient is treated following the best therapeutic option established for the specific diagnosis.

First Step
Baseline screening questionnaire
The baseline screening questionnaire consists of 12 questions, focusing on 11 CTD manifestations such as RP (question 1), mechanic's hands and pitting scars (question 2), cutaneous sclerosis or puffy fingers (question 3), skin lesions such as heliotrope rash, Gottron's papules, malar rash (question 4), arthritis/inflammatory arthralgias (questions 5 and 6), dry eyes

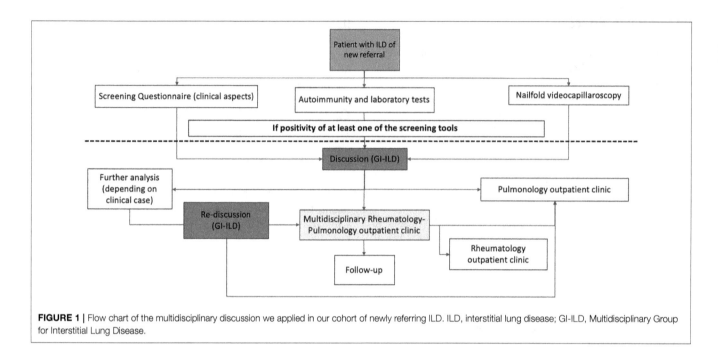

FIGURE 1 | Flow chart of the multidisciplinary discussion we applied in our cohort of newly referring ILD. ILD, interstitial lung disease; GI-ILD, Multidisciplinary Group for Interstitial Lung Disease.

Laboratory questionnaire

☐ ANA Centromere pattern positivity

☐ ANA Nucleolar pattern positivity

☐ ANA > 1/160 titer

    Specify the pattern of ANA test: ....

☐ ANA Cytoplasmic pattern positivity

☐ Rheumatoid Factor

    Titer and laboratory reference values: ....

☐ Anti-CCP positivity

    Titer and laboratory reference values: ....

☐ Anti-ENA positivity

    Specify which Anti-ENA are positive: ....

☐ Myositis specific/associated antibodies positivity

    Specify which Myositis specific/associated antibodies are positive: ....

☐ Systemic sclerosis rare antibodies positivity (test only if history of Raynaud's phenomenon)

    Specify which Systemic sclerosis rare antibodies are positive: ....

☐ p-ANCA positivity (anti-myeloperoxidase antibody)

☐ c-ANCA positivity (anti-proteinase 3 antibody)

☐ Lymphopenia (lymphocytes < 1500/mmc)

☐ Hyperferritinemia

    Value and reference levels: ....

☐ High Creatine-phosphokinase

    Value and reference levels: ....

☐ High aldolase

    Value and reference levels: ....

☐ Nailfold videocapillaroscopy with severe alterations (scleroderma or borderline pattern)

FIGURE 2 | Laboratory tests assessed as a screening tool in newly referring patients with interstitial lung disease.

and dry mouth (question 7), oral ulcers (question 8), dysphagia (question 9), proximal muscle weakness (question 10), cutaneous telangiectasias (question 11), and other CTD (and also vasculitis) features such as deep venous thrombosis, sinusitis, and adult-onset asthma (question 12). As pointed-out, every item explores a single manifestation, except for questions 5 and 6, which should be considered as a single item. The positivity of a single item of the baseline questionnaire is sufficient to enter the MDD.

Autoimmune and laboratory tests

Laboratory tests (**Figure 2**) include the antinuclear antibody (ANA) test (for both classic and cytoplasmic positivity) (HEp-2000®; Immunoconcepts), an extractable nuclear antigen screen test (EliA SymphonyS; Phadia 250), rheumatoid factor (Rheumatoid factor Flex reagent cartridge Dimension Vista; Siemens), anticyclic citrullinated peptide antibodies (EliA CCP; Phadia 250), antineutrophil cytoplasmic antibodies (ANCA) tests (EliA PR3 S and EliA MPO S: Phadia 250), creatine-phosphokinase, aldolase, erythrocyte sedimentation rate and C-reactive protein, and myositis-specific/myositis-associated antibodies (anti-Jo1, anti-PL7, anti-PL12, anti-OJ, anti-EJ, anti-Pm-Scl 75 and 100, anti-SRP, anti-Mi2, anti-MDA5, anti-NXP2, anti-TIF1gamma, anti-Ku, and anti-Ro52) (EUROLINE, Autoimmune Inflammatory Myopathies 16 Ag; EUROIMMUN). Systemic sclerosis rare antibodies (e.g., anti-PDGFR, anti-Ku, anti-Th/T0, anti-NOR90, anti-fibrillarin, anti-RNA polymerase I and III) [EUROLINE: Systemic Sclerosis (Nucleoli) Profile; Immunoblot EUROIMMUN] are tested only in patients with RP and after the negative result of myositis-specific/myositis-associated antibodies. As a reference value for autoimmune tests, we used the IPAF criteria (8), although for ANA without the nucleolar and anticentromere positivity, we considered as significant every pattern with titers higher than 1/160. Among the positive laboratory findings, we considered also hyperferritinemia and lymphopenia because of some reports as negative prognostic factor in patients with anti-MDA5 syndrome and thus potentially linked to the occurrence of CTD-ILD (37–39). Furthermore, on the basis of previous reports, we included also ANCA antibodies, ANA cytoplasmic positivity, and muscle enzymes assessment (15, 23, 40, 41). In case of a single positive result in autoimmune or laboratory tests, the patient is considered eligible for discussion during the GI-ILD.

Nailfold videocapillaroscopy

NVC is performed by the Rheumatology team generally within 10 days from the first pulmonology assessment. A single experienced operator (LC) performs NVC on a VideoCap 13 microscope with 200× magnification. Each exam includes the storage of pictures (three per finger) on a dedicated computer. A second rheumatologist reviews all the stored NVC images and formulates a comment (see Contribution). NVC is systematically performed in all patients according to the consolidated methodology described by Cutolo et al. (42) on each finger of both hands excluding thumbs. Patterns are described as "normal," "aspecific abnormalities," and "scleroderma pattern" (25). Scleroderma anomalies include megacapillaries, specific microhemorrhages, neoangiogenesis, or avascular areas (42). Patients with scleroderma anomalies are discussed during the GI-ILD.

Second Step

Multidisciplinary discussion

The results of the first step are presented during the GI-ILD by the clinician in charge of the patient. HRCT scans are collegially reviewed and discussed, to identify the radiological pattern of lung involvement (43). CT findings are qualitatively analyzed by two radiologists with great expertise on ILD. Similarly, PFTs results are presented, together with other clinically relevant information. In some cases, according to clinical suspicion, further analysis could be asked: muscle magnetic resonance, or muscle biopsy in suspected inflammatory myositis; plan X-rays or Doppler ultrasound of hands and feet in the suspect of arthritis; bronchoscopy with bronchoalveolar lavage fluid examination and cytogram to better characterize alveolitis; and surgical or cryo-biopsies in case of suspected IPF or other forms of fibrosing ILD not otherwise characterizable. Cases for which further analysis are needed enter a rediscussion in the subsequent GI-ILD. After the multidisciplinary discussion, patients diagnosed with a CTD-ILD or IPAF are followed up in the multidisciplinary Rheumatology–Pulmonology outpatient clinic, whereas all the other ILD patients without any rheumatologic involvement continue a regular pulmonology follow-up in a dedicated ILD outpatient clinic. According to the diagnosis, when clinically indicated, specific anti-fibrotic or immunosuppressant therapy is started.

Multidisciplinary rheumatology–pulmonology outpatient clinic

The Rheumatology–Pulmonology outpatient clinic is in charge to FMe (Pulmonologist) and to LC (Rheumatologist). At first assessment, patients generally repeat PFT with DLCO. A pulmonology and rheumatology medical examination is then performed, and all the data from the screening phase and of previous tests are reviewed. If a diagnosis is obtained, the appropriate treatment is started according to international guidelines or expert recommendations, and follow-up is planned. PFT + DLCO are repeated every 6 months. Annual HRCT is performed in patients with fibrotic ILD (with or without CTD) or IPF to follow up the stability/progression of fibrotic lung disease, as well as surveillance for possible neoplastic evolution on fibrotic scars or parenchyma. Timing for HRCT follow-up in non-fibrotic CTD-ILD depends largely on clinical and functional aspects. ILD patients diagnosed with established CTDs are subsequently followed in the CTD outpatient clinic and in the Rheumatology–Pulmonology outpatient clinic, while IPAF patients are followed up only in the Rheumatology–Pulmonology outpatient clinic, to identify patients who will develop an established CTD during follow-up. For every definite diagnosis, we adopt well-established classification criteria (8, 44–49), except for the antisynthetase syndrome, because of the lack of shared definitions (8, 50). In fact, in our cohort, every patient testing positive for antisynthetase antibodies is diagnosed with antisynthetase syndrome, in line with our previous reports (5). In case of ILD patients with clinical or laboratory findings suggestive for CTD but without fulfilling any of the existing classification criteria, the final attributed diagnosis is undifferentiated connective tissue disease (45).

Data collection

Patient's data from January to December 2018 were collected from electronic health records and medical records of GI-ILD. Every patient signed an informed consent during the first clinical evaluation. The screening questionnaire, autoimmune and laboratory tests, and NVC are collected from patient's medical records, while HRCT and PFT performed at the IRCCS Policlinico S. Matteo Foundation are stored in electronic health records. Copies of outside-performed HRCT DICOM files and PFT are recorded during GI-ILD evaluation and stored locally on a dedicated computer. All patient's medical records are stored in the multidisciplinary Rheumatology–Pulmonology outpatient clinic.

Statistical Analysis

Patients' characteristics at screening visit have been reported using median and interquartile range for the quantitative variables and absolute/relative frequency values for the qualitative ones. The population study has been divided in three different groups: *connective tissue disease* (CTD), which includes patients diagnosed with established autoimmune rheumatic diseases; *interstitial pneumonia with autoimmune features* (IPAF); and finally, the "other ILD" group, including all the remaining patients. Overall comparison among groups was performed by the one-way ANOVA or by non-parametric Kruskal–Wallis test for quantitative variables and by the chi-square or Fisher's exact test for categorical variables. Statistical significance was set at $p < 0.05$. Significant differences between groups were further evaluated in a *post-hoc* analysis (head-to-head comparison) with a statistical significance set at $p < 0.025$ (Bonferroni correction). Analyses were performed using STATA software package (2018, release 15.1; StataCorp, College Station, TX).

RESULTS

We retrospectively analyzed the performance of the GI-ILD group from January to December 2018 (**Table 1**). A total of 142 patients were referred to the Pulmonology outpatient clinic for a suspected ILD. Fifteen of them were excluded from the multidisciplinary approach after the first screening visit because an alternative diagnosis out of ILD was reached (five idiopathic pulmonary arterial hypertension, one pulmonary veno-occlusive disease; eight chronic obstructive pulmonary disease with paraseptal emphysema mimicking lung cysts or fibrotic air space enlargements; one lung cancer with carcinomatous lymphangitis). Eight patients entered the GI-ILD multidisciplinary discussion, but a definite diagnosis was not yet established at the end of the period considered for the present study, so they were excluded from analysis (STROBE diagram, **Figure 3**). We thus enrolled 119 patients (59 female and 60 male, 50% each), with a median age at first referral of 70 years (interquartile range, 64–77 years). A CTD was diagnosed in 18 cases (15%: 11 male, 60%; 7 female, 40%) and an IPAF in 39 (33%: 10 male, 26%; 29 female, 74%), together representing 48% of the evaluated cases. The remaining 62 patients (52% of cases: 23 female, 37%; 39 male, 63%) had other forms of ILD (idiopathic, sarcoidosis, exposure related,

rare ILD, other origin, i.e., Langerhans cell histiocytosis and lymphangioleiomyomatosis). Sex prevalence was different across the three groups ($p = 0.036$). In a *post-hoc* analysis, we observed that female patients were more commonly classified as IPAF ($p = 0.010$). The age at first referral was not different between patients with (70 years; interquartile range, 64–77) and without CTD/IPAF (70 years; interquartile range, 63–77) ($p = 0.665$). In addition, when considering the referral age of CTD (median, 69 years; interquartile range, 61–73) vs. IPAF (median, 70 years; interquartile range, 64–78 years), we did not find statistically significant differences ($p = 0.508$). The CTD patients were classified as rheumatoid arthritis in four (3%), systemic sclerosis in three (3%), undifferentiated connective tissue disease in three (2%), and antisynthetase syndrome in two (2%) cases, whereas six patients (5%) were classified one each as polymyositis, dermatomyositis, Sjogren syndrome, scleromyositis, amyopathic dermatomyositis, and granulomatosis with polyangiitis. Although granulomatosis with polyangiitis is not a CTD but a vasculitis, we included this patient in the analysis because identified thanks to screening steps. Patients in the "other ILD" group ($n = 62$) were mainly classified as idiopathic pulmonary fibrosis ($n = 30$, 48%). Interestingly, three of these patients (10%) were also diagnosed with polymyalgia rheumatica. The remaining 32 patients were diagnosed as idiopathic non-specific interstitial pneumonia (NSIP) ($n = 2$; 2%), respiratory bronchiolitis–ILD ($n = 5$; 4%), cryptogenic organizing pneumonia ($n = 2$; 2%), lymphoid interstitial pneumonia ($n = 2$; 2%), hypersensitivity pneumonitis ($n = 5$; 4%), secondary organizing pneumonia (OP) ($n = 3$; 2%), postactinic fibrosis ($n = 1$; 1%), sarcoidosis ($n = 3$; 2%), Langerhans cell histiocytosis ($n = 1$; 1%), lymphangioleiomyomatosis ($n = 1$; 1%), combined pulmonary fibrosis and emphysema ($n = 5$; 4%), pleuroparenchymal fibroelastosis ($n = 2$; 2%).

The results of the first screening step have been reported in **Figure 4**, stratified according to the diagnosis. The screening questionnaire discriminated well between CTD and other groups (CTD vs. IPAF, $p = 0.001$; CTD vs. other ILD, $p < 0.001$). Laboratory screening was less significantly positive in other ILD ($p = 0.002$ vs. CTD and $p < 0.001$ vs. IPAF). ANA test positivity was more common in CTD group ($p = 0.016$ vs. IPAF and $p < 0.001$ vs. other ILD) and in IPAF group (with respect to other ILD, $p = 0.016$), whereas cytoplasmic positivity of ANA test was more common in CTD and IPAF group with respect to other ILD ($p = 0.012$ and $p = 0.003$, respectively). A similar trend was observed for antiextractable nuclear antigen screen ($p < 0.001$ between IPAF and other ILD) and for myositis-specific and myositis-associated antibodies positivity (for both CTD vs. other ILD and for IPAF vs. other ILD, $p < 0.001$). Rheumatoid factor positivity was not different across the groups ($p = 0.791$), anticyclic citrullinated peptide antibodies were more common in CTD patients with respect to other ILD ($p = 0.008$). Finally, NVC was more frequently positive in CTDs ($p = 0.003$) with respect to IPAF and ($p < 0.001$) with respect to other ILD and in IPAF patients ($p = 0.010$) with respect to other ILD.

Regarding the HRCT pattern observed (**Figure 5**), the most prevalent was usual interstitial pneumonia (usual interstitial

TABLE 1 | Results of the GI-ILD multidisciplinary approach in the cohort of patients analyzed (from January to December 2018), see text for details.

ILD category	Specific diagnosis (no of patients and %)	No ILD patients (tot 119)	Median Age (y) and IQR	Male (n = 60; 50%)	Female (n = 59; 50%)	Questionnaire (≥1 item pos)	Scleroderma pattern at NVC	ANA	Cytoplasmic ANA	Anti-ENA	MSA/MAA	RF	anti-CCP	NSIP	NSIP + OP	UIP (def/prob)	OP	Other patterns
						Preliminary screening phase		Laboratory screening						HRCT pattern				
CTD-ILD	SSc	4 (3%)	18 (15%)	69 (61–73)	11 (57%)	7 (43%)	100%	44%	89%	28%	28%	28%	17%	11%	34%	22%	17%	11%	17%
	RA	3 (3%)																	
	ASSD	2 (2%)																	
	UCTD	3 (2%)																	
	Other CTD	6 (5%)																	
IPAF	IPAF	39 (33%)	39 (33%)	70 (64–78)	10 (26%)	29 (74%)	56%	10%	56%	28%	51%	56%	10%	3%	61%	8%	15%	13%	3%
Other ILD — Idiopathic	IPF	30 (25%)	62 (52%)	70 (63–77)	39 (63%)	23 (37%)	52%	0%	32%	6%	10%	0%	3%	0%	10%	2%	61%	6%	21%
	RB-ILD	5 (4%)																	
	idiopathic NSIP	2 (2%)																	
	idiopathic LIP	2 (2%)																	
	COP	2 (2%)																	
Sarcoidosis	Sarcoidosis	2 (2%)																	
Exposure-related	SOP	2 (2%)																	
	Post actinic Fibrosis	1 (1%)																	
Rare ILD	CPFE	5 (4%)																	
	PPFE	2 (2%)																	
Myscellanea	HP	5 (4%)																	
	LAM	1 (1%)																	
	LCH	1 (1%)																	
	p-value		=0.665	=0.036		<0.001	<0.001	<0.001	=0.007	<0.001	<0.001	=0.791	=0.003	<0.001	=0.008	<0.001	=0.005	=0.035

ILD, interstitial lung disease; CTD-ILD, connective tissue disease associated ILD; IPAF, interstitial pneumonia with autoimmune features; SSc, systemic sclerosis; RA, rheumatoid arthritis; ASSD, antisynthetase syndrome; UCTD, undifferentiated connective tissue disease; IPF, idiopathic pulmonary fibrosis; RB-ILD, respiratory bronchiolitis-ILD; NSIP, non-specific interstitial pneumonia; LIP, lymphoid interstitial pneumonia; COP, cryptogenic organizing pneumonia; SOP, secondary organizing pneumonia; CPFE, combined pulmonary fibrosis and emphysema; PPFE, pleuroparenchymal fibroelastosis; HP, hypersensitivity pneumonitis; LAM, lymphangioleiomyomatosis; LCH, Langerhans cell histiocytosis. MSA/MAA, myositis specific antibodies/myositis associated antibodies; RF, rheumatoid factor; anti-CCP, anti-cyclic citrullinated peptide antibodies; NVC, nailfold videocapillaroscopy; NSIP, non-specific interstitial pneumonia; NSIP + OP, non-specific interstitial pneumonia + organizing pneumonia; UIP, usual interstitial pneumonia.

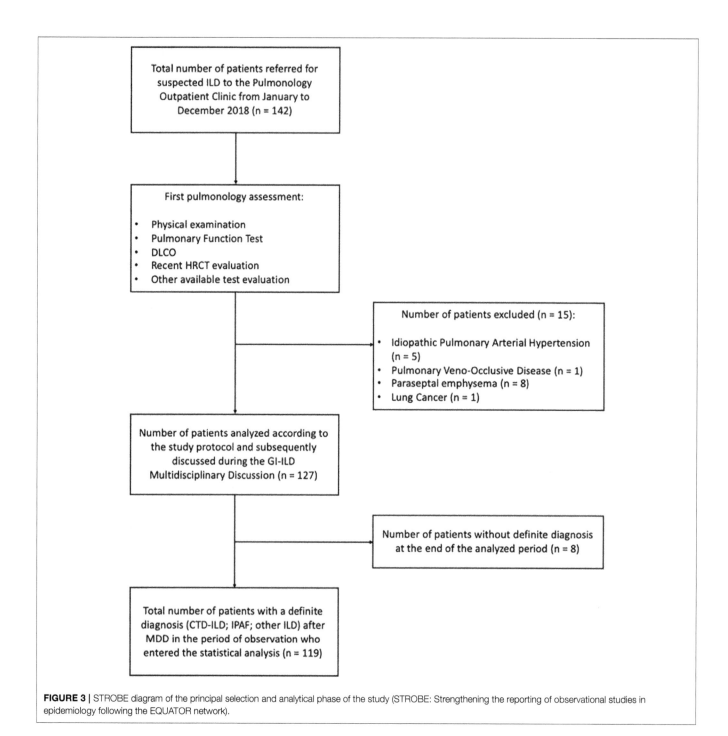

FIGURE 3 | STROBE diagram of the principal selection and analytical phase of the study (STROBE: Strengthening the reporting of observational studies in epidemiology following the EQUATOR network).

pneumonia probable, $n = 47$, 44%) followed by NSIP ($n = 24$, 20%), fibrosing NSIP ($n = 12$, 10%) and OP ($n = 11$, 8%). Some patients had superimposed NSIP and OP ($n = 8$, 7%). The distribution of different patterns across the established groups (CTD, IPAF, and other ILD) was statistically different ($p < 0.001$). In particular (**Figure 5**), NSIP pattern was less common in "other ILD" ($p = 0.013$ vs. CTD and $p < 0.001$ vs. IPAF), the mixed pattern NSIP + OP was more common in CTD than in other ILD ($p < 0.001$), and usual interstitial pneumonia was more common in other ILD ($p \leq 0.001$ with respect to other groups).

DISCUSSION

The multidisciplinary collaborative model we applied in the assessment of newly referred ILD seems to be effective in the *de novo* diagnosis of CTD/IPAF. In fact, we correctly classified more than 45% of patients within the spectrum of autoimmune connective tissue disorders. Interestingly, we did not include three patients with polymyalgia rheumatica in the CTD group, although this exclusion could be discussed, in particular if we

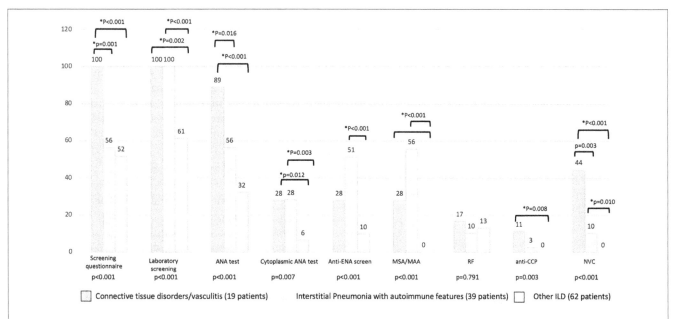

FIGURE 4 | Results (in percentage) of different screening steps according to final patients' classification. *Statistical significance <0.025 for *post-hoc* analysis. MSA/MAA, myositis specific antibodies/myositis associated antibodies; RF, rheumatoid factor; anti-CPP, anti-cyclic citrullinated peptide antibodies; NVC, nailfold videocapillaroscopy.

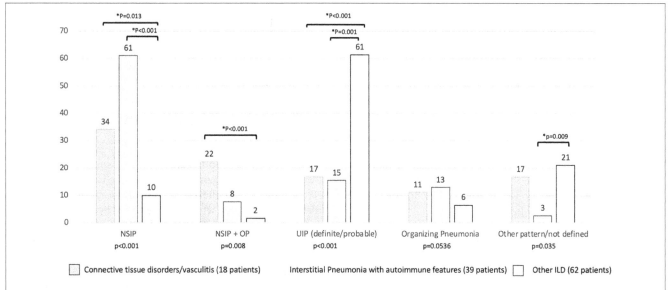

FIGURE 5 | Prevalence (in percentage) of high resolution computed tomography pattern according to final patients' classification. *Statistical significance <0.025 for *post-hoc* analysis. NSIP, non-specific interstitial pneumonia; NSIP + OP, non-specific interstitial pneumonia + organizing pneumonia.

consider the recently described case series of Sambataro et al. (51).

The results we obtained are relevant, even because our model is reproducible and potentially applicable in other centers after an external validation of the entry questionnaire. The model described seems to improve the overall ILD management, increasing the capability to perform a preliminary differential diagnosis of possible rheumatic disorders underlying an ILD. In fact, the identification of subtle CTD signs is not always easy

(52), with the risk to underdiagnose rheumatologic disorders, as we recently showed in a cohort of patients first referring to our hospital with a diagnosis of idiopathic pulmonary arterial hypertension (6). Furthermore, several patients we screened were at the end diagnosed with established CTDs, as a further confirmation that the definition of CTD signs is not rarely troublesome also in ILD patients. The adoption of a self-administered questionnaire seems to represent an added value, allowing the homogeneous evaluation of CTD symptoms in a non-rheumatology setting before the MDD. Moreover, thanks to a well-established collaboration between the Gynecology and the Rheumatology Division of our hospital, a similar approach has been previously applied to a cohort of pregnant women, showing that in patients with positive results, a final diagnosis of CTD was performed in the 25% of cases (16). This is a preliminary confirmation of the potential efficacy of a similar approach in patients referred for ILD, not suspected for but at risk to have a CTD. It is true that continuous clinical exchange within the multidisciplinary team may increase the sensibility of pulmonologist to rheumatology conditions and vice versa, but a standardized preliminary screening for ILD patients may surely reduce the interoperator variability in the assessment of CTD signs. This may be useful, in particular, in smaller secondary centers, were an MDD is not established or feasible. Obviously, as previously suggested, this approach should be validated in other contexts, and support from the National Health Systems and of respective national scientific societies will be necessary for its further application. If the questionnaire is important and generally positive in patients diagnosed with established CTD, in IPAF patients, it is possible to have only laboratory signs of autoimmunity and not clinically relevant features (8). On this basis, during the screening of ILD patients, it is mandatory not only to evaluate the autoimmune profile indicated in the IPAF criteria but also to consider other laboratory tests (15, 23) that have been associated to ILD occurrence, such as the panel we selected. The prototypical example is the cytoplasmic positivity of ANA, which has been linked to the occurrence of antisynthetase syndrome (41). Furthermore, we also enlarged the spectrum of potential rheumatology conditions identified by considering ANCA-associated vasculitis because these conditions are not rarely complicated by the occurrence of ILD (40) and are of primarily interest for both rheumatologists and pulmonologists. One of the patients discussed in the GI-ILD was diagnosed with granulomatosis with polyangiitis, having reported the occurrence of sinusitis together with ANCA positivity at baseline assessment. However, the most useful screening tool we identified was nailfold videocapillaroscopy, which was positive only in case of CTD or IPAF diagnosis, independent to the occurrence of RP, as recently shown in antisynthetase syndrome (25). Although nailfold capillaroscopy should surely enter the routine assessment of every ILD patient, the overall rate of positivity of the test we found in our cohort was quite low.

From the combination of these different domains, during the MDD, we can obtain a series of information that could be helpful in patient's classification, at the same time reducing the number of referral visits before a CTD diagnosis is established.

When an ILD occurs, the early identification of CTD or IPAF is crucial and should be carefully considered for the best therapeutic strategy to apply. In fact, an ILD with an autoimmune origin could benefit from immunosuppressant drugs such as cyclophosphamide, cyclosporine, mycophenolate mofetil, azathioprine, and rituximab (20, 53, 54), whereas until now, these patients were simply excluded from the access to anti-fibrotic drugs, such as Nintedanib and Pirfenidone (55). However, the exclusion of these patients from CTD group could be discussed, in particular, if we consider the recently described case series of Sambataro et al. (51) or the promising results of the INBUILD study (56).

In conclusion, with our study, we confirmed that the multidisciplinary approach we applied may be really useful in the identification of CTD-ILD/IPAF in ILD patients without previous rheumatology diagnosis. We suggest that a rheumatologist is necessary in every ILD multidisciplinary team and that, to optimize the diagnostic pathway, a preliminary screening phase with a dedicated questionnaire could be useful. In our opinion, a targeted autoimmune and laboratory profile evaluation and nailfold capillaroscopy should be part of the routine assessment of ILD patients.

ETHICS STATEMENT

The GI-ILD is approved and recognized by our Foundation. In line with the Declaration of Helsinki, with our national and institutional regulations, and according to our local Institutional Review Board, we obtained from all patients the signed informed consent for the retrospective use of clinical data collected.

AUTHOR CONTRIBUTIONS

TO, RD, AV, FMe, FMa, ZK, PM, and VC organized the GI-ILD. VC, CM, FMe, CS, and LC drafted the screening questionnaire. CA, LC, ZK, CS, FMa, and FMe defined the laboratory test to be searched for in the preliminary phase. LC performed the nailfold videocapillaroscopies, which were reviewed by EM and, in case of conflict, by VC and GZ. AV, RD, and AF performed, analyzed, and discussed CT scans. CT and CL for the pulmonology counterpart. SG, LD, EM, GZ, and VM for the rheumatology counterpart filled the database. LC performed statistical analysis. All Pavia's authors participated to GI-ILD meetings. The paper was mainly drafted by CT, VM, LC, and FMe. CM revised the first draft, and other authors contributed to paper improvement with respect to first version.

REFERENCES

1. Antoniou KM, Margaritopoulos GA, Tomassetti S, Bonella F, Costabel U, Poletti V. Interstitial lung disease. Eur Respir Rev. (2014) 23:40–54. doi: 10.1183/09059180.00009113
2. Kouranos V, Miranda G, Corte TJ, Renzoni EA. New treatment paradigms for connective tissue disease-associated interstitial lung disease. Curr Opin Pulm Med. (2018) 24:453–60. doi: 10.1097/MCP.0000000000000508
3. Maher TM, Wuyts W. Management of fibrosing interstitial lung diseases. Adv Ther. (2019) 36:1518–31. doi: 10.1007/s12325-019-00992-9
4. Cavagna L, Monti S, Grosso V, Boffini N, Scorletti E, Crepaldi G, et al. The multifaceted aspects of interstitial lung disease in rheumatoid arthritis. BioMed Res Int. (2013) 2013:759760. doi: 10.1155/2013/759760
5. Cavagna L, Nuño L, Scirè CA, Govoni M, Longo FJL, Franceschini F, et al. Clinical spectrum time course in anti Jo-1 positive antisynthetase syndrome: results from an international retrospective multicenter study. Medicine. (2015) 94:e1144. doi: 10.1097/MD.0000000000001144
6. Cavagna L, Codullo V, Ghio S, Scirè CA, Guzzafame E, Scelsi L, et al. Undiagnosed connective tissue diseases: high prevalence in

pulmonary arterial hypertension patients. *Medicine.* (2016) 95:e4827. doi: 10.1097/MD.0000000000004827

7. Demoruelle MK, Mittoo S, Solomon JJ. Connective tissue disease-related interstitial lung disease. *Best Pract Res Clin Rheumatol.* (2016) 30:39–52. doi: 10.1016/j.berh.2016.04.006

8. Fischer A, Antoniou KM, Brown KK, Cadranel J, Corte TJ, du Bois RM, et al. An official European Respiratory Society/American Thoracic Society research statement: interstitial pneumonia with autoimmune features. *Eur Respir J.* (2015) 46:976–87. doi: 10.1183/13993003.00150-2015

9. Chartrand S, Swigris JJ, Peykova L, Chung J, Fischer A. A multidisciplinary evaluation helps identify the antisynthetase syndrome in patients presenting as idiopathic interstitial pneumonia. *J Rheumatol.* (2016) 43:887–92. doi: 10.3899/jrheum.150966

10. Chaudhuri N, Spencer L, Greaves M, Bishop P, Chaturvedi A, Leonard C. A review of the multidisciplinary diagnosis of interstitial lung diseases: a retrospective analysis in a single UK specialist centre. *J Clin Med.* (2016) 5:E66. doi: 10.3390/jcm5080066

11. Prasad JD, Mahar A, Bleasel J, Ellis SJ, Chambers DC, Lake F, et al. The interstitial lung disease multidisciplinary meeting: a position statement from the Thoracic Society of Australia and New Zealand and the Lung Foundation Australia. *Respirology.* (2017) 22:1459–72. doi: 10.1111/resp.13163

12. Kalluri M, Claveria F, Ainsley E, Haggag M, Armijo-Olivo S, Richman-Eisenstat J. Beyond idiopathic pulmonary fibrosis diagnosis: multidisciplinary care with an early integrated palliative approach is associated with a decrease in acute care utilization and hospital deaths. *J Pain Symptom Manage.* (2018) 55:420–6. doi: 10.1016/j.jpainsymman.2017.10.016

13. Richeldi L, Launders N, Martinez F, Walsh SLF, Myers J, Wang B, et al. The characterisation of interstitial lung disease multidisciplinary team meetings: a global study. *ERJ Open Res.* (2019) 5:00209–2018. doi: 10.1183/23120541.00209-2018

14. Fischer A, Strek ME, Cottin V, Dellaripa PF, Bernstein EJ, Brown KK, et al. Proceedings of the American College of Rheumatology/Association of Physicians of Great Britain and Ireland Connective Tissue Disease-Associated Interstitial Lung Disease Summit: a multidisciplinary approach to address challenges and opportunities. *Arthritis Rheumatol.* (2019) 71:182–95. doi: 10.1002/art.40769

15. Sambataro G, Sambataro D, Torrisi SE, Vancheri A, Pavone M, Rosso R, et al. State of the art in interstitial pneumonia with autoimmune features: a systematic review on retrospective studies and suggestions for further advances. *Eur Respir Rev.* (2018) 27:170139. doi: 10.1183/16000617.0139-2017

16. Spinillo A, Beneventi F, Epis OM, Montanari L, Mammoliti D, Ramoni V, et al. Prevalence of undiagnosed autoimmune rheumatic diseases in the first trimester of pregnancy. Results of a two-steps strategy using a self-administered questionnaire and autoantibody testing. *BJOG.* (2018) 115:51–7. doi: 10.1111/j.1471-0528.2007.01530.x

17. Sambataro G, Sambataro D, Torrisi SE, Vancheri A, Colaci M, Pavone M, et al. Clinical, serological and radiological features of a prospective cohort of interstitial pneumonia with autoimmune features (IPAF) patients. *Respir Med.* (2019) 150:154–60. doi: 10.1016/j.rmed.2019.03.011

18. Chartrand S, Swigris JJ, Stanchev L, Lee JS, Brown KK, Fischer A. Clinical features and natural history of interstitial pneumonia with autoimmune features: a single center experience. *Respir Med.* (2016) 119:150–4. doi: 10.1016/j.rmed.2016.09.002

19. Jo HE, Corte TJ, Moodley Y, Levin K, Westall G, Hopkins P, et al. Evaluating the interstitial lung disease multidisciplinary meeting: a survey of expert centres. *BMC Pulm Med.* (2016) 16:22. doi: 10.1186/s12890-016-0179-3

20. Cavagna L, Caporali R, Abdì-Alì L, Dore R, Meloni F, Montecucco C. Cyclosporine in anti-Jo1-positive patients with corticosteroid-refractory interstitial lung disease. *J Rheumatol.* (2013) 40:484–92. doi: 10.3899/jrheum.121026

21. Cavagna L, Monti S, Caporali R, Gatto M, Iaccarino L, Doria A. How I treat idiopathic patients with inflammatory myopathies in the clinical practice. *Autoimmun Rev.* (2017) 16:999–1007. doi: 10.1016/j.autrev.2017.07.016

22. Cavagna L, Nuño L, Scirè CA, Govoni M, Longo FJL, Franceschini F, et al. Serum Jo-1 autoantibody and isolated arthritis in the antisynthetase syndrome: review of the literature and report of the experience of AENEAS collaborative group. *Clin Rev Allergy Immunol.* (2017) 52:71–80. doi: 10.1007/s12016-016-8528-9

23. Cavagna L, Gonzalez Gay MA, Allanore Y, Matucci-Cerinic M. Interstitial

pneumonia with autoimmune features: a new classification still on the move. *Eur Respir Rev.* (2018) 27:180047. doi: 10.1183/16000617.0047-2018

24. Gonzalez-Gay MA, Montecucco C, Selva-O'Callaghan A, Trallero-Araguas E, Molberg O, Andersson H, et al. Timing of onset affects arthritis presentation pattern in antisyntethase syndrome. *Clin Exp Rheumatol.* (2018) 36:44–9.

25. Sebastiani M, Triantafyllias K, Manfredi A, González-Gay MA, Palmou-Fontana N, Cassone G, et al. Nailfold capillaroscopy characteristics of antisynthetase syndrome and possible clinical associations: results of a multicenter international study. *J Rheumatol.* (2019) 46:279–84. doi: 10.3899/jrheum.180355

26. Piloni D, Morosini M, Magni S, Balderacchi A, Scudeller L, Cova E, et al. Analysis of long term CD4+CD25highCD127- T-reg cells kinetics in peripheral blood of lung transplant recipients. *BMC Pulm Med.* (2017) 17:102. doi: 10.1186/s12890-017-0446-y

27. Nosotti M, Dell'Amore A, Diso D, Oggionni T, Aliberti S, Study Group for Thoracic Organs Transplantation. Selection of candidates for lung transplantation: the first Italian Consensus Statement. *Transplant Proc.* (2017) 49:702–6. doi: 10.1016/j.transproceed.2017.02.026

28. Aiello M, Bertorelli G, Bocchino M, Chetta A, Fiore-Donati A, Fois A, et al. The earlier, the better: impact of early diagnosis on clinical outcome in idiopathic pulmonary fibrosis. *Pulm Pharmacol Ther.* (2017) 44:7–15. doi: 10.1016/j.pupt.2017.02.005

29. Sverzellati N, Odone A, Silva M, Polverosi R, Florio C, Cardinale L, et al. Structured reporting for fibrosing lung disease: a model shared by radiologist and pulmonologist. *Radiol Med.* (2018) 123:245–53. doi: 10.1007/s11547-017-0835-6

30. Panigada S, Ravelli A, Silvestri M, Granata C, Magni-Manzoni S, Cerveri I, et al. HRCT and pulmonary function tests in monitoring of lung involvement in juvenile systemic sclerosis. *Pediatr Pulmonol.* (2009) 44:1226–34. doi: 10.1002/ppul.21141

31. Cavagna L, Caporali R. Therapeutic options in anti-jo-1 antisynthetase syndrome with interstitial lung disease: comment on the article by Marie et al. *Arthritis Care Res.* (2013) 65:1548. doi: 10.1002/acr.22024

32. Cavagna L, Castañeda S, Sciré C, Gonzalez-Gay MA, AENEAS Collaborative Group Members. Antisynthetase syndrome or what else? Different perspectives indicate the need for new classification criteria. *Ann Rheum Dis.* (2018) 77:e50. doi: 10.1136/annrheumdis-2017-212368

33. Alpini C, Lotzniker M, Valaperta S, Bottone MG, Malatesta M, Montanelli A, et al. Characterization for anti-cytoplasmic antibodies specificity by morphological and molecular techniques. *Auto Immun Highlights.* (2012) 3:79–85. doi: 10.1007/s13317-012-0033-4

34. Bartoloni E, Alunno A, Bistoni O, Bizzaro N, Migliorini P, Morozzi G, et al. Diagnostic value of anti-mutated citrullinated vimentin in comparison to anti-cyclic citrullinated peptide and anti-viral citrullinated peptide 2 antibodies in rheumatoid arthritis: an Italian multicentric study and review of the literature. *Autoimmun Rev.* (2012) 11:815–20. doi: 10.1016/j.autrev.2012.02.015

35. Bizzaro N, Allegri F, Alpini C, Doria A, Gerli R, Lotzniker M, et al. Multicentric evaluation of a second generation assay to detect antiviral citrullinated peptide antibodies: a collaborative study by the Forum Interdisciplinare per la Ricerca nelle Malattie Autoimmuni. *J Clin Pathol.* (2011) 64:1139–41. doi: 10.1136/jclinpath-2011-200308

36. Bizzaro N, Bartoloni E, Morozzi G, Manganelli S, Riccieri V, Sabatini P, et al. Anti-cyclic citrullinated peptide antibody titer predicts time to rheumatoid arthritis onset in patients with undifferentiated arthritis: results from a 2-year prospective study. *Arthritis Res Ther.* (2013) 15:R16. doi: 10.1186/ar4148

37. Osawa T, Morimoto K, Sasaki Y, Matsuda S, Yamana K, Yano R, et al. The Serum ferritin level is associated with the treatment responsivity for rapidly progressive interstitial lung disease with amyopathic dermatomyositis, irrespective of the anti-MDA5 antibody level. *Intern Med.* (2018) 57:387–91. doi: 10.2169/internalmedicine.8335-16

38. Yamada K, Asai K, Okamoto A, Watanabe T, Kanazawa H, Ohata M, et al. Correlation between disease activity and serum ferritin in clinically amyopathic dermatomyositis with rapidly-progressive interstitial lung disease: a case report. *BMC Res Notes.* (2018) 11:34. doi: 10.1186/s13104-018-3146-7

39. Xu Y, Yang CS, Li YJ, Liu XD, Wang JN, Zhao Q, et al. Predictive factors of rapidly progressive-interstitial lung disease in patients with clinically amyopathic dermatomyositis. *Clin Rheumatol.* (2016) 35:113–6. doi: 10.1007/s10067-015-3139-z

40. Alba MA, Flores-Suárez LF, Henderson AG, Xiao H, Hu P, Nachman PH, et al. Interstitial lung disease in ANCA vasculitis. *Autoimmun Rev.* (2017) 16:722–9. doi: 10.1016/j.autrev.2017.05.008

41. Aggarwal R, Dhillon N, Fertig N, Koontz D, Qi Z, Oddis CV. A negative antinuclear antibody does not indicate autoantibody negativity in myositis: role of anticytoplasmic antibody as a screening test for antisynthetase syndrome. *J Rheumatol.* (2017) 44:223–9. doi: 10.3899/jrheum.160618

42. Cutolo M, Pizzorni C, Tuccio M, Burroni A, Craviotto C, Basso M, et al. Nailfold videocapillaroscopic patterns and serum autoantibodies in systemic sclerosis. *Rheumatology.* (2004) 43:719–26. doi: 10.1093/rheumatology/keh156

43. Walsh SLF, Hansell DM. High-resolution CT of interstitial lung disease: a continuous evolution. *Semin Respir Crit Care Med.* (2014) 35:129–44. doi: 10.1055/s-0033-1363458

44. Aletaha D, Neogi T, Silman AJ, Funovits J, Felson DT, Bingham CO, et al. 2010 Rheumatoid arthritis classification criteria: an American College of Rheumatology/European League Against Rheumatism collaborative initiative. *Arthritis Rheum.* (2010) 62:2569–81. doi: 10.1002/art.27584

45. Mosca M, Neri R, Bombardieri S. Undifferentiated connective tissue diseases (UCTD): a review of the literature and a proposal for preliminary classification criteria. *Clin Exp Rheumatol.* (1999) 17:615–20.

46. van den Hoogen F, Khanna D, Fransen J, Johnson SR, Baron M, Tyndall A, et al. 2013 classification criteria for systemic sclerosis: an American college of rheumatology/European league against rheumatism collaborative initiative. *Ann Rheum Dis.* (2013) 72:1747–55. doi: 10.1136/annrheumdis-2013-204424

47. Bohan A, Peter JB. Polymyositis and dermatomyositis (second of two parts). *N Engl J Med.* (1975) 292:403–7. doi: 10.1056/NEJM197502202920807

48. Shiboski CH, Shiboski SC, Seror R, Criswell LA, Labetoulle M, Lietman TM, et al. 2016 American College of Rheumatology/European League Against Rheumatism classification criteria for primary Sjögren's syndrome: a consensus and data-driven methodology involving three international patient cohorts. *Ann Rheum Dis.* (2017) 76:9–16. doi: 10.1136/annrheumdis-2016-210571

49. Dasgupta B, Cimmino MA, Kremers HM, Schmidt WA, Schirmer M, Salvarani C, et al. 2012 Provisional classification criteria for polymyalgia rheumatica: a European League Against Rheumatism/American College of Rheumatology collaborative initiative. *Arthritis Rheum.* (2012) 64:943–54. doi: 10.1016/j.ymed.2012.09.009

50. Castañeda S, Cavagna L, González-Gay MA. New criteria needed for antisynthetase syndrome. *JAMA Neurol.* (2018) 75:258–9. doi: 10.1001/jamaneurol.2017.3872

51. Sambataro G, Sambataro D, Pignataro F, Torrisi SE, Vancheri A, Pavone M, et al. Interstitial lung disease in patients with polymyalgia rheumatica: a case series. *Respir Med Case Rep.* (2019) 26:126–30. doi: 10.1016/j.rmcr.2018.12.014

52. Cottin V. Idiopathic interstitial pneumonias with connective tissue diseases features: a review. *Respirol.* (2016) 21:245–58. doi: 10.1111/resp.12588

53. Bauhammer J, Blank N, Max R, Lorenz HM, Wagner U, Krause D, et al. Rituximab in the treatment of Jo1 Antibody-associated antisynthetase syndrome: anti-Ro52 positivity as a marker for severity and treatment response. *J Rheumatol.* (2016) 43:1566–74. doi: 10.3899/jrheum.150844

54. Denton CP, Khanna D. Systemic sclerosis. *Lancet.* (2017) 390:1685–99. doi: 10.1016/S0140-6736(17)30933-9

55. Raghu G, Remy-Jardin M, Myers JL, Richeldi L, Ryerson CJ, Lederer DJ, et al. Diagnosis of idiopathic pulmonary fibrosis. An official ATS/ERS/JRS/ALAT clinical practice guideline. *Am J Resp Crit Care Med.* (2018) 198:e44–68. doi: 10.1164/rccm.201807-1255ST

56. Flaherty KR, Wells AU, Cottin V, Devaraj A, Walsh SLF, Inoue Y, et al. Nintedanib in progressive fibrosing interstitial lung diseases. *N Engl J Med.* (2019) 381:1718–27. doi: 10.1056/NEJMoa1908681

17

Lung Tissue Microbiome is Associated With Clinical Outcomes of Idiopathic Pulmonary Fibrosis

Hee-Young Yoon, Su-Jin Moon and Jin Woo Song*

Department of Pulmonary and Critical Care Medicine, Asan Medical Center, University of Ulsan College of Medicine, Seoul, South Korea

*Correspondence:
Jin Woo Song
jwsongasan@gmail.com

Background: Several studies using bronchoalveolar lavage fluid (BALF) reported that lung microbial communities were associated with the development and clinical outcome of idiopathic pulmonary fibrosis (IPF). However, the microbial communities in IPF lung tissues are not well known. This study is aimed to investigate bacterial microbial communities in lung tissues and determine their impact on the clinical outcomes of patients with IPF.

Methods: Genomic DNA extracted from lung tissues of patients with IPF ($n = 20$; 10 non-survivors) and age- and sex-matched controls ($n = 20$) was amplified using fusion primers targeting the V3 and V4 regions of the 16S RNA genes with indexing barcodes.

Results: Mean age of IPF subjects was 63.3 yr, and 65% were male. Alpha diversity indices did not significantly differ between IPF patients and controls, or between IPF non-survivors and survivors. The relative abundance of *Lactobacillus*, *Paracoccus,* and *Akkermansia* was increased, whereas that of *Caulobacter*, *Azonexus*, and *Undibacterium* decreased in patients with IPF compared with that in the controls. A decreased relative abundance of *Pelomonas* (odds ratio [OR], 0.352, $p = 0.027$) and *Azonexus* (OR, 0.013, $p = 0.046$) was associated with a diagnosis of IPF in the multivariable logistic analysis adjusted by age and gender. Multivariable Cox analysis adjusted for age and forced vital capacity (FVC) revealed that higher relative abundance of *Streptococcus* (hazard ratio [HR], 1.993, $p = 0.044$), *Sphingomonas* (HR, 57.590, $p = 0.024$), and *Clostridium* (HR, 37.189, $p = 0.038$) was independently associated with IPF mortality. The relative abundance of *Curvibacter* ($r = 0.590$) and *Thioprofundum* ($r = 0.373$) was correlated positively, whereas that of *Anoxybacillus* ($r = -0.509$) and *Enterococcus* ($r = -0.593$) was correlated inversely with FVC. In addition, the relative abundance of the *Aquabacterium* ($r = 0.616$) and *Peptoniphilus* ($r = 0.606$) genera was positively correlated, whereas that of the *Fusobacterium* ($r = -0.464$) and *Phycicoccus* ($r = -0.495$) genera was inversely correlated with distance during the 6-min walking test.

Conclusions: The composition of the microbiome in lung tissues differed between patients with IPF and controls and was associated with the diagnosis, mortality, and disease severity of IPF.

Keywords: idiopathic pulmonary fibrosis, prognosis, respiratory function tests, microbiota, diagnosis

INTRODUCTION

Idiopathic pulmonary fibrosis (IPF) is a chronic progressive fibrosing interstitial lung disease of unknown etiology (1). It is characterized by worsening dyspnea, impaired lung function, decreased quality of life, and a poor prognosis (1). The pathogenesis of IPF involves both genetic (2, 3) and environmental factors (4, 5). Repeated epithelial injuries caused by multiple environmental factors, such as smoking, micro-aspiration, organic and inorganic dust, and viral infection (4, 5), can lead to the abnormal wound healing process, such as epithelial-mesenchymal transition (6) in genetically susceptible individuals who have a mutation in airway defense (*MUC5B*), telomerase function (*TERT*), or immune responses (*TOLLIP*, *TLR3*, and *IL1RN*) (2, 3, 7). Much evidence supports an association between the etiology of several viruses (8–11), and the development or acute exacerbation (AE) of IPF (12, 13). The fact that combined therapy with steroid, azathioprine, and N-acetylcysteine increases the mortality and hospitalization rates of patients with IPF (14) also suggests that infectious organisms are involved in IPF progression.

Along with the development of culture-independent molecular-sequencing techniques, such as 16s ribosomal RNA (16s rRNA) gene sequencing (15), several studies of bronchoalveolar lavage fluid (BALF) have suggested that lung microbial communities are associated with the clinical course of IPF (16–21). The findings of the Correlating Outcomes With Biochemical Markers to Estimate Time-progression in IPF (COMET) study revealed that an increased bacterial burden in BALF from patients with IPF ($n = 65$), compared with controls ($n = 44$), is associated with a 10% decline in forced vital capacity (FVC) at 6 months and mortality (16). On the contrary, a study of explanted lung tissues from patients with IPF ($n = 40$) showed very low bacterial abundance in IPF lung tissues that was similar to that of negative controls (22). These contradictory findings could be attributed to different types of samples or sample collection times. Therefore, the composition and impact of the lung tissue microbiome at diagnosis on clinical outcomes in patients with IPF are not well defined. Our study aimed to identify the diversity and composition of the bacterial microbial communities in lung tissues at the time of diagnosis and determine their association with clinical outcomes, such as survival, disease severity, and progression in patients with IPF.

MATERIALS AND METHODS

Study Population

All participating patients with IPF were diagnosed between January 2011 and December 2013 at Asan Medical Center, Seoul, Republic of Korea and met the diagnostic criteria of the American Thoracic Society (ATS)/European Respiratory Society/Japanese Respiratory Society/Latin American Thoracic Association statement (1). Samples of lung tissues from patients with IPF ($n = 20$; 10 non-survivors [cause of death: AE = 1, disease progression = 2, unknown = 7]) were aseptically obtained at the time of surgical biopsy for diagnosis, and those from age- and gender-matched controls (lung cancer patients;

$n = 20$) with no histological evidence of disease collected aseptically at the time of surgery were obtained from the Bio-Resource Center of Asan Medical Center. None of the patients with IPF or the controls had been treated with antibiotics, steroids, anti-fibrotic agents, or probiotics within 1 month before undergoing surgery. Lung tissues were procured under protocol #2016-1366. This study was conducted in accordance with the Declaration of Helsinki (2013) and was approved by the Institutional Review Board of Asan Medical Center (2018–1096). Written informed consent was obtained from all study participants.

Clinical and survival data of all patients were retrospectively collected from medical records, telephone interviews, and/or the National Health Insurance of Korea. Spirometry, total lung capacity (TLC) determined by plethysmography and diffusing capacity for carbon monoxide (DLco) measured according to published recommendations are expressed as ratios (%) of normal predicted values (23–25). The patients with IPF underwent 6-min walk tests (6MWT) according to the ATS guidelines (26). Baseline clinical data at the time of IPF diagnosis were collected within one month of sample acquisition.

Bacterial 16S rRNA Gene Sequencing

Tissue samples were frozen in liquid nitrogen immediately after collection and stored at $-80°C$. Genomic DNA was extracted from lung tissues using Mo Bio PowerSoil® DNA Isolation Kits (Mo Bio Laboratories, Carlsbad, CA, USA) according to the instructions of the manufacturer. The variable V3 and V4 regions of the 16S rRNA genes were amplified using the following specific forward and reverse primers with overhang adapters: 5′-TCGTCGGCAGCGTCAGATGTGTATA AGAGACAGCCTACG GGNGGCWGCAG-3′ and 5′-GTCTCG TGGGCTCGGAGATGTGTATAAGAGACAGGACTACHVG GGTATCTAATCC-3′, respectively (27). The PCR proceeded using a 5 ng/µl DNA template, 2 × KAPA HiFi HotStart Ready Mix (KAPA Biosystems, Wilmington, MA, USA), and two amplicon PCR forward and reverse primers. The PCR protocol comprised initial incubation at 95°C for 3 min, followed by 25 cycles of 95°C for 30 s, 55°C for 30 s, and 72°C for 30 s, then 72°C for 5 min, and retention at 4°C. After PCR clean-up and index PCR, 300 bp paired-end sequences were pooled on the Illumina MiSeq platform (Illumina Inc., San Diego, CA, USA) as described by the manufacturer for all sample sequencing (28, 29). Distilled water provided in the PCR kit was used as a negative control, and no amplification was identified during the processes.

Reconstruction and Compositional Analysis

Fast Length Adjustment of Short (FLASH) reads, http://ccb.jhu. edu/software/FLASH/), were used for 16S rRNA gene by merging pairs of reads when the original DNA fragments were shortened than two times the length of the reads (30). Pre-processing and clustering were performed using the CD-HIT-operational taxonomic units (OTU; http://weizhongli-lab.org/cd-hit-otu/). Short reads (56,825) were filtered out and extra-long tails were trimmed. After filtering, the remaining reads were clustered

TABLE 1 | Comparison of baseline characteristics between IPF and control groups.

Variables	IPF			Control
	Total	**Survivors**	**Non-survivors**	
Number	20	10	10	20
Age, years	63.3 ± 6.2	62.4 ± 6.4	64.2 ± 6.1	67.3 ± 7.4
Male	13 (65.0)	6 (60.0)	7 (70.0)	17 (85.0)
Ever-Smoker	13 (65.0)	7 (70.0)	6 (60.0)	15 (75.0)
PFT, % predicted				
FVC	64.2 ± 14.7	69.2 ± 15.1	60.2 ± 14.0	91.3 ± 16.0*
DLco	54.8 ± 14.8	58.3 ± 17.5	51.3 ± 11.3	97.4 ± 20.6*
TLC	65.9 ± 11.3	68.7 ± 10.2	63.0 ± 12.2	108.4 ± 17.7*
6MWT				
Distance, m	433.6 ± 63.5	452.8 ± 48.9	434.3 ± 77.1	NA
Resting SpO$_2$, %	96.3 ± 1.6	96.4 ± 1.6	96.2 ± 1.7	NA
Lowest SpO$_2$, %	90.6 ± 5.8	91.5 ± 5.1	89.6 ± 6.5	NA

*Data are presented as means ± SD or number (%), unless otherwise indicated. 6MWT, 6-min walk test; DLco, diffusing capacity of the lungs for carbon monoxide; FVC, forced vital capacity; IPF, idiopathic pulmonary fibrosis; NA, not available; PFT, pulmonary function test; SpO$_2$, peripheral oxygen saturation; TLC, total lung capacity; 6MWD, 6-min walk test distance. *P < 0.05 (IPF vs. control).*

at 100% identity. Chimeric reads (254,891) were filtered, and secondary clusters were recruited into primary clusters. After excluding reads with all other noise (5,292,165), the remaining reads (3,484,551) were clustered algorithm into OTUs at a cutoff of 97% (31, 32). Feature tables, such as abundance and representational sequence files, were created using UCLAST in Quantitative Insights Into Microbial Ecology (QIIME1; https://qiime.org) software (33). Taxonomy was assigned based on information about organisms with the closest similarity to the representative sequence of each OTU in the Basic Local Alignment Search Tool (BLAST), version 2.4.0, the NCBI 16S microbial reference database. Taxonomy was not assigned when the query coverage of the best match in the database was <85%, and the identity of the matched area was <85%.

Statistical Analysis

Continuous data were analyzed using Mann–Whitney U tests, and categorical data were analyzed using Fisher exact tests. The decline rate of lung function and exercise capacity for one year was estimated by linear regression analysis. Correlations between the relative abundance of the microbiome and clinical parameters were assessed using Spearman's correlation coefficients (r). The risk of microbial relative abundance for a diagnosis of IPF was expressed as odds ratio (OR) with 95% CI using binary logistic regression. In addition, the risk of microbial relative abundance for IPF mortality was presented as hazard ratio (HR) with 95% CI using Cox proportional hazards regression analyses. Alpha diversity indices that estimate the number of unique OTU in each sample are represented using four indices; Observed estimated the actual number of different taxa evident in a sample, Chao 1 non-parametrically estimated the richness of the species (34), Shannon estimated richness and evenness of species present in a sample considering the distribution of strains belonging to each species (35), and Inverse Simpson measured the probability that two randomly selected objects in a sample belong to

the same species (36). Principal coordinates analysis (PCoA), based on weighted UniFrac methods to obtain phylogenetic and quantitative indices for assessing abundance differences among groups (IPF vs. controls, survivors vs. non-survivors), was conducted for all samples using QIIME1 (37). The exploratory and differential microbial compositions were analyzed using QIIME1. All data were statistically analyzed using SPSS version 24.0 (IBM Corp., Armonk, NY, USA), and values with $p < 0.05$ (two-tailed) were considered statistically significant.

RESULTS

Microbial Diversity and Composition

Among 20 patients with IPF, the mean age was 63.3 yr, and 65.0% were male (**Table 1**). Lung function (FVC, DLco, and TLC) was worse in the patients with IPF than in the controls, whereas demographics, lung function, and exercise capacity during the 6MWT did not significantly differ between IPF non-survivors and survivors.

Alpha diversity indexes, such as Observed, Chao 1, Shannon, and Inverse Simpson, did not differ between the IPF and control groups (**Supplementary Figure A1**). However, the PCoA plot revealed dissimilarity in the weighted UniFrac distance between the IPF and controls (**Figures 1A–C**), especially between five of the patients with IPF (non-survivors, $n = 3$; **Figures 1A,C** red circles) and controls, indicating more heterogeneity in the microbial distribution.

Among the 10 most frequent taxa, the genus *Ralstonia* was the most prevalent in the IPF and control groups, followed by *Nocardia* and *Pelomonas* (**Supplementary Figure A2**). On the contrary, *Lactobacillus, Enterobacter, Tetragenococcus,* and *Neisseria* were frequently identified in IPF, whereas *Haemophilus, Caulobacter, Bradyrhizobium*, and *Thermomonas* were prevalent in the controls. The relative abundance of *Lactobacillus* (0.91 [IPF] vs. 0.06% [control], $p = 0.009$), *Paracoccus,* (0.13 vs.

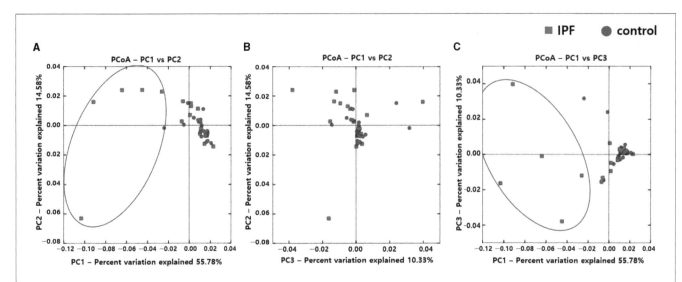

FIGURE 1 | Comparison of principal coordinates analysis using weighted UniFrac method between patients with IPF and controls. Two-dimensional PCoA plots display inter-sample distances by three principal coordinates as PC1 and PC2 **(A)**, PC2 and PC3 **(B)**, and PC1 and PC3 **(C)**. Each dot represents one sample, plotted by a principal component on the X-axis and another principal component on the Y-axis, and colored by the group. The ratio (%) on each axis presents the contribution of values to discrepancies among samples. IPF, idiopathic pulmonary fibrosis; PCoA, principal coordinates analysis.

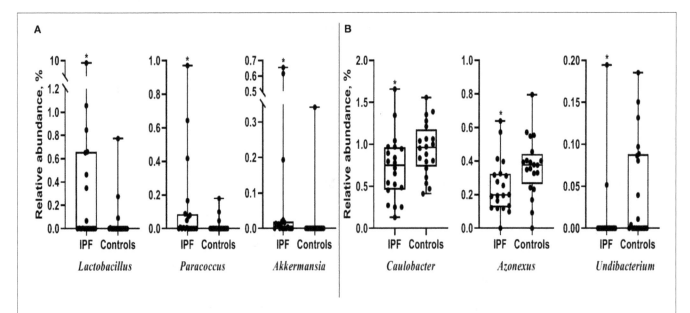

FIGURE 2 | Comparison of relative abundance between patients with IPF and controls. **(A)** Increased and **(B)** decreased in patients with IPF. The box plot shows the minimum, first quartile, median, third quartile, and maximum of relative abundance. *$p < 0.05$. IPF, idiopathic pulmonary fibrosis.

0.02%, $p = 0.013$), and *Akkermansia* (0.08 vs. 0.02%, $p = 0.001$) was higher, whereas that of *Caulobacter* (0.73 vs. 0.95%, $p = 0.040$), *Azonexus* (0.25 vs. 0.37%, $p = 0.021$), and *Undibacterium* (0.01 vs. 0.04%, $p = 0.011$) was lower in patients with IPF than in the controls (**Figure 2**). Logistic analysis adjusted by age and gender independently associated a diagnosis of IPF with lower relative abundance of the genera, *Pelomonas* (OR, 0.352; 95% CI, 0.139–0.891; $p = 0.027$), and *Azonexus* (OR, 0.013; 95% CI, 0.000–0.926; $p = 0.046$; **Table 2**).

Microbial Communities: IPF Non-survivors vs. Survivors

Alpha diversity did not significantly differ between non-survivors and survivors of IPF (**Supplementary Figure A3**). However, the PCoA plot showed that the distribution of microbes differed between non-survivors and survivors (**Figure 3**). Among the 10 most frequent taxa, *Ralstonia* and *Nocardia* were the most common in both groups (**Supplementary Figure A4**). The genus *Streptococcus* was more abundant in non-survivors compared with survivors. In addition, the genera *Neisseria,*

Haemophilus, Rothia, and *Rubrobacter* were frequently detected in non-survivors, while the genera *Tetragenococcus, Enterobacter, Lactobacillus,* and *Caulobacter* were prevalent in survivors. The relative abundance of genera *Bifidobacterium* (2.77 [non-survivors] vs. 0.68% [survivors], $p = 0.003$) and *Olsenella* (0.51 vs. 0.41%, $p = 0.013$) was significantly higher in non-survivors than in survivors (**Figures 4A,B**).

Impact on Survival

The median follow-up period for patients with IPF was 3.0 yr (interquartile range: 1.5–5.4 yr), and the median survival period was 3.1 yr. Unadjusted Cox analysis significantly associated the relative abundance of the *Streptococcus, Sphingomonas, Veillonella,* and *Clostridium* genera with IPF mortality. *Neisseria* and *Granulicatella* were also marginally associated with IPF mortality (**Table 3**). A multivariable model adjusted for age, and FVC selected a higher relative abundance of the *Streptococcus* (HR, 1.993; 95% CI, 1.019–3.901; $p = 0.044$), *Sphingomonas* (HR,

57.590; 95% CI, 1.714–1934.881; $p = 0.024$), and *Clostridium* (HR, 37.189; 95% CI, 1.228–1126.474; $p = 0.038$) genera as independent predictors of IPF mortality.

Association With Disease Severity

The relative abundance of *Curvibacter* and *Thioprofundum* was positively associated with FVC in patients with IPF, whereas *Anoxybacillus, Enterococcus, Akkermansia,* and *Clostridium* negatively correlated with FVC (**Figure 5A** and **Supplementary Table A1**). The relative abundance of *Thermomonas* and *Peptoniphilus* positively correlated with DLco, whereas that of *Granulicatella* and *Rhodoferax* was positively correlated with TLC.

The relative abundance of the *Aquabacterium, Nakamurella,* and *Peptoniphilus* genera was positively correlated, whereas that of the *Fusobacterium, Anaerococcus,* and *Phycicoccus* genera was negatively correlated with distance during the 6MWT (**Figure 5B** and **Supplementary Table A2**). The relative abundance of genus *Rhodoferax* and *Lactococcus* was positively correlated with resting and lowest oxygen saturation (SpO_2) during the 6MWT.

Association With Disease Progression

We estimated the decline rate in lung function and exercise capacity for one yr and compared them between survivors and non-survivors (**Table 4**). Non-survivors had a faster decline rate in DLco, and distance and the lowest SpO_2 during 6MWT compared with survivors. The relative abundance of *Granulicatella* and *Paracoccus* genera was positively correlated, while that of the *Novosphingobium* genus was negatively correlated with the decline rate in FVC (**Figure 6A** and **Supplementary Table A3**). The relative abundance of *Bifidobacterium* was positively associated, whereas *Streptococcus* was negatively associated with the decline rate in DLco.

TABLE 2 | Predictive factors for IPF diagnosis assessed by multivariable logistic regression.

Genus	OR (95% CI)*	P-value
Pelomonas	0.352 (0.139–0.891)	0.027
Dyella	0.277 (0.067–1.139)	0.075
Caulobacter	0.154 (0.021–1.105)	0.063
Lactobacillus	12.881 (0.666–249.192)	0.091
Bradyrhizobium	0.051 (0.002–1.102)	0.058
Azonexus	0.013 (0.000–0.926)	0.046

OR, odds ratio per 1% increase in relative abundance; IPF, idiopathic pulmonary fibrosis.
*Adjusted by age and gender.

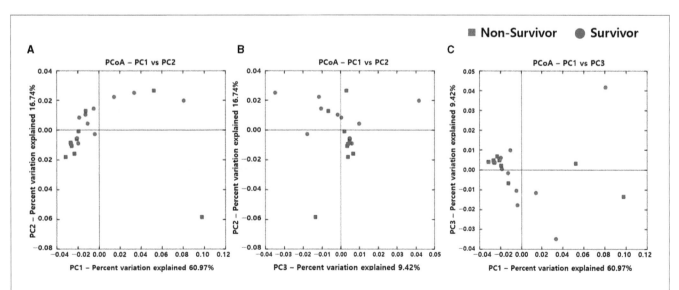

FIGURE 3 | Comparison of principal coordinates analysis outcomes using weighted UniFrac between non-survivors and survivors of IPF. Two-dimensional PCoA plots display inter-sample distances by three principal coordinates as PC1 and PC2 **(A)**, PC2 and PC3 **(B)**, and PC1 and PC3 **(C)**. Each dot represents one sample, plotted by a principal component on the X-axis and another principal component on the Y-axis, and colored by the group. The ratio (%) on each axis presents the contribution of values to discrepancies among samples. IPF, idiopathic pulmonary fibrosis; PCoA, principal coordinates analysis.

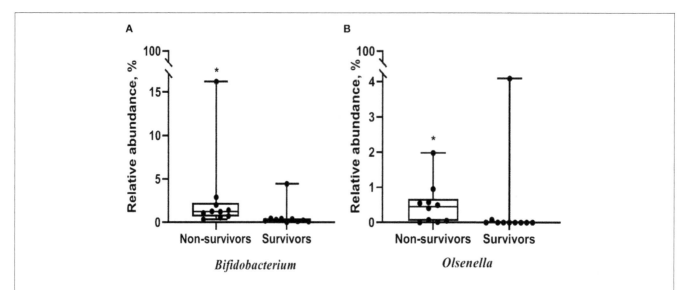

FIGURE 4 | Comparison of relative abundance of microbes between non-survivors and survivors of IPF. **(A)** Genus *Bifidobacterium* **(B)** genus *Olsenella*. The box plot represents minimum, first quartile, median, third quartile, and maximum relative abundance. IPF, idiopathic pulmonary fibrosis. *$p < 0.05$.

TABLE 3 | Risk factors for mortality in patients with IPF assessed using multivariable Cox proportional hazards models.

Genus	Unadjusted		Multivariable*	
	HR (95% CI)	P-value	HR (95% CI)	P-value
Streptococcus	1.389 (1.047–1.842)	0.023	1.993 (1.019–3.901)	0.044
Neisseria	1.500 (0.937–2.400)	0.091	1.500 (0.937–2.400)	0.091
Sphingomonas	57.590 (1.714–1934.881)	0.024	57.590 (1.714–1934.881)	0.024
Veillonella	3.164 (1.026–9.752)	0.045	5.855 (0.821–41.769)	0.078
Granulicatella	14.029 (0.668–294.603)	0.089	14.029 (0.668–294.603)	0.089
Clostridium	37.189 (1.228–1126.474)	0.038	37.189 (1.228–1126.474)	0.038

*CI, confidence interval; HR, hazard ratio. * Adjusted by age and FVC. FVC, forced vital capacity; IPF, idiopathic pulmonary fibrosis.*

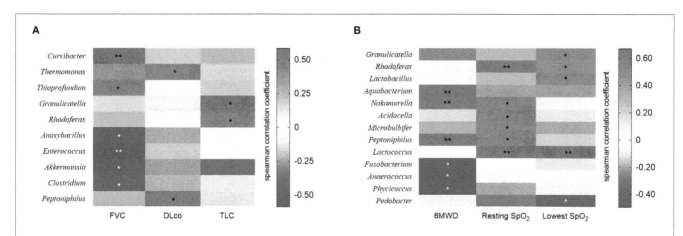

FIGURE 5 | The heatmap showing correlations between relative abundance of bacterial taxa and **(A)** lung function or **(B)** exercise capacity in patients with IPF. Spearman's correlations between the relative abundances of the bacterial genera and lung function and exercise capacity at diagnosis were calculated. Blue: negative correlations; red: positive correlations. *$p < 0.05$, ** $p < 0.01$. DLco, diffusing capacity of the lung for carbon monoxide; FVC, forced vital capacity; IPF, idiopathic pulmonary fibrosis; TLC, total lung capacity. 6MWD, 6-minute walk test distance; SpO$_2$, oxygen saturation.

The relative abundance of *Lactobacillus*, *Staphylococcus*, *Granulicatella*, and *Selenomonas* genera was positively correlated with the decline rate of TLC.

The relative abundance of *Staphylococcus* and *Variovorax* was positively associated, while that of *Legionella*, *Anoxybacillus*, *Acidocella*, and *Hyphomicrobium* genera was negatively associated with the decline rate in distance during 6MWT (**Figure 6B** and **Supplementary Table A4**). The relative abundance of *Beijerinckia*, *Mycobacterium*, and *Microbulbifer* genera was positively correlated, whereas that of *Enterobacter genus was* negatively correlated with the decline rate in resting SpO$_2$. The relative abundance of genus *Staphylococcus* was positively correlated with the lowest SpO$_2$ during 6MWT.

DISCUSSION

The microbial communities in the lung tissues differed between patients with IPF and controls, and between IPF non-survivors and survivors. When adjusted for age and gender, a

decreased relative abundance of genus *Pelomonas* and *Azonexus* was associated with a diagnosis of IPF. A higher relative abundance of the *Streptococcus, Sphingomonas,* and *Clostridium* genera was an independent prognostic factor in patients with IPF and several genera correlated with disease severity and progression.

We found no differences in the alpha diversity of lung tissue microbiomes between patients with IPF and controls, whereas other results of studies of BALF from patients with IPF yielded different results (16, 19). Molineux et al. found a significantly decreased alpha diversity index for the microbiome in BALF samples from 65 patients with IPF at the time of diagnosis (Shannon diversity index, 3.81 ± 0.08 vs. 4.11 ± 0.10; $p = 0.005$) compared with controls ($n = 44$) (16). The Shannon diversity index was also decreased in BALF from mice treated with bleomycin ($n = 6$), compared with control mice ($n = 6$, $p < 0.05$) (19). These contradictory findings could be attributed to differences in baseline demographics and treatment of the subjects in a previous study (16); there were differences in age (68 [IPF] vs. 58.2 years [controls], $p < 0.0001$) and inhaled steroid therapy (6.2 vs. 0.0%, $p = $ not significant) between IPF and controls, and these might affect differences in alpha diversity in microbiome. Our findings were in line with those of Kitsios et al. who identified separate clusters on PCoA plots of Bray-Curtis dissimilarity distances among explanted lung tissues from patients with IPF (n = 40), cystic fibrosis ($n = 5$), and donors ($n = 7$) (22).

The relative abundance of *Lactobacillus* was increased in lung tissues from patients with IPF compared with controls. *Lactobacillus* generally resides in the gastrointestinal and reproductive tract, where it maintains a healthy microecology with lactic acid production (38, 39). However, given the well-known association between IPF and gastroesophageal reflux disease (GERD) (40), the high prevalence of GERD in IPF might contribute to the increase in the relative abundance of *Lactobacillus* in IPF. Moreover, Harata et al.

TABLE 4 | Comparison of changes in lung function and exercise capacity between the survivors and non-survivors among patients with IPF.

	Total	Survivors	Non-survivors
FVC %predicted/year	−0.01 ± 0.04	0.00 ± 0.38	−0.02 ± 0.47
DLco %predicted/year	−0.03 ± 0.05	0.00 ± 0.03	−0.05 ± 0.05*
TLC %predicted/year	0.00 ± 0.04	0.00 ± 0.02	0.00 ± 0.06
6MWD, meter/year	−0.27 ± 0.47	−0.03 ± 0.23	−0.51 ± 0.53*
Resting SpO$_2$, %/year	0.00 ± 0.02	0.00 ± 0.01	0.00 ± 0.02
Lowest SpO$_2$, %/year	−0.01 ± 0.02	0.00 ± 0.02	−0.02 ± 0.02*

*Data are presented as means ± standard, unless otherwise indicated. 6MWT, 6-min walk test; DLco, diffusing capacity of the lungs for carbon monoxide; FVC, forced vital capacity; IPF, idiopathic pulmonary fibrosis; PFT, pulmonary function test; SpO$_2$, peripheral oxygen saturation; TLC, total lung capacity; 6MWD, 6-min walk test distance. *p < 0.05 (survivors vs. non-survivors).*

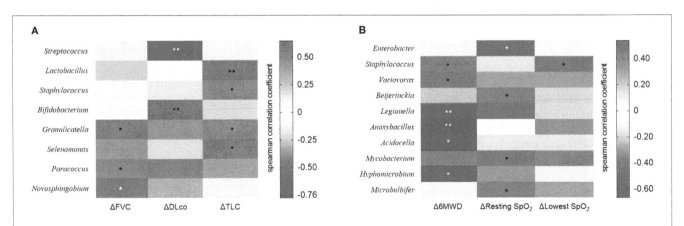

FIGURE 6 | The heatmap showing correlations between relative abundance of bacterial taxa and **(A)** changes in lung function or **(B)** exercise capacity in patients with IPF. Spearman's correlations between the relative abundances of the bacterial genera and decline rate in lung function and exercise capacity for 1 year after diagnosis were calculated. Blue: negative correlations; red: positive correlations. *p < 0.05, ** p < 0.01. DLco, diffusing capacity of the lung for carbon monoxide; FVC, forced vital capacity; IPF, idiopathic pulmonary fibrosis; TLC, total lung capacity. 6MWD, 6-minute walk test distance; SpO$_2$, oxygen saturation; Δ, decline rate for 1 year.

found the increased expression of the mRNA for interleukin-1, tumor necrosis factor, and monocyte chemotactic protein-1 in the respiratory tracts of mice infected with influenza and treated with intranasal *Lactobacillus rhamnosus* than in infected and untreated mice (41). Since proinflammatory cytokines and chemokines are associated with the pathogenesis of IPF (42), the immunoregulatory effect of *Lactobacillus* might contribute to the pathophysiology of IPF. We found a higher relative abundance of *Bifidobacterium* in IPF non-survivors than survivors. *Bifidobacterium* can also produce lactic acid (43, 44), along with *Lactobacillus*. Levels of lactic acid and lactate dehydrogenase-5, which induce the differentiation of fibroblasts into myofibroblasts by activating transforming growth factor (TGF)-ß1, were elevated in lung tissues from patients with IPF ($n = 6$), compared with healthy persons ($n = 6$) (45). Therefore, bacteria that produce lactic acid might also contribute to the progression of IPF.

We independently associated a higher relative abundance of the *Streptococcus* genus with IPF mortality, which is in line with the previous reports (21, 46–48). The COMET-IPF study of 55 patients with IPF found that a higher relative abundance of *Streptococcus* OTU was an independent prognostic factor for disease progression (HR, 1.11; 95% CI, 1.04–1.18; $p = 0.0009$) according to a multivariable Cox proportional hazard analysis adjusted for age, gender, smoking status, and desaturation during the 6MWT (21). Infection with *Streptococcus pneumoniae* significantly increased hydroxyproline levels in lung tissues from mouse models of TGFß1-induced lung fibrosis compared with mock infection (46). In addition, fibrosis and collagen deposition were increased in lung tissues from mice treated with both bleomycin and *Streptococcus pneumoniae* serotype 3 compared with mice that were either treated with bleomycin or infected with *Streptococcus pneumoniae* (48). These results suggested that *Streptococcus* infection could induce IPF disease progression. Furthermore, lung vascular permeability and neutrophil and monocytes counts were increased in BALF from mice treated with pneumolysin (47), which is a pore-forming cytotoxin released by *Streptococcus pneumoniae* that causes alveolar epithelial injury (47).

In this study, the relative abundance of the *Anoxybacillus* genus in IPF lung tissues was correlated with IPF disease severity. The relative abundance of the *Firmicutes* phylum was inversely correlated with FVC in BALF samples from 34 patients with IPF ($r = -0.5514$, $p = 0.0007$) (19). Our results are consistent with these findings because *Anoxybacillus* belongs to the *Firmicutes* phylum and is negatively correlated with FVC. Another study also found an increased relative abundance of *Firmicutes* in BALF from mice treated with bleomycin (19), suggesting that an increased prevalence of the *Anoxybacillus* genus is associated with the pathogenesis of IPF.

This study had some limitations. Although we matched the baseline characteristics, such as age and sex between the IPF and control groups, other confounding factors might have affected the microbial communities. However, we tried not to include patients who had been treated with agents that might affect the microbiota. The number of samples analyzed was not large. Nevertheless, we identified significant differences in the distribution and clinical impact of the microbiomes of patients with IPF compared with controls. Because non-malignant and non-fibrotic lung tissues from lung cancer patients were used as controls, the microbial community in the control group might be affected by lung cancer. However, in studies of lung tissue microbiome of other diseases, it is common to use normal tissue of lung cancer tissue as normal control (49, 50). Even in lung tissue microbiome studies in lung cancer patients, non-cancer tissue from the lung cancer patient was used as a control (50). The cross-sectional design of this study prevented the identification of causal relationships between changes in microbial communities and IPF development. Additional long-term clinical studies should address this issue. Despite these limitations, the strength of our study is that we first revealed the microbial communities in lung tissues from patients when they were initially diagnosed with IPF and the impact of these communities on their survival.

In conclusion, our finding suggests that specific microbial communities in lung tissues from patients with IPF and associations between the relative abundance of some genera and clinical parameters, such as diagnosis, mortality, disease severity, and progression in such patients, imply microbial communities in the lungs play roles in the pathogenesis of IPF.

ETHICS STATEMENT

The studies involving human participants were reviewed and approved by Institutional Review Board of Asan Medical Center (2018-1096). Written informed consent for participation was not required for this study in accordance with the national legislation and the institutional requirements.

AUTHOR CONTRIBUTIONS

JS was the guarantor of the manuscript for designing and supervising the entire study. H-YY and JS took responsibility for the data analysis. S-JM contributed to sample collection and preparation. H-YY and JS drafted the initial manuscript. All the authors discussed the results and reviewed the manuscript.

and Technology (NRF-2019R1A2C2008541), South Korea. The sponsor had no role in the design of the study, the collection and analysis of the data, or the preparation of the manuscript.

ACKNOWLEDGMENTS

We would like to thank Jin-Woo Bae (Kyunghee University, Seoul, South Korea) and Wonyoung Kim (Chung-Ang University, Seoul, South Korea) for their expert advice on interpreting results.

REFERENCES

1. Raghu G, Collard HR, Egan JJ, Martinez FJ, Behr J, Brown KK, et al. An official ATS/ERS/JRS/ALAT statement: idiopathic pulmonary fibrosis: evidence-based guidelines for diagnosis and management. *Am J Respir Crit Care Med.* (2011) 183:788–824. doi: 10.1164/rccm.2009-040GL

2. Baratella E, Ruaro B, Giudici F, Wade B, Santagiuliana M, Salton F, et al. Evaluation of correlations between genetic variants and high-resolution computed tomography patterns in idiopathic pulmonary fibrosis. *Diagnostics.* (2021) 11:762. doi: 10.3390/diagnostics11050762

3. Evans CM, Fingerlin TE, Schwarz MI, Lynch D, Kurche J, Warg L, et al. Idiopathic pulmonary fibrosis: a genetic disease that involves mucociliary dysfunction of the peripheral airways. *Physiol Rev.* (2016) 96:1567–91. doi: 10.1152/physrev.00004.2016

4. Chambers RC, Mercer PF. Mechanisms of alveolar epithelial injury, repair, and fibrosis. *Ann Am Thorac Soc.* (2015) 12:S16–20. doi: 10.1513/AnnalsATS.201410-448MG

5. Wolters PJ, Collard HR, Jones KD. Pathogenesis of idiopathic pulmonary fibrosis. *Annu Rev Pathol.* (2014) 9:157–79. doi: 10.1146/annurev-pathol-012513-104706

6. Salton F, Ruaro B, Confalonieri P, Confalonieri M. Epithelial-mesenchymal transition: a major pathogenic driver in idiopathic pulmonary fibrosis? *Medicina.* (2020) 56:608. doi: 10.3390/medicina56110608

7. Kaur A, Mathai SK, Schwartz DA. Genetics in idiopathic pulmonary fibrosis pathogenesis, prognosis, and treatment. *Front Med.* (2017) 4:154. doi: 10.3389/fmed.2017.00154

8. Yonemaru M, Kasuga I, Kusumoto H, Kunisawa A, Kiyokawa H, Kuwabara S, et al. Elevation of antibodies to cytomegalovirus and other herpes viruses in pulmonary fibrosis. *Eur Respir J.* (1997) 10:2040–5. doi: 10.1183/09031936.97.10092040

9. Vergnon JM, Vincent M, de The G, Mornex JF, Weynants P, Brune J. Cryptogenic fibrosing alveolitis and Epstein-Barr virus: an association? *Lancet.* (1984) 2:768–71. doi: 10.1016/S0140-6736(84)90702-5

10. Bando M, Ohno S, Oshikawa K, Takahashi M, Okamoto H, Sugiyama Y. Infection of TT virus in patients with idiopathic pulmonary fibrosis. *Respir Med.* (2001) 95:935–42. doi: 10.1053/rmed.2001.1151

11. Ueda T, Ohta K, Suzuki N, Yamaguchi M, Hirai K, Horiuchi T, et al. Idiopathic pulmonary fibrosis and high prevalence of serum antibodies to hepatitis C virus. *Am Rev Respir Dis.* (1992) 146:266–8. doi: 10.1164/ajrccm/146.1.266

12. Moore BB, Moore TA. Viruses in idiopathic pulmonary fibrosis. *Etiol Exacerbat Ann Am Thorac Soc.* (2015) 12:S186–92. doi: 10.1513/AnnalsATS.201502-088AW

13. Wootton SC, Kim DS, Kondoh Y, Chen E, Lee JS, Song JW, et al. Viral infection in acute exacerbation of idiopathic pulmonary fibrosis. *Am J Respir Crit Care Med.* (2011) 183:1698–702. doi: 10.1164/rccm.201010-1752OC

14. Raghu G, Anstrom KJ, King TE. Jr., Lasky JA, Martinez FJ. Prednisone, azathioprine, and N-acetylcysteine for pulmonary fibrosis. *New Engl J Med.* (2012) 366:1968–77. doi: 10.1056/NEJMoa1113354

15. Janda JM, Abbott SL. 16S rRNA gene sequencing for bacterial identification in the diagnostic laboratory: pluses, perils, and pitfalls. *J Clin Microbiol.* (2007) 45:2761–4. doi: 10.1128/JCM.01228-07

16. Molyneaux PL, Cox MJ, Willis-Owen SA, Mallia P, Russell KE, Russell AM, et al. The role of bacteria in the pathogenesis and progression of idiopathic pulmonary fibrosis. *Am J Respir Crit Care Med.* (2014) 190:906–13. doi: 10.1164/rccm.201403-0541OC

17. Garzoni C, Brugger SD, Qi W, Wasmer S, Cusini A, Dumont P, et al. Microbial communities in the respiratory tract of patients with interstitial lung disease. *Thorax.* (2013) 68:1150–6. doi: 10.1136/thoraxjnl-2012-202917

18. Friaza V, la Horra C, Rodriguez-Dominguez MJ, Martin-Juan J, Canton R, Calderon EJ, et al. Metagenomic analysis of bronchoalveolar lavage samples from patients with idiopathic interstitial pneumonia and its antagonic relation with Pneumocystis jirovecii colonization. *J Microbiol Methods.* (2010) 82:98–101. doi: 10.1016/j.mimet.2010.03.026

19. Takahashi Y, Saito A, Chiba H, Kuronuma K, Ikeda K, Kobayashi T, et al. Impaired diversity of the lung microbiome predicts progression of idiopathic pulmonary fibrosis. *Respir Res.* (2018) 19:34. doi: 10.1186/s12931-018-0736-9

20. Molyneaux PL, Cox MJ, Wells AU, Kim HC, Ji W, Cookson WO, et al. Changes in the respiratory microbiome during acute exacerbations of idiopathic pulmonary fibrosis. *Respir Res.* (2017) 18:29. doi: 10.1186/s12931-017-0511-3

21. Han MK, Zhou Y, Murray S, Tayob N, Noth I, Lama VN, et al. Lung microbiome and disease progression in idiopathic pulmonary fibrosis: an analysis of the COMET study. *Lancet Respir Med.* (2014) 2:548–56. doi: 10.1016/S2213-2600(14)70069-4

22. Kitsios GD, Rojas M, Kass DJ, Fitch A, Sembrat JC, Qin S, et al. Microbiome in lung explants of idiopathic pulmonary fibrosis: a case-control study in patients with end-stage fibrosis. *Thorax.* (2018) 73:481–4. doi: 10.1136/thoraxjnl-2017-210537

23. Wanger J, Clausen JL, Coates A, Pedersen OF, Brusasco V, Burgos F, et al. Standardisation of the measurement of lung volumes. *Eur Respir J.* (2005) 26:511–22. doi: 10.1183/09031936.05.00035005

24. Miller MR, Hankinson J, Brusasco V, Burgos F, Casaburi R, Coates A, et al. Standardisation of spirometry. *Eur Respir J.* (2005) 26:319–38. doi: 10.1183/09031936.05.00034805

25. Macintyre N, Crapo RO, Viegi G, Johnson DC, van der Grinten CP, Brusasco V, et al. Standardisation of the single-breath determination of carbon monoxide uptake in the lung. *Eur Respir J.* (2005) 26:720–35. doi: 10.1183/09031936.05.00034905

26. Holland AE, Spruit MA, Troosters T, Puhan MA, Pepin V, Saey D, et al. An official European Respiratory Society/American Thoracic Society technical standard: field walking tests in chronic respiratory disease. *Eur Respir J.* (2014) 44:1428–46. doi: 10.1183/09031936.00150314

27. Klindworth A, Pruesse E, Schweer T, Peplies J, Quast C, Horn M, et al. Evaluation of general 16S ribosomal RNA gene PCR primers for classical and next-generation sequencing-based diversity studies. *Nucleic Acids Res.* (2013) 41:e1. doi: 10.1093/nar/gks808

28. Kozich JJ, Westcott SL, Baxter NT, Highlander SK, Schloss PD. Development of a dual-index sequencing strategy and curation pipeline for analyzing amplicon sequence data on the MiSeq Illumina sequencing platform. *Appl Environ Microbiol.* (2013) 79:5112–20. doi: 10.1128/AEM.01043-13

29. Fadrosh DW, Ma B, Gajer P, Sengamalay N, Ott S, Brotman RM, et al. An improved dual-indexing approach for multiplexed 16S rRNA gene sequencing on the Illumina MiSeq platform. *Microbiome.* (2014) 2:6. doi: 10.1186/2049-2618-2-6

30. Magoc T, Salzberg SL, FLASH. fast length adjustment of short reads to improve genome assemblies. *Bioinformatics.* (2011) 27:2957–63. doi: 10.1093/bioinformatics/btr507

31. Li W, Fu L, Niu B, Wu S, Wooley J. Ultrafast clustering algorithms for metagenomic sequence analysis. *Brief Bioinform.* (2012) 13:656–68. doi: 10.1093/bib/bbs035

32. Schloss PD, Westcott SL, Ryabin T, Hall JR, Hartmann M, Hollister EB, et al. Introducing mothur: open-source, platform-independent, community-supported software for describing and comparing microbial communities. *Appl Environ Microbiol.* (2009) 75:7537–41. doi: 10.1128/AEM.01541-09

33. Caporaso JG, Kuczynski J, Stombaugh J, Bittinger K, Bushman FD, Costello EK, et al. QIIME allows analysis of high-throughput community sequencing data. *Nat Methods.* (2010) 7:335. doi: 10.1038/nmeth.f.303

34. Gotelli NJ. Colwell RKJBdfim, assessment. *Estimat Species Richness.* (2011) 12:35. doi: 10.1080/14452294.2011.11649538

35. Magurran AE. *Measuring Biological Diversity.* John Wiley & Sons (2013). p. 108–9.

36. Lande R. Statistics and partitioning of species diversity, and similarity among multiple communities. *Oikos.* (1996) 1996:5–13. doi: 10.2307/3545743

37. Lozupone C, Lladser ME, Knights D, Stombaugh J, Knight R. UniFrac: an effective distance metric for microbial community comparison. *ISME J.* (2011) 5:169–72. doi: 10.1038/ismej.2010.133

38. Aroutcheva A, Gariti D, Simon M, Shott S, Faro J, Simoes JA, et al. Defense factors of vaginal lactobacilli. *Am J Obstet Gynecol.* (2001) 185:375–9. doi: 10.1067/mob.2001.115867

39. Walter J. Ecological role of lactobacilli in the gastrointestinal tract: implications for fundamental and biomedical research. *Appl Environ Microbiol.* (2008) 74:4985–96. doi: 10.1128/AEM.00753-08

40. Raghu G, Freudenberger TD, Yang S, Curtis JR, Spada C, Hayes J, et al. High prevalence of abnormal acid gastro-oesophageal reflux in idiopathic pulmonary fibrosis. *Eur Respir J.* (2006) 27:136–42. doi: 10.1183/09031936.06.00037005

41. Harata G, He F, Hiruta N, Kawase M, Kubota A, Hiramatsu M, et al. Intranasal

administration of Lactobacillus rhamnosus GG protects mice from H1N1 influenza virus infection by regulating respiratory immune responses. *Lett Appl Microbiol.* (2010) 50:597–602. doi: 10.1111/j.1472-765X.2010.02844.x

42. Agostini C, Gurrieri C. Chemokine/cytokine cocktail in idiopathic pulmonary fibrosis. *Proc Am Thorac Soc.* (2006) 3:357–63. doi: 10.1513/pats.200601-010TK

43. Van der Meulen R, Adriany T, Verbrugghe K, De Vuyst LJAEM. Kinetic analysis of bifidobacterial metabolism reveals a minor role for succinic acid in the regeneration of NAD+ through its growth-associated production. *Appl Environ Microbiol.* (2006) 72:5204–10. doi: 10.1128/AEM.00146-06

44. Smith SM, Eng RH, Buccini F. Use of D-lactic acid measurements in the diagnosis of bacterial infections. *J Infect Dis.* (1986) 154:658–64. doi: 10.1093/infdis/154.4.658

45. Kottmann RM, Kulkarni AA, Smolnycki KA, Lyda E, Dahanayake T, Salibi R, et al. Lactic acid is elevated in idiopathic pulmonary fibrosis and induces myofibroblast differentiation via pH-dependent activation of transforming growth factor-beta. *Am J Respir Crit Care Med.* (2012) 186:740–51. doi: 10.1164/rccm.201201-0084OC

46. Knippenberg S, Ueberberg B, Maus R, Bohling J, Ding N, Tort Tarres M, et al. Streptococcus pneumoniae triggers progression of pulmonary fibrosis through pneumolysin. *Thorax.* (2015) 70:636–46. doi: 10.1136/thoraxjnl-2014-206420

47. Maus UA, Srivastava M, Paton JC, Mack M, Everhart MB, Blackwell TS, et al. Pneumolysin-induced lung injury is independent of leukocyte trafficking into the alveolar space. *J Immunol.* (2004) 173:1307–12. doi: 10.4049/jimmunol.173.2.1307

48. Cho SJ, Moon JS, Nikahira K, Yun HS, Harris R, Hong KS, et al. GLUT1-dependent glycolysis regulates exacerbation of fibrosis via AIM2 inflammasome activation. *Thorax.* (2020) 75:227–36. doi: 10.1136/thoraxjnl-2019-213571

49. Sze MA, Dimitriu PA, Hayashi S, Elliott WM, McDonough JE, Gosselink JV, et al. The lung tissue microbiome in chronic obstructive pulmonary disease. *Am J Respir Crit Care Med.* (2012) 185:1073–80. doi: 10.1164/rccm.201111-2075OC

50. Greathouse KL, White JR, Vargas AJ, Bliskovsky VV, Beck JA, von Muhlinen N, et al. Interaction between the microbiome and TP53 in human lung cancer. *Genome Biol.* (2018) 19:123. doi: 10.1186/s13059-018-1501-6

18

Lung Involvement in Primary Sjögren's Syndrome—An Under-Diagnosed Entity

Georgios Sogkas [1†], Stefanie Hirsch [1†], Karen Maria Olsson [2,3], Jan B. Hinrichs [4],
Thea Thiele [1], Tabea Seeliger [5], Thomas Skripuletz [5], Reinhold Ernst Schmidt [1],
Torsten Witte [1], Alexandra Jablonka [1†] and Diana Ernst [1*†]

[1] Department of Immunology and Rheumatology, Medical School Hannover, Hanover, Germany, [2] Department of Respiratory Medicine, Hannover Medical School, Hanover, Germany, [3] BREATH German Centre for Lung Research (DZL), Hanover, Germany, [4] Department of Diagnostic and Interventional Radiology, Hannover Medical School, Hanover, Germany, [5] Department of Neurology, Hannover Medical School, Hanover, Germany

*Correspondence:
Diana Ernst
ernst.diana@mh-hannover.de

† These authors have contributed equally to this work

Interstitial lung disease (ILD) represents a frequent extra-glandular manifestation of primary Sjögren's Syndrome (pSS). Limited published data regarding phenotyping and treatment exists. Advances in managing specific ILD phenotypes have not been comprehensively explored in patients with coexisting pSS. This retrospective study aimed to phenotype lung diseases occurring in a well-described pSS-ILD cohort and describe treatment course and outcomes. Between April 2018 and February 2020, all pSS patients attending our Outpatient clinic were screened for possible lung involvement. Clinical, laboratory and high-resolution computed tomography (HRCT) findings were analyzed. Patients were classified according to HRCT findings into five groups: usual interstitial pneumonia (UIP), non-specific interstitial pneumonia (NSIP), desquamative interstitial pneumonia (DIP), combined pulmonary fibrosis and emphysema (CPFE), and non-specific-ILD. Lung involvement was confirmed in 31/268 pSS patients (13%). One-third (10/31) of pSS-ILD patients were Ro/SSA antibody negative. ILD at pSS diagnosis was present in 19/31 (61%) patients. The commonest phenotype was UIP $n = 13$ (43%), followed by NSIP $n = 9$ (29%), DIP $n = 2$ (6 %), CPFE $n = 2$ (6 %), and non-specific-ILD $n = 5$ (16%). Forced vital capacity (FVC) and carbon monoxide diffusion capacity (D_{LCO}) appeared lower in UIP and DIP, without reaching a significant difference. Treatment focused universally on intensified immunosuppression, with 13/31 patients (42%) receiving cyclophosphamide. No anti-fibrotic treatments were used. Median follow-up was 38.2 [12.4–119.6] months. Lung involvement in pSS is heterogeneous. Better phenotyping and tailored treatment may improve outcomes and requires further evaluation in larger prospective studies.

Keywords: interstitial lung disease (ILD), lung fibrosis, sicca syndrome, ESSDAI—EULAR Sjögren's Syndrome Disease Activity Index, Sjögren's Syndrome (SS)

INTRODUCTION

Primary Sjögren's Syndrome (pSS) is an increasingly recognized autoimmune disease, primarily affecting secretory gland tissue. Its prevalence is estimated at ~60 cases per 1,00,000 population. The clinical hallmarks are xerophthalmia and xerostomia, however ~30–50% of patients will develop extra-glandular manifestations in a variety of organ systems (1, 2). Lung involvement is relatively common, affecting 9–22% and confers major adverse effects on both life quality and mortality, resulting in a 4-fold increase in 10 years mortality (3, 4).

Lung involvement typically presents with exertional dyspnea and a persisting dry cough. Pulmonary function testing (PFT) is recommended, commonly revealing a reduced carbon monoxide lung diffusion capacity (D_{LCO}), and a disproportional loss in forced vital capacity (FVC) (5–7). Abnormalities may be apparent on a standard chest x-ray (CXR), but their absence should not discourage further evaluation for interstitial lung disease (ILD). Pulmonary symptoms can be the first manifestation of pSS. Nannini et al. reported on 105 pSS patients, 10% of whom displayed respiratory manifestations at diagnosis or within the 1st year. At 5 years, prevalence had risen to 20% (+/– 4%) (8). Dry cough was the predominating symptom, affecting 41–61% of patients, with higher than anticipated rates for respiratory infections and pneumonia at 10–35% (3, 9).

Efforts have been made to characterize the relationship between various pSS and interstitial lung diseases, with emphasis upon idiopathic pulmonary fibrosis (IPF). HRCT has been advocated, with a recent systematic evaluation in 527 unselected pSS patients confirming significant interstitial lung changes in 39%. By far the commonest pattern of involvement was non-specific interstitial pneumonia (NSIP), which was observed in 42% of those affected. Usual interstitial pneumonia (UIP), similar in character to IPF, occurred in 11%. Organizing pneumonia (OP) and lymphocytic interstitial pneumonia (LIP) both accounted for <4% of cases. In 82 patients (40%), mixed disease patterns were observed on HRCT (4). The commonest recognized entity is combined pulmonary fibrosis and emphysema (CPFE), which typically consists of upper lobe pan-lobular lung emphysema and basal interstitial features similar to UIP. Usually occurring in smokers, it has also been observed in never smokers (5). LIP has been reported in 10–15% of pSS ILD cases. HRCT imaging reveals thickening of broncho-vascular bundles and interlobular septa, as well as interstitial nodules, ground-glass opacities, and cysts in up to 82% (6, 7, 10).

Within pSS cohorts, ILD has traditionally been linked to smoking, older age, hypergammaglobulinemia, increased rheumatoid factor (RF), or antinuclear antibody titers, anti-SSA or -SSB antibody positivity, elevated C-reactive protein (CRP), and reduced serum C3 levels (10–13). Regarding treatment for pSS ILD, few studies have considered the nature of lung involvement when evaluating efficacy of immunosuppressive drugs, with most being derived from case studies. Corticosteroids together with azathioprine or cyclophosphamide are common in treating pSS-ILD. Many patients, particularly those with UIP, do not appear to benefit from this approach (14–16). Rituximab has been suggested as a universal agent to control pSS-ILD irrespective of form, but data from large studies remains elusive (17).

There is little published information regarding ILD and the typical pSS serological markers and disease activity. No data exists for correlations between biomarkers and the ILD response to immunosuppressive regiments. The primary aim of this study was to systematically evaluate the incidence and characterize ILD phenotype in a well-defined pSS-ILD cohort and summarize

outcomes in terms of survival, pulmonary function, serial HRCT scans and response to treatment.

METHODS

Study Design

A retrospective observational cohort study at a single tertiary care institution was performed.

Setting

Patients were recruited *a priori* from attendances at both the Rheumatology or Pulmonology outpatient departments of Hannover Medical School between April 2018 and February 2020. Preliminary clinical screening involved identifying patients with new-onset persisting cough and/or exertional dyspnoea New York Heart Association (NYHA) ≥2 associated with any combination of sicca symptoms, myalgia and/or arthralgia or already known patients with pSS and ILD. Patients fulfilling clinical criteria underwent PFT and assessment of various serum markers for autoimmune disease. Based upon these findings, patients suspected of having ILD were referred for HRCT chest imaging in keeping with EULAR Sjögren's syndrome disease activity score (ESSDAI) recommendations (11). Patients fulfilling diagnostic criteria for pSS without pathological lung function and/or imaging formed the control group (**Figure S1**). All study participants provided written informed consent and the study received Institutional Review Board approval by Hannover Medical School (8179_BO_S_2018).

Participants

Diagnosis of pulmonary involvement in pSS reflected American College Rheumatology (ACR) and European League Against Rheumatism (EULAR) criteria (12), with a minimum score of 10, which includes shortness of breath or dry cough accompanying abnormal PFT or pathological findings on HRCT scans. pSS classification criteria were applied to all patients reporting either dry eyes or mouth, or those fulfilling at least one positive domain of the ESSDAI with suspected pSS (ESSDAI) (11).

ESSDAI score was calculated for all patients with lung involvement. pSS criteria were met if the combined score for the following items was ≥4: focal lymphocytic sialadenitis and focus score ≥1 (three points) in the labial minor salivary gland biopsy (13), positive anti-SSA (Ro) antibodies (three points), Schirmer test ≤ 5 mm/5 min in at least one eye, or stimulated whole saliva flow rate increase in weight <2.75 g/2 min (one point). In our institute the Saxon test continues to be used to measure xerostomy. It is defined as a stimulated salivary flow test, an increase in weight <2.75 g/2 min is defined as pathological (14). Stimulated and unstimulated salivary flow tests seem to be comparable (15) and the stimulated salivary flow test is still recommended by EULAR in their latest pSS management recommendations (16). Patients presenting with secondary Sjögren's syndrome or possible secondary Sjögren's syndrome with overlap to dermatomyositis or scleroderma were excluded of the study.

Regarding peripheral neuropathy, the same criteria as in a recently published pSS cohort were used (2). All patients underwent Saxon and Schirmer tests, as well as testing for Ro52 and Ro60 antibodies, which were measured quantitatively using EliA by Thermo Fisher (Freiburg, device Phadia250). Patients with one positive test and suspected pSS, underwent a labial minor salivary gland biopsy. Biopsies exhibiting focal lymphocytic sialadenitis with a focus score ≥1, were considered diagnostic of pSS. Patients with biopsies revealing a focus score of <1 did not meet the classification criteria for pSS, and were excluded from the study.

Variables

Analyses of PFT, HRCT, ESSDAI score, and diagnostic criteria were collated. Furthermore, all treatments for pSS-ILD was documented.

Data Collection

Non-contrast, HRCT scans were performed using volumetric acquisition, with thin-section reconstruction using maximum 1.5 mm slices, as recommended in the American Thoracic Society/European Respiratory Society (ATS/ERS) guidelines (17). Images were reviewed by a blinded thoracic radiologist, and classified according to Fleischner Society criteria for interstitial lung disease (18, 19).

PFTs were performed on all patients in a dedicated laboratory, consisting of either standard spirometry or body plethysmography in cases with FVC loss suspected of having restrictive ventilatory defects. Diffusion capacity was measured using single-breath determination of carbon monoxide uptake. All tests were performed according to ATS/ERS guidelines (20–22) and results interpreted by blinded pulmonologists. In case of abnormal FVC and or low diffusion capacity (DLCO) chest X-ray (CXR) and in 36 cases HRCT of the chest were performed. Only patients with pathological HRCT scans were included into the analyses.

Follow up PFTs were considered improved if they increased ≥10% of level at treatment initiation, or progressive disease if they decreased ≥10% over treatment baseline. Values remaining between ±10% corridor of baseline were considered stable.

Participants completed a structured questionnaire regarding symptoms, including EULAR Sjögren's syndrome patient reported index (ESSPRI). Furthermore, Saxon and Schirmer tests, salivatory gland biopsy, if necessary, as well as diagnostic work up for ESSDAI scoring were performed (11). In keeping with routine departmental protocols, all clinical and diagnostic data were prospectively archived in a customized Microsoft® Access database (Microsoft Corporation, Redmond, WA, USA).

Statistical Analysis

Descriptive statistics were calculated using R version 3.6.0 (Foundation for Statistical Computing, Vienna, Austria) in conjunction with "Hmisc" (Frank E. Harrell Jr. (2020). Hmisc: Harrell Miscellaneous. R package version 4.3-1.), "dplyr" (Hadley Wickeam, Romain Fracois, Lionel Henry, and Kirill Müller (2020). Dplyr: A Grammar of Data Manipulation. R package version 0.8.5.) and "ggplot2" (H. Wickam. ggplot2: Elegant graphics for data analysis. Springer-Verlag New York, 2016)

packages. To compare age of pSS onset between ILD and non-ILD controls, a non-parametric age distribution was assumed and a two-sided Wilcoxon signed-rank test was used, $p < 0.05$ were considered statistically significant. Values reported are median [inter-quartile range] unless otherwise reported.

RESULTS

Two-hundred and sixty-eight patients with pSS were identified, of whom 51/268 had clinical symptoms like dry cough or shortness of breath. All symptomatic patients underwent PFT, 36/51 had pathological findings defined as FVC ≤ 80% predicted and/or DLCO ≤ 70% predicted. HRCTs were performed on all 36 patients. Of these, 31/36 (86%) exhibited pathological findings possibly related to pSS. Five patients had no changes suggestive of ILD and were excluded from the analysis. In total 31/268 (13%) pSS patients had ILD. Demographics for pSS-ILD patients are summarized in **Table 1**. The majority of patients were never-smoking females, presenting in their seventh decade. All were Caucasian. Compared to non-ILD patients ($n = 237$), pSS-ILD patients were significantly older (59.0 [50.4–68.5] vs. 53.3 [40.9–63.9] years; Wilcoxon Rank Sum $p = 0.0044$, **Figure 1**) at time of pSS diagnoses. Median follow-up was 38.2 [12.4–119.6] months.

At ILD diagnosis, the median ESSDAI was 19.0 [14.3–24.8]. After lung involvement, the most common domains of disease activity were hematological (15/31, 48%), joints (12/31, 39%), and biological (9/31, 29%). The latter derived from hypergammaglobulinemia and or hypocomplementemia or presence of cryoglobulinemia. In nine patients (29%), both the Saxon and Schirmer tests were pathological, with one or other being positive in 22/31 patients (71%). Of the 10 SSA (Ro)-antibody negative patients (31%), whilst half were also Saxon test negative all had salivary gland biopsies ≥ Chisholm Mason grade 3. Four patients without objective xeropthalmia and xerostomia were diagnosed with pSS due to positive anti-SSA(Ro) antibodies and focal sialadenitis.

At ILD diagnosis PFTs demonstrated impaired ventilation and diffusion in almost all patients, with median forced vital capacity (FVC) being 65 [52–88]% predicted and median DLCO of 48 [41–80]% predicted. Patients demonstrating UIP and in particular desquamative interstitial pneumonia (DIP) were most severely affected with FVC of 60 [−46-65]% predicted and 50 [45–55]% predicted at diagnosis, along with DLCO of 53 [36–71]% predicted, and 35 [29–41]% predicted respectively (**Table 2**).

Analysis of the CT imaging revealed that UIP was the predominating pattern of disease ($n = 13$, 42%), with NSIP also proving common ($n = 9$, 29%). Similar numbers of the much more aggressive DIP and multi-factorial CPFE were observed (both $n = 2$, 6%).

The remaining five patients exhibited various different patterns of lung involvement including bronchiectasis, tree in bud phenomena suggestive of bronchiolitis, and in one patient cystic changes suggestive of LIP. Due to the small numbers these cases were amalgamated into non-specific disease for the purposes of analysis (**Figure 2**).

TABLE 1 | Summary of patient demographics.

Cohort demographics (*n* = 31)		
Female, *n* (%)	22	(71)
Never smoking, *n* (%)	23	(74)
Initial manifestation (ILD), *n* (%)	17	(71)
Age 1st manifestation, years	58.9	[49.6–68.4]
– ILD as 1st manifestation, *n* (%)	19	(61)
– Time to pSS diagnosis in ILD first, months	6.2	[3.1–44.1]
– Time to ILD diagnosis in pSS first, months	3.1	[0.0–38.8]
Follow up, months	38.2	[12.4–119.6]
EULAR Sjögren's Syndrome Disease Activity Index (ESSDAI)		
Constitutional Symptoms, *n* (%)	1	(3)
Lymphadenopathy, *n* (%)	1	(3)
Glandular involvement, *n* (%)	2	(7)
Articular involvement, *n* (%)	12	(39)
Cutaneous involvement, *n* (%)	3	(10)
Pulmonary involvement, *n* (%)	31	(100)
Renal involvement, *n* (%)	1	(3)
Muscular involvement, *n* (%)	1	(3)
Peripheral nervous system involvement, *n* (%)	6	(19)
Central nervous system involvement, *n* (%)	1	(3)
Hematological involvement, *n* (%)	15	(48)
Biological involvement, *n* (%)	9	(29)
Laboratory values at ILD diagnosis		
CRP >10 mg/l, *n* (%)	13	(42)
Rheumatoid factor positive, *n* (%)	16	(52)
ANA >1:160, *n* (%)	28	(90)
Presence of SSA (Ro) antibody, *n* (%)	21	(68)
Presence of SSB (La) antibody, *n* (%)	7	(23)
xANCA positive, *n* (%)	3	(10)
Xerostomia tests		
Saxon test pathological, *n* (%)	12[a]	(41)
Schirmer test pathological, *n* (%)	27[a]	(87)
Salivary gland biopsy		
Chisholm Mason- grade ≥3, *n* (%)	11[b]	(85)
Lung function at ILD diagnosis		
% Predicted forced vital capacity (FVC)	65	[52–88]
% Predicted diffusing capacity (D_{LCO})	48	[41–80]
CT patterns of lung disease		
Usual interstitial pneumonia, *n* (%)	13	(42)
Non-specific interstitial pneumonia, *n* (%)	9	(29)
Desquamative interstitial pneumonia, *n* (%)	2	(7)
Combined pulmonary fibrosis and emphysema, *n* (%)	2	(7)
Unspecific interstitial change, *n* (%)	5	(16)
Treatment		
1st line DMARD		
– *Cyclophosphamide, n (%)*	13	(42)
– *Azathioprine, n (%)*	8	(26)
– *Methotrexate, n (%)*	5	(16)
– *Hydroxychloroquine, n (%)*	2	(7)
– *Rituximab, n (%)*	1	(3)
– *Mycophenolate mofetil, n (%)*	1	(3)
Number of treatment modalities attempted per patient	3	[2–3]

Clinical, laboratory, pulmonary function, and computer tomography findings at the time of original diagnosis have been included.
[a]*Results available for 29/31 patients included in the cohort.*
[b]*Results available for 13/31 patients included in the cohort.*
Values represent median [inter-quartile range] unless otherwise stated.
ILD, interstitial lung disease; pSS, primary Sjögren's Syndrome; CRP, C reactive protein; ANA, antinuclear antibody; xANCA, atypical anti-neutrophil cytoplasmic antibodies; DMARD, disease modifying anti-rheumatic drug.

Subgroup analysis revealed a persisting female predominance across all forms of lung involvement. Patients exhibiting a DIP pattern presented much earlier. Lung function revealed more profound ventilatory impairment in UIP and DIP compared to other phenotypes. A similar, albeit less obvious, pattern was observed in diffusion coefficients. Regarding 1st line treatment, no clear patterns reflecting pulmonary phenotype were identified and again the small numbers prevented statistical appraisal. During the 29.0 [8.9–80.5] months of follow-up after ILD diagnosis, 24/31 patients achieved stabilized or improved FVC after commencing treatment (**Figure 3**). One patient died during follow-up due to an unrelated cancer. It should be noted however, that follow-up in the predominant pulmonary phenotypes remains limited (UIP 18.0 [9.5–97.8] months; NSIP 12.0 [8.9–49.7] months).

In general terms, 1st line treatment consisted of systemic corticosteroids in conjunction with disease modifying anti-rheumatic drugs (DMARDs). Cyclophosphamide was most commonly used (*n* = 13, 42%), followed by azathioprine and methotrexate (*n* = 8, 26% and *n* = 5, 16%). In 26/31 patients (84%) the 1st line DMARD was changed. The median numbers of different DMARDs used was 3 [2–3], with the maximum used in an individual patient being seven.

Evaluating 1st line treatment choice, patients commenced on cyclophosphamide tended to be younger at median 58.4 [47.6–67.2] years and have poorer lung function (median FVC 64 [44–88]% predicted) compared to the other DMARDs used. Given the limited data available no statistical analysis has been performed.

In terms of initial treatment response, across all groups and independent of treatment received, a gradual slowing in FVC loss was observed, with a suggestion of some recovery among those patients with the longest follow-up. These trends were more apparent in the larger NSIP and UIP subgroups but the limited follow-up prevents meaningful interpretation of these preliminary findings (**Figure S2**). Follow-up HRCT Thorax has to date been performed in 13/31 patients (42%) at a median 7.0 [4.1–17.8] months after the first scans. A small minority of patients (6/13, 46%) demonstrated radiological progression. This included both DIP patients who had received cyclophosphamide, as well as 2/9 (22%) NSIP patients who received hydroxychloroquine or cyclophosphamide respectively, a CPFE patient (1/2, 50%) who received methotrexate and a single UIP patient (1/13, 8%) who initially received mycophenolate. Nonetheless none of the patients have died due to their lung disease or required lung transplantation during ongoing follow-up, or have been commenced on additional anti-fibrotic therapies, such as pirfenidone or nintedanib.

DISCUSSION

Our data raises a number of important aspects regarding ILD and pSS despite small cohort size and limited follow-up. Firstly, symptomatic lung involvement was identified in 13% of pSS patients attending our institution. This corroborates previously reported prevalence ranging from 9–22% (23, 24) and supports initiating structured screening for lung disease in pSS patients.

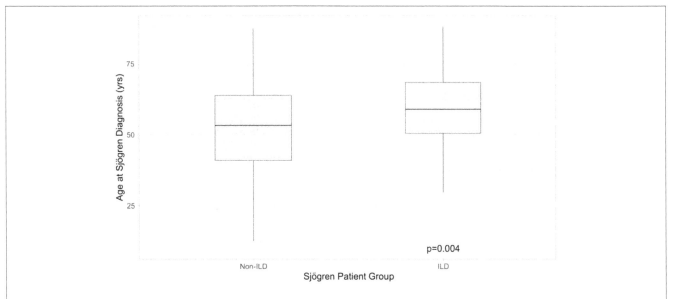

FIGURE 1 | Boxplot illustrating age at which Sjögren's syndrome was diagnosed in patients with (n = 31) and without (n = 268) lung involvement. The former were older at presentation. ILD, interstitial lung disease.

Normal lung physiology features inherent functional reserves and inevitably significant pathology exists before patients become symptomatic. This is common in many lung diseases, partially accounting for disappointing outcomes in chronic respiratory conditions including ILD.

The second important implication is the need for effective pSS screening in patients presenting with apparently idiopathic ILD. Reliance upon antibody testing for anti-SSA (Ro) and anti-SSB (La) appears inadequate for screening, with our results suggesting that up to one-third of patients could be missed. Potential advantages of augmenting screening with testing for dry eyes and mouth and in equivocal cases proceeding to salivary gland biopsy requires further careful evaluation.

Rheumatologists regularly evaluate ILD patients on respiratory wards or as outpatient pulmonology referrals. Interdisciplinary cooperation may explain the high percentage of ILD patients, in whom pSS was subsequently diagnosed on routine screening (9/31, 29%) compared to previous reports. of 10% (8). This raises the possibility that significant numbers of ILD patients with undetected pSS may be missed or managed as IPF instead. Recently, interstitial pneumonia with autoimmune features (IPAF) was defined by the American Thoracic Society (ATS)/European Respiratory Society (ERS) as an interstitial pneumonia with clinical, serological, or morphological features of an autoimmune disease without fulfilling criteria for a specific connective tissue disease (CTD) (25). In such cases, we would advocate additional diagnostic work up for pSS-ILD given the heterogeneity of the latter, which lies well within the IPAF criteria.

Compounding this further, is the diversity of ILD observed in the cohort. A persisting misconception remains, that NSIP is the predominating HRCT phenotype occurring in autoimmune connective tissue diseases (4, 26). Our data could not corroborate this, with UIP actually being the most common manifestation. Unquestionably, the data presented is circumstantial and no causality can be inferred. It remains possible that our results merely reflect different conditions occurring in the same patient. Contradicting this however is the predominance of never-smoking females with UIP. Nevertheless, the data reiterates the need for critical appraisal of ILD phenotypes as a catalyst for further research and potentially, individualized treatment. Current data for UIP in pSS is limited, with case reports suggesting a poor response to augmented immunosuppression (1). Although our data does not support these results, it should be reiterated that our experiences are greatly limited, in terms of both numbers and duration of follow-up. It should be noted however that reports suggesting more favorable outcomes in CTD-associated UIP compared to idiopathic UIP (27).

Contradictory data exists regarding the age of diagnosis in pSS with ILD and without. Whilst Dong et al. report a significant age difference 57.44 (+/− 14.08) years in pSS patients without ILD vs. 61.00 (+/− 11.23) years in patients with ILD, Palm et al. did not see a difference (4, 23, 28). In our cohort pSS patients with ILD were older than patients without ILD at time of diagnosis.

The choice of treatment in our cohort was based on severity of lung involvement and HRCT findings. If alveolitis was detected and severe impairment of lung function was present, glucocorticoids in combination with intravenous cyclophosphamide was used as first line treatment. If possible six courses of cyclophosphamide (15 mg/kg) were given monthly followed by a maintenance therapy of mycophenolate mofetil or azathioprine.

TABLE 2 | Subgroup demographics with respect to interstitial lung disease patterns, as determined in the original CT Thorax.

	UIP		NSIP		DIP		CPFE		Unspecific	
Patient, n (%)	13	(43)	9	(29)	2	(6)	2	(6)	5	(16)
Female, n (%)	9	(69)	5	(56)	2	(100)	1	(50)	3	(60)
Age Onset, years	58.9	[50.6–68.8]	57.3	[50.0–64.3]	36.8	[36.2–37.4]	60.6	[43.5–77.8]	67.8	[63.9–68.3]
Age SS, years	59.0	[50.7–68.8]	57.7	[50.2–68.4]	45.7	[37.5–53.9]	60.7	[43.6–77.9]	67.9	[64.0–68.4]
Age ILD, years	61.9	[54.9–69.3]	57.4	[51.1–64.4]	36.9	[36.2–37.5]	62.7	[47.6–77.9]	68.4	[65.9–70.8]
Never smoker, n (%)	10	(77)	6	(67)	1	(50)	1	(50)	5	(100)
– Pack years	2		9		3		18		-	
ESSDAI score	18	[14–25]	17	[15–22]	19	[13–25]	12	[10–14]	22	[21–25]
Lung function at ILD diagnosis										
FVC, % pred	60	[46–65]	70	[54–76]	50	[45–55]	98	[93–102]	79	[78–98]
D_{LCO}, % pred	53	[36–71]	47	[41–68]	35	[29–41]	70	[55–84]	79	[63–84]
Treatment										
1st line treatment										
CYC, n (%)	6	(45)	5	(56)	2	(100)	0	-	0	-
AZA, n (%)	4	(31)	1	(11)	0	-	1	(50)	2	(40)
MTX, n (%)	1	(8)	1	(11)	0	-	1	(50)	2	(40)
HCQ, n (%)	0	-	1	(11)	0	-	0	-	1	(20)
RTX, n (%)	1	(8)	0	-	0	-	0	-	0	-
MMF, n (%)	1	(8)	0	-	0	-	0	-	0	-
Number treatments	3	[2–4]	3	[2–3]	2	[1–3]	3	[1–4]	2	[2–3]
Treatment outcomes										
FVC										
Improved, n (%)	2	(15)	1	(12)	2	(100)	0	-	0	
Stabilized, n (%)	8	(62)	4	(44)	0	-	2	(100)	3	(100)
Declined, N (%)	3	(23)	4	(44)	0	-	0	-	0	-
D_{LCO}										
Improved, n (%)	3	(23)	1	(11)	2	(100)	0	-	1	(20)
Stabilized, n (%)	9	(69)	5	(56)	0	-	2	(100)	4	(80)
Declined, N (%)	1	(8)	3	(33)	0	-	0	-	0	-
Follow up, months	37	[12–96]	17	[13–50]	113	[9–218]	65	[10–120]	170	[81–182]
Deaths, n (%)	1	(8)	0		0		0		0	

Lung function outcomes based upon ±1% per month change over baseline values at original diagnosis.
UIP, usual interstitial pneumonia; NSIP, non-specific interstitial pneumonia; DIP, desquamative interstitial pneumonia; CPFE, combined pulmonary fibrosis and emphysema; SS, Sjögren's Syndrome; ILD, interstitial lung disease; ESSDAI, EULAR Sjögren's Syndrome Disease Activity Index; FVC, forced vital capacity; D_{LCO}, Carbon monoxide lung diffusion capacity; CYC, cyclophosphamide; AZA, azathioprine; MTX, methotrexate; HCQ, hydroxychloroquine; RTX, rituximab; MMF, mycophenolate mofetil.
Values represent median [inter-quartile range] unless otherwise stated.

In January 2020 EULAR recommendations for the management of pSS have been published, as first line treatment for moderate and high ESSDAI score glucocorticoids 0.5–1 mg/kg are recommended regarding to severity. As second line immunosuppressive agents are suggested, and as a rescue therapy cyclophosphamide and rituximab are recommended. But the task force points out that there are no controlled studies or head to head comparisons of any immunosuppressive agents allowing support of a differentiated organ-guided therapeutic approach (16). Which highlights the necessity of therapy studies in pSS patients with extra-glandular manifestations.

Research into UIP treatments in non-pSS populations has received a great deal of attention in the past decade. Traditional treatments with steroids, azathioprine, and n-acetyl-cysteine, based on IFIGENIA study (29) were called

into question by the extended PANTHER-IPF study (30) which suggested that immunosuppression was actually worsening prognosis in UIP-ILD. This combined with the early results from the CAPACITY (31) and ASCEND (32) trials led to a paradigm shift away from immunosuppression and toward novel anti-fibrotic agents. Beyond idiopathic pulmonary fibrosis, recent data from the SENSCIS study (33) examined the effects of nintedanib in systemic sclerosis associated lung disease. This prospective, randomized, placebo controlled study included over 570 patients and demonstrated clinical benefit. Current publications from this cohort have not yet attempted to describe or phenotype ILD in these patients.

Our cohort included only one patient with HRCT features suggestive of LIP, which may just reflect the small size of our

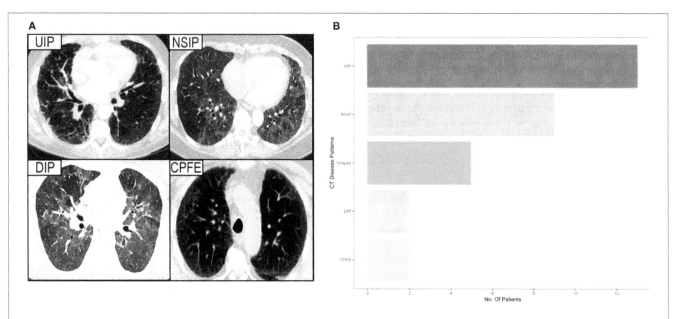

FIGURE 2 | **(A)** Showing the HRCT pattern of the various interstitial lung diseases. **(B)** Showing the prevalence of different forms of interstitial lung disease among patients with a proven Sjögren's syndrome, considered contributory to their lung disease. UIP, usual interstitial pneumonia; NSIP, non-specific interstitial pneumonia; DIP, desquamative interstitial pneumonia; CPFE, combined pulmonary fibrosis and emphysema; Unspez, unspecific interstitial changes.

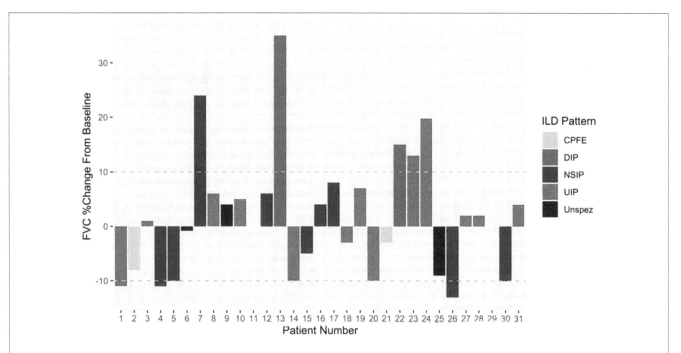

FIGURE 3 | Illustrating %changes in FVC following treatment initiation. Deltas calculated using last available measurement. Disease progression (treatment failure) was defined as a 10% fall in FVC from that recorded at treatment initiation. A 10% improvement symbolized Improved on treatment. Patients within ± 10% baseline were classed as stable.

cohort. Furthermore, LIP is a histological diagnosis, biopsies were performed only in 4/31 patients, so that no meaningful statistical analyses was possible.

Nevertheless, our cumulative findings reinforce the need for continued refinement of disease phenotypes and evaluation of tailored treatment approaches. Due to its limitations, the data presented here is at best preliminary and serves principally as a basis for focusing future research. Our cohort is small, the data collection was entirely retrospective and both evaluation—in terms of lung function and HRCT scanning—contains inevitable selection bias. In certain populations, HRCT in asymptomatic patients have confirmed pathological interstitial findings (4). In our institution performance of HRCT in asymptomatic patients is ethically difficult. To compensate for this, the PFT criteria are intended to allow very early detection, to minimize the number of potential missed cases. Crucially, no reliable screening has been performed in asymptomatic patients. Compounding this further, was the reliance on lung function and HRCT imaging rather than histological confirmation. Regarding PFT, analysis was based on FVC values, rather than lung volumes such as total lung capacity (TLC). FVC has been almost universally employed in large multi-center IPF studies due to logistical concerns. TLC measurements on body plethysmography offer clear advantages in identifying and monitoring ILD, but is both time consuming and expensive. Similar issues exist with transbronchial and open-lung biopsies, notwithstanding the additional patient risk such procedures entail.

In conclusion, our results reveal that pulmonary disease is commonly associated with pSS, manifesting in a variety of different clinical entities. Screening for pSS in patients with unclear lung disease should be performed regardless of subjective sicca symptoms via screening for xeropththalmy or xerostomy and in case of unremarkable antibodies a salivary gland lip biopsy should be performed. Based upon existing data from other disease groups, potential exists for improving outcomes by refining disease recognition strategies and designing appropriate studies with aim of structured surveillance and tailored treatment strategies.

ETHICS STATEMENT

The studies involving human participants were reviewed and approved by ethics committee of Hannover Medical Highschool. The patients/participants provided their written informed consent to participate in this study.

AUTHOR CONTRIBUTIONS

DE, AJ, GS, and SH: conception and design of the study, acquisition and interpretation of data, drafting the article, and final approval of the version to be submitted. TSk, TW, and RS: interpretation of data, revising critically for important intellectual content, and final approval of the version to be submitted. JH: acquisition of data, analyzing all CT reports, revising critically for important intellectual content, and final approval of the version to be submitted. TT and TSe: acquisition and interpretation of data and final approval of the version to be submitted. All authors take responsibility for all aspects of the reliability and freedom from bias of the data presented and their discussed interpretation.

REFERENCES

1. Parambil JG, Myers JL, Lindell RM, Matteson EL, Ryu JH. Interstitial lung disease in primary sjogren syndrome. *Chest.* (2006) 130:1489–95. doi: 10.1378/chest.130.5.1489
2. Seeliger T, Prenzler NK, Gingele S, Seeliger B, Korner S, Thiele T, et al. Neuro-sjogren: peripheral neuropathy with limb weakness in sjogren's syndrome. *Front Immunol.* (2019) 10:1600. doi: 10.3389/fimmu.2019.01600
3. Fairfax AJ, Haslam PL, Pavia D, Sheahan NF, Bateman JR, Agnew JE, et al. Pulmonary disorders associated with sjogren's syndrome. *Q J Med.* (1981) 50:279–95.
4. Dong X, Zhou J, Guo X, Li Y, Xu Y, Fu Q, et al. A retrospective analysis of distinguishing features of chest HRCT and clinical manifestation in primary sjogren's syndrome-related interstitial lung disease in a Chinese population. *Clin Rheumatol.* (2018) 37:2981–8. doi: 10.1007/s10067-018-4289-6
5. Alsumrain M, De Giacomi F, Nasim F, Koo CW, Bartholmai BJ, Levin DL, et al. Combined pulmonary fibrosis and emphysema as a clinicoradiologic entity: characterization of presenting lung fibrosis and implications for survival. *Respir med.* (2019) 146:106–12. doi: 10.1016/j.rmed.2018.12.003
6. Ramos-Casals M, Brito-Zeron P, Seror R, Bootsma H, Bowman SJ, Dorner T, et al. Characterization of systemic disease in primary sjogren's syndrome: EULAR-SS task force recommendations for articular, cutaneous, pulmonary and renal involvements. *Rheumatology.* (2015) 54:2230–8. doi: 10.1093/rheumatology/kev200
7. Swigris JJ, Berry GJ, Raffin TA, Kuschner WG. Lymphoid interstitial pneumonia: a narrative review. *Chest.* (2002) 122:2150–64. doi: 10.1378/chest.122.6.2150
8. Nannini C, Jebakumar AJ, Crowson CS, Ryu JH, Matteson EL. Primary sjogren's syndrome 1976-2005 and associated interstitial lung disease: a population-based study of incidence and mortality. *BMJ Open.* (2013) 3:e003569. doi: 10.1136/bmjopen-2013-003569
9. Papiris SA, Maniati M, Constantopoulos SH, Roussos C, Moutsopoulos HM, Skopouli FN. Lung involvement in primary sjogren's syndrome is mainly related to the small airway disease. *Ann Rheum Dis.* (1999) 58:61–4. doi: 10.1136/ard.58.1.61
10. Hansell DM, Bankier AA, MacMahon H, McLoud TC, Muller NL, Remy J. Fleischner society: glossary of terms for thoracic imaging. *Radiology.* (2008) 246:697–722. doi: 10.1148/radiol.2462070712
11. Seror R, Bootsma H, Saraux A, Bowman SJ, Theander E, Brun JG, et al. Defining disease activity states and clinically meaningful improvement in primary sjogren's syndrome with EULAR primary Sjogren's syndrome disease activity (ESSDAI) and patient-reported indexes (ESSPRI). *Ann Rheum Dis.* (2016) 75:382–9. doi: 10.1136/annrheumdis-2014-206008
12. Shiboski CH, Shiboski SC, Seror R, Criswell LA, Labetoulle M, Lietman TM, et al. (2016). American college of rheumatology/european league against rheumatism classification criteria for primary sjogren's syndrome: a consensus and data-driven methodology involving three international patient cohorts. *Ann Rheum Dis.* (2017) 76:9–16. doi: 10.1136/annrheumdis-2016-210571
13. Daniels TE, Cox D, Shiboski CH, Schiodt M, Wu A, Lanfranchi H, et al. Associations between salivary gland histopathologic diagnoses and phenotypic features of sjogren's syndrome among 1,726 registry participants. *Arthritis Rheum.* (2011) 63:2021–30. doi: 10.1002/art.30381
14. Kohler PF, Winter ME. A quantitative test for xerostomia. The saxon test, an oral equivalent of the Schirmer test. *Arthritis Rheum.* (1985) 28:1128–32. doi: 10.1002/art.1780281008
15. Sanchez-Perez L, Irigoyen-Camacho E, Saenz-Martinez L, Zepeda Zepeda M, Acosta-Gio E, Mendez-Ramirez I. Stability of unstimulated and stimulated whole saliva flow rates in children. *Int J Paediatr Dent.* (2016) 26:346–50. doi: 10.1111/ipd.12206
16. Ramos-Casals M, Brito-Zeron P, Bombardieri S, Bootsma H, De Vita S, Dorner T, et al. EULAR recommendations for the management of sjogren's syndrome with topical and systemic therapies. *Ann Rheum Dis.* (2020) 79:3–18. doi: 10.1136/annrheumdis-2019-216114
17. Raghu G, Remy-Jardin M, Myers JL, Richeldi L, Ryerson CJ, Lederer DJ, et al. Diagnosis of idiopathic pulmonary fibrosis. An official ATS/ERS/JRS/ALAT

clinical practice guideline. *Am J Respir Crit Care Med.* (2018) 198:e44–68. doi: 10.1164/rccm.201807-1255ST

18. Hansell DM, Goldin JG, King TE Jr, Lynch DA, Richeldi L, et al. CT staging and monitoring of fibrotic interstitial lung diseases in clinical practice and treatment trials: a position paper from the fleischner society. *Lancet Respir Med.* (2015) 3:483–96. doi: 10.1016/S2213-2600(15)00096-X

19. Lynch DA, Sverzellati N, Travis WD, Brown KK, Colby TV, Galvin JR, et al. Diagnostic criteria for idiopathic pulmonary fibrosis: a fleischner society white paper. *Lancet Respir Med.* (2018) 6:138–53. doi: 10.1016/S2213-2600(17)30433-2

20. Wanger J, Clausen JL, Coates A, Pedersen OF, Brusasco V, Burgos F, et al. Standardisation of the measurement of lung volumes. *Eur Respir J.* (2005) 26:511–22. doi: 10.1183/09031936.05.00035005

21. Pellegrino R, Viegi G, Brusasco V, Crapo RO, Burgos F, Casaburi R, et al. Interpretative strategies for lung function tests. *Eur Respir J.* (2005) 26:948–68. doi: 10.1183/09031936.05.00035205

22. Macintyre N, Crapo RO, Viegi G, Johnson DC, van der Grinten CP, Brusasco V, et al. Standardisation of the single-breath determination of carbon monoxide uptake in the lung. *Eur Respir J.* (2005) 26:720–35. doi: 10.1183/09031936.05.00034905

23. Palm O, Garen T, Berge Enger T, Jensen JL, Lund MB, Aalokken TM, et al. Clinical pulmonary involvement in primary sjogren's syndrome: prevalence, quality of life and mortality–a retrospective study based on registry data. *Rheumatology.* (2013) 52:173–9. doi: 10.1093/rheumatology/kes311

24. Belenguer R, Ramos-Casals M, Brito-Zeron P, del Pino J, Sentis J, Aguilo S, et al. Influence of clinical and immunological parameters on the health-related quality of life of patients with primary sjogren's syndrome. *Clin Exp Rheumatol.* (2005) 23:351–6.

25. Wilfong EM, Lentz RJ, Guttentag A, Tolle JJ, Johnson JE, Kropski JA, et al. Interstitial pneumonia with autoimmune features: an emerging challenge at the intersection of rheumatology and pulmonology. *Arthritis Rheumatol.* (2018) 70:1901–13. doi: 10.1002/art.40679

26. Gupta S, Ferrada MA, Hasni SA. Pulmonary manifestations of primary sjogren's syndrome: underlying immunological mechanisms, clinical presentation, and management. *Front Immunol.* (2019) 10:1327. doi: 10.3389/fimmu.2019.01327

27. Moua T, Zamora Martinez AC, Baqir M, Vassallo R, Limper AH, Ryu JH. Predictors of diagnosis and survival in idiopathic pulmonary fibrosis and connective tissue disease-related usual interstitial pneumonia. *Respir Res.* (2014) 15:154. doi: 10.1186/s12931-014-0154-6

28. Carmona FD, Mackie SL, Martin JE, Taylor JC, Vaglio A, Eyre S, et al. A large-scale genetic analysis reveals a strong contribution of the HLA class II region to giant cell arteritis susceptibility. *Am J Hum Genet.* (2015) 96:565–80. doi: 10.1016/j.ajhg.2015.02.009

29. Demedts M, Behr J, Buhl R, Costabel U, Dekhuijzen R, Jansen HM, et al. High-dose acetylcysteine in idiopathic pulmonary fibrosis. *N Engl J Med.* (2005) 353:2229–42. doi: 10.1056/NEJMoa042976

30. Wells AU, Behr J, Costabel U, Cottin V, Poletti V. Triple therapy in idiopathic pulmonary fibrosis: an alarming press release. *Eur Respir J.* (2012) 39:805–6. doi: 10.1183/09031936.00009112

31. Noble PW, Albera C, Bradford WZ, Costabel U, Glassberg MK, Kardatzke D, et al. Pirfenidone in patients with idiopathic pulmonary fibrosis (CAPACITY): two randomised trials. *Lancet.* (2011) 377:1760–9. doi: 10.1016/S0140-6736(11)60405-4

32. King TE Jr, Bradford WZ, Castro-Bernardini S, Fagan EA, Glaspole I, et al. A phase 3 trial of pirfenidone in patients with idiopathic pulmonary fibrosis. *N Engl J Med.* (2014) 370:2083–92. doi: 10.1056/NEJMoa1402582

33. Distler O, Highland KB, Gahlemann M, Azuma A, Fischer A, Mayes MD, et al. Nintedanib for systemic sclerosis-associated interstitial lung disease. *N Engl J Med.* (2019) 380:2518–28. doi: 10.1056/NEJMoa1903076

19

Health Related Quality of Life in Interstitial Lung Disease: Can We Use the Same Concepts Around the World?

Kerri I. Aronson[1] and Atsushi Suzuki[2]*

[1] Division of Pulmonary and Critical Care Medicine, Weill Cornell Medicine, New York, NY, United States, [2] Department of Respiratory Medicine, Nagoya University Graduate School of Medicine, Nagoya, Japan

*Correspondence:
Kerri I. Aronson
kia9010@med.cornell.edu

Health-Related Quality of Life (HRQOL) is increasingly viewed as an important patient-centered outcome by leading health organizations, clinicians, and patients alike. This is especially true in the interstitial lung disease community where patients often struggle with progressive and debilitating disease with few therapeutic options. In order to test the effectiveness of new pharmacologic therapies and non-pharmacologic interventions globally in ILD, this will require expansion of clinical research studies to a multinational level and HRQOL will be an important endpoint to many. In order to successfully expand trials across multiple nations and compare the results of studies between different communities we must recognize that there are differences in the concepts of HRQOL across the world and have strategies to address these differences. In this review, we will describe the different global influences on HRQOL both generally and in the context of ILD, discuss the processes of linguistic translation and cross-cultural adaptation of HRQOL Patient Reported Outcome Measures (PROMs), and highlight the gaps and opportunities for improving HRQOL measurement in ILD across the world.

Keywords: HRQOL—health-related quality of life, interstitial lung disease, global, cross cultural adaptation, linguistic validation

INTRODUCTION

Health-related quality of life (HRQOL), or one's quality of life as it relates to health status or disease, is increasingly recognized as an important patient centered-outcome by leading health organizations (1, 2)[1]. HRQOL is a subjective, dynamic, and multidimensional concept that includes domains representative of an individual patients' goals, values, and beliefs (3, 4). Over the past several decades, various conceptual models of HRQOL have contributed to our study of HRQOL in human disease (2, 5–7). These models provide an essential structure for conceptualization of HRQOL, including both the positive and negative aspects, and are often used as a guide for research and practices that promote improved HRQOL in different populations of interest (8). HRQOL frameworks most commonly focus on the physical and psychosocial impacts of health or disease on an individual's ability to live what they consider to be a fulfilling life (9). HRQOL amongst those who share the same or different chronic diseases is often very personal and subjective. This subjectivity will vary even more depending on a person's cultural background and environment. The various domains of HRQOL (e.g., psychosocial, physical etc.) that we intend to measure therefore should ideally be considered in the context of an individual's culture and value system

---

[1] Population Assessment of Health-Related Quality of Life.

(10, 11). This adds a level of complexity to measurement of HRQOL as we are compelled to recognized that these constructs will differ across different cultural, religious, and socioecological contexts (12). The processes of linguistic and cross-cultural adaptation have allowed for improved measurement of HRQOL across different cultures and languages.

During the past decade, HRQOL has gained much traction as a priority endpoint in the Interstitial Lung Disease (ILD) community. ILD is a group of heterogeneous parenchymal lung diseases with various clinical courses, many of which may be progressive, fibrotic, life altering, and eventually fatal (13, 14). Patients and ILD experts alike have vocalized the importance prioritizing HRQOL as a top area of focus in research studies and clinical practice (15, 16). Though a few therapies are documented to slow progression of disease [as measured by forced vital capacity (FVC)] in idiopathic pulmonary fibrosis (IPF) and the progressive fibrotic form of other ILDs, there is now much interest in how our interventions effectively slow deterioration in HRQOL (17, 18).

Patient Reported Outcome Measures (PROMs) that measure HRQOL gather information directly from the patient (without interpretation by a clinician or anyone else) about their perspective of the quality of their life in the context of their disease and it's treatments (19, 20). There are several PROMs that have undergone validation testing to measure HRQOL in ILD. The most commonly used instruments in the past few decades were originally intended for use in other respiratory diseases, while a handful of newer instruments have been developed for use specifically in ILD and pulmonary fibrosis (21). These "condition" or "disease-specific" PROMs are intended to capture more nuanced information about the impact of living with ILD that is most pertinent to patients with this particular chronic respiratory disease (e.g., breathlessness, cough, fatigue, aspects of psychological well-being) (22). Despite the ILD-targeted items in these instruments, one must be cognizant of the interpretation of the wording of these items for those from other cultures or countries in which the instrument was not developed. For example, dyspnea, or breathlessness is a common ILD symptom that impacts HRQOL. There are various qualitative aspects of this symptom are interpreted differently across different languages and cultures (23–25).

Here we introduce the concept of measuring HRQOL around the world, and as it pertains to specifically to ILD with a focus on linguistics, regional and environmental factors, health literacy and health-care systems, and race, ethnicity, religion and spirituality. We will describe the process of cross-cultural adaptation, the work that has been performed to cross-culturally validate PROMs in ILD, and the potential challenges and opportunities for the future study of HRQOL in ILD on a global scale.

GLOBAL INFLUENCES ON HRQOL

HRQOL generally reflects each individual's perspective on their own health and is widely accepted as one of the most important patient-centered outcomes. HRQOL measures the impact a chronic disease and its treatment have on several domains of one's life and is largely influenced by cultural and spiritual backgrounds. Therefore, it is expected that the concept of HRQOL will differ across communities within a nation, as well as between countries. Given the growing number of international clinical trials and large population health studies it is increasingly important to recognize the global factors that influence accurate measurement of HRQOL, and how to potentially address them. This section focuses on general considerations for assessing HRQOL in chronic illness, which is pertinent when we consider measurement in ILDs.

Language Diversity

Linguistic differences are an important consideration when measuring HRQOL. Historically, most HRQOL instruments have been developed in the English Language. Over the past few decades, various HRQOL scales have been internationally translated and standardized across different languages. Translation approaches are traditionally performed by qualified academicians or language experts. With advancements in technology, online translation has also been made available. Despite the availability, convenience, and cost effectiveness of online translation (e.g., google translate), there is controversy related to the validity of this approach when used as the sole method of translation. It has been suggested that if one were to consider using an online program, a more valid approach is a hybrid method with traditional translation by experts with high-level degrees in linguistics in combination with an online program (26). Whatever approach is chosen, researchers must ultimately decide on the translation and adaptation procedures that are most appropriate for their scope of work with consideration of time constraints and available resources.

In order to use a HRQOL instrument appropriately in a new country or culture, the instrument must not only possess linguistic equivalence, but must also capture the cultural differences in disease expression and perception of HRQOL (27, 28). We will expand upon this process of "cross cultural adaptation" later in this review.

Regional and Environmental Differences

An individual's region of origin and environmental context are important considerations during HRQOL assessment. The built environment, defined as the space in which people spend their time in daily life (e.g., home, neighborhood, transportation, or workplace), is closely associated with their health status (29). Seasonal and weather conditions affect physical activity and psychological states (e.g., winter season, unfavorable weather, or decreased sunlight exposure vs. the more positive alternative) (30). Air pollution represented by particulate matter ($PM_{2.5}$) is associated with increased respiratory symptoms and worsened HRQOL (31, 32). There is also evidence to suggest that habitat may influence HRQOL. For example, there are reported differences in HRQOL scores between those in rural vs. urban environments (33–36). These environmental contextual factors may play a role in our interpretation of HRQOL scores amongst different populations and more work is needed to formulate an approach to addressing this issue. Few clinical studies have corrected for the various potential regional and environmental effects on HRQOL, and this is an important area of potential investigation in the future.

Health Literacy and Diversity of Healthcare Systems

Health literacy is defined as the ability to access, understand, and effectively use health information (37, 38). Patients with low health literacy have less of an understanding about their medical conditions and treatments. This is associated with the potential to worsen health status and disease outcomes (39, 40). A recent study revealed that older age, higher body mass index, residence far from medical institutions, lower monthly income, and lower education levels are associated with a lower health literacy (41). The access to primary care systems and the presence of reliable, understandable, and comprehensive native language medical information websites also contribute to global differences in health literacy (42). The same intervention for a particular chronic disease may be interpreted differently by two patients depending on their comprehension, which may drastically impact patient decision making. Healthcare professionals have made a large effort to improve the impact of low health literacy, including establishment of universal education systems, but many inequalities still exist (42). While mobile health applications may help to enhance interactive patient-provider communication, there is more investigation needed to creatively adapt this technology for use in more remote and resource-limited parts of the world (17, 43–45).

Race, Ethnicity, Religion, and Spirituality

There is a growing body of literature that reveals the association between race, ethnicity, religion, spirituality and HRQOL. A recent study showed that racial and ethnic differences were associated with differences in HRQOL even within the same community (46). If the prevalence of a certain chronic disease is low in a particular race or ethnic group, the negative impact on HRQOL may become greater (47). A lack of familiarity with a chronic disease in a patient's community may lead to social discrimination, with a negative downstream impact on HRQOL (48). A systematic review focused on the relationship between religiosity/spirituality and quality of life (QOL) in patients with cardiovascular disease found a positive association between mental and emotional well-being, spiritual well-being, intrinsic religiousness, and frequency of church attendance (49). While it is important to recognize that these factors play an important role in HRQOL, there is controversy over the extent to which patients should be subdivided by spiritual and religious beliefs for clinical and epidemiological research (50). In order to address these differences, one potential approach is to focus on the longitudinal relative changes in each individual's HRQOL score, rather than comparing cross-sectional absolute values between different patients, but more work is needed to better define and operationalize this approach.

CROSS CULTURAL ADAPTATION

In the past several decades, the measurement of HRQOL has garnered significant attention as an important endpoint in clinical trials and public health research (51). With the increasing number of multi-country, multi-center trials that are conducted in clinical research there is a growing need for HRQOL measures that can be administered in countries with various languages of origin and amongst different cultural groups where disease expression and health-care system usage may vary (52). In order to administer an HRQOL instrument appropriately in a new country or culture, the instrument must not only possess linguistic equivalence, but must also capture the cultural differences in disease expression and perception of HRQOL (27, 28). This allows investigators to collect accurate information about HRQOL of the whole population in one study (when several countries are represented) and to compare results across different studies both nationally and internationally (53). Development of a new PROM is a rigorous and time intensive process (20). It may take years to gather enough data to prove the instrument possesses adequate validity to use in a clinical trial, often with stringent regulatory approval criteria that must be met (54). Rather than develop a brand-new instrument for each distinct language and culture, current practice is to perform "cross cultural adaptation." This process facilitates the translation of existing and well-validated instruments in a manner that allows the instrument to retain its psychometric properties in a culturally distinct population (55).

There is overwhelming agreement that an instrument should not be simply translated word for word into another linguistic context, as this can compromise the cultural integrity and equivalence of the findings (56). However, there is not a standardized protocol for linguistic validation or cross cultural adaptation, therefore risking poor translation and compromised research data (57, 58).

Several approaches to cross cultural adaptation have been suggested with the goal of maximizing validity and reliability of the instrument that is to be translated into the "target" (or new) language. The Translation and Cultural Adaptation Group (TCA) of the International Society for Pharmacoeconomics and Outcomes Research (ISPOR) task force put forth recommendations for translation and cultural adaptation of PROs in the research community based upon review of the literature and multidisciplinary expert consensus (59). Their recommended approach includes stages of translation and validations testing that require both forward and backwards translation, harmonization that allows for concept equivalence between the source and target language versions of the instrument, review by an expert committee, and cognitive debriefing to assess comprehensibility and cognitive equivalence of the translation by interviewing patients from the target population (60, 61). While the ISPOR task force guidelines provide a rigorous approach to translation, they provide less guidance on further psychometric testing to perform beyond translation and assessment of content validity.

In 1991, the international quality of life assessment (IQOLA) project was established to translate and validate the short-form 36-item health survey (SF-36) (28, 62, 63). The IQOLA project group guidelines encompass a three-stage process that incorporates further psychometric testing; (1) rigorous translation and evaluation process, (2) formal psychometric testing of the assumptions underlying item scoring and construction of multi-item scales, and (3) studies evaluating the equivalence of interpretations across countries (64, 65). Their project with the SF-36 transferred an existing generic HRQOL questionnaire to another culture, a process termed "sequential development". On the other hand, in 1990s, the World Health Organization (WHO) developed the WHO Quality of Life assessment instrument (WHOQOL) simultaneously in fifteen different centers worldwide (2). This type of approach helps to ensure equivalence of concepts at each stage as the questionnaire is developed in multiple languages at the same time, a process termed "simultaneous development". In the 1980-1990s, the European Organization for Research and Treatment of Cancer (EORTC) and the EuroQol Group developed the quality of life questionnaire (QLQ-C30), and the EuroQol-5 dimensions (EQ-5D), respectively (66–68). These questionnaires were generated in one language and then forward and backward translated into multiple languages by multinational discussions, a "parallel development" approach. With these historical developments, various HRQOL questionnaire translations are available for clinical trials, daily clinical practice, population studies, and health economic evaluations around the world.

CROSS CULTURAL ADAPTATION IN ILD

Several patient-reported outcome measures (PROMs) have been adapted for use in ILDs. The PROMs utilized in ILD research and practice are mainly categorized into three groups: (1) disease-specific HRQOL, (2) generic HRQOL, and (3) domain-specific instruments (69). These instruments are ideally chosen as endpoints in research according to the objective of the study and characteristics of the study population. Each of the most common PROMs administered in ILD are at different stages of validation, translation, cross-cultural adaptation, and level of use in clinical trials (**Table 1**). Here we provide an overview of the current state of cross-cultural adaptation of PROMs in ILD.

Disease-Specific HRQOL PROMs

Disease-specific HRQOL PROMs in ILD often provide information about the impact of the patient's lung disease on their quality of life. The St George's Respiratory Questionnaire (SGRQ), which was originally developed for patients with chronic obstructive pulmonary diseases (COPD), is one of the most extensively used PROMs for patients with ILDs (70–92). The SGRQ is relatively well-validated in ILD, however there are concerns regarding the applicability of several of the items to patients with ILD. While the SGRQ length and complicated scoring algorithm may pose some challenges for use in daily clinical practice, it has been translated into a wide range of languages making it a potentially attractive option when conducting multinational studies. The cross-sectional

reliability of an IPF-specific version of SGRQ (SGRQ-I), has been reported for patients with IPF, however longitudinal data, language translations, and experiences in clinical trials are limited (93, 94). The COPD Assessment Test (CAT) is a short and simple questionnaire developed for COPD and is reported to correlate well with the SGRQ in IPF and connective tissue disease-associated ILD (CTD-ILD), but experiences in clinical trials is limited (96–98). The King's Brief ILD (K-BILD), is a disease-specific instrument developed in the UK for use in ILD and has been tested in patients with a large number of ILDs (99–102). There is translation and cultural adaptation data for the K-BILD available for several European and South American countries (149, 150), and it is available in multiple languages for use across the globe. Additionally, A tool to Assess the quality of life in Idiopathic Pulmonary Fibrosis (ATAQ-IPF) which was developed initially in the United States to measure HRQOL in Pulmonary Fibrosis has published data on reliability and validity in Chinese patients (cATAQ-IPF) (105, 151).

The Living with IPF questionnaire (L-IPF) (107), developed in the English language, has published initial validation data in a cohort of patients with IPF and has recently expanded applicability as the Living with Pulmonary Fibrosis questionnaire (L-PF) (108). The Patient Experiences and Satisfaction with Medications questionnaire (PESaM) is a unique instrument evaluating patients' expectations, experiences, and satisfaction with disease-modifying drugs (109, 110). This instrument was developed in the Netherlands and provides systematic evaluation of patient experiences and expectations that may allow for improved shared-decision making. For these more newly developed instruments, more data is needed on the applicability across different languages and cultures.

Generic HRQOL PROMs

Generic HRQOL measures are designed to assess the overall health status across the general population, regardless of a specific type of chronic disease that one may have. Many of these instruments have been well-translated into a wide range of languages and well-validated in various ways as mentioned above. These instruments allow us to compare the health status between patients with different chronic diseases and healthy people. They are valued as key secondary endpoints in many clinical trials.

The SF-36 is the most widely used generic HRQOL measure. The validity of the SF-36 in ILDs has been established since the 1990s, with various studies reporting the cross-sectional and longitudinal validity in IPF, and has been used in many clinical trials of patients with ILD (73, 80, 81, 86, 90, 119, 137–141). As the minimal clinically importance difference (MCID) for the SF-36 in IPF varies depending on the cohort, further global validation studies are required. The EuroQol-5 dimensions 5-level (EQ-5D-5L) is also a well-known and widely-translated generic HRQOL measure. EQ-5D-5L was developed by the EuroQol Group to improve the instrument's sensitivity as compared with the previous version (142, 143). The scores obtained from EQ-5D-5L can be used to calculate quality-adjusted life years (QALY), a generic measure of disease burden. QALY measurements enable investigators to assess both the quality and the quantity of life lived and to examine the value of medical interventions (144).

TABLE 1 | Cross-cultural adaptation and linguistic validation of PROMs in ILD.

Patient-reported outcome measure	Validated IDL	Originally development and translations	Multi-center/country clinical trial use in IDL	MCID	References
DISEASE-SPECIFIC					
SGRQ	IPF CTD-ILD	Developed in 1991 English for the UK 170 translations	Yes	IPF: 4–8 CTD-ILD: 4–13	(70–92)
SGRQ-I	IPF	Developed in 2010 English for the UK 1 translation	No	IPF: 4–5	(93–95)
CAT	IPF CTD-ILD	Published in 2009 English for the UK 62 translations	No	IPF: N/A CTD-ILD: 1–4	(96–98)
K-BILD	IPF ILD	Published in 2012 English for the UK 6 translations	Yes	IPF/ILD: 4–8	(83, 99–104)
ATAQ-IPF	IPF	Published in 2010 English for the USA 2 translations	Yes	N/A	(105, 106)
L-IPF (L-PF)	IPF PF-ILD	Published in 2020 English for the USA In translations process	Not yet	Validation process	(107, 108)
PESaM	IPF	Published in 2017 Dutch for Belgium and the Netherlands 1 translation	Not yet	Validation process	(109–111)
CHP-HRQOL	HP	Development and Content Validity Published in 2021 English for the USA Undergoing further validation	Not Yet	Validation process	(112)
DOMAIN-SPECIFIC					
Dyspnea					
UCSD-SOBQ	IPF CTD-ILD	Developed in 1987 English for the USA 53 translations	Yes	IPF: 8 CTD-ILD: N/A	(80, 81, 83, 84, 87, 91, 92, 113–116)
mMRC	IPF ILD	Modified in 1976, 1986 English for the UK 12 translations	No	N/A	(71, 117, 118)
BDI-TDI	IPF SSc-ILD	Published in 1984 English for the USA 96 translations	Yes	IPF: N/A SSc-ILD: 1.5	(90, 119–121)
Cough					
LCQ	IPF	Published in 2003 English for the UK 23 translations	Yes	Chronic cough: 1.3	(91, 122–124)
CQLQ	IPF	Developed in 2002 English for the USA 4 translations	No	IPF: 5	(125)
Fatigue					
FAS	IPF Sarcoidosis	Developed in 2003 Dutch for the Netherlands 2 translations	No	IPF: N/A Sarcoidosis: 4	(126–129)
Anxiety/depression					
HADS	IPF	Developed in 1983 English for the UK 118 translations	Yes	N/A	(130–133)

(Continued)

TABLE 1 | Continued

Patient-reported outcome measure	Validated IDL	Originally development and translations	Multi-center/country clinical trial use in IDL	MCID	References
Sleep disorders					
ESS	IPF	Developed in 1983, and revised in 1997 English for Australia 95 translations	No	N/A	(134–136)
Generic HRQOL questionnaires					
SF-36	IPF SSc-ILD	Developed in 1998 (current version) English for the USA 191 translations	Yes	IPF: 2–4 SSc-ILD: N/A	(73, 80, 81, 86, 90, 119, 137–141)
EQ-5D-5L	ILD	Developed in 2011 Dutch for the Netherlands, English for the UK, Finnish for Finland, Norwegian for Norway, Swedish for Sweden 181 translations	Yes (including EQ-5D)	ILD: 0.005–0.095	(142–145)
PROMIS-29	IPF SSc-ILD	Published in 2005 English for the USA 47 translations	Not yet	N/A	(146–148)

ATAQ-IPF, A Tool to Assess Quality of life in IPF; BDI-TDI, Baseline Dyspnea Index-Transition Dyspnea Index; CAT, Chronic obstructive pulmonary disease Assessment Test; CHP-HRQOL, Chronic Hypersensitivity Pneumonitis Health Related Quality of Life; CQLQ, Cough Quality of Life Questionnaire; CTD-ILD, connective tissue disease associated interstitial lung disease; EQ-5D-5L, EuroQol-5 Dimension-5 Level; ESS, Epworth sleepiness scale; FAS, Fatigue Assessment Scale; GAD-7, Generalized Anxiety Disorder-7; HADS, Hospital Anxiety and Depression Scale; ILD, interstitial lung disease; IPF, idiopathic pulmonary fibrosis; K-BILD, King's Brief Interstitial Lung Disease health status questionnaire; LCQ, Leicester Cough Questionnaire; L-IPF, Living with IPF; L-PF, Living with Pulmonary Fibrosis; MCID, minimal clinically important difference; MFI, multidimensional fatigue inventory; mMRC, modified Medical Research Council dyspnea scale; PESaM, Patient Experiences and Satisfaction with Medication; PF-ILD, progressive fibrosing ILD; PROMIS, Patient Reported Outcome Measurement Information System; SF-36, Short Form-36; SGRQ, St George's Respiratory Questionnaire, SGRQ-I, IPF-specific version of the St George's Respiratory Questionnaire; SSc-ILD, systemic sclerosis related interstitial lung disease; UCSD-SOBQ, University of California San Diego-Shortness of Breath Questionnaire.
The number of translations was referred from ePROVIDE™ from MAPI RESEARCH TRUST (https://eprovide.mapi-trust.org) and EQ-5D from EuroQol group (https://euroqol.org).

A recent large cohort study demonstrated the construct validity and MCID of EQ-5D-5L in patients with a variety of fibrotic ILD subtypes (145). The Patient-Reported Outcomes Measurement Information System (PROMIS) is a research initiative launched by the National Institutes of Health to develop the PROMs for clinical research and practice across a wide variety of chronic diseases (146). Some studies have shown that PROMIS-29 accurately reflects the deficit in HRQOL of patients with IPF and systemic sclerosis-associated ILD (SSc-ILD), but it is still not widely used in the field of ILD (147, 148).

Domain-Specific PROMs

Domain-specific PROMs focus heavily on specific symptoms that patients may experience, which in ILD often include dyspnea, cough, fatigue, anxiety/depression, and sleep disturbance. While these PROMs do not measure HRQOL per say, they are important to mention as we know that many of these physical and psychologic symptoms are larger drivers of HRQOL in ILD. Among these, dyspnea and cough are most often assessed in ILD studies.

The University of California San Diego-Shortness of Breath Questionnaire (UCSD-SOBQ), the modified Medical Research Council dyspnea scale (mMRC), the Baseline Dyspnea Index-Transition Dyspnea Index (BDI-TDI), and the dyspnea-12 (D-12) are common questionnaires administered to assess dyspnea

in ILD. The UCSD-SOBQ has been administered in different ILD clinical trials and is well-translated in other languages aside from English. The MCID for IPF has been assessed (80, 81, 83, 84, 87, 91, 92, 113–116). The mMRC is a simple and easy tool for use in daily clinical practice and is reported as a useful predictor of mortality. Experience administering the mMRC in clinical trials and the number of linguistic translations is limited (71, 117, 118). The BDI-TDI assesses both baseline and change measures over time. It is well-translated into multiple languages, however there is little reported experience in clinical trials (90, 119–121). The D-12 is a brief and reliable instrument with positive validation data in ILDs but experience in clinical trials and the number of linguistic translations are limited (113, 152, 153).

The Leicester Cough Questionnaire (LCQ) and the Cough Quality of Life Questionnaire (CQLQ) have been used to assess severity, frequency, and impact of cough in patients with ILD. LCQ is a reliable and relatively easy to complete measure, and there is some experience using it in clinical trials. The responsiveness and MCID are not yet reported in ILD (91, 122–124). CQLQ is a comprehensive and responsive measure, and has good cross-sectional validity in IPF, however our experience using this questionnaire in ILD is still limited (125). More studies are needed to assess the validity of cross-culturally adapted versions of these instruments.

REMAINING GAPS AND OPPORTUNITIES

Despite the great strides that have been made to highlight the importance of HRQOL in ILD in the past two decades, there are still many opportunities to internationally and cross culturally improve its measurement. The ILD-specific HRQOL questionnaires (e.g., K-BILD, ATAQ-IPF, or L-IPF/L-PF) are designed to measure the nuanced impacts of ILD on HRQOL more precisely than generic instruments. A limited number of translations and cross-cultural adaptations have been performed on these instruments making them less generalizable for use in a larger international study compared to others that may be less ILD specific, but have been around longer and are more widely established (99–102, 105, 107, 108, 149). For example, questionnaires developed for COPD (e.g., SGRQ) are not specific to ILD, but have a large number of translations and are relatively-well-validated in ILD (70–92). More studies are needed to continue to linguistically validate and cross culturally adapt the new ILD disease-specific instruments. To standardize this process internationally, it will require global consensus and a collaborative approach (95).

There is little information on the international equivalence of the methods we use to validate PROMs, e.g., how we calculate internal consistency, construct validity including correlation with other parameters, and responsiveness. The various global concepts that impact HRQOL have the potential to affect the interpretation of PROMs. These diversities may contribute to different interpretation of the items in a single questionnaire amongst various communities and countries. Although no formal method has been established to address this possibility, subgroup analyses of multinational clinical trials may support the validity of each questionnaire across these communities and nations if similar results are obtained (154–156). We must also recognize that a PROM is ideally chosen to measure a certain outcome based upon the context and objective of the research study. This means that one questionnaire that is deemed appropriate for one trial design may not be the same questionnaire that is ideal for another, even if they are both measuring HRQOL. This adds another layer of complexity for multi-national studies as one must not only choose an instrument that will capture information about HRQOL in multiple languages and cultures, but they must also be comfortable that the instrument is measuring the constructs that are important to answer their particular question.

To date, trials testing medications developed for use in fibrotic ILDs have overwhelmingly targeted the halt of disease progression as reflected by pulmonary function, exercise tolerance, or progression-free survival (82, 103, 115, 157). As disease-specific HRQOL PROMs generally reflect changes in these parameters, these have characteristically been chosen for use in those clinical trials (77, 98, 100). As patient-centered research in ILD expands, future interventions may target the more disease-specific symptoms (e.g., cough, dyspnea, fatigue) (158–160). For these clinical trials, domain-specific PROMs focusing on each symptom may likely be chosen as the primary endpoint and therefore these instruments will need to be adapted for use cross-culturally.

The guidelines for development of PROMs are not internationally unified. Regulatory agencies such as the US Food and Drug Administration (FDA) and the European Medicines Agency (EMA) have released PROM development guidance as we increasingly recognize the importance of including these measures in clinical trials (161, 162). Recent PROMs including the K-BILD and L-IPF/L-PF adhered strictly to their guidelines during the process of developments (99, 107). Although there is no question that these guidelines are well-established and rigorous, it is necessary to verify whether the same methodology can be adapted in non-English speaking countries where there are different cultural components as well as potentially different resources available.

Finally, we need to consider the international inequalities of HRQOL itself. As discussed in this review, many individual factors are closely associated with a patient's health status. In fact, the global burdens of ILD measured by disability-adjusted life years (DALYs), which is calculated as the number of years lost due to disability or early death, are known to greatly vary across the countries (163). The level of HRQOL impairment may differ in each country, even if the disease severity assessed by pulmonary function is the same. Therefore, an understanding of the baseline health status in any individual country is important. If there is a large difference in the baseline health status between groups, then the evaluation of relative change in each individual or group should be considered. Multinational consortia of researchers with expertise in PROMs and who study HRQOL are needed in order to begin to address some of these gaps on an international level.

CONCLUSION

HRQOL is an increasingly important end point in ILD amongst patients, clinicians, and researchers alike. As our understanding of the disease and its possible therapies expands, we are rapidly accelerating opportunities for clinical trial conduct across the globe. While we have made great strides in the measurement of HRQOL in ILD, we have many opportunities to improve our measurement across cultures and countries. We have identified several ways in which HRQOL may be interpreted differently across the globe and highlighted potential mechanisms for translation and cross-cultural adaptation of HRQOL PROMs, both in general and in ILD. By recognizing these important differences and working together with our colleagues and patients across the globe we have the opportunity to improve the way we study and report HRQOL which will have a substantial impact on the conduct of multinational studies and interventions in the future.

AUTHOR CONTRIBUTIONS

KA and AS contributed equally to the conception and writing of this manuscript. Both authors contributed to the article and approved the submitted version.

REFERENCES

1. Institute of Medicine. *The Future of the Public's Health in the 21st Century.* Washington, DC: National Academies Press (US) (2002).

2. The WHOQOL Group. The World Health Organization Quality of Life assessment (WHOQOL): position paper from the World Health Organization. *Soc Sci Med.* (1995) 41:1403–9. doi: 10.1016/0277-9536(95)00112-K

3. Skevington SM, Lotfy M, O'Connell KA. The World Health Organization's WHOQOL-BREF quality of life assessment: psychometric properties and results of the international field trial. A Report from the WHOQOL Group. *Qual Life Res.* (2004) 13:299–310. doi: 10.1023/B:QURE.0000018486.91360.00

4. The World Health Organization Quality of Life Assessment (WHOQOL): development and general psychometric properties. *Soc Sci Med.* (1998) 46:1569–85. doi: 10.1016/S0277-9536(98)00009-4

5. Wilson IB, Cleary PD. Linking clinical variables with health-related quality of life. a conceptual model of patient outcomes. *JAMA.* (1995) 273:59–65. doi: 10.1001/jama.273.1.59

6. Ferrans CE, Zerwic JJ, Wilbur JE, Larson JL. Conceptual model of health-related quality of life. *J Nurs Scholarsh.* (2005) 37:336–42. doi: 10.1111/j.1547-5069.2005.00058.x

7. Burckhardt CS, Anderson KL, Archenholtz B, Hägg O. The Flanagan Quality Of Life Scale: evidence of construct validity. *Health Qual Life Outcomes.* (2003) 1:59. doi: 10.1186/1477-7525-1-59

8. Bakas T, McLennon SM, Carpenter JS, Buelow JM, Otte JL, Hanna KM, et al. Systematic review of health-related quality of life models. *Health Qual Life Outcomes.* (2012) 10:134. doi: 10.1186/1477-7525-10-134

9. Haraldstad K, Wahl A, Andenæs R, Andersen JR, Andersen MH, Beisland E, et al. A systematic review of quality of life research in medicine and health sciences. *Qual Life Res.* (2019) 28:2641–50. doi: 10.1007/s11136-019-02214-9

10. O'Connell KA, Skevington SM. To measure or not to measure? Reviewing the assessment of spirituality and religion in health-related quality of life. *Chronic Illn.* (2007) 3:77–87. doi: 10.1177/1742395307079195

11. O'Connell KA, Skevington SM. The relevance of spirituality, religion and personal beliefs to health-related quality of life: themes from focus groups in Britain. *Br J Health Psychol.* (2005) 10(Pt 3):379–98. doi: 10.1348/135910705X25471

12. Ashing-Giwa KT. The contextual model of HRQoL: a paradigm for expanding the HRQoL framework. *Qual Life Res.* (2005) 14:297–307. doi: 10.1007/s11136-004-0729-7

13. Cottin V, Hirani NA, Hotchkin DL, Nambiar AM, Ogura T, Otaola M, et al. Presentation, diagnosis and clinical course of the spectrum of progressive-fibrosing interstitial lung diseases. *Eur Respir Rev.* (2018) 27:180076. doi: 10.1183/16000617.0076-2018

14. Kolb M, Vašáková M. The natural history of progressive fibrosing interstitial lung diseases. *Respir Res.* (2019) 20:57. doi: 10.1186/s12931-019-1022-1

15. Bajwah S, Colquitt J, Loveman E, Bausewein C, Almond H, Oluyase A, et al. Pharmacological and nonpharmacological interventions to improve symptom control, functional exercise capacity and quality of life in interstitial lung disease: an evidence synthesis. *ERJ Open Res.* (2021) 7:00107-2020. doi: 10.1183/23120541.00107-2020

16. Lammi MR, Baughman RP, Birring SS, Russell A-M, Ryu JH, Scholand M, et al. Outcome measures for clinical trials in interstitial lung diseases. *Curr Respir Med Rev.* (2015) 11:163–74. doi: 10.2174/1573398X11666150619183527

17. Rajala K, Lehto JT, Sutinen E, Kautiainen H, Myllärniemi M, Saarto T. Marked deterioration in the quality of life of patients with idiopathic pulmonary fibrosis during the last two years of life. *BMC Pulm Med.* (2018) 18:172. doi: 10.1186/s12890-018-0738-x

18. Brown KK, Martinez FJ, Walsh SLF, Thannickal VJ, Prasse A, Schlenker-Herceg R, et al. The natural history of progressive fibrosing interstitial lung diseases. *Eur Respir J.* (2020) 55:2000085. doi: 10.1183/13993003.00085-2020

19. Kingsley C, Patel S. Patient-reported outcome measures and patient-reported experience measures. *BJA Educ.* (2017) 17:137–44. doi: 10.1093/bjaed/mkw060

20. Food and Drug Administration. *Guidance For Industry Patient-Reported Outcome Measures: Use in Medical Product Development to Support Labeling Claims.* (2009). Available online at: https://www.fda.gov/media/77832/download (accessed 29, 2020).

21. Swigris JJ, Brown KK, Abdulqawi R, Buch K, Dilling DF, Koschel D, et al. Patients' perceptions and patient-reported outcomes in progressive-fibrosing interstitial lung diseases. *Eur Respir Rev.* (2018) 27:180075. doi: 10.1183/16000617.0075-2018

22. Moor CC, Heukels P, Kool M, Wijsenbeek MS. Integrating patient perspectives into personalized medicine in idiopathic pulmonary fibrosis. *Front Med.* (2017) 4:226. doi: 10.3389/fmed.2017.00226

23. O'Donnell DE, Chau LK, Webb KA. Qualitative aspects of exertional dyspnea in patients with interstitial lung disease. *J Appl Physiol.* (1998) 84:2000–9. doi: 10.1152/jappl.1998.84.6.2000

24. Smith J, Albert P, Bertella E, Lester J, Jack S, Calverley P. Qualitative aspects of breathlessness in health and disease. *Thorax.* (2009) 64:713–8. doi: 10.1136/thx.2008.104869

25. Vázquez-García JC, Balcázar-Cruz CA, Cervantes-Méndez G, Mejía-Alfaro R, Cossío-Alcántara J, Ramírez-Venegas A. [Descriptors of breathlessness in Mexican Spanish]. *Arch Bronconeumol.* (2006) 42:211–7. doi: 10.1016/S1579-2129(06)60448-5

26. Goyal AK, Bakshi J, Panda NK, Kapoor R, Vir D, Kumar K, et al. A hybrid method for the cross-cultural adaptation of self-report measures. *Int J Appl Posit Psychol.* (2021) 6:45–54. doi: 10.1007/s41042-020-00039-3

27. Chakka S, Werth VP. Cross-cultural adaptations of health-related quality of life measures. *Br J Dermatol.* (2019) 181:659–60. doi: 10.1111/bjd.18272

28. Beaton DE, Bombardier C, Guillemin F, Ferraz MB. Guidelines for the process of cross-cultural adaptation of self-report measures. *Spine.* (2000) 25:3186–91. doi: 10.1097/00007632-200012150-00014

29. Roof K, Oleru N. Public health: seattle and King County's push for the built environment. *J Environ Health.* (2008) 71:24–7.

30. Tucker P, Gilliland J. The effect of season and weather on physical activity: a systematic review. *Public Health.* (2007) 121:909–22. doi: 10.1016/j.puhe.2007.04.009

31. Pirozzi CS, Mendoza DL, Xu Y, Zhang Y, Scholand MB, Baughman RP. Short-term particulate air pollution exposure is associated with increased severity of respiratory and quality of life symptoms in patients with fibrotic sarcoidosis. *Int J Environ Res Public Health.* (2018) 151077. doi: 10.3390/ijerph15061077

32. Han B. Associations between perceived environmental pollution and health-related quality of life in a Chinese adult population. *Health Qual Life Outcomes.* (2020) 18:198. doi: 10.1186/s12955-020-01442-9

33. Zhou Z, Zhou Z, Gao J, Lai S, Chen G. Urban-rural difference in the associations between living arrangements and the health-related quality of life (HRQOL) of the elderly in China-Evidence from Shaanxi province. *PLoS ONE.* (2018) 13:e0204118. doi: 10.1371/journal.pone.0204118

34. Zhang T, Shi W, Huang Z, Gao D, Guo Z, Liu J, et al. Influence of culture, residential segregation and socioeconomic development on rural elderly health-related quality of life in Guangxi, China. *Health Qual Life Outcomes.* (2016) 14:98. doi: 10.1186/s12955-016-0499-2

35. Wang C, Li H, Li L, Xu D, Kane RL, Meng Q. Health literacy and ethnic disparities in health-related quality of life among rural women: results from a Chinese poor minority area. *Health Qual Life Outcomes.* (2013) 11:153. doi: 10.1186/1477-7525-11-153

36. Sabbah I, Drouby N, Sabbah S, Retel-Rude N, Mercier M. Quality of life in rural and urban populations in Lebanon using SF-36 health survey. *Health Qual Life Outcomes.* (2003) 1:30. doi: 10.1186/1477-7525-1-30

37. Nutbeam D. The evolving concept of health literacy. *Soc Sci Med.* (2008) 67:2072–8. doi: 10.1016/j.socscimed.2008.09.050

38. Liu C, Wang D, Liu C, Jiang J, Wang X, Chen H, et al. What is the meaning of health literacy? A systematic review and qualitative synthesis. *Family Med Commun Health.* (2020) 8:e000351. doi: 10.1136/fmch-2020-000351

39. Health literacy: report of th'e Council on Scientific. *Ad Hoc* Committee on Health Literacy for the Council on Scientific Affairs, American Medical Association. *JAMA.* (1999) 281:552–7.

40. Zheng M, Jin H, Shi N, Duan C, Wang D, Yu X, et al. The relationship between health literacy and quality of life: a systematic review and meta-analysis. *Health Qual Life Outcomes.* (2018) 16:201. doi: 10.1186/s12955-018-1031-7

41. Xie Y, Ma M, Zhang Y, Tan X. Factors associated with health literacy in rural areas of Central China: structural equation model. *BMC Health Serv Res.* (2019) 19:300. doi: 10.1186/s12913-019-4094-1

42. Nakayama K, Osaka W, Togari T, Ishikawa H, Yonekura Y, Sekido A, et al. Comprehensive health literacy in Japan is lower than in Europe: a validated Japanese-language assessment of health literacy. *BMC Public Health.* (2015) 15:505. doi: 10.1186/s12889-015-1835-x

43. Moor CC, van Leuven SI, Wijsenbeek MS, Vonk MC. Feasibility of online home spirometry in systemic sclerosis-associated interstitial lung disease: a pilot study. *Rheumatology.* (2021) 60:2467–71. doi: 10.1093/rheumatology/keaa607

44. Abolfotouh MA, BaniMustafa A, Salam M, Al-Assiri M, Aldebasi B, Bushnak I. Use of smartphone and perception towards the usefulness and practicality of its medical applications among healthcare workers in Saudi Arabia. *BMC Health Serv Res.* (2019) 19:826. doi: 10.1186/s12913-019-4523-1

45. Moor CC, Wapenaar M, Miedema JR, Geelhoed JJM, Chandoesing PP, Wijsenbeek MS. A home monitoring program including real-time wireless home spirometry in idiopathic pulmonary fibrosis: a pilot study on experiences and barriers. *Respir Res.* (2018) 19:105. doi: 10.1186/s12931-018-0810-3

46. Lim E, Davis J, Siriwardhana C, Aggarwal L, Hixon A, Chen JJ. Racial/ethnic differences in health-related quality of life among Hawaii adult population. *Health Qual Life Outcomes.* (2020) 18:380. doi: 10.1186/s12955-020-01625-4

47. Quittner AL, Schechter MS, Rasouliyan L, Haselkorn T, Pasta DJ, Wagener JS. Impact of socioeconomic status, race, and ethnicity on quality of life in patients with cystic fibrosis in the United States. *Chest.* (2010) 137:642–50. doi: 10.1378/chest.09-0345

48. Sentell T, Zhang W, Davis J, Baker KK, Braun KL. The influence of community and individual health literacy on self-reported health status. *J Gen Intern Med.* (2014) 29:298–304. doi: 10.1007/s11606-013-2638-3

49. Abu HO, Ulbricht C, Ding E, Allison JJ, Salmoirago-Blotcher E, Goldberg RJ, et al. Association of religiosity and spirituality with quality of life in patients with cardiovascular disease: a systematic review. *Qual Life Res.* (2018) 27:2777–97. doi: 10.1007/s11136-018-1906-4

50. Ferrell B, Chung V, Koczywas M, Borneman T, Irish TL, Ruel NH, et al. Spirituality in cancer patients on phase 1 clinical trials. *Psychooncology.* (2020) 29:1077–83. doi: 10.1002/pon.5380

51. Guyatt GH, Ferrans CE, Halyard MY, Revicki DA, Symonds TL, Varricchio CG, et al. Exploration of the value of health-related quality-of-life information from clinical research and into clinical practice. *Mayo Clin Proc.* (2007) 82:1229–39. doi: 10.4065/82.10.1229

52. Guillemin F, Bombardier C, Beaton D. Cross-cultural adaptation of health-related quality of life measures: literature review and proposed guidelines. *J Clin Epidemiol.* (1993) 46:1417–32. doi: 10.1016/0895-4356(93)90142-N

53. Herdman M, Fox-Rushby J, Badia X. "Equivalence" and the translation and adaptation of health-related quality of life questionnaires. *Qual Life Res.* (1997) 6:237–47. doi: 10.1023/A:1026410721664

54. Rothrock NE, Kaiser KA, Cella D. Developing a valid patient-reported outcome measure. *Clin Pharmacol Ther.* (2011) 90:737–42. doi: 10.1038/clpt.2011.195

55. da Mota Falcão D, Ciconelli RM, Ferraz MB. Translation and cultural adaptation of quality of life questionnaires: an evaluation of methodology. *J Rheumatol.* (2003) 30:379–85.

56. Gjersing L, Caplehorn JRM, Clausen T. Cross-cultural adaptation of research instruments: language, setting, time and statistical considerations. *BMC Med Res Methodol.* (2010) 10:13. doi: 10.1186/1471-2288-10-13

57. Wang W-L, Lee H-L, Fetzer SJ. Challenges and strategies of instrument translation. *West J Nurs Res.* (2006) 28:310–21. doi: 10.1177/0193945905284712

58. Sechrest L, Fay TL, Zaidi SMH. Problems of translation in cross-cultural research. *J Cross Cult Psychol.* (1972) 3:41–56. doi: 10.1177/002202217200300103

59. Wild D, Grove A, Martin M, Eremenco S, McElroy S, Verjee-Lorenz A, et al. Principles of good practice for the translation and cultural adaptation process for Patient-Reported Outcomes (PRO) Measures: report of the ISPOR task force for translation and cultural adaptation. *Value Health.* (2005) 8:94–104. doi: 10.1111/j.1524-4733.2005.04054.x

60. Hofmeyer A, Sheingold BH, Taylor R. Do you understand what I mean? how cognitive interviewing can strengthen valid, reliable study instruments and dissemination products. *J Int Educ Res.* (2015) 11:261. doi: 10.19030/jier.v11i4.9460

61. Scott K, Gharai D, Sharma M, Choudhury N, Mishra B, Chamberlain S, et al. Yes, no, maybe so: the importance of cognitive interviewing to enhance structured surveys on respectful maternity care in northern India. *Health Policy Plan.* (2020) 35:67–77. doi: 10.1093/heapol/czz141

62. Ware JE, Gandek B. Methods for testing data quality, scaling assumptions, and reliability: the IQOLA Project approach. International Quality of Life Assessment. *J Clin Epidemiol.* (1998) 51:945–52. doi: 10.1016/S0895-4356(98)00085-7

63. Aaronson NK, Acquadro C, Alonso J, Apolone G, Bucquet D, Bullinger M, et al. International quality of life assessment (IQOLA) project. *Qual Life Res.* (1992) 1:349–51. doi: 10.1007/BF00434949

64. Ware JE, Keller SD, Gandek B, Brazier JE, Sullivan M. Evaluating translations of health status questionnaires. Methods from the IQOLA project. International Quality of Life Assessment. *Int J Technol Assess Health Care.* (1995) 11:525–51. doi: 10.1017/S0266462300008710

65. Ware JE, Gandek B. Overview of the SF-36 health survey and the International Quality of Life Assessment (IQOLA) project. *J Clin Epidemiol.* (1998) 51:903–12. doi: 10.1016/S0895-4356(98)00081-X

66. Aaronson NK, Ahmedzai S, Bergman B, Bullinger M, Cull A, Duez NJ, et al. The European Organization for Research and Treatment of Cancer QLQ-C30: a quality-of-life instrument for use in international clinical trials in oncology. *J Natl Cancer Inst.* (1993) 85:365–76. doi: 10.1093/jnci/85.5.365

67. EuroQol Group. EuroQol–a new facility for the measurement of health-related quality of life. *Health Policy.* (1990) 16:199–208. doi: 10.1016/0168-8510(90)90421-9

68. Devlin NJ, Brooks R. EQ-5D and the EuroQol group: past, present and future. *Appl Health Econ Health Policy.* (2017) 15:127–37. doi: 10.1007/s40258-017-0310-5

69. Aronson KI, Danoff SK, Russell A-M, Ryerson CJ, Suzuki A, Wijsenbeek MS, et al. Patient-centered Outcomes Research in Interstitial Lung Disease: an Official American Thoracic Society Research Statement. *Am J Respir Crit Care Med.* (2021) 204:e3–23. doi: 10.1164/rccm.202105-1193ST

70. Jones PW, Quirk FH, Baveystock CM, Littlejohns P. A self-complete measure of health status for chronic airflow limitation. The St. George's Respiratory Questionnaire. *Am Rev Respir Dis.* (1992) 145:1321–7. doi: 10.1164/ajrccm/145.6.1321

71. Tzanakis N, Samiou M, Lambiri I, Antoniou K, Siafakas N, Bouros D. Evaluation of health-related quality-of-life and dyspnea scales in patients with idiopathic pulmonary fibrosis. Correlation with pulmonary function tests. *Eur J Intern Med.* (2005) 16:105–12. doi: 10.1016/j.ejim.2004.09.013

72. Beretta L, Santaniello A, Lemos A, Masciocchi M, Scorza R. Validity of the Saint George's Respiratory Questionnaire in the evaluation of the health-related quality of life in patients with interstitial lung disease secondary to systemic sclerosis. *Rheumatology.* (2007) 46:296–301. doi: 10.1093/rheumatology/kel221

73. Swigris JJ, Brown KK, Behr J, du Bois RM, King TE, Raghu G, et al. The SF-36 and SGRQ: validity and first look at minimum important differences in IPF. *Respir Med.* (2010) 104:296–304. doi: 10.1016/j.rmed.2009.09.006

74. Wallace B, Kafaja S, Furst DE, Berrocal VJ, Merkel PA, Seibold JR, et al. Reliability, validity and responsiveness to change of the Saint George's Respiratory Questionnaire in early diffuse cutaneous systemic sclerosis. *Rheumatology.* (2015) 54:1369–79. doi: 10.1093/rheumatology/keu456

75. Swigris JJ, Esser D, Wilson H, Conoscenti CS, Schmidt H, Stansen W, et al. Psychometric properties of the St George's Respiratory Questionnaire in patients with idiopathic pulmonary fibrosis. *Eur Respir J.* (2017) 49:1601788. doi: 10.1183/13993003.01788-2016

76. Glaspole IN, Chapman SA, Cooper WA, Ellis SJ, Goh NS, Hopkins PM, et al. Health-related quality of life in idiopathic pulmonary fibrosis: data from the Australian IPF Registry. *Respirology.* (2017) 22:950–6. doi: 10.1111/resp.12989

77. Suzuki A, Kondoh Y, Swigris JJ, Ando M, Kimura T, Kataoka K, et al. Performance of the St George's Respiratory Questionnaire in patients with connective tissue disease-associated interstitial lung disease. *Respirology*. (2018). doi: 10.1111/resp.13293. [Epub ahead of print].

78. Kreuter M, Swigris J, Pittrow D, Geier S, Klotsche J, Prasse A, et al. The clinical course of idiopathic pulmonary fibrosis and its association to quality of life over time: longitudinal data from the INSIGHTS-IPF registry. *Respir Res*. (2019) 20:59. doi: 10.1186/s12931-019-1020-3

79. Swigris JJ, Wilson H, Esser D, Conoscenti CS, Stansen W, Kline Leidy N, et al. Psychometric properties of the St George's Respiratory Questionnaire in patients with idiopathic pulmonary fibrosis: insights from the INPULSIS trials. *BMJ Open Respir Res*. (2018) 5:e000278. doi: 10.1136/bmjresp-2018-000278

80. Idiopathic Pulmonary Fibrosis Clinical Research Network, Zisman DA, Schwarz M, Anstrom KJ, Collard HR, Flaherty KR, et al. A controlled trial of sildenafil in advanced idiopathic pulmonary fibrosis. *N Engl J Med*. (2010) 363:620–8. doi: 10.1056/NEJMoa1002110

81. Idiopathic Pulmonary Fibrosis Clinical Research Network, Raghu G, Anstrom KJ, King TE, Lasky JA, Martinez FJ. Prednisone, azathioprine, and N-acetylcysteine for pulmonary fibrosis. *N Engl J Med*. (2012) 366:1968–77. doi: 10.1056/NEJMoa1113354

82. Richeldi L, du Bois RM, Raghu G, Azuma A, Brown KK, Costabel U, et al. Efficacy and safety of nintedanib in idiopathic pulmonary fibrosis. *N Engl J Med*. (2014) 370:2071–82. doi: 10.1056/NEJMoa1402584

83. Visca D, Mori L, Tsipouri V, Fleming S, Firouzi A, Bonini M, et al. Effect of ambulatory oxygen on quality of life for patients with fibrotic lung disease (AmbOx): a prospective, open-label, mixed-method, crossover randomised controlled trial. *Lancet Respir Med*. (2018) 6:759–70. doi: 10.1016/S2213-2600(18)30289-3

84. Kolb M, Raghu G, Wells AU, Behr J, Richeldi L, Schinzel B, et al. Nintedanib plus Sildenafil in patients with idiopathic pulmonary fibrosis. *N Engl J Med*. (2018) 379:1722–31. doi: 10.1056/NEJMoa1811737

85. Demedts M, Behr J, Buhl R, Costabel U, Dekhuijzen R, Jansen HM, et al. High-dose acetylcysteine in idiopathic pulmonary fibrosis. *N Engl J Med*. (2005) 353:2229–42. doi: 10.1056/NEJMoa042976

86. Raghu G, Brown KK, Costabel U, Cottin V, du Bois RM, Lasky JA, et al. Treatment of idiopathic pulmonary fibrosis with etanercept: an exploratory, placebo-controlled trial. *Am J Respir Crit Care Med*. (2008) 178:948–55. doi: 10.1164/rccm.200709-1446OC

87. King TE, Albera C, Bradford WZ, Costabel U, Hormel P, Lancaster L, et al. Effect of interferon gamma-1b on survival in patients with idiopathic pulmonary fibrosis (INSPIRE): a multicentre, randomised, placebo-controlled trial. *Lancet*. (2009) 374:222–8. doi: 10.1016/S0140-6736(09)60551-1

88. Han MK, Bach DS, Hagan PG, Yow E, Flaherty KR, Toews GB, et al. Sildenafil preserves exercise capacity in patients with idiopathic pulmonary fibrosis and right-sided ventricular dysfunction. *Chest*. (2013) 143:1699–708. doi: 10.1378/chest.12-1594

89. Richeldi L, Costabel U, Selman M, Kim DS, Hansell DM, Nicholson AG, et al. Efficacy of a tyrosine kinase inhibitor in idiopathic pulmonary fibrosis. *N Engl J Med*. (2011) 365:1079–87. doi: 10.1056/NEJMoa1103690

90. Raghu G, Behr J, Brown KK, Egan JJ, Kawut SM, Flaherty KR, et al. Treatment of idiopathic pulmonary fibrosis with ambrisentan: a parallel, randomized trial. *Ann Intern Med*. (2013) 158:641–9. doi: 10.7326/0003-4819-158-9-201305070-00003

91. Maher TM, Corte TJ, Fischer A, Kreuter M, Lederer DJ, Molina-Molina M, et al. Pirfenidone in patients with unclassifiable progressive fibrosing interstitial lung disease: a double-blind, randomised, placebo-controlled, phase 2 trial. *Lancet Respir Med*. (2020) 8:147–57. doi: 10.1016/S2213-2600(19)30341-8

92. Behr J, Nathan SD, Wuyts WA, Mogulkoc Bishop N, Bouros DE, Antoniou K, et al. Efficacy and safety of sildenafil added to pirfenidone in patients with advanced idiopathic pulmonary fibrosis and risk of pulmonary hypertension: a double-blind, randomised, placebo-controlled, phase 2b trial. *Lancet Respir Med*. (2021) 9:85–95. doi: 10.1016/S2213-2600(20)30356-8

93. Yorke J, Jones PW, Swigris JJ. Development and validity testing of an IPF-specific version of the St George's Respiratory Questionnaire. *Thorax*. (2010) 65:921–6. doi: 10.1136/thx.2010.139121

94. Prior TS, Hoyer N, Shaker SB, Davidsen JR, Yorke J, Hilberg O, et al. Validation of the IPF-specific version of St. George's Respiratory Questionnaire. *Respir Res*. (2019) 20:199. doi: 10.1186/s12931-019-1169-9

95. Prior TS, Hoyer N, Hilberg O, Shaker SB, Davidsen JR, Bendstrup E. Responsiveness and minimal clinically important difference of SGRQ-I and K-BILD in idiopathic pulmonary fibrosis. *Respir Res*. (2020) 21:91. doi: 10.1186/s12931-020-01359-3

96. Jones PW, Harding G, Berry P, Wiklund I, Chen WH, Kline Leidy N. Development and first validation of the COPD Assessment Test. *Eur Respir J*. (2009) 34:648–54. doi: 10.1183/09031936.00102509

97. Nagata K, Tomii K, Otsuka K, Tachikawa R, Otsuka K, Takeshita J, et al. Evaluation of the chronic obstructive pulmonary disease assessment test for measurement of health-related quality of life in patients with interstitial lung disease. *Respirology*. (2012) 17:506–12. doi: 10.1111/j.1440-1843.2012.02131.x

98. Suzuki A, Kondoh Y, Swigris JJ, Matsuda T, Kimura T, Kataoka K, et al. Performance of the COPD Assessment Test in patients with connective tissue disease-associated interstitial lung disease. *Respir Med*. (2019) 150:15–20. doi: 10.1016/j.rmed.2019.01.017

99. Patel AS, Siegert RJ, Brignall K, Gordon P, Steer S, Desai SR, et al. The development and validation of the King's Brief Interstitial Lung Disease (K-BILD) health status questionnaire. *Thorax*. (2012) 67:804–10. doi: 10.1136/thoraxjnl-2012-201581

100. Nolan CM, Birring SS, Maddocks M, Maher TM, Patel S, Barker RE, et al. King's Brief Interstitial Lung Disease questionnaire: responsiveness and minimum clinically important difference. *Eur Respir J*. (2019) 54:1900281. doi: 10.1183/13993003.00281-2019

101. Patel AS, Siegert RJ, Keir GJ, Bajwah S, Barker RD, Maher TM, et al. The minimal important difference of the King's Brief Interstitial Lung Disease Questionnaire (K-BILD) and forced vital capacity in interstitial lung disease. *Respir Med*. (2013) 107:1438–43. doi: 10.1016/j.rmed.2013.06.009

102. Sinha A, Patel AS, Siegert RJ, Bajwah S, Maher TM, Renzoni EA, et al. The King's Brief Interstitial Lung Disease (KBILD) questionnaire: an updated minimal clinically important difference. *BMJ Open Respir Res*. (2019) 6:e000363. doi: 10.1136/bmjresp-2018-000363

103. Flaherty KR, Wells AU, Cottin V, Devaraj A, Walsh SLF, Inoue Y, et al. Nintedanib in progressive fibrosing interstitial lung diseases. *N Engl J Med*. (2019) 381:1718–27. doi: 10.1056/NEJMoa1908681

104. Wapenaar M, Patel AS, Birring SS, Domburg RT van, Bakker EW, Vindigni V, et al. Translation and validation of the King's Brief Interstitial Lung Disease (K-BILD) questionnaire in French, Italian, Swedish, and Dutch. *Chron Respir Dis*. (2017) 14:140–50. doi: 10.1177/1479972316674425

105. Swigris JJ, Wilson SR, Green KE, Sprunger DB, Brown KK, Wamboldt FS. Development of the ATAQ-IPF: a tool to assess quality of life in IPF. *Health Qual Life Outcomes*. (2010) 8:77. doi: 10.1186/1477-7525-8-77

106. Maher TM, Costabel U, Glassberg MK, Kondoh Y, Ogura T, Scholand MB, et al. Phase 2 trial to assess lebrikizumab in patients with idiopathic pulmonary fibrosis. *Eur Respir J*. (2021) 57:1902442. doi: 10.1183/13993003.02442-2019

107. Swigris JJ, Andrae DA, Churney T, Johnson N, Scholand MB, White ES, et al. Development and initial validation analyses of the living with idiopathic pulmonary fibrosis questionnaire. *Am J Respir Crit Care Med*. (2020) 202:1689–97. doi: 10.1164/rccm.202002-0415OC

108. Swigris J, Cutts K, Male N, Baldwin M, Rohr KB, Bushnell DM. The Living with Pulmonary Fibrosis questionnaire in progressive fibrosing interstitial lung disease. *ERJ Open Res*. (2021) 7:00145-2020. doi: 10.1183/23120541.00145-2020

109. Kimman ML, Rotteveel AH, Wijsenbeek M, Mostard R, Tak NC, van Jaarsveld X, et al. Development and pretesting of a questionnaire to assess patient experiences and satisfaction with medications (PESaM Questionnaire). *Patient*. (2017) 10:629–42. doi: 10.1007/s40271-017-0234-z

110. Kimman ML, Wijsenbeek MS, van Kuijk SMJ, Wijnsma KL, van de Kar NCAJ, Storm M, et al. Validity of the patient experiences and satisfaction with medications (PESaM) questionnaire. *Patient*. (2019) 12:149–62. doi: 10.1007/s40271-018-0340-6

111. Moor CC, Mostard RLM, Grutters JC, Bresser P, Aerts JGJV, Dirksen CD, et al. Patient expectations, experiences and satisfaction with nintedanib and pirfenidone in idiopathic pulmonary fibrosis: a quantitative study. *Respir Res*. (2020) 21:196. doi: 10.1186/s12931-020-01458-1

112. Aronson KI, Ali M, Reshetynak E, Kaner RJ, Martinez FJ, Safford MM, et al. Establishing content-validity of a disease-specific health-related quality of life instrument for patients with chronic hypersensitivity pneumonitis. *J Patient Rep Outcomes*. (2021) 5:9. doi: 10.1186/s41687-020-00282-x

113. Swigris JJ, Yorke J, Sprunger DB, Swearingen C, Pincus T, du Bois RM, et al. Assessing dyspnea and its impact on patients with connective tissue disease-related interstitial lung disease. *Respir Med*. (2010) 104:1350–5. doi: 10.1016/j.rmed.2010.03.027

114. Swigris JJ, Han M, Vij R, Noth I, Eisenstein EL, Anstrom KJ, et al. The UCSD shortness of breath questionnaire has longitudinal construct validity in idiopathic pulmonary fibrosis. *Respir Med*. (2012) 106:1447–55. doi: 10.1016/j.rmed.2012.06.018

115. King TE, Bradford WZ, Castro-Bernardini S, Fagan EA, Glaspole I, Glassberg MK, et al. A phase 3 trial of pirfenidone in patients with idiopathic pulmonary fibrosis. *N Engl J Med*. (2014) 370:2083–92. doi: 10.1056/NEJMoa1402582

116. Noble PW, Albera C, Bradford WZ, Costabel U, Glassberg MK, Kardatzke D, et al. Pirfenidone in patients with idiopathic pulmonary fibrosis (CAPACITY): two randomised trials. *Lancet*. (2011) 377:1760–9. doi: 10.1016/S0140-6736(11)60405-4

117. Nishiyama O, Taniguchi H, Kondoh Y, Kimura T, Kato K, Kataoka K, et al. A simple assessment of dyspnoea as a prognostic indicator in idiopathic pulmonary fibrosis. *Eur Respir J*. (2010) 36:1067–72. doi: 10.1183/09031936.00152609

118. Rajala K, Lehto JT, Sutinen E, Kautiainen H, Myllärniemi M, Saarto T. mMRC dyspnoea scale indicates impaired quality of life and increased pain in patients with idiopathic pulmonary fibrosis. *ERJ Open Res*. (2017) 3:00084-2017. doi: 10.1183/23120541.00084-2017

119. King TE, Brown KK, Raghu G, du Bois RM, Lynch DA, Martinez F, et al. BUILD-3: a randomized, controlled trial of bosentan in idiopathic pulmonary fibrosis. *Am J Respir Crit Care Med*. (2011) 184:92–9. doi: 10.1164/rccm.201011-1874OC

120. Mahler DA, Witek TJ. The MCID of the transition dyspnea index is a total score of one unit. *COPD*. (2005) 2:99–103. doi: 10.1081/COPD-200050666

121. Khanna D, Tseng C-H, Furst DE, Clements PJ, Elashoff R, Roth M, et al. Minimally important differences in the Mahler's Transition Dyspnea Index in a large randomized controlled trial–results from the Scleroderma Lung Study. *Rheumatology*. (2009) 48:1537–40. doi: 10.1093/rheumatology/kep284

122. Birring SS, Prudon B, Carr AJ, Singh SJ, Morgan MDL, Pavord ID. Development of a symptom specific health status measure for patients with chronic cough: LEICESTER Cough Questionnaire (LCQ). *Thorax*. (2003) 58:339–43. doi: 10.1136/thorax.58.4.339

123. Key AL, Holt K, Hamilton A, Smith JA, Earis JE. Objective cough frequency in Idiopathic Pulmonary Fibrosis. *Cough*. (2010) 6:4. doi: 10.1186/1745-9974-6-4

124. Scholand MB, Wolff R, Crossno PF, Sundar K, Winegar M, Whipple S, et al. Severity of cough in idiopathic pulmonary fibrosis is associated with MUC5 B genotype. *Cough*. (2014) 10:3. doi: 10.1186/1745-9974-10-3

125. Lechtzin N, Hilliard ME, Horton MR. Validation of the Cough Quality-of-Life Questionnaire in patients with idiopathic pulmonary fibrosis. *Chest*. (2013) 143:1745–9. doi: 10.1378/chest.12-2870

126. De Vries J, Michielsen H, Van Heck GL, Drent M. Measuring fatigue in sarcoidosis: the Fatigue Assessment Scale (FAS). *Br J Health Psychol*. (2004) 9(Pt 3):279–91. doi: 10.1348/1359107041557048

127. de Kleijn WPE, De Vries J, Wijnen PAHM, Drent M. Minimal (clinically) important differences for the Fatigue Assessment Scale in sarcoidosis. *Respir Med*. (2011) 105:1388–95. doi: 10.1016/j.rmed.2011.05.004

128. Drent M, Lower EE, De Vries J. Sarcoidosis-associated fatigue. *Eur Respir J*. (2012) 40:255–63. doi: 10.1183/09031936.00002512

129. Atkins CP, Gilbert D, Brockwell C, Robinson S, Wilson AM. Fatigue in sarcoidosis and idiopathic pulmonary fibrosis: differences in character and severity between diseases. *Sarcoidosis Vasc Diffuse Lung Dis*. (2016) 33:130–8.

130. Lee YJ, Choi SM, Lee YJ, Cho Y-J, Yoon HI, Lee J-H, et al. Clinical impact of depression and anxiety in patients with idiopathic pulmonary fibrosis. *PLoS ONE*. (2017) 12:e0184300. doi: 10.1371/journal.pone.0184300

131. Matsuda T, Taniguchi H, Ando M, Kondoh Y, Kimura T, Kataoka K, et al. Depression is significantly associated with the health status in patients with idiopathic pulmonary fibrosis. *Intern Med*. (2017) 56:1637–44. doi: 10.2169/internalmedicine.56.7019

132. Glaspole IN, Watson AL, Allan H, Chapman S, Cooper WA, Corte TJ, et al. Determinants and outcomes of prolonged anxiety and depression in idiopathic pulmonary fibrosis. *Eur Respir J*. (2017) 50:1700168. doi: 10.1183/13993003.00168-2017

133. Stern AF. The hospital anxiety and depression scale. *Occup Med*. (2014) 64:393–4. doi: 10.1093/occmed/kqu024

134. Johns MW. A new method for measuring daytime sleepiness: the Epworth sleepiness scale. *Sleep*. (1991) 14:540–5. doi: 10.1093/sleep/14.6.540

135. Lancaster LH, Mason WR, Parnell JA, Rice TW, Loyd JE, Milstone AP, et al. Obstructive sleep apnea is common in idiopathic pulmonary fibrosis. *Chest*. (2009) 136:772–8. doi: 10.1378/chest.08-2776

136. Mermigkis C, Stagaki E, Tryfon S, Schiza S, Amfilochiou A, Polychronopoulos V, et al. How common is sleep-disordered breathing in patients with idiopathic pulmonary fibrosis? *Sleep Breath*. (2010) 14:387–90. doi: 10.1007/s11325-010-0336-5

137. Ware JE, Sherbourne CD. The MOS 36-item short-form health survey (SF-36). I. Conceptual framework and item selection. *Med Care*. (1992) 30:473–83. doi: 10.1097/00005650-199206000-00002

138. Chang JA, Curtis JR, Patrick DL, Raghu G. Assessment of health-related quality of life in patients with interstitial lung disease. *Chest*. (1999) 116:1175–82. doi: 10.1378/chest.116.5.1175

139. Martinez TY, Pereira CA, dos Santos ML, Ciconelli RM, Guimarães SM, Martinez JA. Evaluation of the short-form 36-item questionnaire to measure health-related quality of life in patients with idiopathic pulmonary fibrosis. *Chest*. (2000) 117:1627–32. doi: 10.1378/chest.117.6.1627

140. Tomioka H, Imanaka K, Hashimoto K, Iwasaki H. Health-related quality of life in patients with idiopathic pulmonary fibrosis–cross-sectional and longitudinal study. *Intern Med*. (2007) 46:1533–42. doi: 10.2169/internalmedicine.46.6218

141. Khanna D, Clements PJ, Furst DE, Chon Y, Elashoff R, Roth MD, et al. Correlation of the degree of dyspnea with health-related quality of life, functional abilities, and diffusing capacity for carbon monoxide in patients with systemic sclerosis and active alveolitis: results from the Scleroderma Lung Study. *Arthritis Rheum*. (2005) 52:592–600. doi: 10.1002/art.20787

142. Herdman M, Gudex C, Lloyd A, Janssen M, Kind P, Parkin D, et al. Development and preliminary testing of the new five-level version of EQ-5D (EQ-5D-5L). *Qual Life Res*. (2011) 20:1727–36. doi: 10.1007/s11136-011-9903-x

143. Mulhern B, Feng Y, Shah K, Janssen MF, Herdman M, van Hout B, et al. Correction to: comparing the UK EQ-5D-3L and English EQ-5D-5L value sets. *Pharmacoeconomics*. (2018) 36:727. doi: 10.1007/s40273-018-0648-z

144. Szentes BL, Kreuter M, Bahmer T, Birring SS, Claussen M, Waelscher J, et al. Quality of life assessment in interstitial lung diseases:a comparison of the disease-specific K-BILD with the generic EQ-5D-5L. *Respir Res*. (2018) 19:101. doi: 10.1186/s12931-018-0808-x

145. Tsai APY, Hur SA, Wong A, Safavi M, Assayag D, Johannson KA, et al. Minimum important difference of the EQ-5D-5L and EQ-VAS in fibrotic interstitial lung disease. *Thorax*. (2021) 76:37–43. doi: 10.1136/thoraxjnl-2020-214944

146. Cella D, Yount S, Rothrock N, Gershon R, Cook K, Reeve B, et al. The patient-reported outcomes measurement information system (PROMIS): Progress of an NIH roadmap cooperative group during its first two years. *Med Care*. (2007) 45(5 Suppl. 1):S3–11. doi: 10.1097/01.mlr.0000258615.42478.55

147. Yount SE, Beaumont JL, Chen S-Y, Kaiser K, Wortman K, Van Brunt DL, et al. Health-related quality of life in patients with idiopathic pulmonary fibrosis. *Lung*. (2016) 194:227–34. doi: 10.1007/s00408-016-9850-y

148. Fisher CJ, Namas R, Seelman D, Jaafar S, Homer K, Wilhalme H, et al. Reliability, construct validity and responsiveness to change of the PROMIS-29 in systemic sclerosis-associated interstitial lung disease. *Clin Exp Rheumatol*. (2019) 37(Suppl. 119):49–56.

149. Prior TS, Hilberg O, Shaker SB, Davidsen JR, Hoyer N, Birring SS, et al. Validation of the King's brief interstitial lung disease questionnaire in idiopathic pulmonary fibrosis. *BMC Pulm Med*. (2019) 19:255. doi: 10.1186/s12890-019-1018-0

150. Silveira K, Steidle LJM, Matte DL, Tavares PH, Pincelli MP, Pizzichini MMM, et al. Translation and cultural adaptation of the King's Brief Interstitial Lung Disease health status questionnaire for use in Brazil. *J Bras Pneumol.* (2019) 45:e20180194. doi: 10.1590/1806-3713/e20180194

151. Pan R-L, Swigris JJ, Zhao Y-W, Guo A-M, Wu Q, Li S-J. Reliability and validity of Chinese version of a tool to assess the quality of life in idiopathic pulmonary fibrosis in patients with interstitial lung disease. *Int J Nurs Sci.* (2019) 6:38–42. doi: 10.1016/j.ijnss.2018.11.005

152. Yorke J, Moosavi SH, Shuldham C, Jones PW. Quantification of dyspnoea using descriptors: development and initial testing of the Dyspnoea-12. *Thorax.* (2010) 65:21–6. doi: 10.1136/thx.2009.118521

153. Yorke J, Swigris J, Russell A-M, Moosavi SH, Ng Man Kwong G, Longshaw M, et al. Dyspnea-12 is a valid and reliable measure of breathlessness in patients with interstitial lung disease. *Chest.* (2011) 139:159–64. doi: 10.1378/chest.10-0693

154. Taniguchi H, Xu Z, Azuma A, Inoue Y, Li H, Fujimoto T, et al. Subgroup analysis of Asian patients in the INPULSIS® trials of nintedanib in idiopathic pulmonary fibrosis. *Respirology.* (2016) 21:1425–30. doi: 10.1111/resp.12852

155. Xu Z, Li H, Wen F, Bai C, Chen P, Fan F, et al. Subgroup analysis for chinese patients included in the INPULSIS® trials on nintedanib in idiopathic pulmonary fibrosis. *Adv Ther.* (2019) 36:621–31. doi: 10.1007/s12325-019-0887-1

156. Azuma A, Chung L, Behera D, Chung M, Kondoh Y, Ogura T, et al. Efficacy and safety of nintedanib in Asian patients with systemic sclerosis-associated interstitial lung disease: subgroup analysis of the SENSCIS trial. *Respir Investig.* (2021) 59:252–9. doi: 10.1016/j.resinv.2020.10.005

157. Distler O, Highland KB, Gahlemann M, Azuma A, Fischer A, Mayes MD, et al. Nintedanib for systemic sclerosis-associated interstitial lung disease. *N Engl J Med.* (2019) 380:2518–28. doi: 10.1056/NEJMoa1903076

158. van Manen MJG, Birring SS, Vancheri C, Vindigni V, Renzoni E, Russell A-M, et al. Effect of pirfenidone on cough in patients with idiopathic pulmonary fibrosis. *Eur Respir J.* (2017) 50:1701157. doi: 10.1183/13993003.01157-2017

159. Suzuki A, Sakaguchi H, Sakamoto K, Ebina M, Azuma A, Ogura T, et al. The effect of pirfenidone on the prescription of antibiotics and antitussive drugs in patients with idiopathic pulmonary fibrosis: a *post hoc* exploratory analysis of phase III clinical trial. *Chest.* (2021). doi: 10.1016/j.chest.2021.05.058. [Epub ahead of print].

160. Kronborg-White S, Andersen CU, Kohberg C, Hilberg O, Bendstrup E. Palliation of chronic breathlessness with morphine in patients with fibrotic interstitial lung disease - a randomised placebo-controlled trial. *Respir Res.* (2020) 21:195. doi: 10.1186/s12931-020-01452-7

161. US Department of Health and Human. *Guidance for Industry-Patient-Reported Outcome Measures: Use in Medical Product Development to Support Labeling Claims* (2009). Available online at: http://www.fda.gov (accessed July 19, 2021).

162. Committee for Medicinal Products for Human Use. *European Medicines Agency. Reflection Paper on the Regulatory Guidance for the Use of Health-Related Quality of Life (HRQL) Measures in the Evaluation of Medicinal Products* (2005). Available online at: https://www.ema.europa.eu/en/documents/scientific-guideline/reflection-paper-regulatory-guidance-use-healthrelated-quality-life-hrql-measures-evaluation_en.pdf

163. Sauleda J, Núñez B, Sala E, Soriano JB. Idiopathic pulmonary fibrosis: epidemiology, natural history, phenotypes. *Med Sci.* (2018) 6:110. doi: 10.3390/medsci6040110

20

Predictors and Mortality of Rapidly Progressive Interstitial Lung Disease in Patients With Idiopathic Inflammatory Myopathy: A Series of 474 Patients

Yuhui Li[1†], Xiaojuan Gao[2†], Yimin Li[1†], Xiaohui Jia[3], Xuewu Zhang[1], Yan Xu[4], Yuzhou Gan[1],
Shiming Li[5], Renli Chen[2], Jing He[1*] and Xiaolin Sun[1*]

[1] Beijing Key Laboratory for Rheumatism and Immune Diagnosis (BZ0135), Department of Rheumatology and Immunology,
Peking University People's Hospital, Beijing, China, [2] Department of Rheumatology, Ningde Hospital, Affiliated Hospital of
Fujian Medical University, Ningde, China, [3] Department of Rheumatology, The First Hospital of Hebei Medical University,
Shijiazhuang, China, [4] Department of Neurology, Peking University People's Hospital, Beijing, China, [5] Department of
Endocrinology, People's Hospital of Wushan County, Gansu, China

*Correspondence:
Jing He
hejing1105@126.com
Xiaolin Sun
sunxiaolin_sxl@126.com

[†] These authors have contributed
equally to this work

Objective: This study was conducted to identify the characteristics and prognosis of rapidly progressive interstitial lung disease (RP-ILD) in idiopathic inflammatory myopathy (IIM) and to assess the predictors for poor survival of RP-ILD in IIM.

Methods: A total of 474 patients with IIM were enrolled retrospectively according to medical records from Peking University People's Hospital. Clinical and laboratory characteristics recorded at the diagnosis of patients with RP-ILD and chronic ILD (C-ILD) were compared. The Kaplan–Meier estimator and univariate and multivariate analyses were used for data analysis.

Results: ILD was identified in 65% (308/474) of patients with IIM. Patients with ILD were classified into two groups based on lung features: RP-ILD (38%, 117/308) and C-ILD (62%, 191/308). RP-ILD resulted in significantly higher mortality in IIM compared with C-ILD (27.4 vs. 7.9%, $P < 0.05$). In this study, by comparing IIM patients with and without RP-ILD, a list of initial predictors for RP-ILD development were identified, which included older age at onset, decreased peripheral lymphocytes, skin involvement (periungual erythema, skin ulceration, and subcutaneous/mediastinal emphysema), presence of anti-MDA5 antibody, serum tumor markers, etc. Further multivariate Cox proportional hazards model analysis identified that anti-MDA5 positivity was an independent risk factor for mortality due to RP-ILD ($P < 0.05$), and lymphocytes <30% in BALF might also be associated with poor survival of myositis-associated RP-ILD ($P < 0.05$).

Conclusion: Our study shows that RP-ILD results in increased mortality in IIM. Anti-MDA5 positivity and a lower lymphocyte ratio in BALF might be the predictive factor of mortality due to RP-ILD.

Keywords: myositis, interstitial lung disease, MSAs, rapidly progressive, survival

INTRODUCTION

Idiopathic inflammatory myopathy (IIM) is a group of systemic autoimmune diseases characterized by skin rash, proximal muscle weakness, and extramuscular manifestations, such as arthralgia, fever, and interstitial lung disease (ILD). Dermatomyositis (DM), polymyositis (PM), and clinically amyopathic dermatomyositis (CADM) are the three main subtypes of IIM (1, 2). Myositis-associated ILD is one of the leading extramuscular features, occurring in 20–80% of all PM/DM/CADM patients (3, 4). Rapidly progressive ILD (RP-ILD) in IIM is a life-threatening subtype of myositis-associated ILD, which tends to be resistant to high-dose glucocorticoid treatment and immunosuppressants (4–6). Recently, a study in a European myositis cohort reported that 40–60% of patients with RP-ILD were admitted to the ICU, and hospital mortality was 45–51% (7). Some patients with RP-ILD decline within weeks, but for other patients, the time to ILD-induced deterioration is on the order of years (8), and the 5-year survival rate is more than 85% in myositis-associated ILD (9, 10). However, it is difficult to predict whether patients with myositis-associated ILD will develop fatal disease progression at the early stage of the disease. Therefore, it is necessary to identify potential factors to predict survival of patients with myositis-associated RP-ILD in the early stage of disease development.

The pathogenesis of lung injury in myositis is unclear. Although anti-aminoacyl tRNA synthetase (ARS) and anti-melanoma differentiation-associated 5 (MDA5) antibodies have been described as associated with RP-ILD (11), the exact pathophysiology and diagnostic value of these autoantibodies remain to be elucidated. Previous studies have reported the relationship between poor outcomes of RP-ILD with DM classification, older age, skin ulceration, lack of myositis, and positivity of anti-MDA5 antibody (12–14). Fever, elevated serum CRP, and ferritin levels and ground-glass attenuation on high-resolution CT (HRCT) have been suggested as risk factors for ILD in myositis (14–16). However, due to the heterogeneity of IIM, the prevalence, risk predictors, and survival rates of RP-ILD vary widely among different studies.

In this study, we investigated the clinical and laboratory characteristics at the time of diagnosis of ILD in DM/PM/CADM patients. Moreover, we compared serum biomarkers and pulmonary characteristics of RP-ILD and chronic-ILD (C-ILD) to exploit potential prognostic markers of myositis-associated RP-ILD in a large-scale patient cohort in China.

MATERIALS AND METHODS

Patients

Patients diagnosed with DM/PM/CADM in the department of rheumatology and immunology, Peking University People's Hospital between July 2000 and October 2019 were identified in this retrospective study. Cases satisfied diagnostic criteria suggested by the Bohan & Peter DM/PM classification or Sontheimer's definitions (2, 17). CADM is the combination of amyopathic DM (ADM) and hypomyopathic DM (HDM). Patients with other definite causes of interstitial lung disease, such

as infectious pneumonia, chronic obstructive pulmonary disease (COPD), lung injury, and drug or occupational-environmental exposures were excluded at the initial diagnosis. Patients with complicating conditions, such as an active neoplasm and history of lung cancer, and other identifiable autoimmune diseases, such as systemic lupus erythematosus (SLE), rheumatoid arthritis (RA), or systemic sclerosis (SSc), or that had been treated with systemic corticosteroids and immunosuppressants before referral to our hospital were also excluded. This study was approved by the ethics committee of Peking University People's Hospital.

Methods

Demographic, clinical, and laboratory data at the time of diagnosis and during follow-up were collected from hospital records. Demographic and clinical information, including age at onset, gender, disease duration at diagnosis, initial symptoms associated with the disease, Gottron's sign/papules, skin ulceration, periungual erythema, proximal muscle weakness, malignancy history, and ILD, were assessed. Laboratory data were recorded, including serum levels of creatine kinase (CK), aspartate aminotransferase (AST), lactate dehydrogenase (LDH), and ferritin. Myositis-specific autoantibodies (MSAs, antigens including Jo-1, PL-7, PL-12, EJ, OJ, KS, MDA5, NXP2, SAE, Mi-2, TIF-1γ) and myositis-associated autoantibodies (MAAs, antigens including Ro-52, PM-Scl, Ku) were identified in 207 patients by immunoblotting according to the manufacturers' instructions (Euroimmun, Germany).

Findings on arterial blood gas analysis, pulmonary function tests (PFT, including forced vital capacity, diffusing capacity for carbon monoxide and total lung capacity), chest high-resolution computed tomography (HRCT), and bronchoalveolar lavage fluid (BALF) were recorded at ILD diagnosis when available. Images of ILD on HRCT, including ground-glass attenuation (GGA), consolidations, nodular, reticulonodular, interlobular septal thickening, honeycombing, and traction bronchiectasis, were assessed. Based on the HRCT scan pattern, patients were classified into the following four groups: non-specific interstitial pneumonia (NSIP), lymphocytic interstitial pneumonia (LIP), usual interstitial pneumonia (UIP), and organizing pneumonia (OP). HRCT were reviewed by a panel of experienced radiologists according to 2013 ATS/ERS policies (18). The definition of RP-ILD was rapidly progressive dyspnea and hypoxemia with a worsening of radiologic interstitial lung changes within 3 months after the onset of respiratory symptoms. C-ILD was defined as an asymptomatic, slowly progressive ILD or as non-rapidly progressive over 3 months (19).

BALF was collected during bronchoscopy in clinic. Bronchoscopy was administrated with local anesthesia induced by lidocaine; 100 ml of sterile saline (0.9% NaCL) was instilled through the bronchoscope into the right lung field in two to four aliquots. BALF was collected after administration. Cellular components were separated from BALF by centrifugation (10 min, 1,200 rpm). Cytospin slides of cells in BALF were stained with hematoxylin-eosin for subsequent cell identification. The numbers of macrophages, lymphocytes, and neutrophils were recorded. The data of cytological analyses of BALF were collected from the standardized case record form in the clinical record.

The R Maximal Selected Rank (MaxStat) package was used to determine the optimal cutoff point in lymphocytes in BALF to predict poor survival of RP-ILD.

Statistical Analysis

Categorical variables were presented as frequency (percentages). Continuous data were expressed as the mean ± standard error or medians (interquartile range), and data on RP-ILD vs. C-ILD were compared using Student's t-test or the Mann–Whitney U test. Categorical variables were compared using Fisher's exact test or chi-square test. Outcomes were compared between RP-ILD patients and C-ILD patients. Survival between various groups was analyzed using a Kaplan–Meier curve with log rank test. Univariate and multivariate Cox regression analyses were used to identify predictors of poor survival due to RP-ILD.

RESULTS

Characteristics of ILD in Patients With PM/DM/CADM

The study cohort included 505 patients with myositis and 31 patients with other autoimmune diseases (11 patients overlapped with SLE, 9 patients overlapped with SSc, 9 patients overlapped with RA, 2 patients overlapped with SLE+SSc) were excluded. A total of 474 patients with PM/DM/CADM were enrolled in this study, including 87.6% (369/474) females with a mean age of 49.7 ± 14.0 years (**Table 1**). ILD was found in 65% (308/474) of patients with PM/DM/CADM. ILD was identified to precede IIM clinical manifestations in 10.7% (33/308) of patients; among these patients with isolated ILD, 57.6% (19/33) of them developed myositis within 1 year after ILD diagnosis, 36.4% (12/33) were diagnosed with myositis 1–3 years after ILD diagnosis, and 6.1% (2/33) had myositis after 3 years. ILD onset was identified concurrently with PM/DM/CADM in 57.1% (176/308) of patients and occurred after IIM onset in 32.1% (99/308) of patients. Patients with ILD were divided into two groups according to pulmonary manifestations: RP-ILD (38%, 117/308) and C-ILD (62%, 191/308). The most common pattern of chest HRCT in IIM with ILD was NSIP (67.2%, 207/308), followed by OP (26.0%, 80/308) and UIP (6.8%, 21/308).

Clinical and Laboratory Features in IIM Patients With RP-ILD Compared With C-ILD

Among 117 consecutive patients with RP-ILD, 41% (48/117) of patients had DM, 51.3% (60/117) of patients had CADM, and 7.7% (9/117) of patients had PM (**Table 2**). Patients with RP-ILD were older than those with C-ILD (54.1 ± 12.7 vs. 50.1 ± 12.9 years, P = 0.009). The mean disease duration in the RP-ILD group was significantly shorter than the C-ILD group (2.0 ± 0.9 vs. 31.6 ± 59.4 months, P = 0.000). Additionally, fever, periungual erythema, skin ulceration, and subcutaneous/mediastinal emphysema were significantly more common in patients with RP-ILD compared with C-ILD with incidence rates of 63.2 vs. 37.2%, 22.2 vs. 12.0%, 11.1 vs. 3.1%, and 6.0 vs. 0.0%, respectively. The levels of serum LDH (P = 0.014),

TABLE 1 | Demographics and pulmonary characteristics of 474 patients with IIM.

Variables	n = 474
Female, no. (%)	369 (87.6)
Age at onset, years	49.7 ± 14.0
DIAGNOSIS	
DM, no. (%)	216 (45.6)
CADM, no. (%)	201 (42.4)
PM, no. (%)	57 (12.0)
ILD, no. (%)	308 (65)
Rapidly progressive ILD, no. (%)	117/308 (38.0)
Chronic ILD, no. (%)	191/308 (62.0)
ILD ONSET	
Before IIM onset, no. (%)	33/308 (10.7)
Concomitant with IIM, no. (%)	176/308 (57.1)
After IIM onset, no. (%)	99/308 (32.1)
HRCT PATTERN	
NSIP, no. (%)	207/308 (67.2)
OP, no. (%)	80/308 (26.0)
UIP, no. (%)	21/308 (6.8)

Continuous data are presented as M (mean) ± SEM (standard error of the mean). Binary data are presented as n/total number (percentage) of the patients. IIM, idiopathic inflammatory myositis; ILD, interstitial lung disease; DM, dermatomyositis; PM, polymyositis; CADM, clinically amyopathic dermatomyositis; HRCT, high resolution computerized tomography; NSIP, nonspecific interstitial pneumonia; OP, organizing pneumonia; UIP, usual interstitial pneumonia.

AST (P = 0.029), CRP (P = 0.019), and ferritin (P = 0.001) were significantly higher in the RP-ILD group than in the C-ILD group. Muscle weakness and malignancy were less common in patients with RP-ILD than those with C-ILD with incidence rates of 47.9 vs. 64.9% (P = 0.003) and 3.4 vs. 9.4% (P = 0.047). Moreover, peripheral blood lymphocytes were significantly lower in patients with RP-ILD compared with C-ILD (1.1 ± 0.7 vs. 1.5 ± 0.9, P = 0.000).

In addition, increased CEA, NSE, and CYFRA21-1 in serum were significantly more common in the RP-ILD group than in the C-ILD group with incidence rates of 31.6 vs. 11.5%, 51.2 vs. 36.6%, and 66.7 vs. 38.2%, respectively. On the other hand, tumor markers including AFP, CA199, and CA125 were also screened for IIM patients, and there were no significant differences in these tumor markers between the RP-ILD and C-ILD groups. A total of 66.7% of patients with RP-ILD and 38.2% of patients with C-ILD had at least one of the tumor markers elevated in serum.

Comparison of MSAs/MAAs in IIM Patients With RP-ILD and C-ILD

MSAs/MAAs were detected in 207 patients with ILD in the present study. Prevalence of anti-MDA5 and anti-Ro-52 antibodies were significantly higher in IIM patients with RP-ILD than with C-ILD with respective incidence rates of 39.0 vs. 12.0% (P = 0.000) and 58.5 vs. 40.8% (P = 0.012) (**Table 3**). Anti-ARS antibodies, especially anti-Jo-1 antibody (13.4 vs. 32.0%, P = 0.002) were detected less commonly in patients with RP-ILD compared with patients with C-ILD. There were

TABLE 2 | Comparison of clinical and laboratory characteristics between DM/CADM/PM patients with RP-ILD and C-ILD.

Variables	RP-ILD n = 117	C-ILD n = 191	P-value
DIAGNOSIS			
DM, no. (%)	48 (41.0)	79 (41.4)	0.954
CADM, no. (%)	60 (51.3)	88 (46.1)	0.375
PM, no. (%)	9 (7.7)	24 (12.6)	0.180
DEMOGRAPHICS			
Female, no. (%)	87 (74.4)	145 (75.9)	0.758
Age at onset, years	54.1 ± 12.7	50.1 ± 12.9	0.009*
Duration of ILD, months	2.0 ± 0.9	31.6 ± 59.4	0.000*
CLINICAL VARIABLES			
Fever, no. (%)	74 (63.2)	71 (37.2)	0.000*
Gottron's sign/papules, no. (%)	81 (69.2)	137 (71.7)	0.640
Periungual erythema, no. (%)	26 (22.2)	23 (12.0)	0.018*
Skin ulceration, no. (%)	13 (11.1)	6 (3.1)	0.005*
Muscle weakness, no. (%)	56 (47.9)	124 (64.9)	0.003*
Subcutaneous/mediastinal emphysema, no. (%)	7 (6.0)	0 (0.0)	0.001*
Malignancy, no. (%)	4 (3.4)	18 (9.4)	0.047*
LABORATORY FEATURES			
Lymphocytes, × 10⁹/L	1.1 ± 0.7	1.5 ± 0.9	0.000*
CK, U/L	65 (30.5,274.5)	72 (34,563)	0.448
LDH, U/L	324 (221,501)	281 (193.8,395)	0.014*
AST, U/L	38 (21.5,84.5)	30 (20,60)	0.029*
CRP, mg/dL	7.6 (2.4,31.0)	5.0 (1.9,13.0)	0.019*
Ferritin (ng/mL)[a]	1,065 (584.1,2690)	307.9 (129.8,881.3)	0.001*
Elevated CEA, no. (%)	37 (31.6)	22 (11.5)	0.000*
Elevated NSE, no. (%)	60 (51.2)	70 (36.6)	0.012*
Elevated CYFRA21-1, no. (%)	78 (66.7)	73 (38.2)	0.000*

*Continuous data were expressed as the mean ± standard error or medians (interquartile range). Binary data were presented as n (percentage) of the patients. [a] 49 patients of 117, 68 values missing in RP-ILD group; * <0.05. IIM, idiopathic inflammatory myopathy; ILD, interstitial lung disease; RP-ILD, rapidly progressive ILD; C-ILD, Chronic ILD; CK, creatine kinase; LDH, lactate dehydrogenase; AST, aspartate aminotransferase; CRP, C-reactive protein; CEA, carcinoembryogenic antigen; NSE, neuron-specific enolase; CYFRA21-1, cytokeratin-19 fragment.*

TABLE 3 | Comparison of MSAs/MAAs between IIM patients with RP-ILD and C-ILD.

Variables	RP-ILD n = 82	C-ILD n = 125	P-value
MYOSITIS-SPECIFIC ANTIBODIES			
Anti-synthetase antibodies (+), no. (%)	35 (42.7)	71 (56.8)	0.047*
Anti-Jo-1, no. (%)	11 (13.4)	40 (32.0)	0.002*
Anti-MDA5, no. (%)	32 (39.0)	15 (12.0)	0.000*
Anti-Mi-2, no. (%)	2 (2.4)	3 (2.4)	1.000
Anti-TIF1-γ, no. (%)	3 (3.7)	4 (3.2)	1.000
Anti-NXP2, no. (%)	2 (2.4)	4 (3.2)	1.000
Anti-SAE, no. (%)	2 (2.4)	3 (2.4)	1.000
MYOSITIS-ASSOCIATED ANTIBODIES			
Anti-Ro-52, no. (%)	48 (58.5)	51 (40.8)	0.012*
Anti-PM/Scl-75/100, no. (%)	8 (9.8)	15 (12.0)	0.615
Anti-Ku, no. (%)	3 (3.7)	7 (5.6)	0.743

* <0.05. IIM, idiopathic inflammatory myopathy; ILD, interstitial lung disease; RP-ILD, rapidly progressive ILD; C-ILD, Chronic ILD. ARS include EJ, OJ, PL-7, PL-12, KS. ARS, aminoacyl-tRNA synthetase; MDA5, melanoma differentiation-associated 5; TIF-1γ, translation initiation factor-1a; NXP2, nuclear matrix protein 2; SAE, small ubiquitin-like modifier enzyme; PM/Scl, polymyositis/scleroderma.

no significant differences in prevalence of anti-Mi-2, anti-NXP2, anti-SAE, and other MAAs between the two groups. Out of 207 patients in which MSAs/MAAs were detected, 20 patients were identified without specific, associated myositis antibodies. Among these patients, ANA, RF, anti-SSA, anti-Sm, anti-Scl-70, anti-U1RNP, and ANCA were found in 35% (7/20), 20% (4/20), 5% (1/20), 0% (0/20), 0% (0/20), 5% (1/20), and 5% (1/20) of the patients, respectively.

Pulmonary Characteristics and Mortality of IIM Patients With RP-ILD and C-ILD

OP pattern on HRCT was more common in the RP-ILD group than in the C-ILD group at the initial assessment with incidence

rates of 52.1 vs. 11.0% ($P = 0.000$) (**Table 4**). In contrast, NSIP and UIP patterns were associated with C-ILD as the incidence rates were 47.9 and 0.0% in RP-ILD subjects compared to 78.0 and 11% in C-ILD subjects, respectively. In total, 161 patients finished PFT and arterial blood gas analysis at initial evaluation, and these results were consistent with ILD in all patients. The results of decreased PaO_2 ($P = 0.000$) and PFTs, including lower FVC ($P = 0.000$), DL_{CO} ($P = 0.000$), and TLC ($P = 0.000$) verified severe lung impairment in patients with RP-ILD compared with those with C-ILD. Analysis of cell composition in BALF showed a significantly increased proportion of lymphocytes and decreased macrophage cells in the RP-ILD group compared with the C-ILD group with rates of 38.2 ± 23.2 vs. 20.4 ± 13.1 ($P = 0.000$) and 47.9 ± 22.5 vs. 68.8 ± 16.1 ($P = 0.000$). Out of 117 patients with RP-ILD, 78 received bronchoalveolar lavage immune cell tests, including 12 patients that did not survive and 66 that survived. Lymphocytes in BALF at <30% was found in 83.3% (10/12) of deceased patients compared with only 33.3% (22/66) of patients who survived ($P = 0.003$) (**Supplementary Table S1**). Out of 191 patients with C-ILD, 97 received bronchoalveolar lavage tests. Lymphocytes in BALF at <30% was found in 100% (7/7) of deceased patients with C-ILD compared with 81.1% (73/90) of C-ILD patients that survived, but the difference was not significant ($P = 0.348$) (**Supplementary Table S2**).

The mortality rates in patients with RP-ILD were significantly higher than those in the C-ILD group (27.4 vs. 7.9%, $P = 0.000$, respectively). The median time to death was 0.2 years in RP-ILD subjects compared to 5.7 years in C-ILD subjects. The main cause of death in the RP-ILD group was respiratory failure due to RP-ILD (62.5%, 20/32), and a quarter of patients died from complicating infections. We also compared therapeutic data between the two groups (**Table 4**). Patients in the RP-ILD group

TABLE 4 | Comparison of baseline pulmonary features and initial treatment between IIM patients with RP-ILD and C-ILD.

Variables	RP-ILD n = 117	C-ILD n = 191	P-value
PaO$_2$ < 80 (mmHg)[a]	59 (92.2)	22 (22.7)	0.000*
BASELINE PFTs (% PREDICTED)[a]			
FVC	65.7 ± 16.2	86.9 ± 15.1	0.000*
DLco	48.5 ± 16.0	72.3 ± 16.2	0.000*
TLC	70.6 ± 15.5	88.2 ± 14.4	0.000*
HRCT PATTERN			
NSIP, no. (%)	56 (47.9)	149 (78.0)	0.000*
OP, no. (%)	61 (52.1)	21 (11.0)	0.000*
UIP, no. (%)	0 (0.0)	21 (11.0)	0.000*
BRONCHOALVEOLAR LAVAGE[b]			
Total cell number (× 10^5/ml)	3.0 ± 2.9	3.1 ± 3.2	0.137
Macrophage (%)	47.9 ± 22.5	68.8 ± 16.1	0.000*
Lymphocyte (%)	38.2 ± 23.2	20.4 ± 13.1	0.000*
Neutrophil (%)	12.6 ± 18.3	9.1 ± 10.0	0.084
Mortality, no. (%)	32 (27.4)	15 (7.9)	0.000*
Median time to death, years	0.2 (0.1, 1.5)	5.7 (1.0, 10.1)	0.012*
CAUSE OF DEATH			
Respiratory failure, no. (%)	20 (62.5)	2 (13.3)	0.002*
RF complicated with infection, no. (%)	8 (25.0)	1 (6.7)	0.236
Cancer, no. (%)	0 (0.0)	6 (40.0)	0.000*
Others, no. (%)	4 (12.5)	6 (40.0)	0.054
INITIAL TREATMENT			
CS pulse therapy (0.5 g/d IV 3 days)	103 (88.0)	15 (7.9)	0.000*
IMMUNOSUPPRESSANTS			
CsA	38 (32.5)	22 (11.5)	0.000*
MMF	1 (0.9)	12 (6.3)	0.020*
Tac	3 (2.6)	1 (0.5)	0.155
Intravenous CYC	74 (63.2)	90 (47.1)	0.007*
CsA+CYC	8 (7.3)	1 (0.5)	0.002*
Tofacitinib	4 (3.4)	0 (0.0)	0.020*
Rituximab	2 (1.7)	0 (0.0)	0.144

Data are presented as n (percentage) of the patients. Data of pulmonary function test and bronchoalveolar lavage are presented as mean ± SEM. * <0.05. [a] 64 patients of 117, 53 values of baseline PaO$_2$, FVC, DLco, TLC missing in RP-ILD group; 97 patients of 191, 94 values of baseline PaO$_2$, FVC, DLco, TLC missing in C-ILD group. [b] 78 patients of 117, 39 values of bronchoalveolar lavage immune cell tests missing in RP-ILD group; 97 patients of 191, 94 values of bronchoalveolar lavage immune cell tests missing in C-ILD group. IIM, idiopathic inflammatory myopathy; ILD, interstitial lung disease; RP-ILD, rapidly progressive ILD; C-ILD, chronic ILD; HRCT, high resolution computerized tomography; NSIP, non-specific interstitial pneumonia; UIP, usual interstitial pneumonia; OP, organizing pneumonia; FVC, forced vital capacity; DLco, diffusion capacity for carbon monoxide; TLC, total lung capacity; RF: respiratory failure; IV, intravenous injection; CS, glucocorticoid; CsA, Cyclosporine; MMF, Mycophenolate mofetil; CYC, Cyclophosphamide; Tac, Tacrolimus.

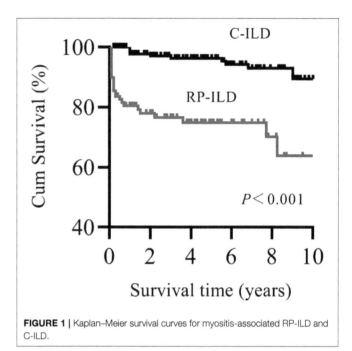

FIGURE 1 | Kaplan–Meier survival curves for myositis-associated RP-ILD and C-ILD.

received more aggressive initial treatment regimes compared with patients in the C-ILD group. A total of 88% of patients with RP-ILD were treated with CS pulse therapy compared with 7.9% of patients with C-ILD at initial treatment ($P = 0.000$). Calcineurin inhibitors, especially cyclosporine, and intravenous cyclophosphamide (0.4–0.6 g every 2 weeks) were preferentially used in the RP-ILD group rather than mycophenolate mofetil; rituximab, tacrolimus, and tofacitinib were seldom used.

Survival Analysis of IIM Patients With RP-ILD

Patients with myositis-associated RP-ILD had significantly lower survival rates than the C-ILD group (1-year survival, 76 vs. 98%; 5-year survival, 73 vs. 94%; $P = 0.000$) (**Figure 1**). Moreover, skin ulceration, LDH > 245 U/L, AST > 40 U/L, lymphocytes in BALF <30%, and anti-MDA5 antibody were associated with mortality on univariate analysis. Multivariate Cox proportional hazards model analysis identified that anti-MDA5 antibody (HR 11.639, [95% CI 1.338–101.240], $P = 0.026$) was an independent risk factor for mortality due to RP-ILD, and lymphocytes at <30% in BALF (HR 12.048, [95% CI 1.466–99.031], $P = 0.021$) might be associated with poor survival of RP-ILD (**Table 5**). Among patients with RP-ILD, anti-MDA5-positivity was significantly associated with poor survival (57% at both 5 and 10 years) compared to the anti-MDA5-negative group (89% at both 5 and 10 years, $P = 0.007$) (**Figure 2A**). Additionally, lymphocytes <30% in BALF might also be associated with poor survival of RP-ILD (87.3% at 5 years and 80.3% at 10 years) compared with lymphocytes at ≥30% in BALF (95.7% at both 5 and 10 years, $P = 0.031$) (**Figure 2B**). Notably, due to lack of data in BALF tests (33.3% in RP-ILD group and 49% in C-ILD group), the statistical power of analysis of the BALF lymphocyte ratio was insufficient, and a probable selection bias existed. Therefore, this result needs to be validated in future studies.

DISCUSSION

RP-ILD, a common complication of IIM, is a poor prognostic factor for patients with IIM (4, 5). Therefore, these patients need careful evaluation of clinical characteristics and radiological features during follow-up (20). The present study retrospectively reviewed 474 cases of IIM and identified initial predictors for myositis-associated RP-ILD from an inpatient rheumatology cohort in China.

TABLE 5 | Survival analysis in myositis-associated RP-ILD (Cox proportional hazards model).

Variables	Hazard ratio	95% CI	P-value
UNIVARIATE			
Fever	2.823	0.730–10.918	0.133
Skin ulceration	3.726	1.554–8.932	0.003*
Subcutaneous/mediastinal emphysema	2.999	0.721–12.475	0.131
LDH > 245 U/L	1.001	1–1.001	0.001*
AST > 40 U/L	1.005	1.002–1.008	0.002*
Anti-Jo-1 antibody	0.040	0–8.705	0.040*
Anti-MDA5 antibody	11.320	1.450–88.356	0.021*
Lymphocytes in BALF<30%	5.281	1.133–24.623	0.034*
MULTIVARIATE			
Anti-MDA5 antibody	11.639	1.338–101.240	0.026*
Lymphocytes in BALF<30%	12.048	1.466–99.031	0.021*
Skin ulceration	1.283	0.240–6.863	0.770

* <0.05. Initial predictors for poor survival of myositis-associated RP-ILD due to respiratory failure were verified by multivariate analysis. MDA5, melanoma differentiation-associated 5; RP-ILD, rapidly progressive interstitial lung disease; BALF, bronchoalveolar lavage fluid.

The prevalence of ILD was 65% in patients with DM/PM/CADM, and nearly 40% of them had RP-ILD in our center. The prevalence of ILD in our center is higher than other historical series (21). The possible reason is that our hospital is a well-known center for myositis and other rheumatic diseases in China, so increased frequency of severe patients with ILD were found in the in-patient clinical records. In addition, all patients received routine examination of HRCT to screen for potential ILD, which might lead to a higher prevalence of ILD in this cohort. However, differences might also exist in different countries. According to several other cohort studies, it seems that the prevalence of ILD in our study was similar with these previous studies and was not extraordinary (22, 23). The present study showed 10.7% of patients diagnosed with ILD before the diagnosis of IIM, so these patients required intensive evaluation during follow-up to reduce the rate of misdiagnosis. NSIP on chest HRCT of IIM patients was reported to be the most common pattern in our study, and this result was consistent with previous studies (24, 25).

Previous studies have identified that survival rates of patients with myositis-associated RP-ILD were lower than in C-ILD (26). Won et al. (27) report a 3-year survival rate for RP-ILD of 27.3%, and Fujisawa et al. (28) report a 5-year survival rate of 52% in the RP-ILD. However, the 5-year survival rate of the RP-ILD group in our study was 73%, which is higher than in previous reports. The potential reason may be the choice of different treatment regimens or different therapeutic effects among racial types. Rapid deterioration and infection secondary to over-immunosuppression were two main causes of death, so appropriate therapy regimens still need to be pursued by clinicians.

This study verified many clinical and laboratory prognostic factors previously reported to be associated with RP-ILD in IIM patients, such as age at onset, fever, periungual erythema, skin ulceration, and decreased peripheral blood lymphocyte cells as well as increased levels of AST, ferritin, LDH, and CRP (29).

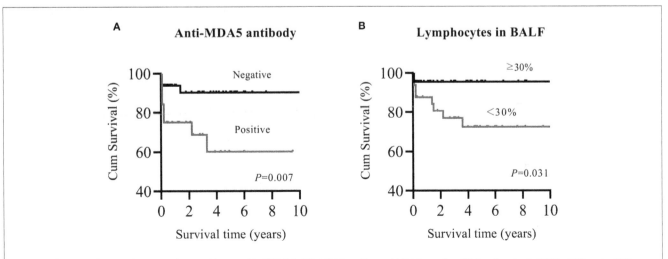

FIGURE 2 | Kaplan–Meier survival curves for myositis-associated RP-ILD. **(A)**, MDA5 positive and MDA5 negative; **(B)**, lymphocytes in BALF <30% and ≥30%. MDA5, melanoma differentiation-associated 5; RP-ILD, rapidly progressive interstitial lung disease; BALF, bronchoalveolar lavage fluid.

Additionally, serum tumor markers, such as CEA, NSE, and CYFRA21-1 were found to be associated with RP-ILD in our study. Although such tumor markers have been used to screen potential cancer in clinical practice, this result has not been reported before. The possible reason is that these tumor markers could be induced by intensive inflammation in lung.

Measurement of MSAs and MAAs are helpful in classifying different subtypes of IIM in clinical practice. Our study demonstrated that anti-MDA5 antibody was a specific biomarker for myositis-associated RP-ILD. Anti-Ro-52 antibody was also associated with RP-ILD in our study. These findings were consistent with previous studies (25, 30–32). In contrast, anti-ARS antibodies, especially anti-Jo-1 antibody, were related to myositis-associated C-ILD in our study, which indicated that anti-ARS antibodies may be a favorable predictor for RP-ILD. The multivariate Cox proportional hazards model analysis used in our study identified anti-MDA5 antibody as an independent predictor of poor outcome in patients with myositis-associated RP-ILD. The importance of anti-MDA5 antibody in the prognosis of myositis has been described by Tanizawa et al. (16), who showed that anti-MDA5 was an independent determinant of overall mortality in DM/PM patients with ILD.

Our analysis verified that low PaO_2, FVC, DL_{CO}, and TLC were associated with RP-ILD. This result confirmed that analyzing arterial blood gas and PFT were useful tests for myositis-associated RP-ILD. FVC and DL_{CO} values have been reported as predictive factors for poor prognosis of ILD in IIM (33, 34). Our study also found that initial low TLC was correlated with the onset of RP-ILD.

Currently, cellular profiles in BALF are used in patients with myositis to rule out infection in clinical practice. The relationship between cellular profiles of BALF and poor prognosis has not been supported by all studies (28, 35). Schnabel et al. (35) report the presence of neutrophils in BALF associated with progressive ILD. In contrast, Fujisawa et al. (28) indicate that a relatively high percentage of lymphocytes in BALF is correlated with myositis-associated ILD. However, our study demonstrates increased lymphocyte infiltration and decreased number of macrophage cells in BALF are associated with onset of RP-ILD in myositis patients. Our study further shows that lymphocytes at <30% in BALF is probably associated with poor survival of myositis-associated RP-ILD. The ATS guidelines (36) indicate that the presence of >15% lymphocytes in BALF represents a lymphocytic cellular pattern such as OP or NSIP.

Takei et al. (37) report that corticosteroids and other immunosuppressants are more effective in the patients with a lymphocyte differential count >15% than in patients with a lymphocyte differential count <15%. According to Takei et al., we speculate that the reason for this association is that patients with a lower lymphocyte ratio in BALF might respond poorly to treatment with corticosteroids or immunosuppressants, which might lead to poorer outcomes. However, due to the rather high percentage of missing data in BALF results (33.3% in RP-ILD group and 49% in C-ILD group), the statistical power of analysis of BALF lymphocyte ratio is insufficient. Only 10.3% (12/117) of patients died in the subgroup of RP-ILD patients with available BALF results compared to the overall mortality of 27.4% (32/117), which suggests a probable selection bias. Therefore, this result needs to be validated in future studies. It should be noted that the cutoff level of lymphocytes <30% in BALF should also be validated in future studies. Further research on lymphocyte subsets and function is also needed in future work to elucidate the immunological mechanism of different lymphocyte phenotypes and functions in myositis-associated RP-ILD.

There are several limitations in the present study. The retrospective nature and the selection of cases from a single center might have caused a selection bias. Because patients were selected from a center for myositis and other rheumatic diseases, more severe forms of disease were recorded. Because the study was retrospective, follow-up time was different among the cases, and some missing data could not be avoided. For example, MSAs, MAAs, lung function, and BALF test (including subsets of lymphocytes) were not performed in all the patients. On the other hand, the strength of the study is that it includes a large cohort of patients with myositis who have undergone HRCT. Further prospective and multicenter studies are needed to overcome these weaknesses.

CONCLUSIONS

Our study highlights that presence of RP-ILD results in an increased rate of mortality in DM/PM/CADM. IIM patients with predictive factors of RP-ILD, including anti-MDA5 antibody and lymphocytes <30% in BALF, should receive intensive follow-up.

ETHICS STATEMENT

Written informed consent was obtained from the individual(s) for the publication of any potentially identifiable images or data included in this article.

AUTHOR CONTRIBUTIONS

YuL, JH, and XS conceived and designed the study and wrote the manuscript. XG, YiL, XJ, YG, YX, XZ, RC, and SL collected the data. YuL, XG, and YiL analyzed the data. All authors contributed to the article and approved the submitted version.

ACKNOWLEDGMENTS

The authors appreciate the assistance of Daojun Hong and Jun Zhang in verification of muscular pathology.

REFERENCES

1. Lundberg IE, Tjärnlund A, Bottai M, Werth VP, Pilkington C, Visser M, et al. 2017 European league against rheumatism/American college of rheumatology classification criteria for adult and juvenile idiopathic inflammatory myopathies and their major subgroups.

Ann Rheum Dis. (2017) 76:1955–64. doi: 10.1136/annrheumdis-2017-211468

2. Sontheimer RD. Would a new name hasten the acceptance of amyopathic dermatomyositis (dermatomyositis sine myositis) as a distinctive subset within the idiopathic inflammatory dermatomyopathies spectrum of clinical illness? *J Am Acad Dermatol.* (2002) 46:626–36. doi: 10.1067/mjd.2002.120621

3. Callen JP. Dermatomyositis. *Lancet.* (2000) 355:53–7. doi: 10.1016/S0140-6736(99)05157-0

4. Jablonski R, Bhorade S, Strek ME, Dematte J. Recognition and management of myositis-associated rapidly progressive interstitial lung disease. *Chest.* (2020) 158:252–63. doi: 10.1016/j.chest.2020.01.033

5. Hervier B, Uzunhan Y. Inflammatory myopathy-related interstitial lung disease: from pathophysiology to treatment. *Front Med.* (2020) 6:326. doi: 10.3389/fmed.2019.00326

6. Morisset J, Johnson C, Rich E, Collard HR, Lee JS. Management of myositis-related interstitial lung disease. *Chest.* (2016) 150:1118–28. doi: 10.1016/j.chest.2016.04.007

7. Vuillard C, Pineton de Chambrun M, de Prost N, Guérin C, Schmidt M, Dargent A, et al. Clinical features and outcome of patients with acute respiratory failure revealing anti-synthetase or anti-MDA-5 dermato-pulmonary syndrome: a French multicenter retrospective study. *Ann Intensive Care.* (2018) 8:87. doi: 10.1186/s13613-018-0433-3

8. Debray M-P, Borie R, Revel M-P, Naccache J-M, Khalil A, Toper C, et al. Interstitial lung disease in anti-synthetase syndrome: initial and follow-up CT findings. *Eur J Radiol.* (2015) 84:516–23. doi: 10.1016/j.ejrad.2014.11.026

9. Obert J, Freynet O, Nunes H, Brillet P-Y, Miyara M, Dhote R, et al. Outcome and prognostic factors in a French cohort of patients with myositis-associated interstitial lung disease. *Rheumatol Int.* (2016) 36:1727–35. doi: 10.1007/s00296-016-3571-7

10. Aggarwal R, Cassidy E, Fertig N, Koontz DC, Lucas M, Ascherman DP, et al. Patients with non-Jo-1 anti-tRNA-synthetase autoantibodies have worse survival than Jo-1 positive patients. *Ann Rheum Dis.* (2014) 73:227–32. doi: 10.1136/annrheumdis-2012-201800

11. Gono T, Kuwana M. Choosing the right biomarkers to predict ILD in myositis. *Nat Rev Rheumatol.* (2016) 12:504–6. doi: 10.1038/nrrheum.2016.120

12. Moghadam-Kia S, Oddis CV, Sato S, Kuwana M, Aggarwal R. Anti-melanoma differentiation-associated gene 5 is associated with rapidly progressive lung disease and poor survival in US patients with amyopathic and myopathic dermatomyositis. *Arthritis Care Res.* (2016) 68:689–94. doi: 10.1002/acr.22728

13. Sato S, Masui K, Nishina N, Kawaguchi Y, Kawakami A, Tamura M, et al. Initial predictors of poor survival in myositis-associated interstitial lung disease: a multicentre retrospective cohort of 497 patients. *Rheumatology.* (2018) 57:1212–21. doi: 10.1093/rheumatology/key060

14. Fujiki Y, Kotani T, Isoda K, Ishida T, Shoda T, Yoshida S, et al. Evaluation of clinical prognostic factors for interstitial pneumonia in anti-MDA5 antibody-positive dermatomyositis patients. *Mod Rheumatol.* (2018) 28:133–40. doi: 10.1080/14397595.2017.1318468

15. Hozumi H, Fujisawa T, Nakashima R, Johkoh T, Sumikawa H, Murakami A, et al. Comprehensive assessment of myositis-specific autoantibodies in polymyositis/dermatomyositis-associated interstitial lung disease. *Respir Med.* (2016) 121:91–99. doi: 10.1016/j.rmed.2016.10.019

16. Tanizawa K, Handa T, Nakashima R, Kubo T, Hosono Y, Ajhara K, et al. The prognostic value of HRCT in myositis-associated interstitial lung disease. *Respir Med.* (2013) 107:745–52. doi: 10.1016/j.rmed.2013.01.014

17. Bohan A, Peter JB. Polymyositis and dermatomyositis(first of the two parts). *N Engl J Med.* (1975) 292:344–7. doi: 10.1056/NEJM197502132920706

18. Travis WD, Costabel U, Hansell DM, King TE Jr, Lynch DA, Nicholson AG, et al. An official American thoracic society/European respiratory society statement: update of the international multidisciplinary classification of the idiopathic interstitial pneumonias. *Am J Respir Crit Care Med.* (2013) 188:733–48. doi: 10.1164/rccm.201308-1483ST

19. American thoracic society. idiopathic pulmonary fibrosis: diagnosis and treatment. International consensus statement. American thoracic society (ATS), and the European respiratory society (ERS). *Am J Respir Crit Care Med.* (2000) 161:646–64. doi: 10.1164/ajrccm.161.2.ats3-00

20. Fathi M, Vikgren J, Boijsen M, Tylen U, Jorfeldt L, Tornling G, et al. Interstitial lung disease in polymyositis and dermatomyositis: longitudinal evaluation by pulmonary function and radiology. *Arthritis Rheum.* (2008) 59:677–85. doi: 10.1002/art.23571

21. Lega JC, Reynaud Q, Belot A, Fabien N, Durieu I, Cottin V. Idiopathic inflammatory myopathies and the lung. *Eur Respir Rev.* (2015) 24:216–38 doi: 10.1183/16000617.00002015

22. Ye S, Chen XX, Lu XY, Wu MF, Deng Y, Huang WQ, et al. Adult clinically amyopathic dermatomyositis with rapid progressive interstitial lung disease: a retrospective cohort study. *Clin Rheumatol.* (2007) 26:1647–54. doi: 10.1007/s10067-007-0562-9

23. Fathi M, Dastmalchi M, Rasmussen E, Lundberg E, Tornling G. Interstitial lung disease, a common manifestation of newly diagnosed polymyositis and dermatomyositis. *Ann Rheum Dis.* (2004) 63:297–301. doi: 10.1136/ard.2003.006122

24. Yura H, Sakamoto N, Satoh M, Ishimoto H, Hanaka T, Ito C, et al. Clinical characteristics of patients with anti-aminoacyl-tRNA synthetase antibody positive idiopathic interstitial pneumonia. *Respir Med.* (2017) 132:189–94. doi: 10.1016/j.rmed.2017.10.020

25. Hozumi H, Enomoto N, Kono M, Fujisawa T, Inui N, Nakamura Y, et al., Prognostic significance of anti-aminoacyltRNA synthetase antibodies in polymyositis/dermatomyositis-associated interstitial lung disease: a retrospective case control study, *PLoS ONE.* (2015) 10:e0120313. doi: 10.1371/journal.pone.0120313

26. Go DJ, Park JK, Kang EH, Kwon HM, Lee YJ, Song YW, et al. Survival benefit associated with early cyclosporine treatment for dermatomyositis-associated interstitial lung disease. *Rheumatol Int.* (2016) 36:125–31. doi: 10.1007/s00296-015-3328-8

27. Won Huh J, Soon Kim D, Keun Lee C, Yoo B, Bum Seo J, Kitaichi M, et al. Two distinct clinical types of interstitial lung disease associated with polymyositisdermatomyositis. *Respir Med.* (2007) 101:1761–9. doi: 10.1016/j.rmed.2007.02.017

28. Fujisawa T, Hozumi H, Kono M, Enomoto N, Hashimoto D, Nakamura Y, et al. Prognostic factors for myositis-associated interstitial lung disease. *PLoS ONE.* (2014) 9:e98824. doi: 10.1371/journal.pone.0098824

29. Xu Y, Yang CS, Li YJ, Liu XD, Wang JN, Zhao Q, et al. Predictive factors of rapidly progressive-interstitial lung disease in patients with clinically amyopathic dermatomyositis. *Clin Rheumatol.* (2016) 35:113–6.doi: 10.1007/s10067-015-3139-z

30. Kishaba T, McGill R, Nei Y, Ibuki S, Momose M, Nishiyama K, et al. Clinical characteristics of dermatomyositis/polymyositis associated interstitial lung disease according to the autoantibody. *J Med Invest.* (2018) 65:251–7. doi: 10.2152/jmi.65.251

31. Yoshida N, Okamoto M, Kaieda S, Fujimoto K, Ebata T, Tajiri M, et al. Association of anti-aminoacyl-transfer RNA synthetase antibody and anti-melanoma differentiation-associated gene 5 antibody with the therapeutic response of polymyositis/dermatomyositis-associated interstitial lung disease. *Respir Investig.* (2017) 55:24–32. doi: 10.1016/j.resinv.2016.08.007

32. Sabbagh S, Pinal-Fernandez I, Kishi T, Targoff IN, Miller FW, Rider LG, et al. Childhood myositis heterogeneity collaborative study group. Anti-Ro-52 autoantibodies are associated with interstitial lung disease and more severe disease in patients with juvenile myositis. *Ann Rheum Dis.* (2019) 78:988–95. doi: 10.1136/annrheumdis-2018-215004

33. Marie I, Hatron PY, Dominique S, Cherin P, Mouthon L, Menard JF. Short-term and long-term outcomes of interstitial lung disease in polymyositis and dermatomyositis: a series of 107 patients. *Arthritis Rheum.* (2011) 63:3439–47. doi: 10.1002/art.30513

34. Fujisawa T, Hozumi H, Kono M, Enomoto N, Nakamura Y, Inui N, et al. Predictive factors for long-term outcome in polymyositis/dermatomyositis-associated interstitial lung diseases. *Respir Investig.* (2017) 55:130–7.doi: 10.1016/j.resinv.2016.09.006

35. Schnabel A, Reuter M, Biederer J, Richter C, Gross WL. Interstitial lung disease in polymyositis and dermatomyositis: clinical course and response to treatment. *Semin Arthritis Rheum.* (2003) 32:273–84. doi: 10.1053/sarh.2002.50012

36. Meyer KC, Raghu G, Baughman RP, Brown KK, Costabel U, du Bois RM, et al. An official American thoracic society clinical practice guideline: the clinical utility of bronchoalveolar lavage cellular analysis in interstitial lung disease. *Am J Respir Crit Care Med.* (2012) 185:1004–14. doi: 10.1164/rccm.201202-0320ST

37. Takei R, Arita M, Kumagai S, Ito Y, Noyama M, Tokioka F, et al. Impact of lymphocyte differential count >15% in BALF on the mortality of patients with acute exacerbation of chronic fibrosing idiopathic interstitial pneumonia. *BMC Pulm Med.* (2017) 17:67. doi: 10.1186/s12890-017-0412-8

21

Variability in Global Prevalence of Interstitial Lung Disease

Bhavika Kaul[1]*, Vincent Cottin[2,3], Harold R. Collard[1] and Claudia Valenzuela[4]

[1] Department of Medicine, University of California, San Francisco, San Francisco, CA, United States, [2] Department of Respiratory Medicine, National Coordinating Reference Center for Rare Pulmonary Diseases, Louis Pradel Hospital, Hospices Civils de Lyon, Lyon, France, [3] IVPC, INRAE, Claude Bernard University Lyon 1, Member of ERN-LUNG, Lyon, France, [4] Interstitial Lung Disease Unit Pulmonology Department, Hospital Universitario de La Princesa, Universidad Autonoma de Madrid, Madrid, Spain

*Correspondence:
Bhavika Kaul
Bhavika.Kaul@ucsf.edu

There are limited epidemiologic studies describing the global burden and geographic heterogeneity of interstitial lung disease (ILD) subtypes. We found that among seventeen methodologically heterogenous studies that examined the incidence, prevalence and relative frequencies of ILDs, the incidence of ILD ranged from 1 to 31.5 per 100,000 person-years and prevalence ranged from 6.3 to 71 per 100,000 people. In North America and Europe, idiopathic pulmonary fibrosis and sarcoidosis were the most prevalent ILDs while the relative frequency of hypersensitivity pneumonitis was higher in Asia, particularly in India (10.7–47.3%) and Pakistan (12.6%). The relative frequency of connective tissue disease ILD demonstrated the greatest geographic variability, ranging from 7.5% of cases in Belgium to 33.3% of cases in Canada and 34.8% of cases in Saudi Arabia. These differences may represent true differences based on underlying characteristics of the source populations or methodological differences in disease classification and patient recruitment (registry vs. population-based cohorts). There are three areas where we feel addition work is needed to better understand the global burden of ILD. First, a standard ontology with diagnostic confidence thresholds for comparative epidemiology studies of ILD is needed. Second, more globally representative data should be published in English language journals as current literature has largely focused on Europe and North America with little data from South America, Africa and Asia. Third, the inclusion of community-based cohorts that leverage the strength of large databases can help better estimate population burden of disease. These large, community-based longitudinal cohorts would also allow for tracking of global trends and be a valuable resource for collective study. We believe the ILD research community should organize to define a shared ontology for disease classification and commit to conducting global claims and electronic health record based epidemiologic studies in a standardized fashion. Aggregating and sharing this type of data would provide a unique opportunity for international collaboration as our understanding of ILD continues to grow and evolve. Better understanding the geographic and temporal patterns of disease prevalence and identifying clusters of ILD subtypes will facilitate improved understanding of emerging risk factors and help identify targets for future intervention.

Keywords: interstitial lung disease, epidemiology—descriptive, global epidemiology, idiopathic pulmonary fibrosis, mortality

INTRODUCTION

Interstitial lung disease (ILD) describes a heterogenous group of disorders that are subclassified based on similar radiographic or pathologic manifestations. Although several classification schemes exist, generally, ILDs can be subcategorized into: (1) those that occur secondary to a known cause such as a culprit drug or connective tissues disease, (2) idiopathic interstitial pneumonias of which idiopathic pulmonary fibrosis (IPF) is the most common, (3) granulomatous parenchymal lung disease such as sarcoidosis or hypersensitivity pneumonitis, (4) occupational pneumoconiosis, and (5) other rarer forms of diffuse parenchymal lung disease (1, 2).

Prior literature describing the epidemiology of ILDs has utilized national registries, health insurance claims, and social security databases to quantify incidence and prevalence, identify risk factors, and describe disease behavior (clinical presentation, natural history, and outcomes) (3, 4), with a growing body of literature focused on the epidemiology of IPF. Very few studies have examined the global burden of ILD or described the between country variability in disease prevalence and subtype. Better quantifying the geographic burden of ILD and understanding the regional variability can lend insight into new risk factors and identify targets for prevention and intervention. It can also help healthcare systems make informed decisions on how best to allocate resources to meet local needs, which is of particular importance in an era of emerging ILD therapies. The objective of this narrative review is to describe what is known from the English language literature about the geographic variability in ILD prevalence and subtype, discuss potential reasons for the observed heterogeneity, and define current knowledge gaps for future investigation.

We queried the PubMed database to identify relevant studies describing ILD epidemiology. Combination of search terms "epidemiology," "interstitial lung disease," "pulmonary fibrosis," and "prevalence" were used to identify English language studies in humans that had the key search terms in their title or abstract. All abstracts were reviewed for relevance. We excluded studies that focused on a single ILD (ex. IPF only) or were intentionally enriched for certain types of ILD as the goal of this review was to describe the comparative frequency of ILD subtypes. References of key articles were reviewed to supplement the electronic search. A total of 17 studies that described incidence, prevalence and relative frequency of ILD subtypes were identified.

COMPARATIVE EPIDEMIOLOGY OF INTERSTITIAL LUNG DISEASE

North America

One of the first epidemiological studies to evaluate the comparative frequencies of ILDs examined the population burden of disease in Bernalillo County, New Mexico between 1988 and 1990 (5). Patients with ILD were identified through a combination of physician referrals, hospital discharge diagnosis, histopathology reports, and death certificates. Electronic health records were reviewed for diagnostic ascertainment. The median age was 69 years and 52.5% of the cohort was male. The

incidence of ILD was 26.1 per 100,000 person-years among women and 31.5 per 100,000 person-years among men (**Table 1**). The prevalence of ILD was 67.2 cases per 100,000 among women and 80.9 cases per 100,000 among men. IPF was the most common ILD, representing 22.5% of prevalent cases, followed by occupational lung disease (14%), connective tissue disease (CTD) ILD (12.8%), and sarcoidosis (11.6%) (**Table 2, Figure 1**). The overall prevalence of ILD was 20% higher in males than females, which was driven in part by a higher prevalence of occupational lung disease among men (20.8 per 100,000) compared to women (0.6 per 100,000). Mining is a major industry in New Mexico, which the authors hypothesized likely contributed to the higher prevalence of pneumoconiosis in the male population.

More recently, a Canadian epidemiologic study evaluated the distribution of ILD subtypes among the indigenous population living in Northern Quebec between 2006 and 2013 (6). Patients were identified using a combination of hospitalization databases, home oxygen use registries and physician surveys. Individual cases were adjudicated *via* multidisciplinary discussion (MDD) and a total of 52 cases were identified as definite ILD. There was a high prevalence of IPF (52%) in the cohort followed by CTD-ILD (11.5%). There was a much lower prevalence of occupational lung disease (1.9%) and sarcoidosis (1.9%) than had been observed in Bernalillo County, likely due to different characteristics and risk factors of the underlying source population.

In contrast to the Bernalillo County and Northern Quebec, which were population-based studies, the Canadian Registry for Pulmonary Fibrosis (CARE-PF), a multi-center, prospective registry that recruited patients from six specialized Canadian ILD clinics between 2016 and 2017, noted a much higher frequency of CTD-ILD (33.3%) followed by IPF (24.7%) and unclassifiable ILD (22.3%) (7). All cases were adjudicated *via* MDD. The mean age of the ILD cohort was 64.8 years with a slightly higher preponderance of females (50.7%). The authors hypothesized that the higher proportion of unclassifiable ILD in their cohort was due to a combination of factors including the complexity of cases seen at tertiary care referral centers and the utilization of strict diagnostic criteria for IPF, chronic hypersensitivity pneumonitis (HP), and idiopathic non-specific interstitial pneumonia (NSIP), the latter of which required biopsy confirmation. Thus, it is possible that the prevalence of IPF, HP and NSIP were under estimated in this cohort because of the diagnostic criteria applied.

Europe

Perhaps the most robust epidemiological data examining comparative frequencies of ILDs comes from national registry studies conducted across Europe, the majority of which have demonstrated a high prevalence of IPF and sarcoidosis.

One of the first prospective registry studies evaluated the epidemiology of ILD in Flanders, the northern region of Belgium, between 1992 and 1996 (8). A total of 362 patients were recruited from 20 centers across 5 provinces *via* enrollment surveys completed by physicians. The mean age of the ILD cohort was 52 years old. There was a high prevalence of sarcoidosis (31% when stage I was included, 22% when stage I was excluded), followed by IPF (20%), HP (13%), and CTD-ILD (7.5%). Approximately

TABLE 1 | Incidence and prevalence of interstitial lung disease subtypes.

		Time Period	ILD (All Subtypes)	IPF	CTD	Sarcoid	HP	Drug	Occupational	Unclassifiable
North America										
New Mexico, USA	Incidence	1988–1990	Male 31.5 Female 26.1	Male 10.7 Female 7.4	Male 2.1 Female 3.0	Male 0.9 Female 3.6	–	Male 1.8 Female 1.1	Male 6.2 Female 0.8	–
New Mexico, USA	Prevalence	1988–1990	Male 80.9 Female 67.2	Male 20.2 Female 13.2	Male 7.1 Female 11.6	Male 8.3 Female 8.8	–	Male 1.2 Female 2.2	Male 20.8 Female 0.6	–
Europe										
Flanders (Belgium)	Incidence	1992–1996	1.0	0.22	0.07	0.26	0.12	0.05	0.07	0.10
Flanders (Belgium)	Prevalence	1992–1996	6.27	1.25	0.47	1.94	0.81	0.21	0.35	0.57
Greece	Incidence	2004	4.63	0.93	0.54	1.07	0.13	0.07	0.14	0.71
Greece	Prevalence	2004	17.3	3.38	2.14	5.89	0.45	0.30	0.36	1.46
Denmark	Incidence	2003–2009	4.1	1.3	–	–	–	–	–	–
Paris, France	Incidence	2012	18.3	2.8	3.3	4.9	0.9	1.2	0.8	1.8
Paris, France	Prevalence	2012	71.0	8.2	12.1	30.2	2.3	2.6	3.5	5.0
Turkey	Incidence	2007–2009	25.8	–	–	4.0	–	–	–	–

Incidence and prevalence defined as cases per 100,000.
ILD, interstitial lung disease; IPF, idiopathic pulmonary fibrosis; CTD, connective tissue disease; HP, hypersensitivity pneumonitis.

9.1% of cases were unclassifiable. Notably, the male to female ratio was variable across disease processes with pneumoconiosis and IPF more prevalent among men (M/F ratio of 2.3 and 1.4, respectively) while CTD-ILD was more common in women (M/F ratio of 0.8). Of the HP cases, the majority (75%) were associated with pigeon breeding, impacting more men than women (M/F ratio of 1.5).

A similar distribution of ILD subtypes was observed in Greece (9). In a multi-center ILD registry study, 967 patients were recruited from pulmonary divisions across the country. There was a slightly higher proportion of females in the cohort (53.6%). The mean age of the male population was 58 years old, and the mean age of the female population was 59.3 years old. Sarcoidosis was the most commonly observed ILD subtype (34.1%), followed by IPF (19.5%) and CTD-ILD (12.4%). The prevalence of HP was relatively low (2.6%) and unclassifiable ILDs comprised 8.5% of the cohort. The Greek cohort, similar to other European studies, included stage I sarcoidosis (isolated hilar adenopathy), which may have contributed to the higher proportion of sarcoid cases relative to North American cohorts, which generally only included sarcoidosis stages II–IV (stage II: hilar adenopathy with parenchymal involvement, stage III: parenchymal involvement without lymphadenopathy, and stage IV: predominantly fibrotic disease) in their registries.

A Danish study that sought to describe the incidence of ILDs in central Denmark recruited 431 patients from a single center between 2003 and 2009 (10). Cases were adjudicated *via* MDD. The mean age of the cohort was 61 years and 55% were male. The overall incidence of ILD was 4.1 cases per 100,000 person-years. The study reported a rising annual incidence rate with a peak of 6.6 cases per 100,000 person-years in 2009. The most common ILD was IPF (28%), followed by CTD-ILD (12.5%) and HP (7%). IPF and HP was more common in men (77% and 63%,

respectively), while CTD-ILD was more common among women (59%). Notably, sarcoidosis was not included in this cohort.

In Spain, a multicenter registry study that enrolled patients *via* surveys completed by 23 pulmonary medicine clinics between 2000 and 2001 noted an estimated ILD incidence of 7.6 per 100,000 person-years (11). IPF was the most common ILD subtype (38.6%), followed by sarcoidosis (14.9%), CTD-ILD (10%) and HP (6.6%). Approximately 5% of the cases were unclassifiable. Among the CTD-ILD cohort, rheumatoid arthritis was the most common etiology. Similar to observations from the Belgium cohort, pigeon breeding was the most common exposure associated with a diagnosis of HP.

In Italy, the Registro Italiano Pneumopatic Infiltrative Diffuse (RIPID) enrolled 3,152 patients *via* surveys completed by 79 centers across 20 regions (12). The mean age at diagnosis was 54 years with a slightly higher proportion of females (50.9%) in the registry. Sarcoidosis was the most frequently reported ILD (33.7%), followed by IPF (27.4%), which together represented more than 60% of cases. 93 cases (2.9%) of HP were identified.

More recent epidemiologic studies in Europe have focused on using large databases (healthcare claims, mortality, social security) as an alternative to hospital-based registries to define the population burden of ILD. In France, a study that described the population burden of chronic ILDs among people living in Seine-Saint-Denis, a multi-ethnic urbanized area of Greater Paris, noted much higher ILD point prevalence rates than prior registry-based studies (13). Patients were recruited from both physicians' offices and the social security system between January and December 2012. A total of 848 cases were reviewed and validated centrally by an expert MDD. The median age was 55.7 years old with an equal distribution of males and females. The overall incidence of ILD was 18.3 per 100,000 person-years and prevalence was 71 per 100,000 people. In

TABLE 2 | Relative frequency of interstitial lung disease subtypes.

N (%)	Source/Case Ascertainment	Time Period	IPF	CTD	Sarcoid	HP	Drug	Occupational	Unclassifiable	Other
North America										
New Mexico, USA 202 (incident cases)	County Chart Review	1988–1990	63 (31.2)	18 (8.9)	16 (7.9)	3 (1.5)	7 (3.5)	21 (10.4)	20 (9.9)	54 (26.7)
New Mexico, USA 258 (prevalent cases)	County Chart Review	1988–1990	58 (22.5)	33 (12.8)	30 (11.6)	–	5 (1.9)	36 (14.0)	29 (11.2)	67 (26.0)
Quebec, Canada 52	Indigenous Population MDD	2006–2013	27 (51.9)	6 (11.5)	1 (1.9)	1 (1.9)	–	1 (1.9)	3 (5.8)	13 (25.0)
Canada 1,285	Multi Center MDD	2016–2017	317 (24.7)	428 (33.3)	41 (3.2)	97 (7.5)	–	–	286 (22.3)	116 (9.0)
Europe										
Flanders (Belgium) 264 (incident cases)	Multi Center Survey	1992–1996	59 (22.3)	19 (7.2)	69 (26.1)	32 (12.1)	12 (4.5)	18 (6.8)	27 (10.2)	28 (10.6)
Flanders (Belgium) 362 (prevalent cases)	Multi Center Survey	1992–1996	72 (20.0)	27 (7.5)	112 (30.9)	47 (13.0)	12 (3.3)	20 (5.5)	33 (9.1)	39 (10.8)
Greece 259 (incident cases)	Multi Center Survey	2004	52 (20.1)	30 (11.6)	60 (23.2)	7 (2.7)	4 (1.5)	8 (3.1)	40 (15.4)	58 (22.4)
Greece 967 (prevalent cases)	Multi Center Survey	2004	189 (19.5)	120 (12.4)	330 (34.1)	25 (2.6)	17 (1.8)	20 (2.0)	82 (8.5)	184 (19.0)
Denmark 431 (incident cases)	Single Center MDD	2003–2009	121 (28.1)	54 (12.5)	–	32 (7.4)	20 (4.6)	–	62 (14.4)	142 (32.9)
Spain 511 (incident cases)	Multi Center Survey	2000–2001	197 (38.6)	51 (10.0)	76 (14.9)	34 (6.6)	17 (3.3)	–	26 (5.1)	110 (21.5)
Italy 3,152	Multi Center Survey	1998–2005	864 (27.4)	–	1,063 (33.7)	93 (2.9)	39 (1.2)	–	–	–
Paris, France 848 (prevalent cases)	County MDD	2012	98 (11.5)	145 (17.1)	361 (42.6)	28 (3.3)	31 (3.7)	42 (5.0)	66 (7.8)	77 (9.1)
Asia										
Turkey 2,245 (incident cases)	Multi Center Survey	2007–2009	408 (18.2)	201 (9.0)	771 (34.3)	82 (3.7)	35 (1.6)	241 (10.7)	99 (4.4)	408 (18.2)
India 566 (incident cases)	Single Center MDD	2015–2017	130 (23.0)	77 (13.6)	217 (38.3)	69 (12.2)	5 (0.9)	6 (1.1)	–	62 (11.0)
India 803 (prevalent cases)	Single Center MDD	2015–2017	170 (21.2)	102 (12.7)	339 (42.2)	86 (10.7)	6 (0.7)	7 (0.9)	7 (0.9)	86 (10.7)
India 1,084 (incident cases)	Multi Center MDD	2012–2015	148 (13.7)	151 (13.9)	85 (7.8)	513 (47.3)	3 (0.3)	33 (3.0)	2 (0.2)	149 (13.7)
Pakistan 253	Single Center Chart Review	2016–2018	95 (37.5)	23 (9.1)	11 (4.3)	31 (12.3)	–	3 (1.2)	4 (1.6)	86 (34.0)
China (Guangzhou) 1,945 (incident cases)	Single Center MDD	2012–2017	395 (20.3)	356 (18.3)	123 (6.3)	59 (3.0)	13 (0.7)	13 (0.7)	285 (14.7)	701 (36.0)
China (Beijing) 2,615 (incident cases)	Single Center Chart Review	2000–2012	692 (26.5)	631 (24.1)	147 (5.6)	62 (2.4)	28 (1.1)	58 (2.2)	344 (13.2)	653 (25.0)
Other										
Saudi Arabia 330 (incident cases)	Single Center MDD	2008–2011	77 (23.3)	115 (34.8)	67 (20)	21 (6.3)	4 (1.2)	–	6 (1.8)	40 (12.1)
Australia 705	Multi Center Survey	2016–2019	240 (34.0)	125 (17.7)	44 (6.2)	66 (9.4)	7 (1.0)	11 (1.6)	51 (7.2)	161 (22.8)

MDD, multidisciplinary discussion; ILD, interstitial lung disease; IPF, idiopathic pulmonary fibrosis; CTD, connective tissue disease; HP, hypersensitivity pneumonitis.

contrast to other European studies, the prevalence of IPF was much lower in this cohort. The most common diagnosis was sarcoidosis (42.6%), followed by CTD-ILD (17.1%), IPF (11.5%) and occupational lung disease (5%). There was a low prevalence of HP (3.3%). The ancestry-standardized prevalence rates noted a higher frequency of sarcoidosis and CTD-ILDs among patients from North Africa (60 and 26.9 per 100,000, respectively) than in Europeans (10.7 and 5.7 per 100,000, respectively). The ancestry-standardized prevalence of IPF was higher among North Africans than Europeans and Afro-Caribbean (26.9, 5.8, and 4.2 per 100,000, respectively). Adjusted multivariable models demonstrated increased risk of sarcoidosis in Afro-Caribbean (OR 2.9) and North Africans (OR 1.9). The risk of CTD-ILDs was also increased in Afro-Caribbean (OR 4.4) relative to their European counterparts. The authors noted that the area of Seine-Saint-Denis is demographically distinct from that of the general French population with a younger mean age and a higher proportion of people of extra-European ancestry and thus may not be generalizable to the French population at-large. The low prevalence of IPF is likely related to the age distribution, which was skewed toward younger patients.

Asia

Compared to Europe and North America, the English language literature on ILD in Asia has until recently been quite limited. In the last few years, several epidemiologic studies evaluating relative frequency of ILDs have emerged from Turkey, India, Pakistan and China.

In a multicenter cohort study involving recruitment from 31 centers in Turkey, a total of 2,245 cases were identified of which 48.2% were males and 51.8% were females. The mean age was 52 years old. The overall incidence of ILD was 25.8 per 100,000 (14). Sarcoidosis was the most common ILD subtype (34.3%) followed by IPF (18.2%), occupational lung disease (10.7%) and CTD-ILD (9%). There was a low prevalence of HP (3.7%) in the cohort. The study also subcategorized disease burden by sex and age. Among females, sarcoid was the most prevalent (53%), followed by an equal distribution of CTD-ILD (15%) and IPF (15%). For men, the proportion of patients with sarcoid, pneumoconiosis and IPF was nearly equivalent (25% sarcoid, 25% IPF, 24% pneumoconiosis) while prevalence of CTD-ILD (6%) was notably lower. With age, the distributions shifted. For men over the age of 50, IPF was the most common ILD (45%) followed by pneumoconiosis (13%) and then sarcoidosis (8%). For men under 50, sarcoidosis was the most prevalent (42%), followed by pneumoconiosis (36%) with a relatively low prevalence of IPF (6%). High rates of pneumoconiosis in Turkey were postulated to be linked to the denim sandblasting profession resulting in a high burden of silicosis among those with occupational lung diseases.

A few large database studies have evaluated the epidemiology of ILD in India. One single center study recruited 803 patients between 2015 and 2017 and adjudicated cases *via* MDD (15). The mean age of the cohort was 50.6 years old with 50.2% women. Sarcoidosis (42.2%) and IPF (21.2%) were the most common ILD subtypes followed by CTD-ILD (12.7%) and HP (10.7%). Most sarcoid patients (63.4%) had stage II or III disease. RA and systemic sclerosis were the most commonly identified CTD-ILD.

Of the patients with HP, the most common exposure was farming (59.3%), followed by exposure to bird feathers (15.1%).

The second epidemiological evaluation of ILD frequencies in India involved a multi-center cohort study, which recruited 1,084 patients from 27 centers between 2012 and 2015 (16). Cases were adjudicated *via* a central MDD. The mean age of registry participants was 55.3 years and 47.2% were male. HP was the final diagnosis in a majority of cases (47.3%), followed by CTD-ILD (13.9%), IPF (13.7%), sarcoidosis (7.8%), and pneumoconiosis (3%). Among patients with HP, 48.1% had been exposed to air coolers, 26.3% to air conditioners, 21.4% to birds and 20.7% to mold in their homes. RA was the most common type of CTD-ILD (38.4%) followed by scleroderma (22.5%). Silicosis was the most common occupational lung disease. The authors noted that compared to other epidemiological studies, a smaller proportion (7.5%) of patients had undergone lung biopsy, which may have led to an underestimation of IPF prevalence, especially as histopathology is often used to differentiate fibrotic HP form IPF. Although the data was presented in aggregate, there was significant within country variability in geographic prevalence of ILD subtypes.

In Pakistan, 253 patients were identified *via* chart review from a single center in Karachi between 2016 and 2018 (17). There was a clear predominance of females (69%) in the registry and the mean age was 49 years old. IPF was the most common disease subtype (37.5%) followed by HP (12.3%), CTD-ILD (9.1%) and sarcoidosis (4.3%). Approximately 37% of patients reported exposure to birds including parakeets, parrots, hens and pigeons.

Two studies examined the epidemiology of ILD in China. The first, retrospectively identified 1,945 patients seen in Guangzhou Institute of Respiratory Health (Southern China) between 2012 and 2017 (18). Case adjudication was done *via* MDD. The mean age at time of diagnosis was 57.9 years and 55.5% of patients were male. The most common ILD subtype was IPF (20.3%), followed by CTD-ILD (18.3%) and interstitial pneumonia with autoimmune features (IPAF) (17.9%). Among the CTD-ILD subgroup, there was a higher proportion of females (60.1%), and RA (32.6%), myositis (25%) and primary Sjogren disease (14%) were the most common CTD subtypes. Although other studies had reported a high percentage of RA-ILD among their CTD-ILD cohorts, the Guangzhou Institute had a much higher prevalence of myositis-ILD than what had been observed in North America, Europe or other parts of Asia. Only 3% of patients were diagnosed with HP. The most common environmental exposure was mold/mildew followed by farming and bird exposure. Relative to other cohorts, especially in Asia, a large number of patients underwent lung biopsy (42.1%).

A second study from China evaluated the distribution of ILD among 2,615 patients of Chinese ancestry admitted to a hospital in Beijing between 2000 and 2012. Patients were identified through chart review. The mean age at diagnosis was 61 years and 59.3% of the cohort was female (19). IPF was the most common ILD subtype (26.5%), followed by CTD-ILD (24.1%) and unclassifiable IIP (13.2%). The most common types of CTD-ILD were

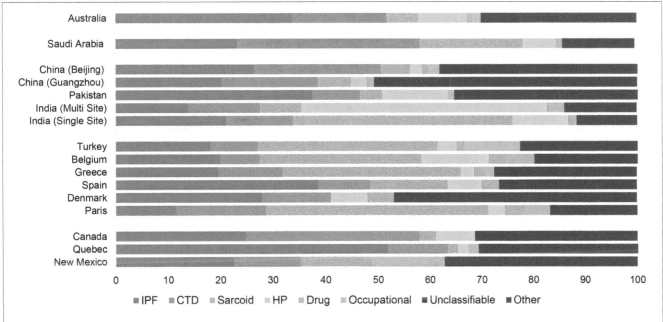

FIGURE 1 | Relative frequency of interstitial lung disease subtype by geography. IPF, idiopathic pulmonary fibrosis; CTD, connective tissue disease; HP, hypersensitivity pneumonitis.

Sjogren disease (11.2%) and RA-ILD (4.6%). Sarcoidosis accounted for 5.6% of cases and pneumoconiosis accounted for 2.2%.

Middle East

There is limited literature on the epidemiology of ILD in the Middle East. One study examined the frequency of ILD subtypes in Saudi Arabia by prospectively recruiting patients with new ILD diagnoses from a single tertiary care center between 2008 and 2011 (20). Cases were adjudicated *via* MDD. A total of 330 patients of native Saudi origin were enrolled with a mean age of 55.4 years and a predominance of females (61.2%) in the cohort. CTD-ILD (34.8%) was the most commonly diagnosed ILD, which included patients diagnosed with IPAF, followed by IPF (23.3%), sarcoidosis (20%), and HP (6.3%). The distribution of sarcoidosis ranged from 12% in stage I, 31% in stage II, 6% in stage III, to 51% in stage IV. The authors postulated that the higher proportion of stage IV sarcoid cases was in part due to referral bias as many patients with stage I and II disease were likely managed in the community. Among patients with HP, an exposure was identified in 66.7% of cases with the most common being birds. Surgical lung biopsies were performed in 22.7% of cases.

Australia

The Australian Interstitial Lung Disease Registry (AILDR) is the largest longitudinal cohort study of ILD in Australia and New Zealand (21). A total of 1,061 patients were recruited from four ILD centers across the continent between 2016 and 2019 *via* surveys distributed to physicians. The mean age of participants was 68.3 years with 54.7% male. The most common diagnosis was IPF (34%) followed by CTD-ILD (17.7%), HP (9.4%) and

sarcoidosis (6.2%). The registry also included cases of IPAF (0.4%), which was significantly lower than the frequency of IPAF cases observed in China and the Middle East.

GLOBAL TRENDS IN INTERSTITIAL LUNG DISEASE MORTALITY

The Global Burden of Disease Study noted that ILDs contributed to 0.26% of all-cause mortality in 2017 and that there had been an 86% increase in ILD-related years of life lost over the past two decades (22). The 5-year survival among patients with ILD has been estimated to be 56% (23). However, there is significant heterogeneity in survival by ILD subtypes. The 5-year survival in a national cohort of Danish patients was 34% among those with IPF, 74% in patients with idiopathic NSIP, and 93% among patients with HP (10). Given this variability, current literature has primarily focused on evaluating global trends in ILD mortality by subtype, with most studies focused on IPF.

IPF is a progressive fibrotic lung disease associated with insidious decline in lung function. Historically, the median survival of IPF has been estimated to range from 2 to 5 years (24, 25). However, there is significant variability by subgroup with longer median survival times among younger patients (26). More recent data suggests that in addition to age-related variability in IPF survival, there may be geographic variability as well. In a review of IPF mortality across 10 countries between 1999 and 2012, the age standardized mortality ranged from 4 to 10 per 100,000 with the lowest mortality rates observed in Sweden, Spain, and New Zealand and the highest mortality rates observed in the United Kingdom and Japan (27).

Within the United States, approximately 0.7% of all deaths that occurred between 2004 and 2016 had a diagnosis of pulmonary fibrosis and mortality rates were lower among women, Black, and Asians. There was significant variability in survival by state (28). The reasons for this variability in outcomes both within countries and between countries is unclear. Notably, the majority of these studies were conducted prior to approval and widespread adoption of antifibrotic therapies (pirfenidone and nintedanib), which have been shown to slow disease progression and improve survival. Thus, newer studies may demonstrate changing disease trajectories.

More recently, there has been increasing interest in understanding the prognosis of patients with non-IPF progressive fibrosing interstitial lung disease (PF-ILD) in light of clinical data suggesting that these patients may also benefit from antifibrotic therapies (29). In France, the median overall survival for patients with non-IPF PF-ILD was 3.7 years. Among this subgroup, patients with sarcoidosis had the longest median survival time (7.9 years) and patients with non-HP exposure related ILD had the shortest (2.4 years). These findings are consistent with prior literature that has suggested that the prognosis for patients with sarcoidosis may be better than other forms of ILD.

DISCUSSION

There are limited epidemiologic studies describing the global burden and relatively geographic heterogeneity of interstitial lung disease subtypes, and there are continents (e.g., South America and Africa) without English language literature on the topic. We found that among seventeen methodologically heterogenous studies that examined the incidence, prevalence and relative frequencies of ILD subtypes, the incidence of ILD ranged from 1 to 31.5 per 100,000 person-years and prevalence ranged from 6.3 to 71 per 100,000 people (**Table 1**). In North America and Europe, IPF and sarcoidosis were generally the most prevalent ILDs with the prevalence of IPF ranging from 1.3 per 100,000 in Belgium to 20.2 per 100,000 among males in Bernalillo County, New Mexico. The prevalence of sarcoidosis ranged from 1.94 per 100,000 in Belgium to 30.2 per 100,000 in Paris, France. The relative frequency of occupational interstitial lung disease was highest among patients in Bernalillo County (14%) and Turkey (10.7%) (**Table 2**, **Figure 1**). The relative frequency of HP was higher in Asia, particularly in India (10.7–47.3%) and Pakistan (12.3%), compared to most of the North American and European cohorts. The relative frequency of CTD-ILD demonstrated the greatest geographic variability, ranging from 7.5% of cases in Belgium to 33.3% of cases in Canada and 34.8% of cases in Saudi Arabia.

The reasons for this geographic heterogeneity is likely due to combination of methodological factors and variability in characteristics of the underlying source populations. Most registry-based epidemiologic studies have historically relied on individual patient recruitment from pulmonary clinics, which can lead to selection bias of the referral base, underestimation of true disease burden, and may not be representative of the general ILD population. This type of recruitment is also more likely to exclude certain types of ILDs like sarcoidosis and CTD-ILD, which may be managed by internal medicine physicians or rheumatologists. The Danish cohort excluded sarcoidosis from its registry for this reason (10).

Changing definitions of ILD subtypes due to evolving society guidelines also pose methodological challenges in quantifying temporal trends and comparing changes in relative frequency of ILDs over time. This is particularly true for idiopathic interstitial pneumonias, specifically IPF, for which there have been multiple iterations of clinical practice guidelines over the last decade (30–32). Additionally, new guidelines describing the entity of interstitial pneumonia with autoimmune features (IPAF) have led newer registries to qualify IPAF as a distinct ILD subtype, while other have collated IPAF under the broader umbrella term idiopathic interstitial pneumonia or alternatively under CTD-ILD itself (18, 20, 21, 33). This may partially explain the geographic variability in frequency of CTD-ILD noted in the literature.

Variable methods for case adjudication and differences in diagnostic confidence thresholds likely also contributed to the geographic heterogeneity noted. Of the 17 studies reviewed, approximately half explicitly reported MDD as a requirement for case adjudication. The remainder, primarily multicenter national registries, relied on enrollment surveys completed by referring physicians. Although these surveys included details about patient demographics, pulmonary function tests, high resolution CT scans and pathology when available, the studies did not uniformly report whether MDD was required prior to a final ILD diagnosis. In addition, as there are no universally agreed upon thresholds for diagnostic confidence, some variability may be explained by the stringency of diagnostic criteria applied. For example, registries like the Canadian national registry, which applied more stringent criteria that required biopsy confirmation for a diagnosis of idiopathic NSIP, may have underestimated the prevalence of some ILDs and had a higher proportion of unclassifiable cases (7). On the other hand, very few cases in the Indian registries had pathology available (16). Biopsies are often used to differentiate HP from IPF. Using history and radiology alone in these registries may have led to higher prevalence of HP in those cohorts.

Despite these methodological limitations, some differences observed between registry-based studies, may represent true differences in the demographics and exposures of the source populations. For example, in the Parisian cohort, which specifically evaluated the epidemiology of ILD among Seine-Saint-Denis, a multi-ethnic county of Greater Paris, the calculated ancestry-standardized incidence and prevalence rates of sarcoidosis and CTD-ILDs were higher among patients of North African descent (13). In India, the high prevalence of HP was partially attributed to widespread use of evaporative air coolers, which are prone to mold growth (16). Cohorts with predominantly younger patients or a higher proportion of women noted higher rates of CTD-ILD and lower rates of IPF. In Turkey and Belgium, the sex-standardized frequency of ILD subtypes favored CTD-ILD among women and pneumoconiosis among men (8, 14). A more complete understanding of these risk factors and the role that genetic ancestry may play in ILD risk can lead to important insight into predisposing factors that contribute to both ILD development and progression. Identification of ILD clusters can shed light on new exposures, their pathogenic mechanisms, and create an opportunity to intervene on modifiable occupation and environmental risk factors.

Mortality data examining the geographic variability in survival by ILD subtype is limited. Current literature suggests that IPF has the worst prognosis. Cohorts with a high proportion of patients with IPF may note higher overall ILD mortality rates associated with high healthcare utilization rates. IPF specific mortality rates may vary by geography. Whether this is due to underlying demographics of source populations or reflective of access to healthcare resources is unclear. Better understanding the reasons for geographic variability in ILD outcomes by subtype can expand our current clinical understanding of disease as well as identify care gaps for potential targeted intervention.

AREAS FOR IMPROVEMENT AND FUTURE DIRECTIONS

There are three areas where we feel additional work is needed to better understand the global burden of interstitial lung diseases. First, a standard ontology with diagnostic confidence thresholds is needed for comparative epidemiology studies of ILD (34). As demonstrated by this review, different authors choose different categorizations schema, employ variable diagnostic thresholds, and utilize different methodologies for establishing diagnosis. A unified set of diagnostic categories and criteria for this work would greatly help aggregate studies into informative reviews.

Second, more globally representative data should be published in English language journals or alternatively be translated into English and made available through open access. Most available epidemiologic studies in English have focused on evaluating disease burden in North America and Europe with only recent data from Asia. There are thus significant knowledge gaps regarding frequency of ILD subtypes in South America and Africa. Japan and South Korea, both major centers for ILD research, are also underrepresented in the English language literature.

Some knowledge gaps may also be due to healthcare infrastructure challenges in developing countries, particularly in South America and Africa, where access to tertiary care referral centers with dedicated chest radiologists and pulmonologists specializing in the diagnosis and management of ILD is limited. In addition, the paucity of data from many developing countries may reflect competing public health priorities, particularly of pulmonary diseases like tuberculosis, which disproportionately impact Asia, South America, and Africa. Multinational collaborative registries between ILD referral centers, like the recently established Latin American Idiopathic Pulmonary Fibrosis Registry (REFIPI), have the potential to consolidate resources and bridge this knowledge gap (35). Building on these types of registries to better understand the burden and relative frequencies of ILD in understudied countries would be informative, especially in light of increasing literature

exploring the complex interplay between genetics, environment and ILD.

Third, the inclusion of larger and more community-based cohorts is needed. Extrapolating regional or national epidemiology from single-center, specialty-based cohorts is likely leading to significant mischaracterization of the true distribution of ILDs. The Bernalillo County, New Mexico registry was among the first to use International Classification of Disease (ICD) codes followed by chart review in an attempt to provide more representative and inclusive data, and this may in part explain the higher incidence and prevalence reported (5). The electronic health record (EHR) is a potentially powerful tool for epidemiologists to address the issue of inclusion and generalizability. To date, most EHR based studies in ILD have focused on describing the epidemiology of individual ILD entities, most commonly IPF (26, 36), rather than evaluating comparative frequencies. One study that explored the epidemiology of IPF in U.S. Medicare claims data reported an annual IPF incidence of 93.7 cases per 100,000 person-years and a cumulative prevalence of 494.5 cases per 100,000 people in 2011 (26). These estimates are much higher than incidence and prevalence estimates noted in the majority of registry-based studies. It is possible that the higher incidence and prevalence noted in EHR-based studies reflects overdiagnosis in the absence of multidisciplinary case validation. Alternatively, it is possible that registry-based studies, many of whom recruit from tertiary care referral centers, underestimate population burden of disease. Future work that can leverage claims data as a screening tool to identify possible ILD cases with additional case validation to verify the accuracy of claims-based algorithms may facilitate more accurate estimates of ILD epidemiology. EHR data could also create an opportunity to recruit patients into national registries by leveraging electronic alerts to encourage referral to subspecialty centers for patients who meet EHR screening criteria for ILD.

Improving the functionality of EHR data for research purposes will require a concerted effort by the broader ILD community. Historically, ICD codes have been the primary means of EHR disease identification. However, ICD codes were developed for billing purposes with less attention given to specificity of diagnosis. This has limited their effectiveness for use in research studies. A concerted effort to adopt standardized codes with an emphasis on diagnostic accuracy has the potential to drastically expand the efficiency and speed with which we are able to draw from large, demographically and clinically diverse population-based cohorts. The opportunity to link EHR data with mortality data as is already done the United States Veterans Affairs Healthcare System, can further accelerate our progress.

We believe the ILD research community should organize a global summit to define a shared ontology for disease classification, set diagnostic confidence thresholds, and commit to conducting global claims and EHR-based epidemiologic studies in a standardized fashion. These data could be published in a shared issue of the major specialty journals. Aggregating and sharing data would provide a unique opportunity for international collaboration as our understanding of ILD continues to grow and evolve. These large, community-based longitudinal cohorts would also allow for tracking of global trends and be a valuable resource for collective study.

CONCLUSIONS

In conclusion, we have summarized the English language literature of the comparative epidemiology of ILD and demonstrated that there is significant geographic heterogeneity in the global disease burden and outcomes. These differences may represent true differences based on demographics and exposures of the source populations or methodological differences in patient recruitment (registry vs. population-based cohorts) and disease classification. Better understanding the geographic and temporal patterns of disease prevalence and identifying clusters of ILD subtypes can facilitate improved understanding of emerging risk factors and help identify targets for intervention. Future work, including a standardized ontology for classification, more globally inclusive studies, and leveraging

EHR data with uniform coding practices to develop more generalizable, community-based cohorts, will help advance our understanding of this important group of diseases. We encourage the international ILD community to organize and address this unmet need.

AUTHOR CONTRIBUTIONS

BK, VC, HC, and CV contributed to conception and design of the review. BK wrote the first draft of the manuscript. VC, HC, and CV provided critical feedback. All authors contributed to manuscript revision, read, and approved the submitted version.

FUNDING

Research reported in this publication was supported by the National Heart Lung and Blood Institute of the NIH under Awards K12HL138046 and K24HL12131.

REFERENCES

1. Larsen BT, Smith ML, Elicker BM, Fernandez JM, de Morvil GAA, Pereira CAC, et al. Diagnostic approach to advanced fibrotic interstitial lung disease: bringing together clinical, radiologic, and histologic clues. *Arch Pathol Lab Med.* (2017) 141:901–15. doi: 10.5858/arpa.2016-0299-SA

2. Travis WD, Costabel U, Hansell DM, King TE, Lynch DA, Nicholson AG, et al. An official American Thoracic Society/European Respiratory Society statement: Update of the international multidisciplinary classification of the idiopathic interstitial pneumonias. *Am J Respir Crit Care Med.* (2013) 188:733–48. doi: 10.1164/rccm.201308-1483ST

3. Demedts M, Wells AU, Anto JM, Costabel U, Hubbard R, Cullinan P, et al. Interstitial lung diseases: an epidemiological overview. *Eur Respir J Suppl.* (2001) 32:2s−16s.

4. Sese L, Khamis W, Jeny F, Uzunhan Y, Duchemann B, Valeyre D, et al. Adult interstitial lung diseases and their epidemiology. *Presse Med.* (2020) 49:104023. doi: 10.1016/j.lpm.2020.104023

5. Coultas DB, Zumwalt RE, Black WC, Sobonya RE. The epidemiology of interstitial lung diseases. *Am J Respir Crit Care Med.* (1994) 150:967–72. doi: 10.1164/ajrccm.150.4.7921471

6. Storme M, Semionov A, Assayag D, Lefson M, Kitty D, Dannenbaum D, et al. Estimating the incidence of interstitial lung diseases in the Cree of Eeyou Istchee, Northern Quebec. *PLoS ONE.* (2017) 12:e0184548. doi: 10.1371/journal.pone.0184548

7. Fisher JH, Kolb M, Algamdi M, Morisset J, Johannson KA, Shapera S, et al. Baseline characteristics and comorbidities in the CAnadian REgistry for Pulmonary Fibrosis. *BMC Pulm Med.* (2019) 19:223. doi: 10.1186/s12890-019-0986-4

8. Thomeer M, Demedts M, Vandeurzen K. Diseases VWGoIL. Registration of interstitial lung diseases by 20 centres of respiratory medicine in Flanders Acta. *Clin Belg.* (2001) 56:163–72. doi: 10.1179/acb.2001.026

9. Karakatsani A, Papakosta D, Rapti A, Antoniou KM, Dimadi M, Markopoulou A, et al. Epidemiology of interstitial lung diseases in Greece. *Respir Med.* (2009) 103:1122–9. doi: 10.1016/j.rmed.2009.03.001

10. Hyldgaard C, Hilberg O, Muller A, Bendstrup E. A cohort study of interstitial lung diseases in central Denmark. *Respir Med.* (2014) 108:793–9. doi: 10.1016/j.rmed.2013.09.002

11. Xaubet A, Ancochea J, Morell F, Rodriguez-Arias JM, Villena V, Blanquer R, et al. Report on the incidence of interstitial lung diseases in Spain. *Sarcoidosis Vasc Diffuse Lung Dis.* (2004) 21:64–70.

12. Tinelli C, De Silvestri A, Richeldi L, Oggionni T. The Italian register for diffuse infiltrative lung disorders (RIPID): a four-year report. *Sarcoidosis Vasc Diffuse Lung Dis.* (2005) 22:S4–8.

13. Duchemann B, Annesi-Maesano I, Jacobe de Naurois C, Sanyal S, Brillet PY, Brauner M, et al. Prevalence and incidence of interstitial lung

diseases in a multi-ethnic county of Greater Paris. *Eur Respir J.* (2017) 50: 1602419. doi: 10.1183/13993003.02419-2016

14. Musellim B, Okumus G, Uzaslan E, Akgun M, Cetinkaya E, Turan O, et al. Epidemiology and distribution of interstitial lung diseases in Turkey. *Clin Respir J.* (2014) 8:55–62. doi: 10.1111/crj.12035

15. Dhooria S, Agarwal R, Sehgal IS, Prasad KT, Garg M, Bal A, et al. Spectrum of interstitial lung diseases at a tertiary center in a developing country: a study of 803 subjects. *PLoS ONE.* (2018) 13:e0191938. doi: 10.1371/journal.pone.0191938

16. Singh S, Collins BF, Sharma BB, Joshi JM, Talwar D, Katiyar S, et al. Interstitial Lung Disease in India. Results of a prospective registry. *Am J Respir Crit Care Med.* (2017) 195:801–13. doi: 10.1164/rccm.201607-1484OC

17. Jafri S, Ahmed N, Saifullah N, Musheer M. Epidemiology and clinico-radiological features of Interstitial Lung Diseases. *Pak J Med Sci.* (2020) 36:365–70. doi: 10.12669/pjms.36.3.1046

18. Guo B, Wang L, Xia S, Mao M, Qian W, Peng X, et al. The interstitial lung disease spectrum under a uniform diagnostic algorithm: a retrospective study of 1,945 individuals. *J Thorac Dis.* (2020) 12:3688–96. doi: 10.21037/jtd-19-4021

19. Ban C, Yan W, Xie B, Zhu M, Liu Y, Zhang S, et al. Spectrum of interstitial lung disease in China from 2000 to 2012. *Eur Respir J.* (2018) 52: 1701554. doi: 10.1183/13993003.01554-2017

20. Alhamad EH. Interstitial lung diseases in Saudi Arabia: A single-center study. *Ann Thorac Med.* (2013) 8:33–7. doi: 10.4103/1817-1737.105717

21. Moore I, Wrobel J, Rhodes J, Lin Q, Webster S, Jo H, et al. Australasian interstitial lung disease registry (AILDR): objectives, design and rationale of a bi-national prospective database. *BMC Pulm Med.* (2020) 20:257. doi: 10.1186/s12890-020-0 1297-2

22. Collaborators GBDCRD. Prevalence and attributable health burden of chronic respiratory diseases, 1990–2017: a systematic analysis for the Global Burden of Disease Study 2017. *Lancet Respir Med.* (2020) 8:585–96. doi: 10.1016/S2213-2600(20)30105-3

23. Hilberg O, Bendstrup E, Lokke A, Ibsen R, Floe A, Hyldgaard C. Co-morbidity and mortality among patients with interstitial lung diseases: a population-based study. *Respirology.* (2018) 23:606–12. doi: 10.1111/resp.13234

24. Ley B, Ryerson CJ, Vittinghoff E, Ryu JH, Tomassetti S, Lee JS, et al. A multidimensional index and staging system for idiopathic pulmonary fibrosis. *Ann Intern Med.* (2012) 156:684–91. doi: 10.7326/0003-4819-156-10-201205150-00004

25. Nathan SD, Shlobin OA, Weir N, Ahmad S, Kaldjob JM, Battle E, et al. Long-term course and prognosis of idiopathic pulmonary fibrosis in the new millennium. *Chest.* (2011) 140:221–9. doi: 10.1378/chest.10-2572

26. Raghu G, Chen SY, Yeh WS, Maroni B, Li Q, Lee YC, et al. Idiopathic pulmonary fibrosis in US Medicare beneficiaries aged 65 years and older:

incidence, prevalence, and survival, 2001–11. *Lancet Respir Med.* (2014) 2:566–72. doi: 10.1016/S2213-2600(14)70101-8

27. Hutchinson J, Fogarty A, Hubbard R, McKeever T. Global incidence and mortality of idiopathic pulmonary fibrosis: a systematic review. *Eur Respir J.* (2015) 46:795–806. doi: 10.1183/09031936.00185114

28. Jeganathan N, Smith RA, Sathananthan M. Mortality trends of idiopathic pulmonary fibrosis in the United States from 2004 through 2017. *Chest.* (2021) 159:228–38. doi: 10.1016/j.chest.2020.08.016

29. Nasser M, Larrieu S, Boussel L, Si-Mohamed S, Bazin F, Marque S, et al. Estimates of epidemiology, mortality and disease burden associated with progressive fibrosing interstitial lung disease in France (the PROGRESS study). *Respir Res.* (2021) 22:162. doi: 10.1186/s12931-021-01749-1

30. Raghu G, Collard HR, Egan JJ, Martinez FJ, Behr J, Brown KK, et al. An official ATS/ERS/JRS/ALAT statement: idiopathic pulmonary fibrosis: evidence-based guidelines for diagnosis and management. *Am J Respir Crit Care Med.* (2011) 183:788–824. doi: 10.1164/rccm.2009-040GL

31. Raghu G, Rochwerg B, Zhang Y, Garcia CA, Azuma A, Behr J, et al. An official ATS/ERS/JRS/ALAT clinical practice guideline: treatment of idiopathic pulmonary fibrosis. an update of the 2011 clinical practice guideline. *Am J Respir Crit Care Med.* (2015) 192:e3–19. doi: 10.1164/rccm.201506-1 063ST

32. Raghu G, Remy-Jardin M, Myers JL, Richeldi L, Ryerson CJ, Lederer DJ, et al. Diagnosis of idiopathic pulmonary fibrosis. An official ATS/ERS/JRS/ALAT clinical practice guideline. *Am J Respir Crit Care Med.* (2018) 198:e44–68. doi: 10.1164/rccm.201807-1255ST

33. Fischer A, Antoniou KM, Brown KK, Cadranel J, Corte TJ, du Bois RM, et al. An official European Respiratory Society/American Thoracic Society research statement: interstitial pneumonia with autoimmune features. *Eur Respir J.* (2015) 46:976–87. doi: 10.1183/13993003.00150-2015

34. Ryerson CJ, Corte TJ, Lee JS, Richeldi L, Walsh SLF, Myers JL, et al. A standardized diagnostic ontology for fibrotic interstitial lung disease. An international working group perspective. *Am J Respir Crit Care Med.* (2017) 196:1249–54. doi: 10.1164/rccm.201702-0400PP

35. Ivette Buendia Roldán FC, Curbelo P, Kairalla R, Mejia M, Noriega L, Paulin F, et al. The Latin American Idiopathic Pulmonary Fibrosis Registry (REFIPI): baseline characteristics. *Eur Respir J.* (2019) 54(suppl 63): PA4699. doi: 10.1183/13993003.congress-2019.PA4699

36. Raghu G. Epidemiology, survival, incidence and prevalence of idiopathic pulmonary fibrosis in the USA and Canada. *Eur Respir J.* (2017) 49:1601504. doi: 10.1183/13993003.02384-2016

22

Lupus and the Lungs: The Assessment and Management of Pulmonary Manifestations of Systemic Lupus Erythematosus

Raj Amarnani[1], Su-Ann Yeoh[1,2], Emma K. Denneny[3,4] and Chris Wincup[1,2]*

[1] Department of Rheumatology, University College London Hospital, London, United Kingdom, [2] Division of Medicine, Department of Rheumatology, University College London, London, United Kingdom, [3] Department of Respiratory Medicine, University College London Hospital, London, United Kingdom, [4] Leukocyte Trafficking Laboratory, Centre for Inflammation and Tissue Repair, UCL Respiratory, University College London, London, United Kingdom

Correspondence:
Chris Wincup
c.wincup@ucl.ac.uk

Pulmonary manifestations of systemic lupus erythematosus (SLE) are wide-ranging and debilitating in nature. Previous studies suggest that anywhere between 20 and 90% of patients with SLE will be troubled by some form of respiratory involvement throughout the course of their disease. This can include disorders of the lung parenchyma (such as interstitial lung disease and acute pneumonitis), pleura (resulting in pleurisy and pleural effusion), and pulmonary vasculature [including pulmonary arterial hypertension (PAH), pulmonary embolic disease, and pulmonary vasculitis], whilst shrinking lung syndrome is a rare complication of the disease. Furthermore, the risks of respiratory infection (which often mimic acute pulmonary manifestations of SLE) are increased by the immunosuppressive treatment that is routinely used in the management of lupus. Although these conditions commonly present with a combination of dyspnea, cough and chest pain, it is important to consider that some patients may be asymptomatic with the only suggestion of the respiratory disorder being found incidentally on thoracic imaging or pulmonary function tests. Treatment decisions are often based upon evidence from case reports or small cases series given the paucity of clinical trial data specifically focused on pulmonary manifestations of SLE. Many therapeutic options are often initiated based on studies in severe manifestations of SLE affecting other organ systems or from experience drawn from the use of these therapeutics in the pulmonary manifestations of other systemic autoimmune rheumatic diseases. In this review, we describe the key features of the pulmonary manifestations of SLE and approaches to investigation and management in clinical practice.

Keywords: systemic lupus erythematosus (SLE), interstitial lung disease (ILD), pleurisy, pleural effusion, shrinking lung syndrome, pulmonary arterial hypertension, acute lupus pneumonitis, pulmonary vasculitis

INTRODUCTION

Systemic lupus erythematosus (SLE) is a chronic, autoimmune disorder that can present with a wide array of clinical and immunological abnormalities (1). Pulmonary manifestations of the disease include disorders of the lung parenchyma, pleura, and pulmonary vasculature. Furthermore, some SLE therapies predispose to an increased risk of respiratory infections (2).

Clinical assessment of patients with SLE should routinely consider careful evaluation for respiratory involvement. Symptoms including dyspnea, pleuritic chest pain, reduced exercise tolerance, cough, and hemoptysis should prompt investigation for potential underlying lung disease (3, 4). However, it is important to consider that some asymptomatic patients may also present with incidental findings of abnormal chest imaging or lung function tests in the absence of overt respiratory symptoms (5). It is also important to consider whether these symptoms are occurring in the context of active SLE involving other organ systems. Serological evidence of increased disease activity including elevated erythrocyte sedimentation rate (ESR), low complement, and increased double-stranded DNA (dsDNA) antibody titers should also prompt the clinician to consider whether new respiratory symptoms are directly attributed to lupus.

The exact prevalence of SLE-related lung disease is unknown and previous studies have varied widely in their estimates. Most report that between 20 and 90% of SLE patients will experience some form of lung involvement during the course of their disease (6, 7). However, more recently it has been suggested that this figure lies between the range of 50–70% (8). Predictors for progression to earlier permanent lung damage, include older age and those positive for anti-RNP antibodies (9). Pulmonary manifestations of SLE are associated with a higher mortality rate (10) and this varies depending upon the exact type and extent of lung involvement seen. More chronic forms of lung disease relating to SLE can have a significant negative affect on patient wellbeing, physical performance status, and are detrimental to quality of life (11).

In this review, we discuss the latest understanding on the ways in which lupus can affect the respiratory system, highlight how these patients may present clinically, and outline current approaches for investigation and management.

DISEASES OF THE LUNG PARENCHYMA

Interstitial Lung Disease (ILD)

The estimated prevalence of SLE-associated interstitial lung diseases (ILD) is suggested to be between 3 and 9% (12, 13). Although ILD is highly prevalent in rheumatoid arthritis and other systemic autoimmune rheumatic diseases (such as scleroderma and anti-synthetase syndrome), it is relatively uncommon in SLE (8). A small study previously reported that clinical progression of ILD in SLE is slow and often stabilizes over time (12). Risk factors for developing SLE-associated ILD include longstanding disease, older age and overlapping clinical features with scleroderma such as Raynaud's phenomenon and sclerodactyly (14–17). Various forms of ILD have been described in SLE including non-specific interstitial pneumonia (NSIP), organizing pneumonia, lymphocytic interstitial pneumonia, follicular bronchitis, and usual interstitial pneumonia (18–21). Bronchiolitis obliterans has also been reported as an initial manifestation of SLE (19).

Patients present similarly in most types of ILD with symptoms such as cough and dyspnea although it is important to consider

that some may be asymptomatic (22). Diagnosis of SLE-associated ILD can be made with high resolution computed tomography (HRCT) and excluding other potential causes of ILD (such as screening for overlap disorders by measuring rheumatoid factor, serum muscle enzymes, an extended myositis panel and anti-centromere autoantibodies) (23). Checking extractable nuclear antigens (ENA) should also be considered as previous studies have demonstrated that patients with anti-La, anti-Scl-70 and anti-U1RNP antibodies were more likely to develop ILD. Interestingly, anti-dsDNA antibody titer do no associate with the development of ILD (24). Lung function tests may show a restrictive pattern of disease and a decrease in diffusing capacity for carbon monoxide (DLCO) (8). Histological studies have reported the presence of lymphocytic and mononuclear interstitial and peribronchiolar infiltrates in biopsies taken from those with SLE-related NSIP (25).

There are a lack of clinical trials assessing the treatment of SLE-related ILD and in particular there are no head-to-head studies. Therefore, recommendations are predominantly based on case reports, small case series, physician expertise, and by applying findings from studies of ILD in other autoimmune rheumatic diseases. Intravenous cyclophosphamide was reported to show significant improvement vital capacity in two SLE patients with ILD in which both patients presented with pleuritic chest pain in the context of active SLE (26). Another case report noted that oral methotrexate resulted in a marked improvement in lung function in a patient with SLE-related ILD (27). An observational study of 14 patients with SLE-associated ILD reported that three patients showed significant improvement with high dose oral steroids (60 mg prednisolone daily for a minimum of 4 weeks). Six of the 14 patients had an improvement in respiratory symptoms and all were treated with systemic steroids (18). Three patients within the cohort died, two of pulmonary fibrosis, and one from infection thus highlighting the clinical challenge posed by immunosuppressive therapy in the context of SLE-related ILD. It is important to consider that this study was published in 1990 and thus predates a number of the newer treatments available for the management of SLE, such as mycophenolate mofetil (MMF), rituximab and belimumab.

Current treatment often includes the use of high dose corticosteroids along with agents such as cyclophosphamide and rituximab in severe cases (28, 29) to induce remission. Steroid-sparing agents such as MMF and azathioprine may be used in milder cases or in maintaining long-term control of the disease (30, 31).

Acute Lupus Pneumonitis

In some cases, chronic ILD may be the long-term sequelae of an acute process, for example acute lupus pneumonitis. This is a rare manifestation of SLE that has been reported to occur in 1–4% of patients (32). Clinically, acute lupus pneumonitis presents in the context of a systemic flare of SLE in addition to dyspnea, cough (including hemoptysis) and pleuritic chest pain. Fever is commonly associated with the acute presentation, thus making it a clinical challenge to differentiate from infection. There is limited data on lung histology in acute lupus pneumonitis, although reports of lymphocytic infiltrates and alveolar damage with associated interstitial edema have been reported in both lung biopsy samples and at post-mortem assessment (24).

Acute lupus pneumonitis may also be the initial presenting symptom of SLE. A case series of five patients in which acute lupus pneumonitis was the first feature of SLE reported that all five were female, aged 14–26 years old. They were all ANA positive, whilst three were also positive for anti-dsDNA antibodies. Fever was present in all cases with cough as a presenting symptom in four of the five patients, with hypoxia noted in three. All patients received corticosteroids and four patients were treated with cyclophosphamide either as monotherapy or in combination with intravenous immunoglobulins (IVIg). The one patient who did not receive cyclophosphamide was treated with azathioprine. Three patients survived but two died as a result of infection (33). Others have also reported the use of IVIg in acute lupus pneumonitis (34, 35). Given that the differential diagnosis in this presentation often includes bacterial pneumonia, and as infection can commonly co-exist with acute lupus pneumonitis, IVIg represents a useful option as it does not convey the high risk of immunosuppression associated with other agents. It is also important to consider using broad spectrum antibiotics (in particular directed against encapsulated organisms) if there are concerns about intercurrent infection. Further, prompt initiation of systemic glucocorticoid therapy has been reported to be of benefit in reducing mortality rates. Additional treatments that have been used in the management of acute lupus pneumonitis are similar to those used in SLE-related ILD, such as high dose glucocorticoids in combination with either MMF, azathioprine, rituximab, or cyclophosphamide. However, in spite of this the outcomes are often poor with associated high mortality rates (33, 36).

PLEURAL DISEASE

Pleural involvement is the most common SLE-related lung disease (37). Clinically, patients often present with pleuritic chest pain, cough and dyspnea due to inflammation of the pleura (38). Patients may have an associated pleural effusion which is often bilateral and exudative in nature (39, 40). Estimates suggest that between 30 and 50% of SLE patients will develop a pleural effusion at some point during their disease course, although often these are small and may not result in obvious symptoms (39, 41).

Diagnosis of pleural involvement in SLE is usually clinical with typical features in the patient history. It is however important to exclude other causes of pleural inflammation that can occur in SLE including infection, pulmonary embolism, malignancy, congestive cardiac failure (37), or pericarditis, which may present in a similar manner. Drug-induced pleuritis from agents such as hydralazine, procainamide and anti-tumor necrosis factor-alpha medications should also be considered (42–44). In such cases, drug cessation is often sufficient to resolve symptoms.

Although not necessary for diagnosis, if there is clinical uncertainty as to the cause of a pleural effusion, aspiration can be performed. Pleural fluid in patients with SLE classically show elevated levels of protein, lactate dehydrogenase (LDH), leukocytes, and in some cases ANA positivity (37, 39).

The mainstay treatment of pleurisy in SLE has traditionally been non-steroidal anti-inflammatory drugs (NSAIDs) with some patients requiring corticosteroids (38). Rarely, other steroid-sparing agents such as azathioprine, methotrexate, cyclosporine, and cyclophosphamide may be indicated (37). In refractory disease, there have been cases showing effective use of pleurodesis (45, 46).

DISORDERS OF THE PULMONARY VASCULATURE

Pulmonary Arterial Hypertension (PAH)

Pulmonary arterial hypertension (PAH) is a progressive disorder characterized by a resting mean pulmonary artery pressure above 25 mmHg and a pulmonary wedge pressure below 15 mmHg (47). There are a number of possible underlying causes that may result in PAH in SLE, including left ventricular dysfunction or congestive cardiac failure that may be a result of the increased risk of atherosclerosis associated with SLE. It may also be a manifestation of the long-term sequelae of parenchymal lung diseases (such as ILD) or chronic thromboembolic disease (48). Studies estimate the prevalence of PAH in SLE to be in the range of 1–43% depending on the cohort (49–54). A recent comprehensive meta-analysis assessing the prevalence of PAH found an estimated pooled prevalence of 8% (55). Despite this, severe PAH is thought to be a rare manifestation in SLE and is not included in the Systemic Lupus Erythematosus Disease Activity Index 2000 (SLEDAI-2K) disease activity score (56).

Clinical symptoms of PAH in SLE are often non-specific and range from generalized fatigue and weakness to chest pain and dyspnea at rest (48). Initial investigations often include an electrocardiogram that may show right ventricular hypertrophy and right axis deviation. Radiographic imaging with computerized tomography may be used to exclude other diseases such as ILD and will often show enlarged pulmonary vessels (57). Echocardiography can estimate systolic pulmonary artery pressure and is therefore a vital non-invasive tool to assist in making a diagnosis. However, even with a suggestive echocardiogram result and high clinical suspicion, right heart catheterization remains the "gold standard" test to confirm the diagnosis (58).

Management of PAH in SLE is similar to that of idiopathic PAH. However, most randomized controlled trials that have specifically analyzed the management of PAH associated with connective tissue diseases often have not included a subgroup analysis of SLE patients (48). Drugs such as phosphodiesterase-5 inhibitors, endothelin receptor antagonists and prostacyclin pathway agonists have all shown to be effective in SLE associated PAH to varying degrees (59–64). More recently, the guanylate cyclase stimulator riociguat has shown to be effective in a small number of SLE-associated PAH cases (65, 66).

Numerous observational cohort studies have also noted benefit with corticosteroids and immunosuppressive therapy including cyclophosphamide, cyclosporine and MMF (67–70). One case report has also described effective use of rituximab in refractory SLE-associated PAH (71). Overall, it is generally thought that a combination of both immunosuppression and traditional PAH treatment should be used together to enhance long-term outcomes (68).

Pulmonary Embolic Disease

Pulmonary embolism (PE) also needs to be considered in the acute setting in any patient with SLE who presents with pleuritic chest pain (especially if associated with acute hypoxia). In the more chronic setting, chronic pulmonary embolic disease can also lead to pulmonary hypertension (chronic thromboembolic pulmonary hypertension). It is particularly important to consider embolic disease in those patients who have secondary anti-phospholipid syndrome (APS), given the obvious increased risk of thrombosis associated with the disease. Previous studies have reported that one-third of patients with SLE will have positive anti-phospholipid antibodies and those with a positive lupus anticoagulant have previously been shown to have a six-fold increased risk of venous thrombosis. In comparison, a positive anti-cardiolipin antibody carried twice the risk when compared with SLE patients without positive anti-cardiolipin antibodies (72). Previous studies have also reported that patients with SLE, even in the absence of APS, are at an increased risk of unprovoked PE when compared with the general population and therefore the absence of positive anti-phospholipid serology should not be falsely reassuring.

The "gold standard" investigation for PE is computed topography pulmonary angiogram (CTPA), which can identify the presence of thrombosis within the pulmonary vasculature. However, it is important to consider that SLE patients presenting with pleuritic chest pain and hypoxia may instead be suffering from pleurisy (as described above). Results from the Michigan Lupus Cohort assessed the outcomes of 182 patients with SLE who had previously undergone a total of 357 CTPA scans. The authors found a significant decrease in the likelihood of confirming PE in patients who had previously had three or more scans, thus suggesting that repeated scanning of patients without a previously proven PE is unlikely to confirm a new diagnosis (73).

In the context of PE associated with APS, lifelong anticoagulation is likely to be recommended. Recent studies investigating direct oral anticoagulants have recommended against their use in arterial thrombosis, such as PE (74).

Pulmonary Vasculitis and Pulmonary Hemorrhage

Pulmonary vasculitis, or diffuse alveolar hemorrhage (DAH), is a rare but severe manifestation of SLE that is associated with a high mortality rate of up to 90% (75). This has been reported to affect <5% of patients with SLE and is more commonly seen concurrently in the context of active lupus nephritis (76). In addition, this manifestation has been reported to be the initial presentation of SLE in ~20% of all cases, which means that it is important to consider lupus in any new case of pulmonary hemorrhage in which an alternate underlying cause is not present (77). It has also been reported that patients with secondary APS may be at increased risk of DAH and that this may also occur *de novo* in patients with SLE who are have anti-phospholipid

antibodies without previous thrombotic events. This suggests that this is not entirely the result of anticoagulant therapy and may represent an as yet unclassified mechanism for pulmonary vasculitis (78). As with other acute pulmonary manifestations of SLE, the symptoms can often mimic infection thus making the diagnosis a challenge.

Findings from small cases series and cohort studies have highlighted that dyspnea and pulmonary infiltrates on thoracic imaging are almost universally in seen. Fever is reported in the majority of cases although occult hemoptysis is only seen in just over half of patients at presentation (79). Many patients will also present with extrapulmonary manifestations of SLE to suggest a generalized systemic flare of the disease. More subtle signs that suggest DAH include pleural effusions and anemia is seen in nearly all cases, and may be present before signs such as hemoptysis are observed (75, 80). Imaging studies often describe classical bilateral alveolar interstitial infiltrates. Many patients are deemed clinically unstable for further dedicated investigation however those that proceed to bronchoscopy are usually found to have high neutrophil count, low lymphocyte count and hemosiderin-laden macrophages within the lavage and occult blood often seen (79, 81). If the patient is able to tolerate pulmonary function tests then an elevated DLCO is usually indicative of alveolar hemorrhage.

Given a lack of clinical trial data from DAH in SLE, treatment recommendations are usually based upon other autoimmune conditions associated with pulmonary hemorrhage (such as ANCA-associated vasculitis) and often include pulsed intravenous steroids in combination with cyclophosphamide (79), rituximab, plasmapheresis, and IVIg (81, 82).

SHRINKING LUNG SYNDROME (SLS)

Shrinking lung syndrome (SLS) is an uncommon manifestation of SLE with an estimated prevalence of ~1–2% (9, 83, 84). The exact cause of SLS is unclear, however it is believed to involve abnormal diaphragmatic strength and may be related to due to impaired phrenic nerve signaling (85).

Patients with SLS often present with symptoms of pleuritic chest pain and progressive dyspnea (86). Due to its rarity, there is no diagnostic criteria for SLS. Lung function tests often show a restrictive defect with a reduction in lung volume and DLCO (84). Radiographic imaging in SLS is often non-specific with occasional elevation of the diaphragm and basal atelectasis with usually no evidence of interstitial lung or pleural disease (87). It is also important to consider other conditions before a diagnosis of SLS is made including central nervous system disorders and diaphragmatic palsies (88).

Evidence for the optimal management of SLS is limited. Corticosteroids and immunosuppressive agents including azathioprine, MMF and rituximab have been used to varying degrees of efficacy (86, 89–92). Some have suggested the use of hematopoietic cell transplantation (93) and beta agonist therapy (94) in SLS. Others have reported some benefit in the use of theophylline thought to be helpful by improving diaphragmatic

TABLE 1 | A summary of the way in which pulmonary manifestations of systemic lupus erythematosus (SLE) may present in clinical practice, the underlying pathogenesis and relevant treatment options.

Diagnosis	Presentation	Pathogenesis	Relevant investigation findings	Histological features	Treatment
Interstitial lung disease	Chronic, often progressive dyspnoea Cough (often non-productive) Possible evidence of scleroderma, anti-synthetase syndrome, or rheumatoid arthritis May be asymptomatic	Poorly understood/unclear Likely a result of the aberrant inflammatory response due to imbalance of pro- and anti-inflammatory cytokine release (96) Possibly the result of repeated alveolar injury resulting in a combination of both impaired apoptosis and abnormal fibroblast proliferation	Infiltrative changes on CXR or HRCT chest Restrictive pattern on pulmonary function tests with reduced DLCO Test for auto-antibodies suggestive of overlap disorder (e.g., RhF, anti-CCP, anti-centromere, anti-Scl-70, anti-RNP) and muscle enzymes (CK, LDH)	Mononuclear or lymphoplasmacytic interstitial and peribronchiolar infiltrates (particularly in NSIP pattern disease) Interstitial fibrosis present. Deposits of IgG, IgM, C1q, and C3 within alveolar septae previously reported (14)	Depends upon severity Severe or rapidly progressive Oral/IV corticosteroids followed by either Cyclophosphamide, Rituximab, MMF, Azathioprine
Acute lupus pneumonitis	Acute dyspnoea Fever Cough (usually non-productive but occasional hemoptysis) Features of extrapulmonary SLE disease activity	Rapid systemic inflammatory response resulting in acute damage to the lung parenchyma. Alveolar injury resulting from direct immune-mediated inflammation	CXR – diffuse bilateral alveolar infiltrates CT thorax – previous reports of ground-glass changes Serological evidence of lupus activity (low complement and elevated anti-dsDNA antibody titers)	Often non-specific: Features can include alveolar wall damage, necrosis, inflammatory infiltrate, oedema, hemorrhage, hyaline membranes (97) Capillary microangitis, fibrin thrombi and necrotic neutrophils have also been described (98)	Systemic corticosteroids (either high dose oral or pulsed IV) plus either Cyclophosphamide, Rituximab, MMF, Azathioprine Possibly IVIg
Pleurisy	Chest pain (often pleuritic in nature) Cough Dyspnoea Physical signs such as pleural rub may be present	Inflammatory infiltration into the pleura	Raised CRP Imaging usually normal CXR ± CT thorax or CTPA helpful to rule out other causes	Non-specific inflammatory changes associated with fibrin deposition along with pleural fibrosis (99)	Mild Oral NSAIDs Moderate Oral corticosteroids Severe (rarely required) IV corticosteroids, Azathioprine, Cyclophosphamide, Rituximab, MMF
Pleural effusion	Dyspnoea Chest pain, usually associated with pleurisy May be asymptomatic Physical signs including reduce basal air entry and decreased resonance	As per "Pleurisy" Excessive inflammation results in exudative fluid secretion between pleural lining resulting in effusion	Effusion(s), usually bilateral, present on CXR or CT thorax Aspirate (if underlying diagnosis in doubt) – elevated protein, LDH, leukocytes, ANA positive in some cases	Predominantly based on cytological features Pleural fluid may show characteristic lupus erythematosus (LE) cells, e.g., neutrophils or macrophages containing intracellular evidence of phagocytosed lymphocyte nuclei (100)	Corticosteroids Drainage if large Pleurodesis in recurrent or refractory cases Cessation of any potential drug causes
Pulmonary arterial hypertension	Can be non-specific (such as fatigue and weakness) Progressive dyspnoea Occasional chest pain Physical signs may show right ventricular heave	Dependent upon underlying cause Left ventricular dysfunction/congestive cardiac failure may result from direct myocardial inflammation from SLE (e.g. myocarditis) or as a result of enhanced atherosclerosis Chronic thromboembolic disease may result from pro-coagulant factors such as aPl antibodies Lung parenchymal disease as the result of direct inflammatory response in lung tissue Dysregulation between vasoconstrictive and vasodilatory mediators	EKG – RVH and right axis deviation Echocardiogram – elevated PASP, TR Right heart catheterization – mean arterial pressure ≥25 mm Hg confirms diagnosis CT thorax – useful to exclude other secondary causes CTPA – useful to rule out chronic embolic disease as a cause Check anti-centromere, anti-Scl-70, anti-U1RNP (to rule out scleroderma and other overlap syndromes)	Limited data Vascular lesions including eccentric and concentric intimal fibrosis and thrombotic lesions Venous occlusive lesions have been reported with pulmonary veins/venules Capillary congestion (101)	Phosphodiesterase-5 inhibitors Endothelin receptor antagonists Prostacyclin agonists Role for immunosuppression not clear
Pulmonary embolic disease	Usually acute onset Dyspnoea Chest pain (often pleuritic) Hypoxia Occasionally hemoptysis	Thromboembolic disease usually as a result of pro-coagulant state This could include secondary antiphospholipid syndrome Severe proteinuria from lupus nephritis may result in anti-thrombin deficiency	Check aPl antibodies (LAC, aCL, anti-B2GPl) Elevated D-dimer CXR usually normal aside from potential wedge infarct CTPA	Evidence of thrombus within pulmonary arterial system	Anti-coagulation (low molecular weight heparin, oral vitamin K antagonist)
Pulmonary vasculitis	Acute dyspnoea Commonly associated with fever and active extrapulmonary manifestations of SLE Hemoptysis May be initial presentation of SLE	Direct immune-mediated inflammatory response of the small vessels of the alveola resulting in increased permeability and eventually structural damage resulting in hemorrhage	CXR – bilateral alveolar interstitial infiltrates Pulmonary function tests – elevated DLCO Drop in Hb Important to check ANCA and urine dip for proteinuria/hematuria (to rule out intercurrent ANCA-associated vasculitis or pulmonary-renal syndrome)	Numerous intra-alveolar or interstitial aggregates that comprise of hemosiderin-laden macrophages Fresh hemorrhagic changes may be present in the context of DAH Capillaritis may be present (26)	IV corticosteroids Cyclophosphamide Rituximab IVIg Plasmapheresis May require mechanical ventilation
Shrinking lung syndrome	Progressive dyspnoea Occasional pleuritic chest pain	Poorly understood Felt to be the result of marked diaphragmatic weakness or immobility. Possibly as a result of pleural adhesions Phrenic neuropathy also previously proposed as a possible mechanism	CXR – often non-specific, elevation of diaphragm and basal atelectasis may be seen Pulmonary function tests – restrictive pattern with reduced lung volume and DLCO	Extremely limited data from lung biopsy with features reported as alveolar microatelectasia and hyaline membrane formation (102) Post-mortem diaphragmatic tissue showing muscle atrophy (85)	Little evidence currently available to support treatment decisions Corticosteroids, Azathioprine, MMF, and Rituximab used with variable success in case reports

CXR, chest x-ray; HRCT, high resolution computerized tomography; NSIP, non-specific interstitial pneumonia; DLCO, diffusing capacity for carbon monoxide; RhF, rheumatoid factor; CCP, cyclic citrullinated peptide; RNP, ribonuclear protein; CK, creatinine kinase; LDH, lactate dehydrogenase; aPl, antiphospholipid; IV, intravenous; MMF, mycophenolate mofetil; CT, computerized tomography; CRP, c-reactive protein; CTPA, computerized tomography pulmonary angiogram; NSAIDs, non-steroidal anti-inflammatory drugs; ANA, anti-nuclear antibody; EKG, electrocardiogram; RVH, right ventricular hypertrophy; PASP, pulmonary artery systolic pressure; TR, tricuspid regurgitation; LAC, lupus anticoagulant; aCL, anti-cardiolipin; B2GPl, beta-2-glyoprotein-l; Hb, hemoglobin; ANCA, anti-neutrophil cytoplasm antibody; DAH, diffuse alveolar hemorrhage.

strength (87, 95). Comprehensive studies have generally shown a good prognosis with treatment in most SLS patients (87, 88).

CONCLUSIONS

Pulmonary manifestations of SLE can present with a wide array of symptoms and can often be difficult to differentiate from other conditions, most notably infection. The key differences between these disorders are summarized in **Table 1**.

It is important to consider that SLE-related lung disorders are likely to be under-represented due to the fact that respiratory involvement may be asymptomatic. Furthermore, serositis (pleurisy/pleural effusion) is the only respiratory symptom included in the revised 1997 American College of Rheumatology (ACR) criteria for SLE (103) and no additional respiratory manifestations were included in the 2019 combined ACR/EULAR criteria (104). In terms of measuring disease activity from pulmonary manifestations of SLE, the British Isles Lupus Assessment Group (BILAG) index includes a subsection on (cardio)respiratory features of the disease, which considers pleurisy, pleural effusion, pulmonary hemorrhage/vasculitis, interstitial lung disease, and shrinking lung syndrome as possible pulmonary manifestations of the disease (105). In comparison, the SLEDAI-2K only accounts for pleurisy as a scorable item of lupus activity involving the lungs (106). In turn, this may result in a number of patients with respiratory complications of SLE (particularly those symptoms considered more mild) to be

falsely considered as either in remission or a low disease activity state (107). In comparison, the Systemic Lupus International Collaborating Clinics (SLICC)/ACR Damage Index for SLE does include a wide array of pulmonary manifestations although these are typically irreversible and thus may not be a useful measure in preventative studies (108). This has important implications for clinical trial design, which may exclude patients who have predominantly respiratory symptoms. As a result, evidence supporting therapeutic options in SLE-related lung disease are often extrapolated from other severe manifestations of the disease. Dedicated studies in the management of pulmonary disorders in SLE are greatly needed and represent a major unmet need.

AUTHOR CONTRIBUTIONS

RA conducted a literature review of relevant respiratory disorders. SAY, EKD, and CW expanded upon this. All authors agreed to the finalized version of this manuscript prior to submission.

ACKNOWLEDGMENTS

CW would like to acknowledge the support he receives from Versus Arthritis and LUPUS UK.

REFERENCES

1. Bakshi J, Segura BT, Wincup C, Rahman A. Unmet needs in the pathogenesis and treatment of systemic lupus erythematosus. *Clin Rev Allergy Immunol.* (2018) 55:352–67. doi: 10.1007/s12016-017-8640-5
2. Cuchacovich R, Gedalia A. Pathophysiology and clinical spectrum of infections in systemic lupus erythematosus. *Rheum Dis Clin North Am.* (2009) 35:75–93. doi: 10.1016/j.rdc.2009.03.003
3. Alamoudi OSB, Attar SM. Pulmonary manifestations in systemic lupus erythematosus: association with disease activity. *Respirology.* (2015) 20:474–80. doi: 10.1111/resp.12473
4. Hellman DB, Kirsch CM, Whiting-O'Keefe Q, Simonson J, Schiller NB, Petri M, et al. Dyspnea in ambulatory patients with SLE: prevalence, severity, and correlation with incremental exercise testing. *J Rheumatol.* (1995) 22:455–61.
5. Nakano M, Hasegawa H, Takada T, Ito S, Muramatsu Y, Satoh M, et al. Pulmonary diffusion capacity in patients with systemic lupus erythematosus. *Respirology.* (2002) 7:45–9. doi: 10.1046/j.1440-1843.2002.00361.x
6. Aguilera-Pickens G, Abud-Mendoza C. Pulmonary manifestations in systemic lupus erythematosus: pleural involvement, acute pneumonitis, chronic interstitial lung disease and diffuse alveolar hemorrhage. *Reumatol Clin.* (2018) 14:294–300. doi: 10.1016/j.reuma.2018.03.012
7. Tselios K, Urowitz MB. Cardiovascular and pulmonary manifestations of systemic lupus erythematosus. *Curr Rheumatol Rev.* (2017) 13:206–18. doi: 10.2174/1573397113666170704102444
8. Hannah JR, D'Cruz DP. Pulmonary complications of systemic lupus erythematosus. *Semin Respir Crit Care Med.* (2019) 40:227–34. doi: 10.1055/s-0039-1685537
9. Bertoli AM, Vila LM, Apte M, Fessler BJ, Bastian HM, Reveille JD, et al. Systemic lupus erythematosus in a multiethnic US Cohort LUMINA XLVIII: factors predictive of pulmonary damage. *Lupus.* (2007) 16:410–7. doi: 10.1177/0961203307079042
10. Kamen DL, Strange C. Pulmonary manifestations of systemic lupus erythematosus. *Clin Chest Med.* (2010) 31:479–88. doi: 10.1016/j.ccm.2010.05.001
11. Fidler L, Keen KJ, Touma Z, Mittoo S. Impact of pulmonary disease on patient-reported outcomes and patient-performed functional testing in systemic lupus erythematosus. *Lupus.* (2016) 25:1004–11. doi: 10.1177/0961203316630818
12. Weinrib L, Sharma OP, Quismorio FP, Jr. A long-term study of interstitial lung disease in systemic lupus erythematosus. *Semin Arthritis Rheum.* (1990) 20:48–56. doi: 10.1016/0049-0172(90)90094-V
13. Wiedemann HP, Matthay RA. Pulmonary manifestations of systemic lupus erythematosus. *J Thorac Imaging.* (1992) 7:1–18. doi: 10.1097/00005382-199203000-00003
14. Eisenberg H, Dubois EL, Sherwin RP, Balchum OJ. Diffuse interstitial lung disease in systemic lupus erythematosus. *Ann Intern Med.* (1973) 79:37–45. doi: 10.7326/0003-4819-79-1-37
15. Mathai SC, Danoff SK. Management of interstitial lung disease associated with connective tissue disease. *BMJ.* (2016) 352:h6819. doi: 10.1136/bmj.h6819
16. ter Borg EJ, Groen H, Horst G, Limburg PC, Wouda AA, Kallenberg CG. Clinical associations of antiribonucleoprotein antibodies in patients with systemic lupus erythematosus. *Semin Arthritis Rheum.* (1990) 20:164–73. doi: 10.1016/0049-0172(90)90057-M
17. Ward MM, Polisson RP. A meta-analysis of the clinical manifestations of older-onset systemic lupus erythematosus. *Arthritis Rheum.* (1989) 32:1226–32. doi: 10.1002/anr.1780321007
18. Frankel SK, Brown KK. Collagen vascular diseases of the lung. *Clin Pulm Med.* (2006) 13:25–36. doi: 10.1097/01.cpm.0000197403.64631.de
19. Min JK, Hong YS, Park SH, Park JH, Lee SH, Lee YS, et al. Bronchiolitis obliterans organizing pneumonia as an initial manifestation in patients with systemic lupus erythematosus. *J Rheumatol.* (1997) 24:2254–7.
20. Tansey D, Wells AU, Colby TV, Ip S, Nikolakoupolou A, du Bois RM, et al. Variations in histological patterns of interstitial pneumonia between connective tissue disorders and their relationship to prognosis. *Histopathology.* (2004) 44:585–96. doi: 10.1111/j.1365-2559.2004.01896.x
21. Yood RA, Steigman DM, Gill LR. Lymphocytic interstitial pneumonitis in a patient with systemic lupus erythematosus. *Lupus.* (1995) 4:161–3. doi: 10.1177/096120339500400217

22. Cheema GS, Quismorio FP, Jr. Interstitial lung disease in systemic lupus erythematosus. *Curr Opin Pulm Med.* (2000) 6:424–9. doi: 10.1097/00063198-200009000-00007

23. Fenlon HM, Doran M, Sant SM, Breatnach E. High-resolution chest CT in systemic lupus erythematosus. *AJR Am J Roentgenol.* (1996) 166:301–7. doi: 10.2214/ajr.166.2.8553934

24. Lian FZJ, Wang Y, Cui W, Chen D, Li H, Qiu Q, et al. Clinical features and independent predictors of interstitial lung disease in systemic lupus erythematosus. *Int J Clin Exp Med.* (2016) 9:4233–42.

25. Vivero M, Padera RF. Histopathology of lung disease in the connective tissue diseases. *Rheum Dis Clin North Am.* (2015) 41:197–211. doi: 10.1016/j.rdc.2014.12.002

26. Eiser AR, Shanies HM. Treatment of lupus interstitial lung disease with intravenous cyclophosphamide. *Arthritis Rheum.* (1994) 37:428–31. doi: 10.1002/art.1780370318

27. Fink SD, Kremer JM. Successful treatment of interstitial lung disease in systemic lupus erythematosus with methotrexate. *J Rheumatol* (1995) 22:967–9.

28. Lim SW, Gillis D, Smith W, Hissaria P, Greville H, Peh CA. Rituximab use in systemic lupus erythematosus pneumonitis and a review of current reports. *Intern Med J.* (2006) 36:260–2. doi: 10.1111/j.1445-5994.2006.01055.x

29. Okada M, Suzuki K, Matsumoto M, Nakashima M, Nakanishi T, Takada K, et al. Intermittent intravenous cyclophosphamide pulse therapy for the treatment of active interstitial lung disease associated with collagen vascular diseases. *Mod Rheumatol.* (2007) 17:131–6. doi: 10.3109/s10165-007-0554-2

30. Koo S-M, Uh S-T. Treatment of connective tissue disease-associated interstitial lung disease: the pulmonologist's point of view. *Korean J Intern Med.* (2017) 32:600–10. doi: 10.3904/kjim.2016.212

31. Swigris JJ, Olson AL, Fischer A, Lynch DA, Cosgrove GP, Frankel SK, et al. Mycophenolate mofetil is safe, well tolerated, and preserves lung function in patients with connective tissue disease-related interstitial lung disease. *Chest* (2006) 130:30–6. doi: 10.1016/S0012-3692(15)50949-5

32. Keane MP, Lynch JP, III. Pleuropulmonary manifestations of systemic lupus erythematosus. *Thorax.* (2000) 55:159–66. doi: 10.1136/thorax.55.2.159

33. Wan SA, Teh CL, Jobli AT. Lupus pneumonitis as the initial presentation of systemic lupus erythematosus: case series from a single institution. *Lupus* (2016) 25:1485–90. doi: 10.1177/0961203316646461

34. Winder A, Molad Y, Ostfeld I, Kenet G, Pinkhas J, Sidi Y. Treatment of systemic lupus erythematosus by prolonged administration of high dose intravenous immunoglobulin: report of 2 cases. *J Rheumatol* (1993) 20:495–8.

35. Chen YJ, Tseng JJ, Yang MJ, Tsao YP, Lin HY. Acute respiratory distress syndrome in a pregnant woman with systemic lupus erythematosus: a case report. *Lupus.* (2014) 23:1528–32. doi: 10.1177/0961203314548713

36. Boulware DW, Hedgpeth MT. Lupus pneumonitis and anti-SSA(Ro) antibodies. *J Rheumatol.* (1989) 16:479–81.

37. Pego-Reigosa JM, Medeiros DA, Isenberg DA. Respiratory manifestations of systemic lupus erythematosus: old and new concepts. *Best Pract Res Clin Rheumatol.* (2009) 23:469–80. doi: 10.1016/j.berh.2009.01.002

38. Wang D-Y. Diagnosis and management of lupus pleuritis. *Curr Opin Pulm Med.* (2002) 8:312–6. doi: 10.1097/00063198-200207000-00012

39. Good JT Jr, King TE, Antony VB, Sahn SA. Lupus pleuritis. Clinical features and pleural fluid characteristics with special reference to pleural fluid antinuclear antibodies. *Chest.* (1983) 84:714–8. doi: 10.1378/chest.84.6.714

40. Hunninghake GW, Fauci AS. Pulmonary involvement in the collagen vascular diseases. *Am Rev Respir Dis.* (1979) 119:471–503.

41. Pines A, Kaplinsky N, Olchovsky D, Rozenman J, Frankl O. Pleuro-pulmonary manifestations of systemic lupus erythematosus: clinical features of its subgroups. Prognostic and therapeutic implications. *Chest* (1985) 88:129–35. doi: 10.1378/chest.88.1.129

42. Ajakumar Menon A, Kirshenbaum D, Burke G. Drug induced lupus presenting as isolated pleural effusion. *Chest.* (2015) 148:884A. doi: 10.1378/chest.2236839

43. Costa MF, Said NR, Zimmermann B. Drug-induced lupus due to anti-tumor necrosis factor alpha agents. *Semin Arthritis Rheum.* (2008) 37:381–7. doi: 10.1016/j.semarthrit.2007.08.003

44. Smith PR, Nacht RI. Drug-induced lupus pleuritis mimicking pleural space infection. *Chest.* (1992) 101:268–9. doi: 10.1378/chest.101.1.268

45. Glazer M, Berkman N, Lafair JS, Kramer MR. Successful talc slurry pleurodesis in patients with nonmalignant pleural effusion. *Chest.* (2000) 117:1404–9. doi: 10.1378/chest.117.5.1404

46. McKnight KM, Adair NE, Agudelo CA. Successful use of tetracycline pleurodesis to treat massive pleural effusion secondary to systemic lupus erythematosus. *Arthritis Rheum.* (1991) 34:1483–4. doi: 10.1002/art.1780341121

47. Hoeper MM, Ghofrani H-A, Grünig E, Klose H, Olschewski H, Rosenkranz S. Pulmonary hypertension. *Dtsch Arztebl Int.* (2017) 114:73–84. doi: 10.3238/arztebl.2016.0073

48. Tselios K, Gladman DD, Urowitz MB. Systemic lupus erythematosus and pulmonary arterial hypertension: links, risks, and management strategies. *Open Access Rheumatol.* (2016) 9:1–9. doi: 10.2147/OARRR.S123549

49. Johnson SR, Gladman DD, Urowitz MB, Ibañez D, Granton JT. Pulmonary hypertension in systemic lupus. *Lupus.* (2004) 13:506–9. doi: 10.1191/0961203303lu1051oa

50. Pan TL, Thumboo J, Boey ML. Primary and secondary pulmonary hypertension in systemic lupus erythematosus. *Lupus.* (2000) 9:338–42. doi: 10.1191/096120300678828361

51. Quismorio FP Jr, Sharma O, Koss M, Boylen T, Edmiston AW, Thornton PJ, et al. Immunopathologic and clinical studies in pulmonary hypertension associated with systemic lupus erythematosus. *Semin Arthritis Rheum.* (1984) 13:349–59. doi: 10.1016/0049-0172(84)90015-5

52. Shen JY, Chen SL, Wu YX, Tao RQ, Gu YY, Bao CD, et al. Pulmonary hypertension in systemic lupus erythematosus. *Rheumatol Int.* (1999) 18:147–51. doi: 10.1007/s002960050074

53. Simonson JS, Schiller NB, Petri M, Hellmann DB. Pulmonary hypertension in systemic lupus erythematosus. *J Rheumatol.* (1989) 16:918–25.

54. Winslow TM, Ossipov MA, Fazio GP, Simonson JS, Redberg RF, Schiller NB. Five-year follow-up study of the prevalence and progression of pulmonary hypertension in systemic lupus erythematosus. *Am Heart J.* (1995) 129:510–5. doi: 10.1016/0002-8703(95)90278-3

55. Lv T-T, Wang P, Guan S-Y, Li H-M, Li X-M, Wang B, et al. Prevalence of pulmonary hypertension in systemic lupus erythematosus: a meta-analysis. *Ir J Med Sci.* (2018) 187:723–30. doi: 10.1007/s11845-017-1727-4

56. Pope J. An update in pulmonary hypertension in systemic lupus erythematosus - do we need to know about it? *Lupus.* (2008) 17:274–7. doi: 10.1177/0961203307087188

57. Dhala A. Pulmonary arterial hypertension in systemic lupus erythematosus: current status and future direction. *Clin Dev Immunol.* (2012) 2012:854941. doi: 10.1155/2012/854941

58. Hoeper MM, Bogaard HJ, Condliffe R, Frantz R, Khanna D, Kurzyna M, et al. Definitions and diagnosis of pulmonary hypertension. *J Am Coll Cardiol.* (2013) 62(25 Suppl.):D42–50. doi: 10.1016/j.jacc.2013.10.032

59. Badesch DB, Hill NS, Burgess G, Rubin LJ, Barst RJ, Galiè N, et al. Sildenafil for pulmonary arterial hypertension associated with connective tissue disease. *J Rheumatol.* (2007) 34:2417–22.

60. Mok MY, Tsang PL, Lam YM, Lo Y, Wong WS, Lau CS. Bosentan use in systemic lupus erythematosus patients with pulmonary arterial hypertension. *Lupus.* (2007) 16:279–85. doi: 10.1177/0961203307076509

61. Oudiz RJ, Schilz RJ, Barst RJ, Galié N, Rich S, Rubin LJ, et al. Treprostinil, a prostacyclin analogue, in pulmonary arterial hypertension associated with connective tissue disease. *Chest.* (2004) 126:420–7. doi: 10.1378/chest.126.2.420

62. Robbins IM, Gaine SP, Schilz R, Tapson VF, Rubin LJ, Loyd JE. Epoprostenol for treatment of pulmonary hypertension in patients with systemic lupus erythematosus. *Chest.* (2000) 117:14–8. doi: 10.1378/chest.117.1.14

63. Rubin LJ, Badesch DB, Barst RJ, Galie N, Black CM, Keogh A, et al. Bosentan therapy for pulmonary arterial hypertension. *N Engl J Med.* (2002) 346:896–903. doi: 10.1056/NEJMoa012212

64. Shirai Y, Yasuoka H, Takeuchi T, Satoh T, Kuwana M. Intravenous epoprostenol treatment of patients with connective tissue disease and pulmonary arterial hypertension at a single center. *Mod Rheumatol.* (2013) 23:1211–20. doi: 10.3109/s10165-012-0828-1

65. Humbert M, Coghlan JG, Ghofrani H-A, Grimminger F, He J-G, Riemekasten G, et al. Riociguat for the treatment of pulmonary arterial hypertension associated with connective tissue disease: results from PATENT-1 and PATENT-2. *Ann Rheum Dis.* (2017) 76:422–6. doi: 10.1136/annrheumdis-2015-209087

66. Kuzuya K, Tsuji S, Matsushita M, Ohshima S, Saeki Y. Systemic sclerosis and systemic lupus erythematosus overlap syndrome with pulmonary arterial hypertension successfully treated with immunosuppressive therapy and riociguat. *Cureus.* (2019) 11:e4327. doi: 10.7759/cureus.4327

67. Gonzalez-Lopez L, Cardona-Muñoz EG, Celis A, García-de la Torre I, Orozco-Barocio G, Salazar-Paramo M, et al. Therapy with intermittent pulse cyclophosphamide for pulmonary hypertension associated with systemic lupus erythematosus. *Lupus.* (2004) 13:105–12. doi: 10.1191/0961203304lu509oa

68. Kommireddy S, Bhyravavajhala S, Kurimeti K, Chennareddy S, Kanchinadham S, Rajendra Vara Prasad I, et al. Pulmonary arterial hypertension in systemic lupus erythematosus may benefit by addition of immunosuppression to vasodilator therapy: an observational study. *Rheumatology.* (2015) 54:1673–9. doi: 10.1093/rheumatology/kev097

69. Prete M, Fatone MC, Vacca A, Racanelli V, Perosa F. Severe pulmonary hypertension as the initial manifestation of systemic lupus erythematosus: a case report and review of the literature. *Clin Exp Rheumatol.* (2014) 32:267–74.

70. Tanaka E, Harigai M, Tanaka M, Kawaguchi Y, Hara M, Kamatani N. Pulmonary hypertension in systemic lupus erythematosus: evaluation of clinical characteristics and response to immunosuppressive treatment. *J Rheumatol.* (2002) 29:282–7.

71. Hennigan S, Channick RN, Silverman GJ. Rituximab treatment of pulmonary arterial hypertension associated with systemic lupus erythematosus: a case report. *Lupus.* (2008) 17:754–6. doi: 10.1177/0961203307087610

72. Wahl DG, Guillemin F, de Maistre E, Perret C, Lecompte T, Thibaut G. Risk for venous thrombosis related to antiphospholipid antibodies in systemic lupus erythematosus—a meta-analysis. *Lupus.* (1997) 6:467–73. doi: 10.1177/096120339700600510

73. Kado R, Siegwald E, Lewis E, Goodsitt MM, Christodoulou E, Kazerooni E, et al. Utility and associated risk of pulmonary embolism computed tomography scans in the michigan lupus cohort. *Arthritis Care Res.* (2016) 68:406–11. doi: 10.1002/acr.22684

74. Pengo V, Denas G, Zoppellaro G, Jose SP, Hoxha A, Ruffatti A, et al. Rivaroxaban vs. warfarin in high-risk patients with antiphospholipid syndrome. *Blood.* (2018) 132:1365–71. doi: 10.1182/blood-2018-04-848333

75. Abud-Mendoza C, Diaz-Jouanen E, Alarcón-Segovia D. Fatal pulmonary hemorrhage in systemic lupus erythematosus. Occurrence without hemoptysis. *J Rheumatol.* (1985) 12:558–61.

76. Zamora MR, Warner ML, Tuder R, Schwarz MI. Diffuse alveolar hemorrhage and systemic lupus erythematosus. Clinical presentation, histology, survival, and outcome. *Medicine.* (1997) 76:192–202. doi: 10.1097/00005792-199705000-00005

77. Cordier JF, Cottin V. Alveolar hemorrhage in vasculitis: primary and secondary. *Semin Respir Crit Care Med.* (2011) 32:310–21. doi: 10.1055/s-0031-1279827

78. Yachoui R, Sehgal R, Amlani B, Goldberg JW. Antiphospholipid antibodies-associated diffuse alveolar hemorrhage. *Semin Arthritis Rheum.* (2015) 44:652–7. doi: 10.1016/j.semarthrit.2014.10.013

79. Santos-Ocampo AS, Mandell BF, Fessler BJ. Alveolar hemorrhage in systemic lupus erythematosus: presentation and management. *Chest.* (2000) 118:1083–90. doi: 10.1378/chest.118.4.1083

80. Koh WH, Thumboo J, Boey ML. Pulmonary haemorrhage in Oriental patients with systemic lupus erythematosus. *Lupus.* (1997) 6:713–6. doi: 10.1177/096120339700600906

81. Masoodi I, Sirwal IA, Anwar SK, Alzaidi A, Balbaid KA. Predictors of mortality in pulmonary haemorrhage during SLE: a single centre study over eleven years. *Open Access Maced J Med Sci.* (2019) 7:92–6. doi: 10.3889/oamjms.2019.038

82. Martínez-Martínez MU, Oostdam DAH, Abud-Mendoza C. Diffuse alveolar hemorrhage in autoimmune diseases. *Curr Rheumatol Rep.* (2017) 19:27. doi: 10.1007/s11926-017-0651-y

83. Borrell H, Narváez J, Alegre JJ, Castellví I, Mitjavila F, Aparicio M, et al. Shrinking lung syndrome in systemic lupus erythematosus: a

84. Deeb M, Tselios K, Gladman DD, Su J, Urowitz MB. Shrinking lung syndrome in systemic lupus erythematosus: a single-centre experience. *Lupus.* (2018) 27:365–71. doi: 10.1177/0961203317722411

85. Laroche CM, Mulvey DA, Hawkins PN, Walport MJ, Strickland B, Moxham J, et al. Diaphragm strength in the shrinking lung syndrome of systemic lupus erythematosus. *Q J Med.* (1989) 71:429–39.

86. Toya SP, Tzelepis GE. Association of the shrinking lung syndrome in systemic lupus erythematosus with pleurisy: a systematic review. *Semin Arthritis Rheum.* (2009) 39:30–7. doi: 10.1016/j.semarthrit.2008.04.003

87. Karim MY, Miranda LC, Tench CM, Gordon PA, D'Cruz DP, Khamashta MA, et al. Presentation and prognosis of the shrinking lung syndrome in systemic lupus erythematosus. *Semin Arthritis Rheum.* (2002) 31:289–98. doi: 10.1053/sarh.2002.32555

88. Duron L, Cohen-Aubart F, Diot E, Borie R, Abad S, Richez C, et al. Shrinking lung syndrome associated with systemic lupus erythematosus: a multicenter collaborative study of 15 new cases and a review of the 155 cases in the literature focusing on treatment response and long-term outcomes. *Autoimmun Rev.* (2016) 15:994–1000. doi: 10.1016/j.autrev.2016.07.021

89. Benham H, Garske L, Vecchio P, Eckert BW. Successful treatment of shrinking lung syndrome with rituximab in a patient with systemic lupus erythematosus. *J Clin Rheumatol.* (2010) 16:68–70. doi: 10.1097/RHU.0b013e3181d0757f

90. Langenskiöld E, Bonetti A, Fitting JW, Heinzer R, Dudler J, Spertini F, et al. Shrinking lung syndrome successfully treated with rituximab and cyclophosphamide. *Respiration.* (2012) 84:144–9. doi: 10.1159/000334947

91. Peñacoba Toribio P, Córica Albani ME, Mayos Pérez M, Rodríguez de la Serna A. Rituximab in the treatment of shrinking lung syndrome in systemic lupus erythematosus. *Reumatol Clin.* (2014) 10:325–7. doi: 10.1016/j.reuma.2013.09.003

92. Walz-Leblanc BA, Urowitz MB, Gladman DD, Hanly PJ. The "shrinking lungs syndrome" in systemic lupus erythematosus–improvement with corticosteroid therapy. *J Rheumatol.* (1992) 19:1970–2.

93. Traynor AE, Corbridge TC, Eagan AE, Barr WG, Liu Q, Oyama Y, et al. Prevalence and reversibility of pulmonary dysfunction in refractory systemic lupus: improvement correlates with disease remission following hematopoietic stem cell transplantation. *Chest.* (2005) 127:1680–9. doi: 10.1378/chest.127.5.1680

94. Muñoz-Rodríguez FJ, Font J, Badia JR, Miret C, Barberà JA, Cervera R, et al. Shrinking lungs syndrome in systemic lupus erythematosus: improvement with inhaled beta-agonist therapy. *Lupus.* (1997) 6:412–4. doi: 10.1177/096120339700600413

95. Van Veen S, Peeters AJ, Sterk PJ, Breedveld FC. The "shrinking lung syndrome" in SLE, treatment with theophylline. *Clin Rheumatol.* (1993) 12:462–5. doi: 10.1007/BF02231771

96. Jindal SK, Agarwal R. Autoimmunity and interstitial lung disease. *Curr Opin Pulm Med.* (2005) 11:438–46. doi: 10.1097/01.mcp.0000170522.71497.61

97. Orens JB, Martinez FJ, Lynch JP III. Pleuropulmonary manifestations of systemic lupus erythematosus. *Rheum Dis Clin North Am.* (1994) 20:159–93.

98. Myers JL, Katzenstein AA. Microangiitis in lupus-induced pulmonary hemorrhage. *Am J Clin Pathol.* (1986) 85:552–6. doi: 10.1093/ajcp/85.5.552

99. Turner-Stokes L, Haslam P, Jones M, Dudeney C, Le Page S, Isenberg D. Autoantibody and idiotype profile of lung involvement in autoimmune rheumatic disease. *Ann Rheum Dis.* (1990) 49:160–2. doi: 10.1136/ard.49.3.160

100. Pandya MR, Agus B, Grady RF. Letter: *In vivo* LE phenomenon in pleural fluid. *Arthritis Rheum.* (1976) 19:962–3. doi: 10.1002/art.1780190526

101. Dorfmüller P, Humbert M, Perros F, Sanchez O, Simonneau G, Müller KM, et al. Fibrous remodeling of the pulmonary venous system in pulmonary arterial hypertension associated with connective tissue diseases. *Hum Pathol.* (2007) 38:893–902. doi: 10.1016/j.humpath.2006.11.022

102. Carmier D, Diot E, Diot P. Shrinking lung syndrome: recognition, pathophysiology and therapeutic strategy. *Expert Rev Respir Med.* (2011) 5:33–9. doi: 10.1586/ers.10.84

103. Hochberg MC. Updating the American College of Rheumatology revised

criteria for the classification of systemic lupus erythematosus. *Arthritis Rheum.* (1997) 40:1725. doi: 10.1002/art.1780400928

104. Aringer M, Costenbader K, Daikh D, Brinks R, Mosca M, Ramsey-Goldman R, et al. 2019 European League Against Rheumatism/American College of Rheumatology Classification Criteria for Systemic Lupus Erythematosus. *Arthritis Rheumatol.* (2019) 71:1400–12. doi: 10.1002/art.40930

105. Yee CS, Farewell V, Isenberg DA, Griffiths B, Teh LS, Bruce IN, et al. The BILAG-2004 index is sensitive to change for assessment of SLE disease activity. *Rheumatology.* (2009) 48:691–5. doi: 10.1093/rheumatology/kep064

106. Gladman DD, Ibañez D, Urowitz MB. Systemic lupus erythematosus disease activity index 2000. *J Rheumatol.* (2002) 29:288–91.

107. Franklyn K, Lau CS, Navarra SV, Louthrenoo W, Lateef A, Hamijoyo L, et al. Definition and initial validation of a Lupus Low Disease Activity State (LLDAS). *Ann Rheum Dis.* (2016) 75:1615–21. doi: 10.1136/annrheumdis-2015-207726

108. Gladman D, Ginzler E, Goldsmith C, Fortin P, Liang M, Urowitz M, et al. The development and initial validation of the Systemic Lupus International Collaborating Clinics/American College of Rheumatology damage index for systemic lupus erythematosus. *Arthritis Rheum.* (1996) 39:363–9. doi: 10.1002/art.1780390303

Permissions

The contributors of this book come from diverse backgrounds, making this book a truly international effort. This book will bring forth new frontiers with its revolutionizing research information and detailed analysis of the nascent developments around the world.

We would like to thank all the contributing authors for lending their expertise to make the book truly unique. They have played a crucial role in the development of this book. Without their invaluable contributions this book wouldn't have been possible. They have made vital efforts to compile up to date information on the varied aspects of this subject to make this book a valuable addition to the collection of many professionals and students.

This book was conceptualized with the vision of imparting up-to-date information and advanced data in this field. To ensure the same, a matchless editorial board was set up. Every individual on the board went through rigorous rounds of assessment to prove their worth. After which they invested a large part of their time researching and compiling the most relevant data for our readers.

The editorial board has been involved in producing this book since its inception. They have spent rigorous hours researching and exploring the diverse topics which have resulted in the successful publishing of this book. They have passed on their knowledge of decades through this book. To expedite this challenging task, the publisher supported the team at every step. A small team of assistant editors was also appointed to further simplify the editing procedure and attain best results for the readers.

Apart from the editorial board, the designing team has also invested a significant amount of their time in understanding the subject and creating the most relevant covers. They scrutinized every image to scout for the most suitable representation of the subject and create an appropriate cover for the book.

The publishing team has been an ardent support to the editorial, designing and production team. Their endless efforts to recruit the best for this project, has resulted in the accomplishment of this book. They are a veteran in the field of academics and their pool of knowledge is as vast as their experience in printing. Their expertise and guidance has proved useful at every step. Their uncompromising quality standards have made this book an exceptional effort. Their encouragement from time to time has been an inspiration for everyone.

The publisher and the editorial board hope that this book will prove to be a valuable piece of knowledge for researchers, students, practitioners and scholars across the globe.

List of Contributors

Cibele Cristine Berto Marques da Silva and Celso R. F. Carvalho
Departament of Physical Therapy, School of Medicine, University of São Paulo, São Paulo, Brazil

Douglas Silva Queiroz
Departament of Physical Therapy, School of Medicine, University of São Paulo, São Paulo, Brazil
Hospital Israelita Albert Einstein, São Paulo, Brazil

Alexandre Franco Amaral, Martina Rodrigues Oliveira, Carlos Roberto Ribeiro Carvalho and Bruno Guedes Baldi
Divisao de Pneumologia, Instituto do Coracao, Hospital das Clínicas da Faculdade de Medicina da Universidade de São Paulo, São Paulo, Brazil

Henrique Takachi Moriya
Biomedical Engineering Laboratory, Escola Politécnica, Universidade de São Paulo, São Paulo, Brazil

Theodoros Karampitsakos
5th Department of Pneumonology, General Hospital for Thoracic Diseases Sotiria, Athens, Greece

Argyro Vraka, Demosthenes Bouros and Argyris Tzouvelekis
First Academic Department of Pneumonology, Hospital for Thoracic Diseases, Sotiria Medical School, National and Kapodistrian University of Athens, Athens, Greece

Stamatis-Nick Liossis
Division of Rheumatology, Department of Internal Medicine, Patras University Hospital, University of Patras Medical School, Patras, Greece

Mauricio Gonzalez-Garcia, Emily Rincon-Alvarez and Mauricio Duran
Fundación Neumológica Colombiana, Bogotá, Colombia

Maria Laura Alberti and Fabian Caro
Hospital María Ferrer, Buenos Aires, Argentina

Maria del Carmen Venero
Hospital Nacional Arzobispo Loayza, Lima, Peru

Yuri Edison Liberato
Hospital Belén de Trujillo, Trujillo, Peru

George E. Fragoulis
First Department of Propaedeutic Internal Medicine, National and Kapodistrian University of Athens, Laiko General Hospital, Athens, Greece

Institute of Infection, Immunity and Inflammation, University of Glasgow, Glasgow, United Kingdom

Elena Nikiphorou
Department of Inflammation Biology, Faculty of Life Sciences & Medicine, Centre for Rheumatic Diseases, School of Immunology and Microbial Sciences, King's College London, London, United Kingdom

Richard Conway
Department of Rheumatology, Blackrock Clinic, Dublin, Ireland

Mouhamad Nasser
Hôpital Louis Pradel, Centre Coordonnateur National de Référence des Maladies Pulmonaires Rares, Hospices Civils de Lyon, UMR754 INRAE and Université Claude Bernard Lyon 1, Member of ERN-LUNG, RespiFil, OrphaLung, Lyon, France

Vincent Cottin
Department of Respiratory Medicine, National Coordinating Reference Center for Rare Pulmonary Diseases, Louis Pradel Hospital, Hospices Civils de Lyon, Lyon, France
IVPC, INRAE, Claude Bernard University Lyon 1, Member of ERN-LUNG, Lyon, France
Hôpital Louis Pradel, Centre Coordonnateur National de Référence des Maladies Pulmonaires Rares, Hospices Civils de Lyon, UMR754 INRAE and Université Claude Bernard Lyon 1, Member of ERN-LUNG, RespiFil, OrphaLung, Lyon, France
National Coordinating Reference Centre for Rare Pulmonary Diseases, Louis Pradel Hospital, Hospices Civils de Lyon, University Claude Bernard Lyon 1, Lyon, France

Sophie Larrieu, Fabienne Bazin and Sébastien Marque
IQVIA – RWS La Défense, Courbevoie, France

Loic Boussel and Salim Si-Mohamed
Département de Radiologie, Hospices Civils de Lyon, Lyon, France
Université Lyon, INSA-Lyon, Université Claude Bernard Lyon 1, UJM-Saint Etienne, CNRS Inserm, CREATIS UMR 5220, Lyon, France

Jacques Massol
AIXIAL – Paris, Paris, France

Françoise Thivolet-Bejui and Lara Chalabreysse
Département d'anatomo-pathologie, Hospices Civils de Lyon, Lyon, France

Delphine Maucort-Boulch
Hospices Civils de Lyon, Pôle Santé Publique, Service de Biostatistique et Bioinformatique, Lyon, France
Université de Lyon, Lyon, France
Université Lyon 1, Villeurbanne, France
CNRS, UMR 5558, Laboratoire de Biométrie et Biologie Évolutive, Équipe Biostatistique-Santé, Villeurbanne, France

Stéphane Jouneau
Centre Hospitalier Universitaire de Rennes, Centre de Compétences pour les Maladies Pulmonaires Rares, Univ Rennes, Inserm, EHESP, IRSET (Institut de recherche en santé, environnement et travail), RespiFil, OrphaLung, Rennes, France

Eric Hachulla
Hôpital Claude Huriez, Centre National de Référence des maladies auto-immunes systémiques rares (CeRAINO), CHU de Lille, Lille, France

Julien Chollet
Boehringer Ingelheim France SAS, Paris, France

Mehdi Mirsaeidi, Pamela Barletta and Marilyn K. Glassberg
Division of Pulmonary, Critical Care, and Sleep Medicine, University of Miami Miller School of Medicine, Miami, FL, United States

Markus Polke
Center for Interstitial and Rare Lung Diseases, Pneumology, Thoraxklinik, University of Heidelberg, Heidelberg, Germany

Yasuhiro Kondoh
Department of Respiratory Medicine and Allergy, Tosei General Hospital, Seto, Japan

Marlies Wijsenbeek and Catharina C. Moor
Department of Respiratory Medicine, Centre for Interstitial Lung Diseases and Sarcoidosis, Erasmus University Medical Centre, Rotterdam, Netherlands

Simon L. F. Walsh
Imperial College, National Heart and Lung Institute, London, United Kingdom

Harold R. Collard
Department of Medicine, University of California, San Francisco, San Francisco, CA, United States

Nazia Chaudhuri
North West Interstitial Lung Disease Unit, Manchester University NHS Foundation Trust, Wythenshawe, Manchester, United Kingdom

Sergey Avdeev
Sechenov First Moscow State Medical University, Moscow, Russia

Jürgen Behr
Medizinische Klinik und Poliklinik V, LMU Klinikum, University of Munich, Munich, Germany
German Center for Lung Research (DZL), Marburg, Germany

Michael Kreuter
Center for Interstitial and Rare Lung Diseases, Pneumology, Thoraxklinik, University of Heidelberg, Heidelberg, Germany
German Center for Lung Research (DZL), Marburg, Germany

Gregory Calligaro
Division of Pulmonology, Department of Medicine, University of Cape Town, Cape Town, South Africa

Tamera J. Corte
Royal Prince Alfred Hospital, University of Sydney, Sydney, NSW, Australia

Kevin Flaherty
Department of Medicine, University of Michigan, Ann Arbor, MI, United States

Manuela Funke-Chambour
Department of Pulmonary Medicine, Inselspital, Bern University Hospital, University of Bern, Bern, Switzerland

Martin Kolb
Department of Medicine, Firestone Institute for Respiratory Health, Research Institute at St Joseph's Healthcare, McMaster University, Hamilton, ON, Canada

Johannes Krisam
Institute of Medical Biometry and Informatics, University of Heidelberg, Heidelberg, Germany

Toby M. Maher
Hastings Centre for Pulmonary Research and Division of Pulmonary, Critical Care, and Sleep Medicine, Keck School of Medicine, University of Southern California, Los Angeles, CA, United States
Interstitial Lung Disease Unit, Imperial College London, National Heart and Lung Institute, Royal Brompton and Harefield NHS Foundation Trust, London, United Kingdom

Maria Molina Molina
Institut d'Investigació Biomèdica de Bellvitge (IDIBELL), University Hospital of Bellvitge, L'Hospitalet de Llobregat, Barcelona, Spain
Centro de Investigación Biomédica en Red Enfermedades Respiratorias (CIBERES), Madrid, Spain

Antonio Morais
Department of Pneumology, Faculdade de Medicina, Centro Hospitalar São João, Universidade do Porto, Porto, Portugal

Julie Morisset
Département de Médecine, Centre Hospitalier de l'Université de Montréal, Montréal, QC, Canada

Carlos Pereira
Lung Disease Department, Paulista School of Medicine, Federal University of São Paulo, São Paulo, Brazil

Silvia Quadrelli
Hospital Británico, Buenos Aires, Argentina
Sanatorio Güemes, Buenos Aires, Argentina

Argyrios Tzouvelekis
Department of First Academic Respiratory, Sotiria General Hospital for Thoracic Diseases, University of Athens, Athens, Greece

Claudia Valenzuela
Interstitial Lung Disease Unit Pulmonology Department, Hospital Universitario de La Princesa, Universidad Autonoma de Madrid, Madrid, Spain

Carlo Vancheri
Regional Referral Centre for Rare Lung Diseases, A.O.U. Policlinico-Vittorio Emanuele, University of Catania, Catania, Italy

Vanesa Vicens-Zygmunt
Unit of Interstitial Lung Diseases, Department of Pneumology, Pneumology Research Group, IDIBELL, L'Hospitalet de Llobregat, University Hospital of Bellvitge, Barcelona, Spain

Julia Wälscher
Center for Interstitial and Rare Lung Diseases, Pneumology, Thoraxklinik, University of Heidelberg, Heidelberg, Germany
Department of Pulmonary Medicine, Centre for Interstitial and Rare Lung Diseases, Ruhrlandklinik University Hospital Essen, Essen, Germany

Wim Wuyts
Unit for Interstitial Lung Diseases, Department of Respiratory Diseases, University Hospitals Leuven, Leuven, Belgium

Elisabeth Bendstrup
Department of Respiratory Diseases and Allergy, Aarhus University Hospital, Aarhus C, Denmark

Federica Furini, Giulio Guerrini, Marcello Govoni and Carlo Alberto Sciré
Section of Rheumatology, Department of Medical Sciences, University of Ferrara and Azienda Ospedaliero-Universitaria Sant'Anna di Ferrara, Cona, Italy

Aldo Carnevale
Department of Radiology, Azienda Ospedaliero-Universitaria Sant'Anna di Ferrara, Cona, Italy

Gian Luca Casoni
Department of Medical Sciences, Research Centre on Asthma and COPD, University of Ferrara, Ferrara, Italy

Marlies S. Wijsenbeek and Iris G. van der Sar
Erasmus Medical Center, Rotterdam, Netherlands

Steve Jones
Action for Pulmonary Fibrosis, Lichfield, United Kingdom

Deborah L. Clarke
Galapagos NV, Mechelen, Belgium

Francesco Bonella
Ruhrlandklinik, University of Duisburg-Essen, Essen, Germany

Jean Michel Fourrier
Association Pierre Enjalran Fibrose Pulmonaire Idiopathique, Meyzieu, France

Katarzyna Lewandowska
Department of Pulmonary Diseases, National Research Institute of Tuberculosis and Lung Diseases, Warsaw, Poland

Guadalupe Bermudo
Hospital Universitari de Bellvitge, Barcelona, Spain

Alexander Simidchiev
Department of Functional Diagnostics, Medical Institute MVR, Sofia, Bulgaria

Irina R. Strambu
Carol Davila University of Medicine and Pharmacy, Bucharest, Romania

Helen Parfrey
Royal Papworth Hospital, Cambridge, United Kingdom

Yaogui Ning
Department of Intensive Care Unit, The First Affiliated Hospital of Xiamen University, Xiamen, China
Medical College, Xiamen University, Xiamen, China

Guomei Yang
Medical College, Xiamen University, Xiamen, China

Yuechi Sun, Shiju Chen, Yuan Liu and Guixiu Shi
Department of Rheumatology and Clinical Immunology, The First Affiliated Hospital of Xiamen University, Xiamen, China

Moises Selman
Instituto Nacional de Enfermedades Respiratorias Ismael Cosío Villegas, Mexico City, Mexico

Ivette Buendia-Roldan
Instituto Nacional de Enfermedades Respiratorias Ismael Cosío Villegas, Ciudad de México, Mexico

Baptiste Hervier
Internal Medicine and Clinical Immunology Department, French Referral Centre for Rare Neuromuscular Disorders, Hôpital Pitié-Salpêtrière, APHP, Paris, France
INSERM UMR-S 1135, CIMI-Paris, UPMC & Sorbonne Université, Paris, France

Yurdagül Uzunhan
Pneumology Department, Reference Center for Rare Pulmonary Diseases, Hôpital Avicenne, APHP, Bobigny, France
INSERM UMR1272, Université Paris 13, Bobigny, France

Abigél Margit Kolonics-Farkas and Veronika Müller
Department of Pulmonology, Semmelweis University, Budapest, Hungary

Martina Šterclová and Martina Vašáková
Department of Respiratory Diseases of the First Faculty of Medicine Charles University, University Thomayer Hospital, Prague, Czechia

Nesrin Mogulkoc
Department of Pulmonary Medicine, Ege University Medical School, Izmir, Turkey

Marta Hájková
Clinic of Pneumology and Phthisiology, University Hospital Bratislava, Bratislava, Slovakia

Mordechai Kramer
Rabin Medical Center, Institute of Pulmonary Medicine, Petah Tikva, Israel

Dragana Jovanovic
Internal Medicine Clinic "Akta Medica", Belgrade, Serbia

Jasna Tekavec-Trkanjec
Pulmonary Department, University Hospital Dubrava, Zagreb, Croatia

Michael Studnicka
Clinical Research Centre Salzburg, Salzburg, Austria

Natalia Stoeva
Tokuda Hospital Sofia, Sofia, Bulgaria

Simona Littnerová
Faculty of Medicine, Institute of Biostatistics and Analyses, Masaryk University, Brno, Czechia

Junyu Liang, Heng Cao, Yini Ke, Chuanyin Sun, Weiqian Chen and Jin Lin
Department of Rheumatology, The First Affiliated Hospital, College of Medicine, Zhejiang University, Hangzhou, China

Silvia Laura Bosello
Rheumatology Unit, A. Gemelli University Hospital Foundation - Istituto di Ricerca e Cura a Carattere Scientifico (IRCCS), Catholic University of the Sacred Heart, Rome, Italy

Lorenzo Beretta
Scleroderma Unit, Istituto di Ricerca e Cura a Carattere Scientifico (IRCCS) Ca' Granda Foundation Ospedale Maggiore Policlinico di Milan, Milan, Italy

Nicoletta Del Papa
Rheumatology Department, Scleroderma Clinic, ASST Pini-CTO, Milan, Italy

Sergio Harari
Department of Medical Sciences, San Giuseppe Hospital MultiMedica Istituto di Ricerca e Cura a Carattere Scientifico (IRCCS), Milan, Italy
Department of Clinical Sciences and Community Health, Università Degli Studi di Milano, Milan, Italy

Stefano Palmucci
Radiology Unit I, Department of Medical Surgical Sciences and Advanced Technologies GF Ingrassia, University Hospital Policlinico "G. Rodolico-San Marco", University of Catania, Catania, Italy

Alberto Pesci
Pneumological Clinic of the University of Milan-Bicocca, ASST-Monza, Monza, Italy

Gilda Rechichi
Radiology Unit, University Hospital San Gerardo, ASST-Monza, Monza, Italy

Francesco Varone
Pneumology Unit, A. Gemelli University Hospital Foundation Istituto di Ricerca e Cura a Carattere Scientifico (IRCCS), Rome, Italy

Marco Sebastiani
Rheumatology Unit, University of Modena and Reggio Emilia, Italy

Claudio Tirelli, Claudia La Carrubba, Tiberio Oggionni, Zamir Kadija, Francesca Mariani and Federica Meloni
Division of Pneumology, University and IRCCS Policlinico S. Matteo Foundation, Pavia, Italy

Valentina Morandi, Giovanni Zanframundo, Silvia Grignaschi, Emiliano Marasco, Ludovico De Stefano, Carlomaurizio Montecucco and Lorenzo Cavagna
Division of Rheumatology, University and IRCCS Policlinico S. Matteo Foundation, Pavia, Italy

Adele Valentini and Andrea Franconeri
Institute of Radiology, University and IRCCS Policlinico S. Matteo Foundation, Pavia, Italy

Roberto Dore
Radiology Unit, Isituti Clinici Città di Pavia, Pavia, Italy

Patrizia Morbini
Pathology Unit, University and IRCCS Policlinico S. Matteo Foundation, Pavia, Italy

Veronica Codullo
Rheumatology Department, Hopital Cochin, Paris, France

Claudia Alpini
Laboratory of Biochemical-Clinical Analyses, IRCCS Policlinico San Matteo Foundation, Pavia, Italy

Carlo Scirè
Division of Rheumatology, Arcispedale Sant'Anna, Ferrara, Italy

Hee-Young Yoon, Su-Jin Moon and Jin Woo Song
Department of Pulmonary and Critical Care Medicine, Asan Medical Center, University of Ulsan College of Medicine, Seoul, South Korea

Georgios Sogkas, Stefanie Hirsch, Thea Thiele, Reinhold Ernst Schmidt, Torsten Witte, Alexandra Jablonka and Diana Ernst
Department of Immunology and Rheumatology, Medical School Hannover, Hanover, Germany

Karen Maria Olsson
Department of Respiratory Medicine, Hannover Medical School, Hanover, Germany
BREATH German Centre for Lung Research (DZL), Hanover, Germany

Jan B. Hinrichs
Department of Diagnostic and Interventional Radiology, Hannover Medical School, Hanover, Germany

Tabea Seeliger and Thomas Skripuletz
Department of Neurology, Hannover Medical School, Hanover, Germany

Kerri I. Aronson
Division of Pulmonary and Critical Care Medicine, Weill Cornell Medicine, New York, NY, United States

Atsushi Suzuki
Department of Respiratory Medicine, Nagoya University Graduate School of Medicine, Nagoya, Japan

Yuhui Li, Yimin Li, Xuewu Zhang, Yuzhou Gan, Jing He and Xiaolin Sun
Beijing Key Laboratory for Rheumatism and Immune Diagnosis (BZ0135), Department of Rheumatology and Immunology, Peking University People's Hospital, Beijing, China

Xiaojuan Gao and Renli Chen
Department of Rheumatology, Ningde Hospital, Affiliated Hospital of Fujian Medical University, Ningde, China

Xiaohui Jia
Department of Rheumatology, The First Hospital of Hebei Medical University, Shijiazhuang, China

Yan Xu
Department of Neurology, Peking University People's Hospital, Beijing, China

Shiming Li
Department of Endocrinology, People's Hospital of Wushan County, Gansu, China

Raj Amarnani
Department of Rheumatology, University College London Hospital, London, United Kingdom

Su-Ann Yeoh and Chris Wincup
Department of Rheumatology, University College London Hospital, London, United Kingdom
Division of Medicine, Department of Rheumatology, University College London, London, United Kingdom

Emma K. Denneny
Department of Respiratory Medicine, University College London Hospital, London, United Kingdom
Leukocyte Trafficking Laboratory, Centre for Inflammation and Tissue Repair, UCL Respiratory, University College London, London, United Kingdom

Index

Printed in the USA
CPSIA information can be obtained
at www.ICGtesting.com
JSHW051400091023
49903JS00006B/217